Essentials of

Aesthetic Surgery

Q&A Companion

Essentials of Aesthetic Surgery

Q&A Companion

Jeffrey E. Janis, MD, FACS
Professor
Department of Plastic and Reconstructive Surgery;
Chief of Plastic Surgery (University Hospital);
Adjunct Professor
Departments of Neurosurgery, Neurology, and Surgery;
Co-Director
Center for Abdominal Core Health, The Ohio State University Wexner Medical Center;
Past President
American Society of Plastic Surgeons, American Council of Academic Plastic Surgeons,
American Hernia Society, and Migraine Surgery Society
Columbus, Ohio, USA

Sammy Sinno, MD
Board-Certified Plastic Surgeon
TLKM Plastic Surgery;
Clinical Professor of Plastic Surgery
Northwestern Memorial Hospital
Division of Plastic Surgery;
Member of The Aesthetic Society
Chicago, Illinois, USA

200 illustrations

Thieme

New York • Stuttgart • Delhi • Rio de Janeiro

Library of Congress Cataloging-in-Publication Data is available with the publisher.

Thieme Publishers New York
333 Seventh Avenue, 18th Floor
New York, NY 10001, USA
www.thieme.com
+1 800 782 3488, customerservice@thieme.com

Cover design: © Thieme
Cover image source: Cover photograph of the sculpture "Surgical Aesthetic Art" provided by the Ronadró Collection

Typesetting by Thomson Digital, India

Printed in India by
Replika Press Pvt. Ltd. 5 4 3 2 1

DOI: 10.1055/b000000370
ISBN: 978-1-68420-135-8

Also available as an e-book:
eISBN (PDF): 978-1-68420-136-5
eISBN (epub): 978-1-63853-669-7

To the field of plastic surgery, filled with amazing talent and innovation, helping to transform lives, restore physical, mental, and emotional health, and serve patients. And most of all to my wife, partner, and best friend, Emily, and our three absolutely incredible children, Jackson, Brinkley, and Holden—for everything and beyond. Nothing is possible without you.

Jeffrey E. Janis, MD, FACS

To my Rosa, Genoa, and Giovanni: thank you always for your patience and support.

Sammy Sinno, MD

Contents

Foreword

It is a great honor and privilege to be invited to write a foreword for *Essentials of Aesthetic Surgery: Q&A Companion* edited by my mentor and friend, Dr. Jeffrey E. Janis, and coedited by Dr. Sammy Sinno, a long-time colleague and friend. I still vividly remember participating in the Parkland Health and Hospital System preoperative rounds as a Chief Resident supervised by Dr. Janis. These were weekly educational sessions that gave the opportunity to the residents to review the treatment plans of patients who were scheduled for surgery. It was immediately clear that Dr. Janis demanded an organized, systematic, and thorough approach to the assessment and treatment planning for each patient. A variety of cases that spanned the whole spectrum of reconstructive and aesthetic plastic surgery were presented. What was most impressive was Dr. Janis' ability to draw from his wealth of knowledge and experience and distill it down to an organized and concise framework, to not only assess the problem and formulate an appropriate plan of care but also teach the fellows, residents, and medical students in attendance. One of the medical students I met during these rounds was Dr. Sinno, who coedited this *Q&A Companion* and who has already contributed to plastic surgery education in an impactful way.

Drs. Janis and Sinno's organized and thoughtful approach is illustrated *in Essentials of Aesthetic Surgery* and the *Q&A Companion*. Aesthetic surgery continues to be difficult to teach as it is the ultimate convergence of the art and science of plastic surgery. Decisions must be made based on the science and clinical evidence, but the outcome is often a subjective measure—beauty. However, Drs. Janis and Sinno have done an excellent job at curating a text that provides a framework to approach aesthetic surgery.

Beyond reading the contents of *Essentials of Aesthetic Surgery*, one of the most useful ways to consolidate the information by the learner is to think through the information with the use of this *Q&A Companion*. The *Q&A Companion* includes 65 chapters with questions and answers to parallel the content in *Essentials of Aesthetic Surgery*. The questions are high yield and accompanied by clear and concise explanations. The *Q&A Companion* will be useful to learners from across the spectrum, from those trainees who are learning the information for the first time to those who are reviewing the information again at any timepoint in their plastic surgery careers. I would like to congratulate Drs. Janis and Sinno on another significant contribution to aesthetic surgery education.

Jamil Ahmad, MD, FRCSC
Director of Research and Education
The Plastic Surgery Clinic;
Assistant Professor
Division of Plastic, Reconstructive, and Aesthetic Surgery
University of Toronto
Toronto, Ontario, Canada

Preface

The first edition of *Essentials of Aesthetic Surgery*, published in 2018, has been a phenomenal success, with thousands of readers across the world. Its popularity stems from its succinct, yet comprehensive, approach to summarizing the highlights and salient points of the spectrum of aesthetic surgery in the "Essentials-style" bullet point fashion, complete with contemporary and classic curated references and key points. Since its release, readers have clamored for a Q&A companion to the parent text, much like what has been published with the *Essentials of Plastic Surgery* title, now in its third edition. Well, your voices have been heard!

We are happy to present the first edition of *Essentials of Aesthetic Surgery: Q&A Companion*. Coedited by Sammy Sinno, a friend, colleague, and private practice plastic surgeon focused on aesthetic surgery, and with invaluable contributions from Anmol Chattha and Simon Moradian, this book boasts 65 chapters that mirror the chapters and content of the parent book. A host of authors, all with dedicated aesthetic surgery interests, have created questions that are specifically designed to test the reader on the content of each source Essentials chapter, with key emphasis on clinical application of the knowledge.

This learning resource is also accompanied by an electronic version (e-book), which means that it can be readily accessed on smartphones and tablets.

For those who prefer traditional books, the format is both compact and portable and presented with high-quality production.

We hope that readers find this companion book to be helpful, practical, and useful as you test your knowledge contained in the parent book. Together, these books are meant to be invaluable resources, whether you are interested in the field, training to become a plastic surgeon, or already in practice. After all, one never stops being a student!!

Jeffrey E. Janis, MD, FACS
Sammy Sinno, MD

Acknowledgments

Like the parent book, *Essentials of Aesthetic Surgery* (first edition), this *Q&A Companion* truly is a labor of love that simply could not have come to life without the tremendous time and effort invested in it by so many people.

First credit must go to the editorial group of Sammy Sinno, Simon Moradian, and Anmol Chattha as well as the chapter authors across the country who have spent a significant amount of time to help create the questions and their rationales based on the parent book to help the reader truly understand the source literature on which these are based. This is certainly no easy task, but I am sure the readers will appreciate the time and effort put into every question, both during the writing phase and during the meticulous editing phase. To them, I am sincerely grateful for their time and for the fruit of their efforts.

This entire project would not be possible without the expertise and experience of Judith Tomat, developmental editor, whom I have partnered with on many other Essentials projects. She, actually, is the definition of "essential"!! Simply put, this could not have been done without her.

Distinct recognition also must go to Karen Edmonson from Thieme, who believed in this project and supported, adding yet another quality title to the Essentials family.

Most of all, with tremendous sincerity, I want to thank my wonderful wife, Emily, and our beautiful children Jackson, Brinkley, and Holden for their understanding and patience, and above all else, their unconditional love and support. Without them, this book would not be possible, and my life would be empty.

Jeffrey E. Janis, MD, FACS

Contributors

Anmol Chattha, MD
Plastic Surgery Resident
Section of Plastic & Reconstructive Surgery
University of Chicago Hospitals
Pleasanton, California,
USA

Cameron R. Erickson, MD
Department of Plastic and Reconstructive Surgery
University of Texas Southwestern
Dallas, Texas, USA

Shervin Etemad, MD
Resident Physician
Department of Surgery
Division of Plastic and Reconstructive Surgery
University of Southern California
Los Angeles, California, USA

Jacob Nathaniel Grow, MD
Plastic Surgeon
Southern Indiana Aesthetic & Plastic Surgery
Columbus, Indiana, USA

Adam Jacoby, MD
Assistant Professor of Surgery (Plastic Surgery)
Department of General Surgery
Division of Plastic Surgery
Weill Cornell Medical College/New York Presbyterian Hospital
New York, New York, USA

Salam Kassis, MD
Associate Professor
Department of Plastic and Reconstructive Surgery
Vanderbilt University Medical Center
Nashville, Tennessee,
USA

Aaron M. Kearney, MD
Plastic Surgeon
Chicago, Illinois, USA

Joseph A. Kelling, MD
Plastic Surgeon
Kelling Plastic Surgery, PA
Dallas, Texas, USA

Nima Khosravani, MD
Chief Resident
Department of Surgery
University of Miami/JFK Medical Center
Atlantis, Florida, USA

Michael R. Lee, MD
Assistant Professor
Department of Plastic Surgery
University of Texas Southwestern
Dallas, Texas, USA

Simon Moradian, MD
Resident
Department of Northwestern Medicine, Plastic, Reconstructive, & Cosmetic Surgery
Northwestern Memorial Hospital
Chicago, Illinois, USA

Michael E. Nissan, MD
Department of Plastic Surgery
University of Texas Southwestern
Dallas, Texas, USA

Jeremie Oliver Piña, MD
Medical Student
Mayo Clinic School of Medicine
Mayo Clinic
Rochester, Minnesota, USA

Anup Patel, MD, MBA, FACS
Plastic, Reconstructive and Hand Surgeon
Orlando Plastic Surgery Institute
Orlando, Florida, USA

Juan L. Rendon, MD, PhD
Plastic Surgeon
South Bay Plastic Surgeons
Torrance, California, USA

Ara A. Salibian, MD
Assistant Professor
Division of Plastic & Reconstructive Surgery
University of California
Davis School of Medicine
Sacramento, California, USA

Ira L. Savetsky, MD
Private Practice
New York, New York, USA

Sammy Sinno, MD
Board-Certified Plastic Surgeon
TLKM Plastic Surgery;
Clinical Professor of Plastic Surgery
Northwestern Memorial Hospital
Division of Plastic Surgery;
Member of The Aesthetic Society
Chicago, Illinois, USA

David A. Sterling, MD
Assistant Professor
Division of Plastic Surgery, Department of Surgery
University of Arkansas for Medical Sciences (UAMS)
Little Rock, Arkansas, USA

Christopher C. Surek, MD, DO FACS
Private Practice
Surek Plastic Surgery
Overland Park, Kansas, USA

Jacob G. Unger, MD
Plastic Surgeon
Nashville Plastic Surgery Institute;
Clinical Assistant Professor of Plastic Surgery
Vanderbilt University
Nashville, Tennessee, USA

Elbert E. Vaca, MD
Doctor
Private Practice
Boca Raton, Florida, USA

Stelios C. Wilson, MD
Clinical Assistant Professor
Department of Surgery
Donald and Barbara Zucker School of Medicine
Hofstra University/Northwell Health
New York, New York, USA

Part I

Basic Considerations

1. The Aesthetic Surgery Patient

Sammy Sinno, Jeremie Oliver Piña
See *Essentials of Aesthetic Surgery*, pp. 3–12

DEMOGRAPHICS AND STATISTICS

1. *Approximately what percentage of aesthetic surgery patients undergo multiple procedures (either simultaneously or consecutively)?*

A. 20%.
B. 32%.
C. 57%.
D. 71%.
E. 95%.

DEMOGRAPHICS AND STATISTICS

2. *In evaluating a patient's candidacy for aesthetic surgical procedures, which of the following should weigh most heavily on the decision to pursue surgery?*

A. Age <20.
B. Age >60.
C. History of prior aesthetic surgical procedures.
D. Body habitus.
E. Overall health.

DEMOGRAPHICS AND STATISTICS

3. *Which of the following has been positively correlated with greater patient satisfaction, shorter recovery times, and less postoperative pain?*

A. Desire to change appearance in order to advance in career.
B. Desire to salvage a romantic relationship.
C. Consultation with at least four other aesthetic surgeons.
D. A high level of internal motivation for change.
E. History of multiple aesthetic surgical procedures.

DEMOGRAPHICS AND STATISTICS

4. *Which of the following scenarios depicts a "red flag" for undergoing an aesthetic surgical procedure?*

A. The patient keeps referring to wanting to look like their 20-year-old self.
B. The patient has been planning a particular aesthetic procedure only for a few weeks.
C. The patient is currently being treated for multiple psychiatric illnesses and/or has a history of several psychiatric hospital admissions.
D. The patient has an anatomic flaw that is visible to the surgeon but not the patient.
E. The patient has an anatomic flaw but is not terribly preoccupied by it.

DEMOGRAPHICS AND STATISTICS

5. *Under which circumstance should an aesthetic surgeon agree to operate on a patient with body dysmorphic disorder?*

A. The patient is overly concerned with the appearance of only one anatomical region.
B. The physical flaw the patient perceives is significantly disrupting the daily life of the patient.
C. The symptoms of body dysmorphic disorder are accompanied by an eating disorder, and the patient feels the aesthetic procedure would alleviate the associated symptoms.
D. The patient does not want to obsess over the physical flaw any longer.
E. Aesthetic surgery is not indicated in patients with active body dysmorphic disorder.

DEMOGRAPHICS AND STATISTICS

6. *Which of the following is an indication for an aesthetic surgeon to refuse to proceed with surgery?*
A. The patient is currently taking a selective serotonin receptor inhibitor (SSRI).
B. The patient has a history of major depressive disorder.
C. The patient shows signs of neuroticism.
D. The patient was under the impression that aesthetic surgery did not produce postoperative scars.
E. The surgeon feels persistently uneasy about the patient or the procedure.

DEMOGRAPHICS AND STATISTICS

7. *Considering the emotional response of the "healing curve," at which postoperative time point would you expect the patient to be most critical, nit-picky, scared, impatient, or complaining?*
A. Day 1.
B. Week 2.
C. Week 4.
D. Week 8.
E. Week 12.

DEMOGRAPHICS AND STATISTICS

8. *Which of the following is considered an essential adjunct to any facial rejuvenation procedure?*
A. Following a strict low-carb diet.
B. Exercising five times per week.
C. Losing 10 pounds prior to the operation.
D. A consistent skin care regimen.
E. Physical therapy.

DEMOGRAPHICS AND STATISTICS

9. *Which of the timeframes listed below is the most appropriate to undergo a revision procedure following primary rhinoplasty?*
A. At least 3 months.
B. Between 3 and 6 months.
C. At least 6 months.
D. At least 12 months.
E. At least 18 months.

Answers

DEMOGRAPHICS AND STATISTICS

1. ***Approximately what percentage of aesthetic surgery patients undergo multiple procedures (either simultaneously or consecutively)?***

   C. 57%.

   Approximately 57% of aesthetic surgery patients have multiple procedures performed. Specifically, 44% of patients who have a cosmetic procedure will return for another one and 57% of patients have multiple procedures performed simultaneously.[1]

REFERENCE

1. Plastic Surgery Statistics Report. American Society of Plastic Surgeons. Available at https://www.plasticsurgery.org/documents/News/Statistics/2020/plastic-surgery-statistics-full-report-2020.pdf

DEMOGRAPHICS AND STATISTICS

2. ***In evaluating a patient's candidacy for aesthetic surgical procedures, which of the following should weigh most heavily on the decision to pursue surgery?***

   E. Overall health.

   As part of the preoperative evaluation for aesthetic surgery candidacy, baseline health, comorbidities, tobacco use, prior surgeries, and prior pregnancies are fully discussed. Surgical risk is often dependent upon general health at consultation, as well as the specific desired procedure. As a general rule, health criteria for aesthetic surgery should be at least as stringent as those for reconstructive cases given the strictly elective nature of aesthetic cases. Thus, aesthetic surgery may be deemed inappropriate for unhealthy patients as well as those with a high risk of post- or intraoperative complications. Age should not be considered a significant determinant of aesthetic surgical candidacy. Rather, overall health should be the primary factor to consider in evaluating any patient's candidacy to undergo aesthetic surgery.[1]

REFERENCE

1. Gorney M. Recognition and management of the patient unsuitable for aesthetic surgery. Plast Reconstr Surg 2010;126:2268

DEMOGRAPHICS AND STATISTICS

3. ***Which of the following has been positively correlated with greater patient satisfaction, shorter recovery times, and less postoperative pain?***

   D. A high level of internal motivation for change.

   Both internal and external motives can be driving patients' desire for aesthetic surgical procedures. Intensity of motivation has been shown to positively correlate with satisfaction and shorter recovery, while negatively correlating with postoperative pain. Patients with primarily internal motives tend to be greater surgical candidates overall, while patients with substantial external motives (e.g., desire to change appearance to salvage a romantic relationship, satisfy a relative, advance in their career, etc.) tend to display greater dissatisfaction with aesthetic surgical results.[1,2] These patients may be pressured into undergoing surgery, thus demonstrating less motivation, often predicating a more difficult postoperative course.

REFERENCES

1. Ferraro GA, Rossano F, D'Andrea F. Self-perception and self-esteem of patients seeking cosmetic surgery. Aesthetic Plast Surg 2005;29:184
2. Nahai F. Evaluating the cosmetic patient on antidepressants. Aesthet Surg J 2014;34:326

DEMOGRAPHICS AND STATISTICS

4. *Which of the following scenarios depicts a "red flag" for undergoing an aesthetic surgical procedure?*

C. The patient is currently being treated for multiple psychiatric illnesses and/or has a history of several psychiatric hospital admissions.

Psychological indicators are important for the aesthetic surgeon to consider when evaluating a patient's surgical candidacy. A thorough evaluation of a patient's motivation and mental state is essential and a predictor of patient's behavior postoperatively. While turning down or referring patients for psychological evaluation is rare, when this is indicated, it must be handled delicately. In patients currently being treated for multiple psychiatric conditions and/or those who have an extensive history of hospital admission for psychiatric illness, it is warranted to first seek psychological evaluation and perhaps delay the surgery until the mental state is more controlled.[1]

REFERENCE

1. Nahai F. Evaluating the cosmetic patient on antidepressants. Aesthet Surg J 2014;34:326

DEMOGRAPHICS AND STATISTICS

5. *Under which circumstance should an aesthetic surgeon agree to operate on a patient with body dysmorphic disorder?*

E. Aesthetic surgery is not indicated in patients with active body dysmorphic disorder.

Patients with body dysmorphic disorder are rarely satisfied, and symptoms of this disorder may actually be exacerbated with aesthetic surgery. Therefore, aesthetic surgical procedures are contraindicated, and patients should be referred for the appropriate psychiatric care.[1,2,3]

REFERENCES

1. Rohrich RJ. Streamlining cosmetic surgery patient selection—just say no! Plast Reconstr Surg 1999;104:220
2. Gorney M. Recognition and management of the patient unsuitable for aesthetic surgery. Plast Reconstr Surg 2010;126:2268
3. Nahai F. Evaluating the cosmetic patient on antidepressants. Aesthet Surg J 2014;34:326

DEMOGRAPHICS AND STATISTICS

6. *Which of the following is an indication for an aesthetic surgeon to refuse to proceed with surgery?*

E. The surgeon feels persistently uneasy about the patient or the procedure.

Aesthetic surgeons should not disregard their "gut" feeling. They should listen to their instincts and not proceed with surgery if they are uneasy about the patient or the surgery. For patients with unrealistic aesthetic goals, surgeons should attempt to clarify that these results are not achievable. To prevent confrontation, if a patient insists on proceeding even when the surgeon feels uneasy, the surgeon can claim that he or she is not able to achieve the patient's desired results.[1] SSRI use, major depressive disorder in the past that is now controlled, and patients with psychiatric conditions are not absolute contraindications for a procedure. However, surgeons should tread carefully. Patients who have wanted a procedure for a long time are good candidates to proceed with surgery. Patients who impulsively want a cosmetic surgery are not suitable candidates.

REFERENCE

1. Rohrich RJ. Streamlining cosmetic surgery patient selection—just say no! Plast Reconstr Surg 1999;104:220

DEMOGRAPHICS AND STATISTICS

7. *Considering the emotional response of the "healing curve," at which postoperative time point would you expect the patient to be most critical, nit-picky, scared, impatient, or complaining?*

B. Week 2.

Patients commonly feel a wide range of emotions in the postoperative period. There are certain time points, which typically display common emotional reactions in patients following surgery,[1] as follows:

- Week 1: "I wish it was a month from now."
  - Days 1 to 3: "I'm beat." Patient is exhausted, sleepy.
  - Days 4 to 7: "What did I do?" Patient is sad, irritated, angry.

- Week 2: "You should have told me about…." Patient is critical, nitpicky, scared, impatient, and complaining.
- Week 3: "Not too bad…." Patient begins to normalize and see results.
- Weeks 4 to 5: "You look great." Patient notices others' reactions and compliments and begins to feel good about surgery.
- Weeks 6 to 8: "But what about…." As most of the swelling and bruising resolve, some focal areas may lag in recovery or may not appear as expected.
- Weeks 8 to 12: "Wow, I love it."
- After 3 to 6 months: "What's next?"

REFERENCE

1. Nahai F, ed. The Art of Aesthetic Surgery: Principles and Techniques. 2nd ed. New York: Thieme Publishers; 2010

DEMOGRAPHICS AND STATISTICS

8. *Which of the following is considered an essential adjunct to any facial rejuvenation procedure?*

D. A consistent skin care regimen.

A consistent skin care regimen for facial procedures in particular is essential in enhancing the desired results and preserving longevity of the surgical intervention.[1] Otherwise a good diet including low alcohol use and decreased salt intake in the first few months is helpful but not a requirement. Exercise, weight loss, and physical therapy are helpful but not essential.

REFERENCE

1. Nahai F, ed. The Art of Aesthetic Surgery: Principles and Techniques. 2nd ed. New York: Thieme Publishers; 2010

DEMOGRAPHICS AND STATISTICS

9. *Which of the timeframes listed below is the most appropriate to undergo a revision procedure following primary rhinoplasty?*

D. At least 12 months.

A clear, documented revision policy should be agreed upon prior to surgery. Adequate time should be allowed for healing and resolution of edema before considering any revision. The operating surgeon should have a thorough understanding of the indications for and expectations of revision surgery. The following timeframes (while not absolute) are useful guidelines[1] for different types of aesthetic procedures:

- Breast: Wait for at least 3 months.
- Blepharoplasty: Wait for 3 to 6 months.
- Body contouring: Wait for at least 6 months.
- Facelift: Wait for 6 to 12 months.
- Rhinoplasty: Wait for at least 12 months.

REFERENCE

1. Nahai F, ed. The Art of Aesthetic Surgery: Principles and Techniques. 2nd ed. New York: Thieme Publishers; 2010

2. The Artistry of Plastic Surgery

Sammy Sinno, Jeremie Oliver Piña
See *Essentials of Aesthetic Surgery*, pp. 13–20

AESTHETICS AND ITS ASSOCIATION

1. ***Which of the following best explains the evolving social acceptance of aesthetic medicine and surgery in various cultures around the world?***
   A. "Ideal" beauty is a constant.
   B. Caucasian beauty standards have influenced social acceptance of plastic surgery.
   C. Clinical studies have failed to show positive outcomes after aesthetic procedures.
   D. There is an increasing relationship between the science of aesthetic medicine and the safety of invasive and noninvasive procedures.
   E. Aesthetic surgeons are more skilled today than they were 20 years ago.

BEAUTY AND ITS CONCEPTS

2. ***Which of the following is an example of documented measures taken by the ancient Egyptians to enhance appearance?***
   A. Use of kohl (lead-based mineral) as eye makeup.
   B. Creation of Pythagorean theorem.
   C. Creation of architecture symbolizing both symmetry and proportion.
   D. Development of the "golden ratio."
   E. Living a virtuous lifestyle.

BEAUTY AND ITS CONCEPTS

3. ***The famous Greek statue "Venus de Milo" (formerly, the logo of PRS and the seal of ASPS) best represents which form of beauty?***
   A. Classical beauty.
   B. Mankind's ideal.
   C. Manufactured beauty.
   D. Natural beauty.
   E. Mythical beauty.

BEAUTY AND ITS CONCEPTS

4. ***Vitruvius was quoted,* "Just so the parts of Temples should correspond with each other, and with the whole." *How can this best apply to an aesthetic surgeon's practice?***
   A. One external aesthetic ideal guiding the surgeon's practice.
   B. The golden ratio is critical in plastic surgery and should not be deviated from.
   C. Making a compromise between what is desired and what is achievable, individualized to each patient.
   D. Strictly follow canons set forth by neoclassical artists and philosophers.
   E. Strive for greater variation in surgical technique.

BEAUTY AND ITS CONCEPTS

5. ***Although objective studies have consistently failed to confirm the applicability of many neoclassical canons to aesthetic surgery practice, which of the following choices lists three components of facial attractiveness considered to be critical?***
   A. Uniqueness, symmetry, skin tone.
   B. Averageness, interalar width, neoteny.
   C. Intercanthal distance, malar projection, defined jawline.
   D. Averageness, symmetry, neoteny.
   E. Pigmentation, symmetry, bone structure.

BEAUTY AND ITS CONCEPTS

6. *Which of the following anatomical features is most concordant with an aesthetic male dimorphic trait?*

A. Less prominent cheek bones.
B. Thicker lips.
C. Supraorbital ridges.
D. Smaller noses.
E. Smaller eyes.

BEAUTY AND ITS CONCEPTS

7. *In women, sexual dimorphism toward the aesthetic ideal implies which of the following?*

A. Lower set eyebrows.
B. Smaller eyes.
C. Thinner lips.
D. Smaller jaw.
E. Longer nose.

Answers

AESTHETICS AND ITS ASSOCIATION

1. ***Which of the following best explains the evolving social acceptance of aesthetic medicine and surgery in various cultures around the world?***

   D. There is an increasing relationship between the science of aesthetic medicine and the safety of invasive and noninvasive procedures.

   The rise in social acceptance and popularity of aesthetic medicine and surgery in the sexes and in various cultures around the world is thought to be intrinsically connected with the increasing relationship between the science of aesthetic medicine and the safety of invasive and noninvasive procedures. The standard of care in aesthetic medicine and surgery is founded upon evidence-based practice, born from clinical and psychological studies, which have shown an overall sense of well-being of patients who seek aesthetic procedures.[1,2,3]

REFERENCES

1. Saariniemi KM, Helle MH, Salmi AM, et al. The effects of aesthetic breast augmentation on quality of life, psychological distress, and eating disorder symptoms: a prospective study. Aesthetic Plast Surg 2012;36:1090
2. Saariniemi KM, Salmi AM, Peltoniemi HH, et al. Does liposuction improve body image and symptoms of eating disorders? Plast Reconstr Surg Glob Open 2015;3:e461
3. Saariniemi KM, Salmi AM, Peltoniemi HH, et al. Abdominoplasty improves quality of life, psychological distress, and eating disorder symptoms: a prospective study. Plast Surg Int 2014;2014:197232

BEAUTY AND ITS CONCEPTS

2. ***Which of the following is an example of documented measures taken by the ancient Egyptians to enhance appearance?***

   A. Use of kohl (lead-based mineral) as eye makeup.

   Ancient Egyptians left behind vast evidence suggesting that both sexes went to great lengths to improve their appearance. Based upon ubiquitous beauty products left by ancient Egyptians in burial settings, much of what is perceived as symbolic of beauty is influenced by what we think was considered beautiful in ancient Egypt. For example, kohl, a mineral base composed of lead, was used as eye makeup in ancient Egypt, which may have given rise to the smoky eye makeup worn today. Also, it is thought that kohl may have antibacterial properties and was utilized as a protectant from the glare of the sun, thus providing not only enhanced beauty, but also function.[1]

REFERENCE

1. Al-Kaff A, Al-Rajhi A, Tabbara K, El-Yazigi A. Kohl—the traditional eyeliner: use and analysis. Ann Saudi Med 1993;13(1):26–30

BEAUTY AND ITS CONCEPTS

3. ***The famous Greek statue "Venus de Milo" (formerly, the logo of PRS and the seal of ASPS) best represents which form of beauty?***

   A. Classical beauty.

   The idea of "classical beauty" arose from the Renaissance referring to re-adoption of ancient Greek idealism and the study of nature. This is symbolized by a woman who conforms to the standard Greek classical ideal, with proportion and symmetry as it relates to nature's ideal, and not necessarily "mankind's ideal."[1]

REFERENCE

1. Brent B. The reconstruction of Venus: following our legacy. Plast Reconstr Surg 2008;121:2170

BEAUTY AND ITS CONCEPTS

4. *Vitruvius was quoted,* "Just so the parts of Temples should correspond with each other, and with the whole." *How can this best apply to an aesthetic surgeon's practice?*

C. Making a compromise between what is desired and what is achievable, individualized to each patient.

As aesthetic surgeons, we hardly ever work with the anatomy that we would like, but rather the anatomy that we have been given. To that end, in practice, the surgeon is guided by the principles described by Vitruvius' quotation of aligning internal aesthetic goals with external aesthetic ideals but must also reach a compromise between what is desired and what is achievable.[1,2]

REFERENCES

1. Bashour M. History and current concepts in the analysis of facial attractiveness. Plast Reconstr Surg 2006;118:741
2. Bashour M. An objective system for measuring facial attractiveness. Plast Reconstr Surg 2006;118:757

BEAUTY AND ITS CONCEPTS

5. Although objective studies have consistently failed to confirm the applicability of many neoclassical canons to aesthetic surgery practice, which of the following choices lists three components of facial attractiveness considered to be critical?

D. Averageness, symmetry, neoteny.

Averageness indicates similarity to a typical phenotype for a group and therefore signals genetic diversity, which has presumable links to greater health and disease resistance.

Symmetry seems obvious as a characteristic of attractiveness; in fact, studies across a number of species have shown that greater symmetry is associated with both fitness and fertility.

Neoteny (juvenile features in an adult) is not simply youthfulness in the aging adult face. A baby's features (large eyes, small nose, round cheeks, smooth skin, glossy hair, and lighter skin tones) correlate with greater perceived attractiveness, more paternal attention, and even a lower incidence of childhood abuse. The preference for childlike facial features appears consistently across ethnic populations, regardless of sexual orientation.[1,2]

REFERENCES

1. Bashour M. History and current concepts in the analysis of facial attractiveness. Plast Reconstr Surg 2006;118:741
2. Bashour M. An objective system for measuring facial attractiveness. Plast Reconstr Surg 2006;118:757

BEAUTY AND ITS CONCEPTS

6. Which of the following anatomical features is most concordant with an aesthetic male dimorphic trait?

C. Supraorbital ridges.

Attractiveness is also related to sexual dimorphism—that is, the degree to which a particular face resembles the prototype of his or her sex. In men, this means larger jaws and supraorbital ridges; more prominent cheekbones; smaller eyes; thinner lips; and wider, larger noses. Although facial attractiveness may not always conform to algorithmic or mathematical proportions, it still derives from species-specific psychological adaptations.[1]

REFERENCE

1. Constantian MB. Rhinoplasty: Craft and Magic. New York: Thieme Publishers; 2009

BEAUTY AND ITS CONCEPTS

7. In women, sexual dimorphism toward the aesthetic ideal implies which of the following?

D. Smaller jaw.

The prototype of the female sex portrays facial features including prominent cheekbones; smooth, hairless skin; wider eyes; higher, thinner eyebrows; smaller jaws; fuller lips; and shorter, smaller noses. The other answer choices depict the aesthetic ideal for males.[1,2,3]

REFERENCES

1. Bashour M. History and current concepts in the analysis of facial attractiveness. Plast Reconstr Surg 2006;118:741
2. Bashour M. An objective system for measuring facial attractiveness. Plast Reconstr Surg 2006;118:757
3. Constantian MB. Rhinoplasty: Craft and Magic. New York: Thieme Publishers; 2009

3. Photography for the Aesthetic Surgeon

Ara A. Salibian, Anmol Chattha
See *Essentials of Aesthetic Surgery*, pp. 21–42

ELEMENTS OF STANDARDIZED CLINICAL PATIENT PHOTOGRAPHY

1. ***What does the focal length of a lens determine?***
   A. How the lens brings an object into focus.
   B. The distance from the camera to the subject.
   C. The width of the image plane.
   D. The sensor type.
   E. The type of flash utilized.

VARIABLES TO CONSIDER IN FACE OR NECK SERIES

2. ***Which of the following areas can be distorted when photographing a patient's face in the lateral view using the Frankfort plane as a reference instead of the natural horizontal plane?***
   A. Nasal tip.
   B. Malar eminence.
   C. Cerviocomental angle.
   D. Upper lip height.
   E. Brow position.

VARIABLES TO CONSIDER IN FACE OR NECK SERIES

3. ***A patient is at her preoperative visit for a facelift and necklift. When taking preoperative photos for this procedure, which of the following pairs of landmarks should be aligned for the most appropriate oblique view of the patient's face?***
   A. Dorsal nose and medial canthus.
   B. Lateral commissure and mandibular angle.
   C. Helix and lateral canthus.
   D. Menton and gonial angle.
   E. Ala and lateral canthus.

STANDARD BROW AND EYELID SERIES

4. ***When taking postoperative photographs of a blepharoplasty patient, a lens with which of the following focal lengths is the most appropriate?***
   A. 20 mm.
   B. 40 mm.
   C. 60 mm.
   D. 80 mm.
   E. 200 mm.

STANDARD RHINOPLASTY SERIES

5. ***When taking a worm's eye or basal view photograph of the nose, what reference points should be used to ensure an appropriate angle?***
   A. Nasal tip and hairline.
   B. Lower lip and nasal base.
   C. Nasal dorsum and forehead.
   D. Nasal tip and glabella.
   E. Chin and lower lip.

STANDARD BODY SERIES

6. ***A patient presents for preoperative consultation for abdominoplasty and truncal lipocontouring. Standard body series photographs are taken for evaluation. What additional view will further help evaluate abdominal soft tissue laxity?***
   A. Swimmer's view.
   B. Diver's view.
   C. Worm's eye view.
   D. Lateral view.
   E. Posterior view.

STANDARD MASSIVE-WEIGHT-LOSS BRACHIOPLASTY AND LATERAL CHEST EXCISION SERIES

7. ***In a massive-weight-loss patient planned to undergo brachioplasty and chest wall skin excision, which of the following arm positions is best for evaluating soft tissue excess of the upper arm?***
   A. Arms at the sides.
   B. Arms straight out with palms up.
   C. Arms straight vertical with palms inward.
   D. Arms straight out with elbows bent at 90 degrees and hands forwards.
   E. Arms on patient's hip.

INFORMED CONSENT

8. ***Which of the following methods is the most appropriate way of ensuring that a photograph of a patient's face used for educational purposes is compliant with Health Insurance Portability and Accountability Act (HIPAA) regulations?***
   A. Blur out the patient's eyes.
   B. Place a black bar over the patient's eyes.
   C. Hide any distinctive birthmarks or lesions.
   D. Obtain full written authorization from the patient.
   E. Only show the upper half of the face.

Answers

ELEMENTS OF STANDARDIZED CLINICAL PATIENT PHOTOGRAPHY

1. ***What does the focal length of a lens determine?***

   A. How the lens brings an object into focus.

   The focal length of a lens is the distance between the lens and the image sensor of the camera when the subject being photographed is in focus. This length is typically measured in millimeters. Using a lens with the appropriate focal length for a particular subject is important to prevent unwanted distortion of the image. With a shorter focal length, the angle of view will be wider and a larger area will be captured. A longer focal length, on the other hand, will have a smaller angle of view, and will make the subject appear larger. The Cardiff Scales of Reproduction recommend using a lens with a focal length equal to at least twice the diagonal of the image plane to avoid distortion.[1]

REFERENCE

1. Roos O, Cederblom S. A standardized system for patient documentation. J Audiov Media Med 1991;14:135

VARIABLES TO CONSIDER IN FACE OR NECK SERIES

2. ***Which of the following areas can be distorted when photographing a patient's face in the lateral view using the Frankfort plane as a reference instead of the natural horizontal plane?***

   C. Cerviocomental angle.

   The Frankfort horizontal plane is formed by a line connecting the porion, or the upper margin of the external auditory meatus, and the orbitale, or infraorbital rim. This plane is a commonly utilized landmark in cephalometric measurements. It can be utilized to orient lateral photographs and the face and neck; however, it can distort the submental tissue and change the jawline contour in certain patients. An alternative reference for facial photography is the natural horizon facial plane, which is based on the patient gazing straight as if looking at himself or herself in a mirror at eye level (**Fig. 3.1a,b**).[1,2]

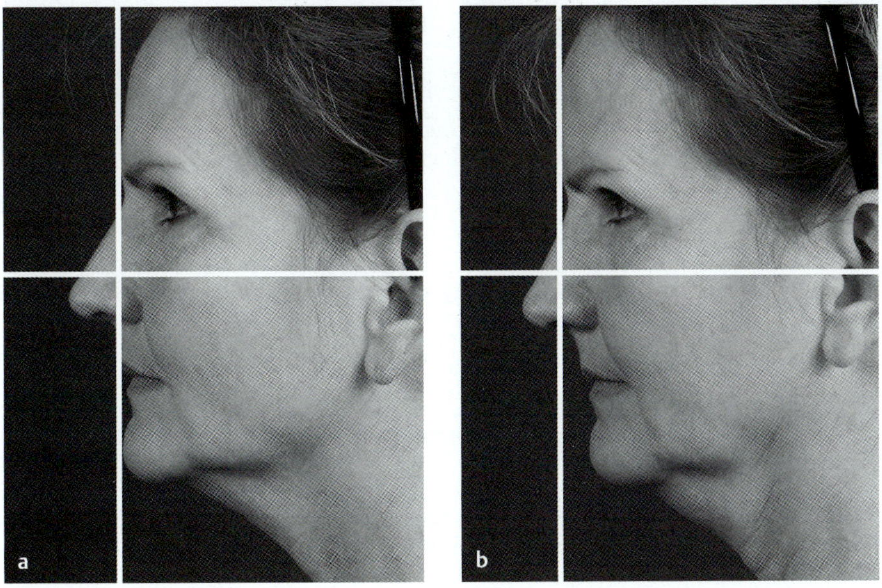

Fig. 3.1 Head positioning. **(a)** Patient shown in the Frankfort plane. Neck retraction can overemphasize the degree of submental soft tissue. **(b)** Patient shown in the natural horizontal facial plane. (Source: Head Positioning. In: Janis J, ed. Essentials of Aesthetic Surgery. 1st Edition. New York: Thieme; 2018.)

References

1. Sommer D. Pitfalls of nonstandardized photography in facial plastic surgery patients. Plast Reconstr Surg 2004;114:10
2. Galdino GM, DaSilva D, Gunter JP. Digital photography for rhinoplasty. Plast Reconstr Surg 2002;109:1421

VARIABLES TO CONSIDER IN FACE OR NECK SERIES

3. *A patient is at her preoperative visit for a facelift and necklift. When taking preoperative photos for this procedure, which of the following pairs of landmarks should be aligned for the most appropriate oblique view of the patient's face?*

A. Dorsal nose and medial canthus.

Different standards are accepted for oblique photographs of the head and neck. The patient should be positioned to have the same degree of neck flexion or head retraction, as well as the same posture as the anterior and lateral photographs. A preferred angle for the oblique photograph is when the dorsum of the nose is touching the medial aspect of the eye. The other accepted angle is taken when the nasal tip touches the opposite side of the cheek (particularly for rhinoplasty series). Whichever angle the surgeon prefers, effort should made to keep these standards consistent in the photography (**Fig. 3.2a,b**).

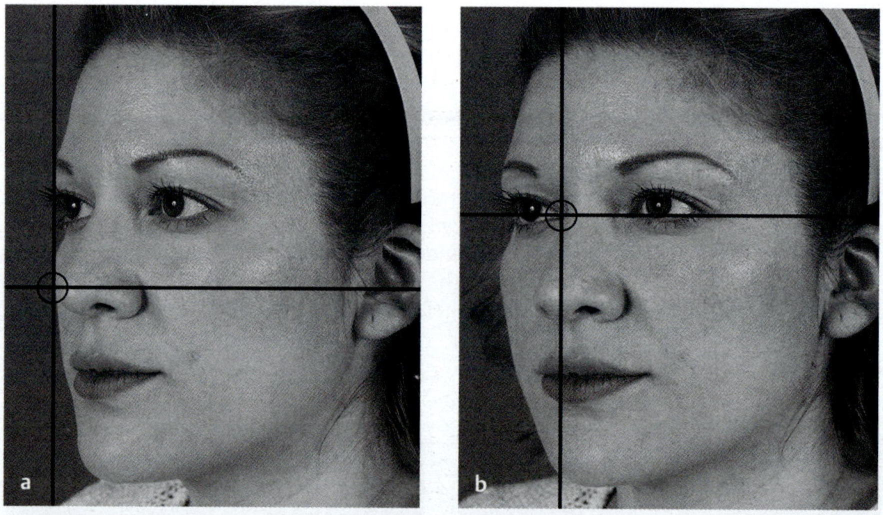

Fig. 3.2 Options for oblique views. **(a)** Tip of the nose touching the side of the far cheek for a rhinoplasty series. **(b)** Dorsum touching the medial eye. (Source: Focal Lengths and Distances. In: Janis J, ed. Essentials of Aesthetic Surgery. 1st Edition. New York: Thieme; 2018.)

Reference

1. Sommer D. Pitfalls of nonstandardized photography in facial plastic surgery patients. Plast Reconstr Surg 2004;114:10

STANDARD BROW AND EYELID SERIES

4. *When taking postoperative photographs of a blepharoplasty patient, a lens with which of the following focal lengths is the most appropriate?*

D. 80 mm.

Post-blepharoplasty patients will have close-up photographs of the eye and periorbit. In these cases, a lens with a longer focal length is more appropriate to prevent distortion and narrowing of the image. These focal lengths typically can be around 80 to 105 mm and are designed for close-up or macro photography.[1]

REFERENCE

1. DiBernadino BE, Adams RL, Krause J, et al. Photographic standards in plastic surgery. Plast Reconstr Surg 1998;102:559

STANDARD RHINOPLASTY SERIES

5. *When taking a worm's eye or basal view photograph of the nose, what reference points should be used to ensure an appropriate angle?*

D. Nasal tip and glabella.

The basal view of the nose is a critical view in rhinoplasty to assess nasal projection, nostril length, columellar proportions, width of the alar base, and flaring of the crura. The angle of this photograph should be standardized for accurate preoperative assessment and analysis of postoperative results. A standard reference point involves aligning the nasal tip between the eyebrows, or at the glabella, to determine appropriate cephalo-caudal angle for the photograph. However, the surgeon must note that this angle may vary in patients with extremes in tip underprojection or upper lip projection that can obstruct the view of the alar base.[1]

REFERENCE

1. Galdino GM, DaSilva D, Gunter JP. Digital photography for rhinoplasty. Plast Reconstr Surg 2002;109:1421

STANDARD BODY SERIES

6. *A patient presents for preoperative consultation for abdominoplasty and truncal lipocontouring. Standard body series photographs are taken for evaluation. What additional view will further help evaluate abdominal soft tissue laxity?*

B. Diver's view.

Standard photographs for truncal procedures should have the patient standing with the midpoint of the body centered in the frame. The lens axis should be parallel to the patient at all times and positioning of the patient's feet should be consistent. The diver's view that can additionally assist in evaluation of abdominal skin laxity involves oblique views of the patient bending forward at the hip while relaxing the abdomen (**Fig. 3.3a–c**).[1]

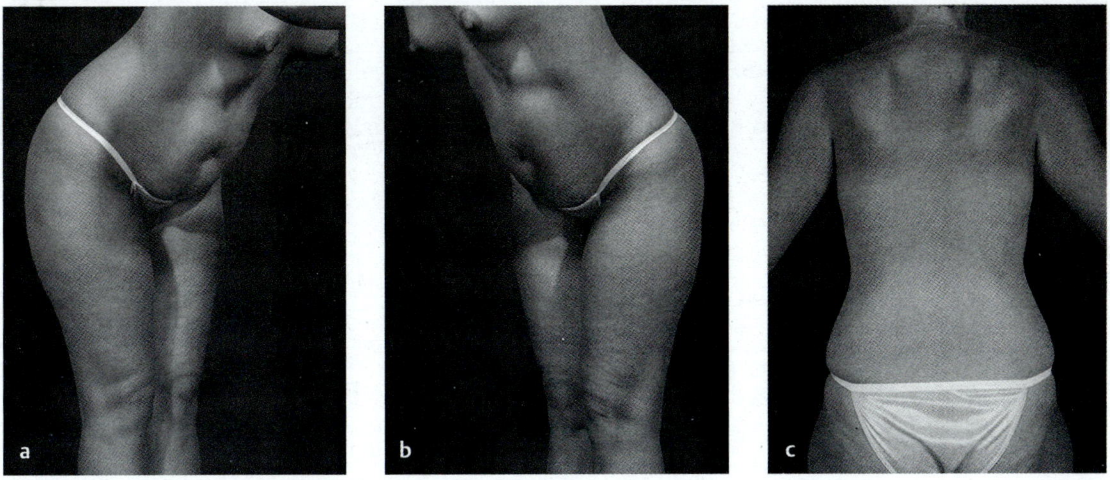

Fig. 3.3 Supplemental views for body contouring. **(a,b)** A diver's view is an oblique view with the patient bending over while relaxing the abdomen. **(c)** Back view. (Source: Supplemental Views for the Body Contouring Series. In: Janis J, ed. Essentials of Aesthetic Surgery. 1st Edition. New York: Thieme; 2018.)

REFERENCE

1. Gherardini G. Standardization in photography for body contour surgery and suction-assisted lipectomy. Plast Reconstr Surg 1997;100:227

STANDARD MASSIVE-WEIGHT-LOSS BRACHIOPLASTY AND LATERAL CHEST EXCISION SERIES

7. *In a massive-weight-loss patient planned to undergo brachioplasty and chest wall skin excision, which of the following arm positions is best for evaluating soft tissue excess of the upper arm?*

D. Arms straight out with elbows bent at 90 degrees and hands forwards.

Photographs of massive-weight-loss patients should demonstrate the proportional relationships of the body while highlighting skin laxity and areas of contour irregularities. When evaluating soft tissue excess and skin laxity of the upper arm, photographs with the patients' arms positioned straight out and elbows bent at 90 degrees will provide an efficient and standardized way of qualifying skin excess in relation to the other structure of the arm. This is also a common position that can be used for marking the skin excess in brachioplasty and designing incisions.[1,2]

REFERENCES

1. Gherardini G. Standardization in photography for body contour surgery and suction-assisted lipectomy. Plast Reconstr Surg 1997;100:227
2. Williams AR. Clinical and operating room photography. In: Vetter JP, ed. Biomedical Photography. Boston: Focal Press; 1992

INFORMED CONSENT

8. *Which of the following methods is the most appropriate way of ensuring that a photograph of a patient's face used for educational purposes is compliant with Health Insurance Portability and Accountability Act (HIPAA) regulations?*

D. Obtain full written authorization from the patient.

According to HIPAA guidelines, patient authorization is *not* required for photographs that are fully de-identified of patient information. However, full-facial photographs cannot be de-identified, and subsequently always require authorization from the patient. Furthermore, editing of the photo, including hiding the patient's eyes, does not qualify as de-identification of the patient and written authorization from the patient should still be obtained. Although masking the eyes is not explicitly addressed in the HIPAA guidelines, it is highly recommended to obtain written authorization from the patient preemptively for any facial photographs.[1,2]

REFERENCES

1. Department of Health and Human Services. Standards for privacy of individually identifiable health information: final rule. 45 CFR Parts 160 and 164. Federal Register 65, no. 250 (December 28, 2000).
2. Roach WH Jr, Hoban RG, Broccolo BM, et al, eds. Medical Records and the Law. Gaithersburg, MD: Aspen Publishers; 1994

4. Medicolegal Considerations in Aesthetic Surgery

Sammy Sinno, Jeremie Oliver Piña
See *Essentials of Aesthetic Surgery*, pp. 43–56

PATIENT SELECTION

1. *What is the best first step in preventing malpractice claims?*

A. Hire a good lawyer.
B. Become well-versed in state and local malpractice laws.
C. Proper patient selection.
D. Transition to a noninvasive practice.
E. Work for an academic hospital.

PATIENT SELECTION

2. *Why is a patient's familial disapproval for undergoing aesthetic surgery a relative contraindication to proceed?*

A. The family may not support the patient postoperatively.
B. The risk of an "I told you so" reaction from the disapproving family.
C. The patient may regret disappointing the family.
D. They may not have the funds to pay for the procedure(s).
E. The family may not refer patient to the surgeon in the future.

PATIENT COMMUNICATION

3. *Which of the following is an example of a communicative measure aesthetic surgeons can implement into their practice to prevent inflated expectations and decrease litigations?*

A. Take notes while the patient is speaking.
B. Highlighting only objective facts from the patient's history.
C. Limiting interactions to essential conversation topics.
D. Strive for repetition in explaining procedures during patient encounters.
E. Sit between the patient and the door in the examination room.

PATIENT COMMUNICATION

4. *Which of the following is considered good standard of practice for documentation in aesthetic surgery?*

A. Minimal documentation in order to avoid unnecessary charting errors.
B. Enter all patient information in electronic chart during the patient encounter.
C. Enter thorough details of all discussion points shortly after patient encounter.
D. Hire a scribe to complete all charting duties.
E. Rely on "smart text" entries to complete clinical notes.

PATIENT COMMUNICATION

5. *A physician would be most likely to lose a jury trial if:*

A. Despite demonstrating compassionate care, the surgical outcome was not optimal due to a postoperative infection from incomplete dressing coverage.
B. The physician chose one standard therapy, which turned out not to be the best choice for the patient.
C. The patient claims to have had a lengthy conversation with the physician, even though the physician had previously documented that no such conversation took place.
D. The physician wrote a handwritten note for a patient encounter, which is illegible, even though there is no evidence that the physician was blatantly negligent.
E. Despite the physician's best judgment in the operating room, the patient experiences a complication due to the surgical technique.

PATIENT COMMUNICATION

6. *A local plastic surgeon was involved in a lawsuit. Which of the following did not help the plastic surgeon's case when it went to court?*

A. Performing a good history of physical.
B. Eligible documentation.
C. Obtaining multiple medical consults with other subspecialities.
D. Attempting to help the patient by addressing her gynecologic concerns.
E. Letting the patient know all the foreseeable risks of the surgery.

PATIENT COMMUNICATION

7. *Which of the following is always a predictable consequence of any surgical procedure?*

A. Loss of neuronal sensitivity.
B. Wound dehiscence.
C. Skin sloughing.
D. Scarring.
E. Swelling.

PATIENT COMMUNICATION

8. *Which of the following aesthetic procedures has the highest degree of unpredictability?*

A. Breast augmentation.
B. Facelift.
C. Rhinoplasty.
D. Blepharoplasty.
E. Brow-lift.

PATIENT COMMUNICATION

9. *Pulmonary embolism is most commonly associated with which of the following procedures?*

A. Breast reduction.
B. Augmentation mastopexy.
C. Rhytidectomy.
D. Abdominoplasty.
E. Suction-assisted lipectomy.

Answers

PATIENT SELECTION

1. ***What is the best first step in preventing malpractice claims?***

   C. Proper patient selection.

   It is crucial as an aesthetic surgeon to be cognizant of the various "red flags" evident in some patients seeking procedures. Some examples of these could include patients who have excessively high expectations for the outcomes of the procedure; excessively demanding patients; indecisive patients; immature patients; secretive patients; patients who do not get along with other physicians; patients with body dysmorphic disorder; or patients who have undergone excessive previous aesthetic procedures. These patients end up more likely to sue their physician. The other answer choices can all help but are not the best first step in preventing a malpractice claim. The best first step in preventing a malpractice claim is operating on the right patients.[1]

REFERENCE

1. Gorney M. Medical liability in plastic and reconstructive surgery. In: Anderson RE, ed. Medical Malpractice: A Physician's Sourcebook. Totowa, NJ: Humana Press; 2005

PATIENT SELECTION

2. ***Why is a patient's familial disapproval for undergoing aesthetic surgery a relative contraindication to proceed?***

   B. The risk of an "I told you so" reaction from the disapproving family.

   Although family approval is not a requirement to undergo aesthetic surgery, familial disapproval is a relative contraindication to proceed with surgery, as less-than-optimal results may produce an untimely "I told you so..." reaction from the disapproving family members. Such a reaction may deepen a patient's feelings of guilt, regret, or dissatisfaction. The other options do not target the underlaying reason.[1]

REFERENCE

1. Gorney M. Medical liability in plastic and reconstructive surgery. In: Anderson RE, ed. Medical Malpractice: A Physician's Sourcebook. Totowa, NJ: Humana Press; 2005

PATIENT COMMUNICATION

3. ***Which of the following is an example of a communicative measure aesthetic surgeons can implement into their practice to prevent inflated expectations and decrease litigations?***

   D. Strive for repetition in explaining procedures during patient encounters.

   It is estimated that the average patient retains only **35%** of what is said; repetition can increase patient comprehension, which can prevent inflated expectations and decrease litigations. Repetition and increasing points of contact help. Taking notes can be helpful; however, surgeons should listen to and make eye contact with patients, then jot down the key words needed to reconstruct the conversation shortly after the consultation. The other options are not communication styles that can be helpful to avoid litigation.[1,2]

REFERENCES

1. Gorney M. Communication and patient safety. In: Anderson RE, ed. Medical Malpractice: A Physician's Sourcebook. Totowa, NJ: Humana Press; 2005
2. Nichols R. Are You Listening? New York: McGraw Hill; 1957

PATIENT COMMUNICATION

4. *Which of the following is considered good standard of practice for documentation in aesthetic surgery?*

C. Enter thorough details of all discussion points shortly after patient encounter.

The digital age poses many new problems for physicians. Interacting with a laptop or notebook and not with the patient can significantly interfere with the doctor–patient relationship. There must be a balance of efficiency, accuracy, and attention paid to the patient. Do not rely on "smart text" entries that default to a response, as they can often be inaccurate.

A lack of evidence is powerful evidence, as scant documentation because of a busy lifestyle will allow the plaintiff attorney to allege that patient care was equally scant and rushed. Remember, a physician's duty to patients includes not only good patient care, but thorough, accurate documentation of such care.

Minimal documentation can hurt the surgeon and make a legal team think the surgeon provides sloppy care. Having an electronic medical record system or a scribe is not required to provide good documentation and sometimes relying on "smart text" entries can actually impact documentation negatively.[1]

REFERENCE

1. Gorney M. Medical liability in plastic and reconstructive surgery. In: Anderson RE, ed. Medical Malpractice: A Physician's Sourcebook. Totowa, NJ: Humana Press; 2005

PATIENT COMMUNICATION

5. *A physician would be most likely to lose a jury trial if:*

D. The physician wrote a handwritten note for a patient encounter, which is illegible, even though there is no evidence that the physician was blatantly negligent.

Good trial attorneys have catchy themes or theatrical ploys that they run throughout their trials. One such medical malpractice theme is: "Sloppy at documentation is sloppy at practice." The duty of the responsible physician is to read and correct everything entered before signing the document, and to confirm that all is legible. Fortunately, handwritten patient notes are becoming less common with the advent of electronic medical records. However, with the electronic world of charting comes a whole host of other potential drawbacks and precautions, which must be addressed.[1]

REFERENCE

1. Gorney M. Medical liability in plastic and reconstructive surgery. In: Anderson RE, ed. Medical Malpractice: A Physician's Sourcebook. Totowa, NJ: Humana Press; 2005

PATIENT COMMUNICATION

6. *A local plastic surgeon was involved in a lawsuit. Which of the following did not help the plastic surgeon's case when it went to court?*

D. Attempting to help the patient by addressing her gynecologic concerns.

Aesthetic plastic surgeons have a duty to the patient but only within the scope of our practice. If a patient has a generalized medical problem, we should have the patient follow-up with the primary care physician. The other answer choices are things that help the plastic surgeon's case. Documenting a thorough history and physical, as well as obtaining medical consults with other providers when in doubt, and documenting eligibly are important considerations. Also, we have an affirmative duty to disclose in detail the benefits, risks, alternatives, possible complications, and unpleasant side effects for any procedure or surgery.[1]

REFERENCE

1. Gorney M. Medical liability in plastic and reconstructive surgery. In: Anderson RE, ed. Medical Malpractice: A Physician's Sourcebook. Totowa, NJ: Humana Press; 2005

PATIENT COMMUNICATION

7. *Which of the following is always a predictable consequence of any surgical procedure?*

D. Scarring.

This should always be included in the informed consent process preoperatively: No healing can occur without a scar! Although scarring qualities differ based on genetics and skin properties, *everyone* scars to some extent. As such, scar formation is a major genesis of patient dissatisfaction, and should be thoroughly discussed preemptively. The consequence in the other options can occur but do not consistently take place with open surgery.[1,2]

REFERENCES

1. Horton JB, Reece EM, Broughton G II, Janis JE, Thornton JF, Rohrich RJ. Patient safety in the office-based setting. Plast Reconstr Surg 2006;117:61e
2. Iverson RE. Patient safety in office-based surgery facilities: I. Procedures in the office-based surgery setting. Plast Reconstr Surg 2002;110:1337; discussion 1343

PATIENT COMMUNICATION

8. *Which of the following aesthetic procedures has the highest degree of unpredictability?*

C. Rhinoplasty.

Asymmetry, continued breathing difficulties (septorhinoplasty), allegations of improper functional capacity, and evolving structural settling can all contribute to the unpredictability in rhinoplasty outcomes. It is advisable to avoid inappropriate use of "brag books" containing only excellent results; also, strictly counsel patients that these results cannot always be obtained.[1]

REFERENCE

1. Gorney M. Medical liability in plastic and reconstructive surgery. In: Anderson RE, ed. Medical Malpractice: A Physician's Sourcebook. Totowa, NJ: Humana Press; 2005

PATIENT COMMUNICATION

9. *Pulmonary embolism is most commonly associated with which of the following procedures?*

E. Suction-assisted lipectomy.

Suction-assisted lipectomy (liposuction) is the most commonly performed elective aesthetic procedure in the United States.[1,2] Liposuction is typically performed in the outpatient setting (outside regulatory control) and by a variety of practitioners (many of whom are unqualified).[3] Mortality increases significantly when liposuction is combined with other procedures,[1] or when a patient endures anesthesia for more than 6 hours.[3] Although certainly not common, the risk of potential mortality associated with this procedure should always be discussed during the informed consent process.

REFERENCES

1. Horton JB, Reece EM, Broughton G II, Janis JE, Thornton JF, Rohrich RJ. Patient safety in the office-based setting. Plast Reconstr Surg 2006;117:61e
2. Iverson RE. Patient safety in office-based surgery facilities: I. Procedures in the office-based surgery setting. Plast Reconstr Surg 2002;110:1337; discussion 1343
3. Gorney M. Medical liability in plastic and reconstructive surgery. In: Anderson RE, ed. Medical Malpractice: A Physician's Sourcebook. Totowa, NJ: Humana Press; 2005

PART II

Anesthesia

5. Basics of Anesthesia for the Aesthetic Surgery Patient

Aaron M. Kearney, Sammy Sinno, Anmol Chattha
See *Essentials of Aesthetic Surgery*, pp. 59–84

SURGICAL JUDGMENT

1. *What is one of the advantages of total intravenous anesthesia (TIVA)?*
- A. Simple administration.
- B. Lower cost.
- C. Easier titration of depth.
- D. Reduced incidence of postoperative nausea and vomiting (PONV).
- E. Does not require an anesthesiologist to be present.

RISK FACTORS

2. *Which of the following comorbidities indicates a patient who is not suitable for general anesthesia in an ambulatory surgical center or office?*
- A. End-stage renal disease (ESRD).
- B. Atrial fibrillation.
- C. Paraplegia.
- D. Peripheral vascular disease.
- E. Mild obstructive sleep apnea (OSA).

PREOPERATIVE TESTING

3. *Which of the following is an accurate statement regarding hCG testing in females undergoing aesthetic surgery?*
- A. Urine hCG must be obtained for all premenopausal females prior to undergoing surgery.
- B. Anesthetic exposure in pregnant females is significantly linked to spontaneous abortion and premature birth.
- C. The American Society of Anesthesiologists recommends "offering" rather than "requiring" hCG testing.
- D. A point of care (POC) urine hCG test is not a reliable test before surgery.
- E. Preoperative hCG testing is positive in 4% of cases.

RISK FACTORS

4. *Which of the following factors is a reason to obtain a preoperative electrocardiogram (ECG) in a patient?*
- A. Any patient over the age of 60.
- B. Diabetes mellitus on metformin.
- C. Renal insufficiency.
- D. End-stage liver disease.
- E. Patient with body mass index (BMI) of 33.

RISK FACTORS

5. *Which of the following is one of the Revised Cardiac Risk Index (RCRI) risk factors?*
- A. Peripheral artery disease with history of bypass.
- B. Cerebral vascular disease with history of stroke or transient ischemic attack.
- C. Poorly controlled hypertension.
- D. Obesity.
- E. Active smoking.

RISK FACTORS

6. ***What is the threshold level of metabolic equivalents (METs), below which functional status is considered poor?***
A. 2 METs.
B. 4 METs.
C. 6 METs.
D. 8 METs.
E. 10 METs.

RISK FACTORS

7. ***Which of the following tasks approximates 4 METs, if the patient can carry out the task without becoming short of breath?***
A. Eating, dressing, or using the toilet.
B. Climbing a flight of stairs.
C. Walking two blocks on level ground at 2 to 3 miles per hour.
D. Participating in moderate recreational activities, such as golf or bowling.
E. Running a marathon.

PHARMACOLOGY

8. ***To which class of drugs does dexmedetomidine belong?***
A. Opiate agonist-antagonist.
B. Benzodiazepine.
C. Phencyclidine.
D. Alpha-2-adrenergic agonist.
E. Alkylphenols.

SURGICAL JUDGMENT

9. ***Which of the following responses to stimulation indicates "moderate sedation"?***
A. Normal response to verbal stimulation.
B. Reflex withdrawal to pain.
C. Purposeful response to verbal or tactile stimulation.
D. Purposeful response with repeated or painful stimulation.
E. Swallow or gag reflex present.

SURGICAL JUDGMENT

10. ***Which of the following is the most common injury in the operating room related to positioning?***
A. Thermal injury.
B. Corneal abrasion.
C. Pressure sore.
D. Peripheral neuropathy.
E. Postoperative vision loss (POVL).

RISK FACTORS

11. ***Which of the following is a risk factor for postoperative nausea and vomiting (PONV)?***
A. Male gender.
B. Female gender.
C. Smoking.
D. Total intravenous anesthesia.
E. High BMI patients.

PHARMACOLOGY

12. ***Which of the following is the drug of choice for malignant hyperthermia?***
A. Sodium bicarbonate.
B. Sodium dantrolene.
C. Flumazenil.
D. Furosemide.
E. Naloxone.

Answers

SURGICAL JUDGMENT

1. *What is one of the advantages of total intravenous anesthesia (TIVA)?*

D. Reduced incidence of postoperative nausea and vomiting (PONV).

Total intravenous anesthesia can be helpful in patients with a history of severe postoperative nausea and vomiting. However, it is more complex to administer and is more expensive than traditional general anesthesia. Usually, it has a better patient experience after surgery. However, it still requires an anesthesiologist to administer.[1,2]

REFERENCES

1. Blakely KR, Klein KW, White PF, et al. A total intravenous anesthetic technique for outpatient facial laser resurfacing. Anesth Analg 1998;87:827
2. Barinholtz D. Intravenous anesthesia for cosmetic surgery. In: Friedberg BL, ed. Anesthesia in Cosmetic Surgery. New York: Cambridge University Press; 2007

RISK FACTORS

2. *Which of the following comorbidities indicates a patient who is not suitable for general anesthesia in an ambulatory surgical center or office?*

A. End-stage renal disease (ESRD).

ESRD is a contraindication to undergoing general anesthesia in an ambulatory surgical center or office. Patients with well-controlled atrial fibrillation (as opposed to those with higher-grade arrhythmias or who have permanent pacemakers/implantable cardioverter-defibrillators), paraplegia, peripheral vascular disease, and those with mild OSA may be appropriate to undergo general anesthesia in these settings. Severe OSA would be a red flag to undergoing general anesthesia in an ambulatory surgical center or office.[1]

REFERENCE

1. Kataria K, Cutter TW, Apfelbaum JL. Patient selection in outpatient surgery. Clin Plast Surg 2013;40:371

PREOPERATIVE TESTING

3. *Which of the following is an accurate statement regarding hCG testing in females undergoing aesthetic surgery?*

C. The American Society of Anesthesiologists recommends "offering" rather than "requiring" hCG testing.

hCG testing is institution dependent. The American Society of Anesthesiologists does not specifically recommend obtaining hCG testing in all females but does recommend offering the test to patients. Evidence is mixed regarding the effect of anesthetics on pregnant females. A POC urine hCG test is a reliable preoperative test. Positive pregnancy tests have been reported in 0.3 to 1.3% of premenopausal menstruating females.[1,2]

REFERENCES

1. Committee on Standards and Practice Parameters, et al. Practice Advisory for Preanesthetic Evaluation. An updated report by the American Society of Anesthesiologists Taskforce on Preanesthesia Evaluation. Anesthesiology 2012;116:522
2. Choosing wisely: an initiative of the ABIM Foundation. Available at www.choosingwisely.org

RISK FACTORS

4. *Which of the following factors is a reason to obtain a preoperative electrocardiogram (ECG) in a patient?*

C. Renal insufficiency.

Renal insufficiency is a component of the Revised Cardiac Risk Index and is an indication to obtain a preoperative electrocardiogram (ECG) within 6 months of surgery. Age alone is not a reason to obtain an ECG. Diabetes on insulin is another reason to obtain an ECG, but diabetes controlled with oral medication is not. Obesity is not a direct indication to obtain an ECG as well.[1,2]

References

1. Cohn SL, Fleisher LA. Evaluation of cardiac risk prior to noncardiac surgery. Available at https://www.uptodate.com/contents/evaluation-of-cardiac-risk-prior-to-noncardiac-surgery
2. Committee on Standards and Practice Parameters, et al. Practice Advisory for Preanesthetic Evaluation. An updated report by the American Society of Anesthesiologists Taskforce on Preanesthesia Evaluation. Anesthesiology 2012;116:522

RISK FACTORS

5. *Which of the following is one of the Revised Cardiac Risk Index (RCRI) risk factors?*

B. Cerebral vascular disease with history of stroke or transient ischemic attack.

Cerebral vascular disease is one of the components of the RCRI. The rest of the above are not.[1]

Reference

1. Cohn SL, Fleisher LA. Evaluation of cardiac risk prior to noncardiac surgery. Available at https://www.uptodate.com/contents/evaluation-of-cardiac-risk-prior-to-noncardiac-surgery

RISK FACTORS

6. *What is the threshold level of metabolic equivalents (METs), below which functional status is considered poor?*

B. 4 METs.

Patients with less than 4 METs are considered to have poor functional status with increased risk of cardiopulmonary complications.[1,2]

References

1. Kataria K, Cutter TW, Apfelbaum JL. Patient selection in outpatient surgery. Clin Plast Surg 2013;40:371
2. Cohn SL, Fleisher LA. Evaluation of cardiac risk prior to noncardiac surgery. Available at https://www.uptodate.com/contents/evaluation-of-cardiac-risk-prior-to-noncardiac-surgery

RISK FACTORS

7. *Which of the following tasks approximates 4 METs, if the patient can carry out the task without becoming short of breath?*

B. Climbing a flight of stairs.

Climbing a flight of stairs is the approximate equivalent of 4 METs. The rest of the mentioned activities require more or less effort. 1 MET = 3.5 mL O_2 uptake/kg/min which is the resting oxygen uptake in sitting position. Eating, dressing, or using the toilet is equivalent to 1 MET. Walking two blocks at 2 to 3 mph is a little less than 4 METs. Moderate recreational activity is approximately 8 METs and strenuous activity such as a marathon is >10 METs. It is a proxy to assess for cardiac risk and <4 METs is a concern for poor functional risk with worse cardiopulmonary complications perioperatively.[1,2]

References

1. Kataria K, Cutter TW, Apfelbaum JL. Patient selection in outpatient surgery. Clin Plast Surg 2013;40:371
2. Cohn SL, Fleisher LA. Evaluation of cardiac risk prior to noncardiac surgery. Available at https://www.uptodate.com/contents/evaluation-of-cardiac-risk-prior-to-noncardiac-surgery

PHARMACOLOGY

8. *To which class of drugs does dexmedetomidine belong?*

D. Alpha-2-adrenergic agonist.

Dexmedetomidine is an alpha-2-adrenergic agonist commonly used for sedation. The other classes of drugs are also used in sedation with different goals and responses.[1]

Reference

1. ASA continuum of depth of sedation: definition of general anesthesia and level of sedation/analgesia. Available at www.asahq.org.

SURGICAL JUDGMENT

9. *Which of the following responses to stimulation indicates "moderate sedation"?*

C. Purposeful response to verbal or tactile stimulation.

Moderate sedation is defined by a purposeful response to verbal or tactile stimulation. Normal response implies minimal sedation, whereas repeated or painful stimulation implies that the patient is under deep sedation. Swallow or gag reflex is present in minimal sedation.[1]

REFERENCE

1. ASA continuum of depth of sedation: definition of general anesthesia and level of sedation/analgesia. Available at www.asahq.org.

SURGICAL JUDGMENT

10. *Which of the following is the most common injury in the operating room related to positioning?*

D. Peripheral neuropathy.

Peripheral neuropathies are the most common intraoperative injury related to positioning. Corneal abrasions are the most common intraoperative injury overall but are not related to positioning. Nerve injuries are the second most frequent liability claim in anesthesia practice. The other options are all rare or "never" events related to the perioperative period.[1,2]

REFERENCES

1. Hansen J, Botney R. Safe patient positioning. In: Young VL, Botney R, eds. Patient Safety in Plastic Surgery. New York: Thieme Publishers; 2009
2. Cheney FW, Domino KB, Kaplan RA, et al. Nerve injury associated with anesthesia: a closed claim analysis. Anesthesiology 1999;90:1062

RISK FACTORS

11. *Which of the following is a risk factor for postoperative nausea and vomiting (PONV)?*

B. Female gender.

Females are at higher risk for postoperative nausea and vomiting. Additional risk factors include non-smokers, prior history of PONV or motion sickness, postoperative opioids, age less than 50 years, and general anesthesia. Total intravenous anesthesia is protective against PONV. The literature does not support that high BMI patients are more likely to be at risk for PONV.[1]

REFERENCE

1. Le TP, Gan TJ. Update on the management of postoperative nausea and vomiting and postdischarge nausea and vomiting in ambulatory surgery. Anesthesiol Clin 2010;28:225

PHARMACOLOGY

12. *Which of the following is the drug of choice for malignant hyperthermia?*

B. Sodium dantrolene.

Dantrolene, or the new preparation Ryanodex, is the only effective treatment for malignant hyperthermia. Flumazenil is used to reverse benzodiazepine overdose. Naloxone is used to reverse narcotic overdose. It is important to know that these two drugs have half-lives shorter than the offending agent so watch out for re-narcotization or re-sedation. Sodium bicarbonate is used for multiple other indications but not for malignant hyperthermia. Furosemide is a diuretic.[1]

REFERENCE

1. Litman RL, Flood CD, Kaplan RF, et al. Postoperative malignant hyperthermia: an analysis of cases from the North American Malignant Hyperthermia Registry. Anesthesiology 2008;109:825

6. Perioperative Anesthesia Considerations for the Aesthetic Surgery Patient

Aaron M. Kearney, Sammy Sinno
See *Essentials of Aesthetic Surgery*, pp. 85–94

HOME MEDICATION CONTINUATION IN THE PERIOPERATIVE PERIOD

1. ***Which of the following medications should patients continue to take on the morning of surgery?***
A. Metoprolol.
B. Metformin.
C. Furosemide.
D. Hydrochlorothiazide.
E. Estradiol.

IMPLANTABLE CARDIOVERTER-DEFIBRILLATOR PREOPERATIVE EVALUATION

2. ***Within what time frame should patients with implantable cardioverter-defibrillators (ICDs) have their device checked prior to elective surgery?***
A. 1 month.
B. 3 months.
C. 6 months.
D. 12 months.
E. 24 months.

PREOPERATIVE ANESTHESIOLOGY EVALUATION

3. ***Which of the following patients may benefit from an evaluation by an anesthesiologist prior to the day of surgery?***
A. A 76-year-old female with coronary artery disease.
B. A 24-year-old male smoker with Hashimoto's thyroiditis.
C. A 55-year-old male with hypertension and obesity class II.
D. A 60-year-old female with diabetes mellitus and stage I chronic kidney disease.
E. An 87-year-old male with well-controlled asthma.

HEMOGLOBIN A1c AND COMPLICATIONS

4. ***Which hemoglobin A1c threshold would be optimal to reduce complications?***
A. ≤4.0.
B. ≤7.4.
C. ≤8.4.
D. ≤9.4.
E. ≤10.4.

MEDICAL RISK FACTORS FOR ANESTHESIA

5. ***Which of the following is a strong contraindication to undergoing elective cosmetic surgery?***
A. Coronary artery disease with drug-eluting stent placed 14 months ago.
B. Severe pulmonary hypertension.
C. End-stage renal disease.
D. Hepatic cirrhosis.
E. 40 pack-year smoking history.

PREVALENCE OF HERBAL SUPPLEMENT USE

6. *Which of the following statements regarding herbal supplements is true?*
A. They are regulated by the US Food and Drug Administration (FDA).
B. They can be continued perioperatively without concern.
C. They are taken regularly by over 30% of the US population.
D. Their ingredients are standardized.
E. More than 60% patients reveal use of herbal supplements at their preoperative appointment.

PREOPERATIVE SMOKING CESSATION

7. *The Centers for Disease Control (CDC) recommends smoking cessation for at least how long before and after surgery?*
A. 5 days.
B. 2 weeks.
C. 30 days.
D. 6 weeks.
E. 8 weeks.

OBSTRUCTIVE SLEEP APNEA SCREENING

8. *Which of the following is a recommended screening method to detect obstructive sleep apnea in patients undergoing surgery?*
A. STOP-BANG questionnaire.
B. Nasal examination by an otolaryngologist.
C. SLEEP questionnaire.
D. Family history of sleep apnea.
E. Assessing oropharynx width.

HERBAL SUPPLEMENT RISKS

9. *Which of the following is true regarding herbal supplements?*
A. Most lead to low-grade kidney failure.
B. They can increase the risk of bleeding.
C. Fish oil supplementation is safe up until the day of surgery.
D. Aesthetic surgery patients are least likely type of plastic surgery patients to use supplements.
E. Kava kava is not one of the herbs that are considered to impact surgery.

Answers

HOME MEDICATION CONTINUATION IN THE PERIOPERATIVE PERIOD

1. *Which of the following medications should patients continue to take on the morning of surgery?*

A. Metoprolol.

Beta blockers taken as a home medication should be continued on the day of surgery. Oral hypoglycemics and diuretics should generally be held. Estradiol and other oral contraceptive pills should generally be stopped for at least 2 weeks.[1]

REFERENCE

1. Levin N. Preanesthetic assessment of the cosmetic patient. In: Friedberg BL, ed. Anesthesia in Cosmetic Surgery. New York: Cambridge University Press; 2007

IMPLANTABLE CARDIOVERTER-DEFIBRILLATOR PREOPERATIVE EVALUATION

2. *Within what time frame should patients with implantable cardioverter-defibrillators (ICDs) have their device checked prior to elective surgery?*

C. 6 months.

Patients with ICDs should have their device checked within the 6 months prior to undergoing elective surgery. Patients with pacemakers can have their device checked within 12 months. One should consider doing these cases in a hospital setting.[1]

REFERENCE

1. American Society of Anesthesiologists. Practice advisory for the perioperative management of patients with cardiac implantable electronic devices: pacemakers and implantable cardioverter-defibrillators: an updated report by the American Society of Anesthesiologists task force on perioperative management of patients with cardiac implantable electronic devices. Anesthesiology 2011;114:247

PREOPERATIVE ANESTHESIOLOGY EVALUATION

3. *Which of the following patients may benefit from an evaluation by an anesthesiologist prior to the day of surgery?*

C. A 55-year-old male with hypertension and obesity class II.

This patient has four of the STOP-BANG criteria used for screening patients to determine the risk of obstructive sleep apnea (OSA). Patients with three or more risk factors have a high risk of OSA. Patients with known or presumptive OSA can benefit from preoperative evaluation by an anesthesiologist to reduce the risk of postoperative respiratory compromise (**Fig. 6.1**).

1. Do you **S**nore loudly? Yes/No
2. Do you feel **T**ired, fatigued, or sleep during the daytime? Yes/No
3. Has anyone **O**bserved you stop breathing during your sleep? Yes/No
4. Have you been or are you now being treated for high blood **P**ressure? Yes/No
5. Is your **B**ody Mass Index greater than 35 kg/m^2? Yes/No
6. Are you over 50 years of **A**ge? Yes/No
7. Is your **N**eck circumference greater than 40 cm? Yes/No
8. **G**ender (male)? Yes/No

Fig. 6.1 STOP-BANG questionnaire used for screening patients to determine the risk of OSA. Fewer than three questions positive = low risk of OSA; three or more questions positive = high risk of OSA; five to eight questions positive = high probability of moderate to severe OSA. (Source: Adapted from Chung F, Yegneswaran B, Liao P, et al. STOP questionnaire: a tool to screen patients for obstructive sleep apnea. Anesthesiology 18:812, 2008.)

REFERENCE

1. Joshi GP, Saravanan PA, Gan TJ, et al. Society of Ambulatory Anesthesia consensus statement of preoperative selection of adult patients with obstructive sleep apnea scheduled for ambulatory surgery. Anesth Analg 2012;115:1060

HEMOGLOBIN A1c AND COMPLICATIONS

4. *Which hemoglobin A1c threshold would be optimal to reduce complications?*

B. ≤7.4.

Patients with a hemoglobin A1c of 7.4 or less have a reduced risk for infectious complications. Hemoglobin A1c greater than 7.4 puts patients at increased risk of complications. Low hemoglobin A1c (<4.0%) was associated with an increased risk of all-cause mortality.[1,2]

REFERENCES

1. Braithwaite SS. Perioperative glucose control and diabetes management. In: Young VL, Botney R, eds. Patient Safety in Plastic Surgery. New York: Thieme Publishers; 2009
2. Joshi GP, Chung F, Vann MA, et al. Society for Ambulatory Anesthesia consensus statement on perioperative blood glucose management in diabetic patients undergoing ambulatory surgery. Anesth Anal 2010;111:1378

MEDICAL RISK FACTORS FOR ANESTHESIA

5. *Which of the following is a strong contraindication to undergoing elective cosmetic surgery?*

B. Severe pulmonary hypertension.

Patients with severe pulmonary hypertension are very high-risk patients for general anesthesia and should not undergo elective cosmetic surgery. The other comorbidities listed can confer increased risk but may be safe if they are optimized appropriately.[1,2]

REFERENCES

1. Levin N. Preanesthetic assessment of the cosmetic patient. In: Friedberg BL, ed. Anesthesia in Cosmetic Surgery. New York: Cambridge University Press; 2007
2. Kataria K, Cutter TW, Apfelbaum JL. Patient selection in outpatient surgery. Clin Plast Surg 2013;40:371

PREVALENCE OF HERBAL SUPPLEMENT USE

6. *Which of the following statements regarding herbal supplements is true?*

C. They are taken regularly by over 30% of the US population.

Herbal supplements are taken by over 32% of the US population. About 70% of these patients do not reveal their use to their doctor. These supplements are not regulated by the FDA and do not have standardized ingredients. Their effects on surgery and their interactions with drugs used perioperatively are generally unknown, so surgeons should consider having patients discontinue them 2 to 3 weeks prior to surgery.[1,2]

REFERENCES

1. Levin N. Preanesthetic assessment of the cosmetic patient. In: Friedberg BL, ed. Anesthesia in Cosmetic Surgery. New York: Cambridge University Press; 2007
2. Abe A, Kaye AD, Gritsenko K, et al. Perioperative analgesia and the effects of dietary supplements. Best Pract Res Clin Anesthesiol 2014;28:183

PREOPERATIVE SMOKING CESSATION

7. *The Centers for Disease Control (CDC) recommends smoking cessation for at least how long before and after surgery?*

C. 30 days.

The CDC recommends 30 days of smoking cessation before and after surgery. The other time frames are incorrect.[1]

Reference

1. Cereda M, Neligan PJ. Managing the risk of perioperative pulmonary complications. In: Young VL, Botney R, eds. Patient Safety in Plastic Surgery. New York: Thieme Publishers; 2009

OBSTRUCTIVE SLEEP APNEA SCREENING

8. *Which of the following is a recommended screening method to detect obstructive sleep apnea in patients undergoing surgery?*

A. STOP-BANG questionnaire.

The STOP-BANG questionnaire is a commonly used screening method to detect patients who may have obstructive sleep apnea. Those who answer three or more questions positively have a high risk of OSA and may benefit from preoperative evaluation by an anesthesiologist.[1,2]

References

1. Stephan PJ, Mercier D, Coleman J, et al. Obstructive sleep apnea: implications for the plastic surgeon and ambulatory surgery centers. Plast Reconstr Surg 2009;125:652
2. American Society of Anesthesiologists Task Force on Perioperative Management of Patients with Obstructive Sleep Apnea. Practice guidelines for the perioperative management of patients with obstructive sleep apnea: an updated report by the American Society of Anesthesiologists Task Force on Perioperative Management of patients with obstructive sleep apnea. Anesthesiology 2014;120:268

HERBAL SUPPLEMENT RISKS

9. *Which of the following is true regarding herbal supplements?*

B. They can increase the risk of bleeding.

Herbal supplements can increase risk of bleeding and hematomas. It is inconclusive whether herbal supplements cause kidney damage. Fish oil supplementation can be a blood thinner and should be stopped 2 to 3 weeks before surgery. Consideration should be given to holding all supplements for 2 to 3 weeks prior to elective surgery.[1,2]

References

1. Broughton G, Crosby MA, Coleman J, et al. Use of herbal supplements and vitamins in plastic surgery: a practical review. Plast Reconstr Surg 2007;119:48e
2. Jalili J, Askeroglu U, Alleyne B, et al. Herbal products that may contribute to hypertension. Plast Reconstr Surg 2013;131:168

7. Procedure-Specific Anesthesia Guidelines for the Aesthetic Surgery Patient

Anmol Chattha, Sammy Sinno, Aaron M. Kearney
See *Essentials of Aesthetic Surgery*, pp. 95–106

RHYTIDECTOMY

1. ***A 52-year-old female with no past medical history undergoes an uncomplicated rhytidectomy. As the patient is being extubated, she experiences a rise in her systolic pressure to 180 mmHg that is sustained for a few minutes. What complication is she most at risk for?***
   A. Intraoperative stroke.
   B. Hematoma.
   C. Seroma.
   D. Postoperative nausea and vomiting (PONV).
   E. Uncontrollable pain.

RHYTIDECTOMY

2. ***A 43-year-old male with a past medical history of moderate asthma and class I obesity is undergoing a rhytidectomy under total intravenous sedation (TIVA). Which of the following is the biggest risk factor for him to potentially develop hematoma postoperatively?***
   A. Male gender.
   B. History of asthma.
   C. Class I obesity.
   D. Undergoing the procedure under TIVA.
   E. Judicious use of IV fluids in the case.

FIRE SAFETY

3. ***A 21-year-old female is about to undergo full-face CO_2 laser resurfacing. A timeout was performed. Intraoperatively, there is a combustion in the operating room near the patient's face; however, she is not harmed. What would have been the best solution to minimize the combustion risk?***
   A. Use of open-circuit oxygen delivery.
   B. Utilizing supplemental narcotic analgesia instead of propofol.
   C. Decreasing FiO_2 to the lowest level that supports adequate oxygenation.
   D. Using supplemental oxygen.
   E. The patient avoiding a chlorhexidine gluconate (CHG) the night before the surgery.

SURGICAL DURATION

4. ***A 56-year-old female patient who has had massive weight loss plans to undergo liposuction of flanks, back, hips as well as bilateral mastopexy and abdominoplasty. She calls the office 2 weeks before the surgery asking if she can have a blepharoplasty as well. The surgeon is trying to calculate the surgical duration to see whether staged procedures should be recommended. After how many hours of surgery it is recommended to stage the procedures?***
   A. 4 hours.
   B. 6 hours.
   C. 8 hours.
   D. 10 hours.
   E. 12 hours.

LIPOSUCTION

5. *What is a commonly accepted threshold for liposuction that indicates when liposuction should be performed in an acute care hospital, or a facility with the capability for overnight observation?*

A. 2 liters total aspirate.
B. 4 liters total aspirate.
C. 5 liters total aspirate.
D. 6 liters total aspirate.
E. 8 liters total aspirate.

LIPOSUCTION

6. *What is the suggested fluid management protocol for liposuction with total aspirate >5 liters?*

A. Maintenance fluids alone.
B. Maintenance fluids + 1 L Lactated Ringer's.
C. Maintenance fluids + 10 mL/kg of albumin.
D. Maintenance + replacement of 0.25 mL of IV crystalloid per mL of aspirate >5 liters.
E. Twice the maintenance rate.

LIPOSUCTION

7. *In tumescent infiltration, what is the American Society of Plastic Surgery (ASPS) recommended maximum dose of lidocaine?*

A. 7.0 mg/kg.
B. 15.0 mg/kg.
C. 35.0 mg/kg.
D. 55.0 mg/kg.
E. 60.0 mg/kg.

LIPOSUCTION

8. *How long after tumescent infiltration do plasma concentrations of lidocaine peak?*

A. 30 minutes.
B. 90 minutes.
C. 5 hours.
D. 12 hours.
E. 30 hours.

LIPOSUCTION

9. *A 32-year-old female undergoes 5 liters of liposuction with 9 liters of tumescent. The circulating nurse accidently infused each tumescent bag with double the normal amount of lidocaine. What would be one of the first clinical signs the patient develops postoperatively in PACU that would denote lidocaine toxicity?*

A. Seizure.
B. A-V block.
C. Hypotension.
D. Metallic taste in mouth.
E. Generalized ulcerative rash.

TREATMENT

10. *What is a helpful adjunct to resuscitation (in addition to standard BLS and ACLS protocols) specifically in patients with lidocaine toxicity?*

A. IV fluid bolus.
B. Lipid emulsion therapy.
C. Giving epinephrine subcutaneously to tissues to prevent excess lidocaine migrating intravenously.
D. Correcting acidosis.
E. Dantrolene.

Answers

RHYTIDECTOMY

1. *A 52-year-old female with no past medical history undergoes an uncomplicated rhytidectomy. As the patient is being extubated, she experiences a rise in her systolic pressure to 180 mmHg that is sustained for a few minutes. What complication is she most at risk for?*

B. Hematoma.

Specifically, when a patient undergoes a facelift, optimal hemodynamic control is critical. Perioperative systolic BP control is important, with BP > 150 mmHg serving as a major risk factor for a postoperative hematoma. An increase in blood pressure would not cause a seroma, PONV, or uncontrollable pain. An increase in intraoperative blood pressure could lead to an increased risk of stroke; however, it would not be the most common complication.[1]

REFERENCE

1. Ramanadham SR, Mapula S, Costa C, Narasimhan K, Coleman JE, Rohrich RJ. Evolution of hypertension management in face lifting in 1089 patients: optimizing safety and outcomes. Plast Reconstr Surg 2015;135(4):1037–1043

RHYTIDECTOMY

2. *A 43-year-old male with a past medical history of moderate asthma and class I obesity is undergoing a rhytidectomy under total intravenous sedation (TIVA). Which of the following is the biggest risk factor for him to potentially develop hematoma postoperatively?*

A. Male gender.

Male gender is the biggest risk factor for hematoma formation after preoperative high blood pressure. History of asthma, obesity, and IV fluids are notable risk factors for hematoma formation. Performing the case under TIVA may confer some advantages such as improved blood pressure control and may possibly be protective against hematoma formation.[1,2,3]

REFERENCES

1. Desai M. General inhalation anesthesia for cosmetic surgery. In: Friedberg BL, ed. Anesthesia in Cosmetic Surgery. New York: Cambridge University Press; 2007
2. Ramanadham SR, Mapula S, Costa C, Narasimhan K, Coleman JE, Rohrich RJ. Evolution of hypertension management in face lifting in 1089 patients: optimizing safety and outcomes. Plast Reconstr Surg 2015;135(4):1037–1043
3. Lau WC, Eagle KA. Managing cardiovascular risk and hypertension. In: Young VL, Botney R, eds. Patient Safety in Plastic Surgery. New York: Thieme Publishers; 2009

FIRE SAFETY

3. *A 21-year-old female is about to undergo full-face CO_2 laser resurfacing. A timeout was performed. Intraoperatively, there is a combustion in the operating room near the patient's face; however, she is not harmed. What would have been the best solution to minimize the combustion risk?*

C. Decreasing FiO_2 to the lowest level that supports adequate oxygenation.

Decreasing FiO_2 to the lowest level that supports adequate oxygenation is the best solution that would minimize combustion risk. Open-circuit oxygen delivery and use of supplemental oxygen both would increase the risk of combustion. Supplemental narcotic use and a CHG bath the night before would not have any effect on combustion risk intraoperatively. In addition, CHG is typically not used on the face/around the eyes.[1,2]

REFERENCES

1. Blakely KR, Klein KW, White PF, et al. A total intravenous anesthetic technique for outpatient facial laser resurfacing. Anesth Analg 1998;87:827
2. Friedberg BL. The dissociative effect and preemptive analgesia. In: Friedberg BL, ed. Anesthesia in Cosmetic Surgery. New York: Cambridge University Press; 2007

SURGICAL DURATION

4. *A 56-year-old female patient who has had massive weight loss plans to undergo liposuction of flanks, back, hips as well as bilateral mastopexy and abdominoplasty. She calls the office 2 weeks before the surgery asking if she can have a blepharoplasty as well. The surgeon is trying to calculate the surgical duration to see whether staged procedures should be recommended. After how many hours of surgery it is recommended to stage the procedures?*

B. 6 hours.

In general, in massive weight loss body contouring patients, if surgery will take more than 6 hours staging the operations should be considered. The other time frames are incorrect.[1]

REFERENCE

1. Whizar-Lugo VM, Cisneros-Corral R, Reyes-Alveleyra MA, et al. Anesthesia for plastic surgery procedures in previously morbidly obese patients. Anestesia en México 2009;21:186

LIPOSUCTION

5. *What is a commonly accepted threshold for liposuction that indicates when liposuction should be performed in an acute care hospital, or a facility with the capability for overnight observation?*

C. 5 liters total aspirate.

Liposuction of over 5 liter total aspirate is considered large volume and should be performed in a hospital or other facility with the capability for overnight observation. This level of liposuction has an increased risk for fluid shifts and electrolyte imbalance, and attention to volume status is necessary.[1,2]

REFERENCES

1. Berry MG, Davies D. Liposuction: a review of principles and techniques. J Plast Reconstr Aesthet Surg 2011;64:985
2. American Society of Plastic Surgeons. Practice advisory on liposuction: executive summary. Available at www.plasticsurgery.org.

LIPOSUCTION

6. *What is the suggested fluid management protocol for liposuction with total aspirate >5 liters?*

D. Maintenance + replacement of 0.25 mL of IV crystalloid per mL of aspirate >5 liters.

For patients undergoing large-volume liposuction, the suggested fluid management is to give a maintenance rate of fluid plus 0.25 mL of crystalloid per mL of aspirate over 5 liters.[1,2]

REFERENCES

1. Berry MG, Davies D. Liposuction: a review of principles and techniques. J Plast Reconstr Aesthet Surg 2011;64:985
2. American Society of Plastic Surgeons. Practice advisory on liposuction: executive summary. Available at www.plasticsurgery.org

LIPOSUCTION

7. *In tumescent infiltration, what is the American Society of Plastic Surgery (ASPS) recommended maximum dose of lidocaine?*

C. 35.0 mg/kg.

In tumescent infiltration, the ASPS has recommended a maximum dose of lidocaine of 35.0 mg/kg.[1,2]

REFERENCES

1. Klein JA. The tumescent technique for liposuction surgery. AM J Cosmetic Surg 1987;4:1124
2. Neal JL, Bernards CL, Butterworth JF IV, et al. ASRA practice advisory on local anesthetic systemic toxicity. Reg Anesth Pain Med 2010;35:152

LIPOSUCTION

8. *How long after tumescent infiltration do plasma concentrations of lidocaine peak?*

D. 12 hours.

Plasma levels of lidocaine typically peak from 12 hours following tumescent infiltration.[1,2]

REFERENCES

1. Klein JA. The tumescent technique for liposuction surgery. AM J Cosmetic Surg 1987;4:1124
2. Neal JL, Bernards CL, Butterworth JF IV, et al. ASRA practice advisory on local anesthetic systemic toxicity. Reg Anesth Pain Med 2010;35:152

LIPOSUCTION

9. *A 32-year-old female undergoes 5 liters of liposuction with 9 liters of tumescent. The circulating nurse accidently infused each tumescent bag with double the normal amount of lidocaine. What would be one of the first clinical signs the patient develops postoperatively in PACU that would denote lidocaine toxicity?*

D. Metallic taste in mouth.

The first signs of lidocaine toxicity occur at plasma levels of 5 to 10 μg/mL and include central nervous system symptoms such as perioral numbness, confusion, lethargy, restlessness, metallic taste, vertigo, slurred speech, and tinnitus. The other answer choices all occur at plasma levels >10 μg/mL. Seizures, coma, and delirium occur between 10 and 20 μg/mL. A-V block, hypotension, and other cardiac manifestations occur >20 μg/mL of lidocaine.[1,2]

REFERENCES

1. Klein JA. The tumescent technique for liposuction surgery. AM J Cosmetic Surg 1987;4:1124
2. Neal JL, Bernards CL, Butterworth JF IV, et al. ASRA practice advisory on local anesthetic systemic toxicity. Reg Anesth Pain Med 2010;35:152

TREATMENT

10. *What is a helpful adjunct to resuscitation (in addition to standard BLS and ACLS protocols) specifically in patients with lidocaine toxicity?*

B. Lipid emulsion therapy.

Lipid emulsion therapy specifically is helpful in patients with lidocaine toxicity. Dantrolene is used in the treatment of malignant hyperthermia. Giving epinephrine to the local tissue would not prevent worsening intravenous lidocaine toxicity. The remaining options are all used commonly in resuscitation of patients in general.[1,2]

REFERENCES

1. Klein JA. The tumescent technique for liposuction surgery. AM J Cosmetic Surg 1987;4:1124
2. Neal JL, Bernards CL, Butterworth JF IV, et al. ASRA practice advisory on local anesthetic systemic toxicity. Reg Anesth Pain Med 2010;35:152

8. Multimodal Analgesia for the Aesthetic Surgery Patient

Anmol Chattha, Sammy Sinno, Aaron M. Kearney
See *Essentials of Aesthetic Surgery*, pp. 107–115

COMPLICATIONS

1. ***A 45-year-old opioid-naïve female patient is undergoing an abdominoplasty. She experiences intense, uncontrolled postoperative pain over the following week. Which of the following will have an increased incidence?***
   A. Nausea.
   B. Hernia formation.
   C. Psychiatric illness.
   D. Delayed wound healing.
   E. Deep vein thrombosis.

NERVE BLOCKS

2. ***Which of the following technical factors of nerve block administration has the greatest impact on block efficiency?***
   A. Use of a large-bore needle.
   B. Timing of the nerve block (preincision vs. postincision).
   C. Volume of dose.
   D. Concentration of dose.
   E. Total dose.

MEDICATION SIDE EFFECTS

3. ***What is one potential disadvantage of using gabapentin in multimodal analgesia?***
   A. Sedation.
   B. Hypoglycemia.
   C. Urinary retention.
   D. Bradycardia.
   E. Nausea.

MEDICATION SIDE EFFECTS

4. ***What is one potential side effect of ketamine?***
   A. Nausea and vomiting.
   B. Tachycardia.
   C. Hypertension.
   D. Hallucinations and nightmares.
   E. Decreases time to first analgesic.

CHRONIC OPIOID USE

5. ***What percentage of elective hand surgery patients continue to take opioids 90 days after surgery?***
   A. 1%.
   B. 10%.
   C. 20%.
   D. 40%.
   E. 80%.

CHRONIC OPIOID USE

6. *A 45-year-old opioid naïve female is undergoing a routine abdominoplasty with rectus plication. Which of the following risk factors would most likely be a risk factor for opioid abuse in this patient?*

A. High socioeconomic background.
B. Female sex.
C. Family history of substance abuse.
D. Psychiatric illness.
E. Opioid naïve status.

Answers

COMPLICATIONS

1. *A 45-year-old opioid-naïve female patient is undergoing an abdominoplasty. She experiences intense, uncontrolled postoperative pain over the following week. Which of the following will have an increased incidence?*

D. Delayed wound healing.

Postsurgical pain intensity was associated with delayed wound healing. Postsurgical pain decreases surgical outcomes, increases cost of care, decreases patient satisfaction, and has no change on the possibility of a patient developing a deep vein thrombosis. Postoperative pain was not associated with hernia formation or psychiatric illness.[1]

REFERENCE

1. Joshi GP, Beck DE, Emerson RH, et al. Defining new directions for more effective management of surgical pain in the United States: highlights of the inaugural Surgical Pain Congress. Am Surg 2014;80:219

NERVE BLOCKS

2. *Which of the following technical factors of nerve block administration has the greatest impact on block efficiency?*

E. Total dose.

Total dose of anesthetic affects the efficiency of the block. However, the volume and concentration do not seem to be key contributors. Use of a large- or small-bore needle does not impact the efficiency either, and the timing of the nerve block does not seem to make a difference in the efficiency of action of the block.[1,2,3]

REFERENCES

1. Lovich-Sapola J, Smith CE, Brandt CP. Postoperative pain control. Surg Clin North Am 2015;95:301
2. Golembiewski J, Dasta J. Evolving role of local anesthetics in managing postsurgical analgesia. Clin Ther 2015;37:1354
3. Joshi GP, Janis JE, Haas EM, et al. Surgical site infiltration for abdominal surgery: a novel neuro-anatomical-based approach. Plast Recon Surg Glob Open 2016;4:e1181

MEDICATION SIDE EFFECTS

3. *What is one potential disadvantage of using gabapentin in multimodal analgesia?*

A. Sedation.

Sedation and dizziness are occasional side effects of gabapentin that may affect discharge from the surgical facility. The other answer choices are not side effects of using gabapentin.[1,2]

REFERENCES

1. Adam F, Menigaux C, Sessler DI, et al. A single preoperative dose of gabapentin (800 milligrams) does not augment postoperative analgesia in patients given interscalene brachial plexus blocks for arthroscopic shoulder surgery. Anesth Analg 2006;103:1278
2. Paech MJ, Goy R, Chua S et al. A randomized, placebo-controlled trial of preoperative oral pregabalin for postoperative pain relief after minor gynecological surgery. Anesth Analg 2007;105:1449

MEDICATION SIDE EFFECTS

4. *What is one potential side effect of ketamine?*

D. Hallucinations and nightmares.

Hallucinations and nightmares can occur, particularly when ketamine provides effective analgesia. The other answer choices are not side effects of ketamine. Ketamine actually reduces nausea and vomiting, increases time to first analgesic, and reduces pain scores when VAS >4.[1]

REFERENCE

1. Lovich-Sapola J, Smith CE, Brandt CP. Postoperative pain control. Surg Clin North Am 2015;95:301

CHRONIC OPIOID USE

5. *What percentage of elective hand surgery patients continue to take opioids 90 days after surgery?*

B. 10%.

Two studies of elective hand surgery patients showed that 3.1 to 13% of patients were still taking opioids 90 days after surgery. Older patients (>66 years old) following low-risk surgery have a 44% increased likelihood of chronic use at 1 year compared with controls. There is a risk of persistent opioid use following exposure to opioid medications in the perioperative period, even in opioid naïve patients.[1,2]

REFERENCES

1. Johnson SP, Chung KC, Zhong L, et al. Risk of prolonged opioid use among opioid-naïve patients following common hand surgery procedures. J Hand Surg 2016;41:947
2. Clarke H, Soneji N, Ko DT, et al. Rates and risk factors for prolonged opioid use after major surgery: population-based cohort study. BMJ 2014;348:g1251

CHRONIC OPIOID USE

6. *A 45-year-old opioid naïve female is undergoing a routine abdominoplasty with rectus plication. Which of the following risk factors would most likely be a risk factor for opioid abuse in this patient?*

D. Psychiatric illness.

Psychiatric illness along with male sex, history of prior substance abuse, and low socioeconomic background is a risk factor for opioid abuse. Having a family history of substance abuse can put one at a higher risk, but it is not most likely to be a risk factor in this case. Opioid naïve status has no bearing on being a risk factor for opioid abuse.[1,2,3]

REFERENCES

1. Johnson SP, Chung KC, Zhong L, et al. Risk of prolonged opioid use among opioid-naïve patients following common hand surgery procedures. J Hand Surg 2016;41:947
2. Clarke H, Soneji N, Ko DT, et al. Rates and risk factors for prolonged opioid use after major surgery: population-based cohort study. BMJ 2014;348:g1251
3. Sun EC, Darnall BD, Baker LC, et al. Incidence of and risk factors for chronic opioid use among opioid-naive patients in the postoperative period. JAMA Intern Med 2016;176:1286

Part III

Safety

9. Safety Considerations in Aesthetic Surgery

Adam Jacoby, Anmol Chattha
See *Essentials of Aesthetic Surgery*, pp. 119–141

ANTIBIOTICS

1. ***What is the ideal timing of administration of prophylactic antibiotics prior to surgery?***
   A. At the time of incision.
   B. <30 minutes before incision.
   C. 30 to 59 minutes of incision.
   D. 60 to 120 minutes before incision.
   E. >120 minutes before incision.

VENOUS THROMBOEMBOLISM (VTE) MANAGEMENT

2. ***A 59-year-old female is undergoing 5-hour body contouring surgery with concomitant mastopexy. Her past medical history consists of preexisting coronary artery disease, obstructive sleep apnea, body mass index of 34, and high cholesterol. Which of the following is a biggest risk factor for developing deep vein thrombosis (DVT) for this patient?***
   A. BMI >30.
   B. Coronary artery disease.
   C. Patient's age.
   D. Undergoing concomitant breast surgery during body contouring.
   E. 5 hours of surgery.

VENOUS THROMBOEMBOLISM (VTE) MANAGEMENT

3. ***Using the Caprini score, which of the following is the greatest risk factor for developing a DVT?***
   A. Age >60.
   B. Pregnancy.
   C. Oral contraceptive use.
   D. Genetic hypercoagulable disorder.
   E. BMI >30.

COMPLICATIONS

4. ***After liposuction, what is the most common cause of death?***
   A. Anesthesia-related complications.
   B. Thromboembolism.
   C. Fat embolism.
   D. Gastrointestinal perforations.
   E. Massive infection.

COMPLICATIONS

5. ***What is the most common cause of patient dissatisfaction after aesthetic plastic surgery procedures?***
   A. Postoperative hematoma.
   B. Surgical site infection.
   C. Irregular body contour.
   D. Postoperative nausea and vomiting (PONV).
   E. Reoccurring seromas.

ANTIBIOTICS

6. ***Prior to which of the following surgical procedures is administration of prophylactic antibiotics suggested?***
   A. Carpal tunnel release.
   B. Breast reduction.
   C. Liposuction.
   D. Blepharoplasty.
   E. Lipoma excision.

PREOPERATIVE MANAGEMENT

7. ***In the postbariatric body contouring patient population, what is the most common vitamin or mineral deficiency seen preoperatively?***
   A. Vitamin B12.
   B. Folate.
   C. Iron.
   D. Calcium.
   E. Magnesium.

COMPLICATION MANAGEMENT

8. ***What is most effective strategy to decrease infection rates?***
   A. Shave patient's hair to remove hair before prepping patient.
   B. Giving preoperative prophylactic antibiotics at the time incision is made.
   C. Double gloving instead of single gloving.
   D. Use betadine instead of chlorhexidine/alcohol for skin prep.
   E. Have the patient take a multivitamin daily a week before surgery.

VENOUS THROMBOEMBOLISM (VTE) MANAGEMENT

9. ***Hormone replacement therapy increases DVT risk through which of the following mechanisms?***
   A. Decreased levels of protein S.
   B. Decreased levels of protein C.
   C. Inducing factor V Leiden deficiency.
   D. Binds to antithrombin III.
   E. Activating plasminogen.

Answers

ANTIBIOTICS

1. ***What is the ideal timing of administration of prophylactic antibiotics prior to surgery?***
   C. 30 to 59 minutes of incision.
   Several trials have found this to be the optimal window of administering prophylactic antibiotics for preventing surgical site infections (SSIs). Time frames outside of this window are associated with a higher risk of developing a surgical site infection (**Table 9.1**).[1]

Table 9.1 *Relationship to SSI Rates: European Data*

Time Administered	RR	OR	*p* Value
<30 minutes before incision	2.0	2.0	0.02
30–59 minutes before incision	1.0	1.0	*
60–120 minutes before incision	1.8	1.7	0.05

Abbreviations: OR, odds ratio; RR, relative risk.
Note: * No *p* value is listed for antibiotic infusion times from 59 to 30 minutes before incision because that timing had the lowest risk of SSI and therefore serves as the reference or standard to which all other infusion times are compared.

REFERENCE

1. Steinberg JP, Braun BI, Hellinger WC, et al; Trial to Reduce Antimicrobial Prophylaxis Errors (TRAPE) Study Group. Timing of antimicrobial prophylaxis and the risk of surgical site infections: results from the Trial to Reduce Antimicrobial Prophylaxis Errors. Ann Surg 2009;250:10

VENOUS THROMBOEMBOLISM (VTE) MANAGEMENT

2. ***A 59-year-old female is undergoing 5-hour body contouring surgery with concomitant mastopexy. Her past medical history consists of preexisting coronary artery disease, obstructive sleep apnea, body mass index of 34, and high cholesterol. Which of the following is a biggest risk factor for developing deep vein thrombosis (DVT) for this patient?***
   A. BMI >30.
   The answer is A, BMI >30, which is a statistically significant risk factor for developing DVT. Other risk factors include increased operative time (>6 hours), increased pain, large excisional procedures, and hormone replacement/birth control. Coronary artery disease, age, and breast surgery are not risk factors for postoperative DVT.[1,2]

REFERENCES

1. McDevitt NB. Deep vein thrombosis prophylaxis. Plast Reconstr Surg 1999;104:1923
2. Seruya M, Baker SB. MOC-PS CME article: venous thromboembolism prophylaxis in plastic surgery patients. Plast Reconstr Surg 2008;122:1

VENOUS THROMBOEMBOLISM (VTE) MANAGEMENT

3. ***Using the Caprini score, which of the following is the greatest risk factor for developing a DVT?***
   D. Genetic hypercoagulable disorder.
   The answer is D, genetic hypercoagulable disorder, which represents 3 risk scores on the Davison-Caprini risk assessment. Age >40, pregnancy, and malignancy are all risk factors described in the Davison-Caprini risk assessment but carry less of a weight than genetic hypercoagulable disorder. Fractures of the hip, stroke, and spinal cord injuries are other factors that place patients at the highest risk of developing DVT (**Table 9.2**).[1]

Table 9.2 *Exposing and Predisposing Risk Factors (Davison-Caprini)*

Exposing Risk Factors	Predisposing Risk Factors
1 Risk Factor (each item represents one risk score)	**1 Risk Factor**
Minor surgery	Age 40–60
	Obesity >20% IBW
	Pregnancy or <10 months postpartum
	Oral contraceptive/hormone replacement therapy
2 Risk Factors (each item represents two risk scores)	**2 Risk Factors**
Major surgery	Age >60
Immobilization	Malignancy
Patients confined to bed for more than 72 hours	
Central venous access	
3–4 Risk Factors (each item represents three risk scores)	**3 Risk Factors**
Previous myocardial infarction	History of DVT/PE
Congestive heart failure	Any genetic hypercoagulable disorder
Severe sepsis	Lupus anticoagulant
Free flap	Antiphospholipid antibodies
	Myeloproliferative disorders
	Heparin-induced thrombocytopenia
	Hyperviscosity
	Homocystinemia
5 Risk Factors (each item represents five risk scores)	
Fracture of the hip, pelvis, or leg	
Stroke	
Multiple trauma	
Acute spinal cord injury	

Abbreviations: DVT/PE, deep vein thrombosis/pulmonary embolism; IBW, ideal body weight.

REFERENCE

1. Davison SP, Venturi ML, Attinger CE, et al. Prevention of venous thromboembolism in the plastic surgery patient. Plast Reconstr Surg 2004;114:43e

COMPLICATIONS

4. *After liposuction, what is the most common cause of death?*

B. Thromboembolism.

The answer is B, thromboembolism, which can lead to pulmonary embolism and death. After thromboembolism, gastrointestinal perforation is the second most common cause of fatality, followed by anesthesia-related complications, and finally fat embolism (**Table 9.3**).[1,2]

Table 9.3 *Fatal Outcomes from Liposuction*

Cause of Death	Number of Deaths	Percentage
Fat embolism	11	8.5
Anesthesia-related complications	13	10.0
Hemorrhage	6	4.6
Thromboembolism	30	23.1
Cardiorespiratory failure	7	5.4
Gastrointestinal perforations	19	14.6
Massive infection	7	5.4
Unknown or confidential	37	28.5
Total	**130**	**~100**

REFERENCES

1. Grazer FM, DeJong R. Fatal outcomes from liposuction: census survey of cosmetic surgeons. Plast Reconstr Surg 2000;105:436
2. Hughes CE III. Reduction of lipoplasty risks and mortality: an ASAPS survey. Aesthet Surg J 2001;21:120

COMPLICATIONS

5. *What is the most common cause of patient dissatisfaction after aesthetic plastic surgery procedures?*

D. Postoperative nausea and vomiting (PONV).

The answer is D, postoperative nausea and vomiting, which is also a major factor in delayed discharge and unplanned postoperative hospital admissions. Upwards of 10% of patients experience postoperative nausea and vomiting in the recovery room. Multimodal pain management, avoiding long-acting narcotics, and inhalational anesthetics are the best ways of preventing and treating nausea and vomiting after surgery.[1,2]

REFERENCES

1. Iverson RE, Lynch DJ. Practice advisory on pain management and prevention of postoperative nausea and vomiting. Plast Reconstr Surg 2006;118:1060
2. Watcha MF. Postoperative nausea and emesis. Anesthesiol Clin North Am 2002;20:709

ANTIBIOTICS

6. *Prior to which of the following surgical procedures is administration of prophylactic antibiotics suggested?*

B. Breast reduction.

The answer is B, breast reduction, as surgery crosses the ductal architecture of the breast which contains bacteria. Carpal tunnel release, standard liposuction, lipoma excision, and blepharoplasty are clean cases and evidence does not support the use of prophylactic antibiotics. Antibiotics are also recommended for contaminated cases, clean contaminated cases where the aerodigestive track is entered, and cases that may involve an implant.[1]

REFERENCE

1. Ariyan S, Martin J, Lal A, et al. Antibiotic prophylaxis for preventing surgical-site infection in plastic surgery: an evidence-based consensus conference statement from the American Association of Plastic Surgeons. Plast Reconstr Surg 2015;135(6):1723–1739

PREOPERATIVE MANAGEMENT

7. *In the postbariatric body contouring patient population, what is the most common vitamin or mineral deficiency seen preoperatively?*

C. Iron.

The answer is C, iron, which is associated with iron-deficiency anemia seen in up to 50% of postbariatric patients. Vitamin B12 and folate deficiencies are commonly seen in this population after malabsorptive procedures but are still not as common as iron deficiency. Hypocalcemia can be seen in this patient population but is not as common.[1,2,3]

References

1. Rhode BM, Maclean LD. Vitamin and mineral supplementation after gastric bypass. In: Deitel M, Cowan GM Jr, eds. Update: Surgery for the Morbidly Obese Patient: The Field of Extreme Obesity Including Laparoscopy and Allied Care. Toronto, Ontario: FD Communications; 2000
2. Brolin RE, Gorman JH, Gorman RC, et al. Are vitamin B12 and folate deficiency clinically important after roux-en-Y gastric bypass? J Gastrointest Surg 1998;2:436
3. Rohrich RJ. Body contouring surgery after massive weight loss. Plast Reconstr Surg 2006;117:S1

COMPLICATION MANAGEMENT

8. *What is most effective strategy to decrease infection rates?*

C. Double gloving instead of single gloving.

Double gloving reduces perforation of the inner glove and reduces risk of contamination. Analysis of 655 cases revealed that 31% of surgical gloves had a perforation by the end of the case. Glove perforations raises the risk of surgical site infection (SSI) (odds ratio [OR] = 2.0). Double gloving is associated with less perforation of the inner glove (OR = 0.10). Shaving increases the risk of infection 2.4-fold. Hypothermia is a risk factor for worsening infection. Preoperative antibiotics should be given 30 to 59 minutes before skin incision, but not immediately before the incision is made. Chlorhexidine/alcohol preps are more effective than betadine in skin decontamination and SSI reduction. Vitamin supplementation in an otherwise healthy patient does not improve wound healing or decrease infection (it is only effective in vitamin-deficient patients).[1,2,3]

References

1. Anderson DJ. Surgical site infections. Infect Dis Clin North Am 2011;25:135
2. Seropian R, Reynolds BM. Wound infections after preoperative depilatory versus razor preparation. Am J Surg 1971;121:251
3. Alexander JW, Solomkin JS, Edwards MJ. Updated recommendations for control of surgical site infections. Ann Surg 2011;253:1082

VENOUS THROMBOEMBOLISM (VTE) MANAGEMENT

9. *Hormone replacement therapy increases DVT risk through which of the following mechanisms?*

A. Decreased levels of protein S.

The answer is A, decreased levels of protein S, which is part of the anticoagulation pathway. Protein C is not affected by exogenous estrogen. Factor V Leiden is associated with deep vein thrombosis (DVT) but is caused by activated protein C resistance. Finally, heparin and not estrogen binds to antithrombin III, which is part of the anticoagulation cascade. Tissue plasminogen activator (tPA) activates plasminogen and is fibrinolytic.[1]

Reference

1. Seruya M, Baker SB. MOC-PS CME article: venous thromboembolism prophylaxis in plastic surgery patients. Plast Reconstr Surg 2008;122:1

10. Decreasing Complications in Aesthetic Surgery

Sammy Sinno, Jeremie Oliver Piña
See *Essentials of Aesthetic Surgery*, pp. 143–159

PREOPERATIVE MEASURES TO REDUCE COMPLICATIONS

1. ***A female patient with multiple comorbidities including diabetes, chronic obstructive pulmonary disorder, hypertension, and an underlying coagulopathy requires preoperative medical clearance by the patient's primary care physician. Which of the following comorbidities places the patient at an increased risk for delayed wound healing?***
   A. Diabetes.
   B. Chronic obstructive pulmonary disorder.
   C. Hypertension.
   D. Female gender.
   E. Coagulopathy.

PREOPERATIVE MEASURES TO REDUCE COMPLICATIONS

2. ***When conducting a preoperative consultation, you find out that your Caucasian female patient has had a history of multiple blood clots during unsuccessful pregnancies resulting in spontaneous abortions. Which of the following hematologic coagulopathy is she most likely to have?***
   A. Factor V Leiden deficiency.
   B. Von Willebrand disease.
   C. Factor X deficiency.
   D. Glanzman disease.
   E. Hemophilia A.

PREOPERATIVE MEASURES TO REDUCE COMPLICATIONS

3. ***The use of herbal medicines and supplements is more prevalent in the aesthetic surgery patient population than in the general population at large. How many weeks prior to and following the procedure should patients stop taking any herbal medicines and/or supplements?***
   A. 2 days.
   B. 1 week.
   C. 2 weeks.
   D. 8 weeks.
   E. 12 weeks.

PREOPERATIVE MEASURES TO REDUCE COMPLICATIONS

4. ***If planning to proceed with an aesthetic procedure on a patient who is an active smoker, how long before and after the operation should the patient refrain from smoking?***
   A. 2 days.
   B. 1 week.
   C. 4 weeks.
   D. 10 weeks.
   E. 12 weeks.

PREOPERATIVE MEASURES TO REDUCE COMPLICATIONS

5. ***Which of the following is a potential effect(s) of alcohol consumption?***
   A. Decreased hemostasis and cardiac function.
   B. Poor wound healing.
   C. Risk of infection.
   D. Increased blood pressure.
   E. Altered mental status.

PREOPERATIVE MEASURES TO REDUCE COMPLICATIONS

6. *A patient comes to your office to request a bilateral silicone implant breast augmentation. The patient is a good surgical candidate but works as a night float nurse at a local community hospital. How would you proceed with preoperative precautions to avoid surgical site infection in this patient?*

A. Have her wash with soap and water twice daily.
B. Prescribe PO antibiotics for 5 to 7 days prior to the operation.
C. Screen for *S. aureus* nasal carriage.
D. Consult infectious disease specialist.
E. Advise her to switch her shifts to day time to improve circadian rhythm 2 weeks before surgery.

PREOPERATIVE MEASURES TO REDUCE COMPLICATIONS

7. *A patient is curious about what they can do about the scars after aesthetic surgery. Which of the following is the best option regarding postoperative early scar treatments?*

A. Silicone gel ointments.
B. Cocoa butter.
C. Mederma.
D. Silicone gel sheeting.
E. Topical vitamin E.

PREOPERATIVE MEASURES TO REDUCE COMPLICATIONS

8. *Which of the following antimicrobial agents has been shown to be most effective?*

A. 2% chlorhexidine gluconate (CHG).
B. 4% CHG (Hibiclens).
C. 70% isopropyl alcohol (IPA).
D. 2% CHG combined with IPA (ChloraPrep).
E. 4% CHG with 70% IPA.

Answers

PREOPERATIVE MEASURES TO REDUCE COMPLICATIONS

1. *A female patient with multiple comorbidities including diabetes, chronic obstructive pulmonary disorder, hypertension, and an underlying coagulopathy requires preoperative medical clearance by the patient's primary care physician. Which of the following comorbidities places the patient at an increased risk for delayed wound healing?*

A. Diabetes.

Poor glycemic control places diabetic patients seeking any aesthetic surgery procedure at increased risk of surgical site infection and delayed wound healing.[1,2] Patients with diabetes must obtain a preoperative medical clearance from their primary care or medical specialist provider in order to undergo elective aesthetic surgery. The other answer choices are not risk factors for wound healing-based complications.

REFERENCES

1. Guyuron B, Raszewski R. Undetected diabetes and the plastic surgeon. Plast Reconstr Surg 1990;86:471
2. Harrison B, Khansa I, Janis JE. Evidence-based strategies to reduce postoperative complications in plastic surgery. Plast Reconstr Surg 2016;137:351

PREOPERATIVE MEASURES TO REDUCE COMPLICATIONS

2. *When conducting a preoperative consultation, you find out that your Caucasian female patient has had a history of multiple blood clots during unsuccessful pregnancies resulting in spontaneous abortions. Which of the following hematologic coagulopathy is she most likely to have?*

A. Factor V Leiden deficiency.

Factor V Leiden gene is found as a heterozygous mutation in 3 to 7% of white females and results in a sixfold increase in the risk of venous thromboembolism (VTE). VTE risk is increased if combined with cancer, travel, immobilization, use of oral contraceptives, hormone replacement therapy, and estrogen receptor antagonists. Factor X deficiency is also a clotting disorder; however, it is rarer. Von Willebrand disease, Glanzman disease, and hemophilia A are all abnormal clotting disorders along different pathways where patients are more likely to bleed and have a difficult time forming a clot.[1]

REFERENCE

1. Fischer JP, Shang EK, Nelson JA, et al. Patterns of preoperative laboratory testing in patients undergoing outpatient plastic surgery procedures. Aesthet Surg J 2014;34:133

PREOPERATIVE MEASURES TO REDUCE COMPLICATIONS

3. *The use of herbal medicines and supplements is more prevalent in the aesthetic surgery patient population than in the general population at large. How many weeks prior to and following the procedure should patients stop taking any herbal medicines and/or supplements?*

C. 2 weeks.

Although it has been shown that aesthetic surgery patients are more likely than the general population to be taking herbal medicines and/or supplements,[1] these patients also tend to be less likely to disclose that they use such supplements.[2] Thus, aesthetic plastic surgeons should discuss cessation of herbal medicines and supplements to all patients at least 2 to 3 weeks prior to and immediately following any operation, as many of these supplements are cited for adverse perioperative reactions.[3]

REFERENCES

1. Broughton G II, Crosby MA, Coleman J, et al. Use of herbal supplements and vitamins in plastic surgery: a practical review. Plast Reconstr Surg 2007;119:48e
2. Zwiebel SJ, Michelle L, Brendan A, et al. The incidence of vitamin, mineral, herbal, and other supplement use in facial cosmetic patients. Plast Reconstr Surg 2013;132:78
3. Heller J, Gabbay JS, Ghadjar K, et al. Top-10 list of herbal and supplemental medicines used by cosmetic patients: what the plastic surgeon needs to know. Plast Reconstr Surg 2006;117:436

PREOPERATIVE MEASURES TO REDUCE COMPLICATIONS

4. *If planning to proceed with an aesthetic procedure on a patient who is an active smoker, how long before and after the operation should the patient refrain from smoking?*

C. 4 weeks.

Cigarette smoking negatively affects surgical outcomes, having a well-established negative effect on the wound-healing process, resulting in tissue hypoxia and ischemia from microvascular insufficiency.[1] As a buffer, smoking cessation is recommended 4 weeks prior to and immediately after the procedure.

REFERENCE

1. Jensen JA, Goodson WH, Hopf H, et al. Cigarette smoking decreases tissue oxygen. Arch Surg 1991;126:1131

PREOPERATIVE MEASURES TO REDUCE COMPLICATIONS

5. *Which of the following is a potential effect(s) of alcohol consumption?*

A. Decreased hemostasis and cardiac function.

Alcohol consumption has been shown to negatively affect multiple systems and processes within the human body, including the liver, pancreas, nervous system, cardiovascular system, and metabolism. There is a dose-dependent response to perioperative morbidity, such that the complication rate is about **50% higher** in patients who drink **3 to 4 times per day** compared with 0 to 2 per day.[1] A common recommendation to alleviate the effects of alcohol consumption on surgical outcomes is to ask the patient to decrease or abstain from consumption about 1 to 2 weeks prior to and following the operation.

REFERENCE

1. Tønnesen H, Nielsen PR, Lauritzen JB, et al. Smoking and alcohol intervention before surgery: evidence for best practice. Br J Anaesth 2009;102:297

PREOPERATIVE MEASURES TO REDUCE COMPLICATIONS

6. *A patient comes to your office to request a bilateral silicone implant breast augmentation. The patient is a good surgical candidate but works as a night float nurse at a local community hospital. How would you proceed with preoperative precautions to avoid surgical site infection in this patient?*

C. Screen for *S. aureus* nasal carriage.

An association between nasal carriage of *S. aureus* and subsequent surgical site infection is well established.[1,2] Screening is a relatively easy and inexpensive way to identify patients at potentially higher risk (i.e., health care workers) for developing postoperative infections. If the patient's screen is positive for *S. aureus*, instruct the patient to apply 2% mupirocin nasal ointment twice daily to both nares and to bathe with chlorhexidine (40 mg/mL Hibiclens) daily for 5 days immediately before the scheduled surgery.

REFERENCES

1. Bode LG, Kluytmans JA, Wertheim HF, et al. Preventing surgical-site infections in nasal carriers of Staphylococcus aureus. N Engl J Med 2010;362:9
2. Wenzel RP, Perl TM. The significance of nasal carriage of Staphylococcus aureus and the incidence of postoperative wound infection. J Hosp Infect 1995;31:13

PREOPERATIVE MEASURES TO REDUCE COMPLICATIONS

7. *A patient is curious about what they can do about the scars after aesthetic surgery. Which of the following is the best option regarding postoperative early scar treatments?*

D. Silicone gel sheeting.

Taping or silicone gel sheeting is probably the most effective and proven means to modulate scar maturation favorably. There is less evidence that silicone gel ointments (e.g., Kelo-cote) are as effective in preventing scarring. Topical vitamin E, cocoa butter, onion extract cream (e.g., Mederma), allantoin-sulfomucopolysaccharide gel, glycosaminoglycan gel, and creams containing extracts from plants such as *Bulbine frutescens* and *Centella asiatica* have not been shown to consistently improve scar appearance as single agents.[1]

Reference

1. Khansa I, Harrison B, Janis JE. Evidence-based scar management: how to improve results with technique and technology. Plast Reconst Surg 2016;138:1655

PREOPERATIVE MEASURES TO REDUCE COMPLICATIONS

8. *Which of the following antimicrobial agents has been shown to be most effective?*

E. 4% CHG with 70% IPA.

It has been demonstrated that 2% chlorhexidine gluconate (CHG) and 4% CHG (Hibiclens) have inferior antimicrobial activity to isopropyl alcohol (IPA) (70%) or 2% CHG combined with IPA (ChloraPrep).[1] Also, a Cochrane analysis suggested 4% CHG with 70% IPA likely has the highest probability of being effective.[2] Alcohol-based antiseptics are likely more effective than those with an aqueous base.

WORD OF CAUTION: Alcohol-based antiseptics have been associated with surgical fires and should be allowed to dry before draping.

Note: ChloraPrep has been shown to be superior to povidone-iodine for preoperative cleansing.

References

1. Hibbard JS. Analyses comparing the antimicrobial activity and safety of current antiseptic agents: a review. J Infus Nurs 2005;28:194
2. Dumville JC, McFarlane E, Edwards P, et al. Preoperative skin antiseptics for preventing surgical wound infections after clean surgery. Cochrane Database Syst Rev 2015;2015:CD003949

11. Venous Thromboembolism and the Aesthetic Surgery Patient

Ara A. Salibian, Anmol Chattha
See *Essentials of Aesthetic Surgery*, pp. 160–167

WHAT DO THE GUIDELINES SAY?

1. ***A 62-year-old obese massive-weight-loss patient is undergoing a 6-hour belt lipectomy and bilateral brachioplasty under general anesthesia at the hospital with postoperative plans to be on bed rest for 72 hours. The patient's venous thromboembolism (VTE) risk is calculated using the 2005 Caprini Risk Assessment Model (RAM) and is determined to be 7. Which of the following regimes is the most appropriate method of VTE prophylaxis in this patient?***
   A. Placement of sequential compression devices (SCDs) prior to surgery.
   B. Placement of SCDs prior to surgery and postoperative screening by lower extremity ultrasound.
   C. Chemoprophylaxis prior to surgery for 3 days.
   D. Placement of SCDs prior to surgery and chemoprophylaxis for 1 month after surgery.
   E. Chemoprophylaxis for 10 weeks after surgery.

WHAT DO THE GUIDELINES SAY?

2. ***Which of the following recommendations is true for plastic surgery patients undergoing aesthetic surgery as stated by the American Association of Plastic Surgery (AAPS)?***
   A. All patients undergoing body contouring should receive postoperative VTE chemoprophylaxis.
   B. All plastic surgery patients should be risk-stratified for VTE using the 2005 Caprini RAM.
   C. All patients should have elastic compression stockings for mechanical VTE prophylaxis.
   D. Patients with a Caprini score of >5 should be considered for chemoprophylaxis on an individualized basis.
   E. All plastic surgery patients should receive general anesthesia.

WHAT DO THE GUIDELINES SAY?

3. ***A 66-year-old female is undergoing abdominoplasty and bilateral brachioplasty. The patient has past medical history of breast cancer and prior lower extremity deep vein thrombosis (DVT) after a 6-hour plane flight 5 years ago. What is the patient's total risk factor score based on the 2005 Caprini RAM?***
   A. 3.
   B. 4.
   C. 5.
   D. 6.
   E. 7.

WHAT DO THE GUIDELINES SAY?

4. ***Which of the following procedures has the highest risk of VTE?***
   A. Medial thigh lift.
   B. Truncal liposuction.
   C. Circumferential abdominoplasty.
   D. Bilateral brachioplasty.
   E. Facelift.

WHAT DO THE GUIDELINES SAY?

5. ***A patient undergoing panniculectomy with a planned postoperative inpatient stay has a preoperative Caprini risk score of 8. What is the 60-day risk for VTE for this patient if VTE chemoprophylaxis is not given?***
   A. 0.3%.
   B. 1%.
   C. 2.5%.
   D. 5%.
   E. 10%.

WHAT DO THE GUIDELINES SAY?

6. ***Which of the following factors has been shown to decrease the risk of VTE?***
   A. Having plastic surgery in a different country.
   B. Performing multiple procedures at the same time to limit number of operations.
   C. Wearing below-knee compression stockings.
   D. Taking aspirin before and after the procedure.
   E. A patient between 41 and 60 years old.

WHAT DO THE GUIDELINES SAY?

7. ***A 62-year-old female is undergoing a facelift, necklift, and bilateral upper blepharoplasty. She has a past medical history of breast cancer that was treated with bilateral mastectomy and implant reconstruction 10 years ago as well as varicose veins. Which of the following measures can be done to decrease the risk of perioperative VTE in this patient without significantly increasing the risk of other complications?***
   A. Have the patient start 81 milligrams of aspirin 1 month prior to the procedure.
   B. Administer 40 milligrams of enoxaparin, 30 minutes prior to starting the case.
   C. Perform a subcutaneous instead of a dual-plane facelift.
   D. Perform the procedure under sedation instead of general anesthesia.
   E. Monitor the patient in the hospital the night after surgery.

Answers

WHAT DO THE GUIDELINES SAY?

1. ***A 62-year-old obese massive-weight-loss patient is undergoing a 6-hour belt lipectomy and bilateral brachioplasty under general anesthesia at the hospital with postoperative plans to be on bed rest for 72 hours. The patient's venous thromboembolism (VTE) risk is calculated using the 2005 Caprini Risk Assessment Model (RAM) and is determined to be 7. Which of the following regimes is the most appropriate method of VTE prophylaxis in this patient?***

   D. Placement of SCDs prior to surgery and chemoprophylaxis for 1 month after surgery.

   The American Society of Plastic Surgeons (ASPS) VTE Task Force made recommendations in 2012 for aesthetic surgery patients undergoing general anesthesia based on the 2005 Caprini RAM:
   - For patients with a Caprini score ≥3, mechanical prophylaxis should be considered.
   - For patients with a Caprini score of 3 to 6, postoperative low-molecular-weight or unfractionated heparin should be considered.
   - For patients with a Caprini score of ≥6, extended-duration low-molecular-weight heparin should be considered.

   This patient has a Caprini risk score of 7; therefore, both mechanical prophylaxis and postoperative extended chemoprophylaxis should be considered (1–4 weeks).[1,2]

REFERENCES

1. Caprini JA. Thrombosis risk assessment as a guide to quality patient care. Dis Mon 2005;51:70
2. Murphy RX Jr, Alderman A, Gutowski K, et al. Evidence-based practices for thromboembolism prevention: summary of the ASPS Venous Thromboembolism Task Force Report. Plast Reconstr Surg 2012;130:168e

WHAT DO THE GUIDELINES SAY?

2. ***Which of the following recommendations is true for plastic surgery patients undergoing aesthetic surgery as stated by the American Association of Plastic Surgery (AAPS)?***

   B. All plastic surgery patients should be risk-stratified for VTE using the 2005 Caprini RAM.

   In 2016, the AAPS published recommendations for venous thromboembolism (VTE) prophylaxis based on a systematic review and meta-analysis, as well as a consensus panel. The reviewed data was mainly based on inpatient surgery, but the recommendations are largely applicable to aesthetic surgery patients. The panel recommended stratifying all plastic surgery patients for VTE risk based on the 2005 Caprini RAM. Routine chemoprophylaxis in the general non-risk-stratified plastic surgery population was not recommended. The use of intermittent pneumatic compression stockings in plastic surgery patients was recommended as a superior means of mechanical prophylaxis compared to compression stockings. Patients with a Caprini score >8 were recommended to be considered for chemoprophylaxis on an individualized basis. The AAPS also recommended using local anesthesia for procedures, when appropriate.[1]

REFERENCE

1. Pannucci CJ, Barta RJ, Portschy PR, et al. Assessment of postoperative venous thromboembolism risk in plastic surgery patients using the 2005 and 2010 Caprini Risk score. Plast Reconstr Surg 2012;130:343

WHAT DO THE GUIDELINES SAY?

3. ***A 66-year-old female is undergoing abdominoplasty and bilateral brachioplasty. The patient has past medical history of breast cancer and prior lower extremity deep vein thrombosis (DVT) after a 6-hour plane flight 5 years ago. What is the patient's total risk factor score based on the 2005 Caprini RAM?***

   E. 7.

   The 2005 Caprini RAM is a venous thromboembolism (VTE) risk assessment model that has been validated in more than 20,000 patients. The simple one-page questionnaire assigns an aggregate risk factor score based on a patient's personal medical history and family history (**Fig. 11.1**). The described patient has several risk factors that should be taken into consideration. She is between the age of 60 and 74 years (2 points), has a prior history of malignancy (2 points), and most importantly has a prior history of DVT (3 points) constituting a total risk factor score of 7.[1]

Each Risk Factor Represents 1 Point

- ☐ Age 41-60 years
- ☐ Minor surgery planned
- ☐ History of prior major surgery (<1 month)
- ☐ Varicose veins
- ☐ History of inflammatory bowel disease
- ☐ Swollen legs (current)
- ☐ Obesity (BMI >25)
- ☐ Acute myocardial infarction
- ☐ Congestive heart failure (<1 month)
- ☐ Sepsis (<1 month)
- ☐ Serious lung disease incl. pneumonia (<1 month)
- ☐ Abnormal pulmonary function (COPD)
- ☐ Medical patient currently at bed rest
- ☐ Other risk factors ______________

Each Risk Factor Represents 2 Points

- ☐ Age 60-74 years
- ☐ Arthroscopic surgery
- ☐ Malignancy (present or previous)
- ☐ Major surgery (>45 minutes)
- ☐ Laparoscopic surgery (>45 minutes)
- ☐ Patient confined to bed (>72 hours)
- ☐ Immobilizing plaster cast (<1 month)
- ☐ Central venous access

Each Risk Factor Represents 3 Points

- ☐ Age over 75 years
- ☐ History of DVT/PE
- ☐ **Family history of thrombosis***
- ☐ Positive Factor V Leiden
- ☐ Positive Prothrombin 20210A
- ☐ Elevated serum homocysteine
- ☐ Positive lupus anticoagulent
- ☐ Elevated anticardiolipin antibodies
- ☐ Heparin-induced thrombocytopenia (HIT)
- ☐ Other congenital or acquired thrombophilia

If yes:
Type ______________

***most frequently missed risk factor**

Each Risk Factor Represents 5 Points

- ☐ Elective major lower extremity arthroplasty
- ☐ Hip, pelvis, or leg fracture (<1 month)
- ☐ Stroke (<1 month)
- ☐ Multiple trauma (<1 month)
- ☐ Acute spinal cord injury (paralysis) (<1 month)

For Women Only (Each Represents 1 Point)

- ☐ Oral contraceptives or hormone replacement therapy
- ☐ Pregnancy or postpartum (<1 month)
- ☐ History of unexplained stillborn infant, recurrent spontaneous abortion (≥3), premature birth with toxemia or growth-restricted infant

Fig. 11.1 Caprini risk assessment model. (Source: Reprinted from Disease of the Month, Vol. 51, Caprini JA, Thrombosis risk assessment as a guide to quality patient care, 2005, with permission from Elsevier.)

Reference

1. Caprini JA. Thrombosis risk assessment as a guide to quality patient care. Dis Mon 2005;51:70

WHAT DO THE GUIDELINES SAY?

4. *Which of the following procedures has the highest risk of VTE?*

C. Circumferential abdominoplasty.

Risk for venous thromboembolism (VTE) is multifactorial and includes a combination of patient- and procedure-specific variables. Abdominoplasty, alone or in combination with other procedures, has been found to have the highest risk of VTE among cosmetic surgery procedures. Circumferential abdominoplasty in particular has been shown to have the absolute highest risk of VTE at 3.40%. Importantly, both the number of surgical procedures and the length of the surgery has been associated with a higher risk of VTE.[1,2,3]

References

1. Hatef DA, Trussler AP, Kenkel JM. Procedural risk for venous thromboembolism in abdominal contouring surgery: a systematic review of the literature. Plast Reconstr Surg 2010;125:352
2. Kim JY, Khavanin N, Rambachan A, et al. Surgical duration and risk of venous thromboembolism. JAMA Surg 2015;150:110
3. Howland WS, Schweizer O. Complication associated with prolonged operation and anesthesia. Clin Anesth 1972;9:1

WHAT DO THE GUIDELINES SAY?

5. *A patient undergoing panniculectomy with a planned postoperative inpatient stay has a preoperative Caprini risk score of 8. What is the 60-day risk for VTE for this patient if VTE chemoprophylaxis is not given?*

C. 2.5%.

The Plastic Surgery Foundation–sponsored Venous Thromboembolism Prevention Study compared venous thromboembolism (VTE) rates in patients with a Caprini score of 3 or higher who received postoperative enoxaparin prophylaxis to historical control patients. The study included 3,334 patients and demonstrated that postoperative enoxaparin prophylaxis was protective against 6-day VTE in high-risk plastic surgery patients. Patients who did not receive chemoprophylaxis and had a Caprini risk of 7 to 8 had around a 2.55% risk of VTE.[1]

REFERENCE

1. Pannucci CJ, Dreszer G, Wachtman CF, et al. Postoperative enoxaparin prevents symptomatic venous thromboembolism in high-risk plastic surgery patients. Plast Reconstr Surg 2011;128:1093

WHAT DO THE GUIDELINES SAY?

6. *Which of the following factors has been shown to decrease the risk of VTE?*

C. Wearing below-knee compression stockings.

During air travel, the risk of deep vein thrombosis (DVT) has been shown to be significantly decreased by wearing below-knee compression stockings (4.5 to 0.24%). Plastic surgery tourism actually increases the risk of venous thromboembolism (VTE) due to air travel. Performing multiple procedures at the same time also increases the risk of VTE. For example, combining abdominoplasty with different procedures can increase the risk of VTE multifold.[1,2]

REFERENCES

1. Hatef DA, Trussler AP, Kenkel JM. Procedural risk for venous thromboembolism in abdominal contouring surgery: a systematic review of the literature. Plast Reconstr Surg 2010;125:352
2. Philbrick JT, Shumate R, Siadaty MS, et al. Air travel and venous thromboembolism: a systematic review. J Gen Intern Med 2007;22:107

WHAT DO THE GUIDELINES SAY?

7. *A 62-year-old female is undergoing a facelift, necklift, and bilateral upper blepharoplasty. She has a past medical history of breast cancer that was treated with bilateral mastectomy and implant reconstruction 10 years ago as well as varicose veins. Which of the following measures can be done to decrease the risk of perioperative VTE in this patient without significantly increasing the risk of other complications?*

D. Perform the procedure under sedation instead of general anesthesia.

Using the 2005 Caprini RAM, this patient has a risk score of around 5 (2 points for age, 2 points for history of malignancy, and 1 point for history of varicose veins). General anesthesia has been shown to increase the risk of venous thromboembolism (VTE), likely primarily due to loss of muscle tone in the posterior compartment of the lower leg and subsequent venous stasis. Procedures under IV sedation have a lower risk of VTE. Facelift, necklift, and blepharoplasty can all be performed under sedation with good local anesthesia. The use of perioperative chemoprophylaxis has been shown to decrease the rate of VTE. However, the use of preoperative or intraoperative chemoprophylaxis has been shown to significantly increase the risk of bleeding in facelift surgery as well as body contouring surgery. Although increased operative time has been shown to raise the risk of VTE, elevating a superficial musculoaponeurotic system(SMAS) flap is unlikely to add a significantamount of operative time to the case and is an important component for achieving and maintaining long-term facial rejuvenation. When performed efficiently, all three components of this case should be accomplished in under 6 hours, a time limit recommended by the American Society of Plastic Surgeons (ASPS).[1,2,3,4]

REFERENCES

1. Hafezi F, Naghibzadeh B, Nouhi A H, et al. Epidural anesthesia as a thromboembolic prophylaxis modality in plastic surgery. Aesthet Surg J 2011;31:821

2. Haeck PC, Swanson JA, Iverson RE, et al. Evidence-based patient safety advisory: patient selection and procedures in ambulatory surgery. Plast Reconstr Surg 2009;124(4, Suppl):S6
3. Hatef DA, Kenkel JM, Nguyen MQ, et al. Thromboembolic risk assessment and the efficacy of enoxaparin prophylaxis in excisional body contouring surgery. Plast Reconstr Surg 2008;122:269
4. Đurnig P, Jungwirth W. Low-molecular-weight heparin and postoperative bleeding in rhytidectomy. Plast Reconstr Surg 2006;118:502; discussion 508

Part IV

Skin Care

12. The Medi Spa and Other Practice Considerations

Sammy Sinno, Jeremie Oliver Piña
See *Essentials of Aesthetic Surgery*, pp. 143–159

PRACTICE BASICS

1. ***The Code of Federal Regulations requires that ambulatory surgical centers participate in Medicare through the Center for Medicare and Medicaid (CMS). This entails limiting Medicare-covered surgical procedures to those with duration of <90 minutes or <4 hours of postsurgical recovery and type of surgery in which scenario?***
   A. Procedures that can generally result in extensive bleeding.
   B. Procedures that generally require major or prolonged invasion into body cavities.
   C. Procedures that directly involve major blood vessels.
   D. Procedures that do not involve major blood vessels.
   E. Procedures that are not generally an emergency or life-threatening in nature.

PRACTICE BASICS

2. ***An aesthetic surgeon has accepted a position in a new city. What is a useful strategy to market and establish his or her practice early on?***
   A. Create a website only after you have started the new position.
   B. Avoid speaking engagements, local radio, or television shows until you have become established in the community.
   C. The surgeon should establish a niche and identify the community's needs or what is lacking in other aesthetic surgeons in order to stand out.
   D. Patient referral patterns should be studied once every 1 to 2 years.
   E. Minimize complementary services, like peels for facelift patients, or offering packages that combine surgical and nonsurgical treatments, as this is a nonfavorable internal branding strategy.

PRACTICE BASICS

3. ***What is a good timeline to renew the practice website?***
   A. Never.
   B. Once a month.
   C. Every 6 months.
   D. Every 2 to 3 years.
   E. Rarely change, as consistency is important to patients.

PRACTICE BASICS

4. ***Which of the following is the best strategy to capitalize on growth and expansion of the practice?***
   A. Hire outside services.
   B. Add a partner or nonphysician provider to the practice.
   C. Carefully project goals and finances often.
   D. Invest in new equipment and products.
   E. Spend more on marketing than other aesthetic providers in your area.

AMBULATORY SURGERY FACILITY CERTIFICATION AND STANDARDS

5. ***Which type of practice setting would require American Association for Accreditation of Ambulatory Surgery Facilities, Inc. (AAAASF) accreditation?***
   A. Any practice offering aesthetic services.
   B. Only practices in the state of California.
   C. Only practices in the state of Texas.
   D. Any practice offering procedures under sedation or general anesthesia.
   E. Any practice offering invasive procedures of any kind.

AMBULATORY SURGERY FACILITY CERTIFICATION AND STANDARDS

6. *An ambulatory surgery facility has a class A accreditation; which of the following is allowed at this facility?*
A. IV and parenteral sedation only.
B. Oral medications producing minimal or moderate sedation.
C. Regional blocks.
D. Spinal or epidural anesthesia.
E. LMA or endotracheal intubation.

LEGAL CONSIDERATIONS

7. *As per mandate by the American Society of Plastic Surgeons (ASPS), American Society of Plastic Surgeons (ASAPS) (The Aesthetic Society), American Medical Association (AMA), and Center for Medicare Services (CMS), all practices offering procedures requiring more than just local anesthesia or oral sedation must comply with which of the following accreditation councils?*
A. Medicaid certification.
B. Federal licensure.
C. American Association of Plastic Surgeons (AAPS).
D. American College of Surgeons (ACS).
E. Accreditation Association for Ambulatory Health Care (AAAHC).

LEGAL CONSIDERATIONS

8. *Which of the following statements is true regarding nonphysician aesthetic providers?*
A. Very few states allow for nonphysicians to administer aesthetic services.
B. A board-certified physician must be in the room observing nonphysician providers.
C. It is difficult to train nonphysician providers to perform aesthetic office services.
D. They are able to offer nonsurgical aesthetic services when competent, trained, and licensed.
E. Nonphysician providers are fully responsible for complications of treatment they provide.

PATIENT SELECTION AND PATIENT SAFETY

9. *Which of the following aesthetic procedures, when combined with an additional procedure, puts patients at greatest risk of postoperative complication?*
A. Rhinoplasty.
B. Blepharoplasty.
C. Facelift.
D. Breast augmentation.
E. Abdominoplasty.

Answers

PRACTICE BASICS

1. ***The Code of Federal Regulations requires that ambulatory surgical centers participate in Medicare through the Center for Medicare and Medicaid (CMS). This entails limiting Medicare-covered surgical procedures to those with duration of <90 minutes or <4 hours of postsurgical recovery and type of surgery in which scenario?***

D. Procedures that do not involve major blood vessels.

The Code of Federal Regulations requires that ambulatory surgical centers participate in Medicare through the Center for Medicare and Medicaid (CMS). This entails limiting Medicare-covered surgical procedures to those with duration of <90 minutes or <4 hours of postsurgical recovery, and to those type of surgeries that: Do not generally result in extensive bleeding, do not require any major or prolonged invasion into body cavities, do not involve major blood vessels, and are generally an emergency or life-threatening in nature.[1]

REFERENCE

1. U.S. Government Publishing Office. Electronic Code of Federal Regulations, Title 42, Part 416. Available at www.ecfr.gov

PRACTICE BASICS

2. ***An aesthetic surgeon has accepted a position in a new city. What is a useful strategy to market and establish his or her practice early on?***

C. The surgeon should establish a niche and identify the community's needs or what is lacking in other aesthetic surgeons in order to stand out.

Depending on the landscape of the community of practice, an aesthetic surgeon will be most successful if he or she can establish a special niche area, which may be lacking in other aesthetic practices in that geographic region. Although it is always wise to maintain a broad, comprehensive skillset in all that aesthetic services have to offer, a niche area can identify why your practice and medi spa are unique or novel. Having an attractive and informative website should start early, even months before the doors open and would be best created by a web designer. External marketing strategies such as community outreach and engagement of referral sources should also be a priority early on. Additionally, noninvasive cosmetic procedures or suggestion of complementary services are powerful tools to garnish direct patient referrals.[1]

REFERENCE

1. Nahai F, Colon GA, Lewis W, et al. The practice: models, management, and marketing. In: Nahai F, ed. The Art of Aesthetic Surgery: Techniques and Principles. 2nd ed. New York: Thieme Publishers; 2010

PRACTICE BASICS

3. ***What is a good timeline to renew the practice website?***

D. Every 2 to 3 years.

With advances in technology, internet sources, referral bases, and patient preferences, it is advisable to plan to update the practice website every 2 to 3 years at a minimum. Hire a full-time social media/website manager to thoroughly study the trends in marketing and advertisement of the practice.

PRACTICE BASICS

4. ***Which of the following is the best strategy to capitalize on growth and expansion of the practice?***

C. Carefully project goals and finances often.

Aesthetic surgeons should set goals for themselves and their practice for financial growth, practice expansion, patient management, and experience. Although projections and goal calculations can certainly be time consuming, goals may go unfulfilled if this is not done. Careful planning and research will allow surgeons to balance their income and assets with expenses and future goals.[1]

Reference

1. Kuechel MC. The practice: staffing, services, and financial planning. In: Nahai F, ed. The Art of Aesthetic Surgery: Techniques and Principles. 2nd ed. New York: Thieme Publishers; 2010

AMBULATORY SURGERY FACILITY CERTIFICATION AND STANDARDS

5. ***Which type of practice setting would require American Association for Accreditation of Ambulatory Surgery Facilities, Inc. (AAAASF) accreditation?***

   D. Any practice offering procedures under sedation or general anesthesia.

   Initially established by plastic surgeons, the American Association for Accreditation of Ambulatory Surgery Facilities, Inc. (AAAASF, formerly the American Association for Accreditation of Plastic Surgery Facilities) helps promote quality control and patient safety in ambulatory surgery centers all around the country. Today, most state departments of health accept accreditation through the AAAASF instead of state licensure, as well as offer Medicare certification.[1,2,3]

References

1. American Association for Accreditation of Ambulatory Surgery Facilities. Regular Standards and Checklist for Accreditation of Ambulatory Surgery Facilities. Available at www.aaaasf.org
2. American Society of Plastic Surgeons and American Society for Aesthetic Plastic Surgery, Inc. Policy Statement on Accreditation of Office Facilities. Available at www.plasticsurgery.org
3. American Medical Association. Office-based Surgery Core Principles. Available at www. ama-assn.org

AMBULATORY SURGERY FACILITY CERTIFICATION AND STANDARDS

6. ***An ambulatory surgery facility has a class A accreditation; which of the following is allowed at this facility?***

   B. Oral medications producing minimal or moderate sedation.

   Accreditation of ambulatory surgery facilities can vary based on safety precautions and resources available at each surgery center. Class A accreditation allows for oral medications producing minimal or moderate sedation as well as topical or local anesthesia. The classification system allows for the most to be administered at Class C facilities, and the least to be offered at Class A facilities. Both Class C and Class C-M accredited surgery facilities are permitted to administer propofol and spinal/epidural anesthetic agents. The differentiator between Class C-M and Class C is that Class C certification allows for inhalational agents to be administered to patients, as well as use of laryngeal mask airway (LMA) or endotracheal intubation. In general, there are more mandates as the anesthesia becomes more invasive.[1]

Reference

1. American Association for Accreditation of Ambulatory Surgery Facilities. Regular Standards and Checklist for Accreditation of Ambulatory Surgery Facilities. Available at www.aaaasf.org

LEGAL CONSIDERATIONS

7. ***As per mandate by the American Society of Plastic Surgeons (ASPS), American Society of Plastic Surgeons (ASAPS) (The Aesthetic Society), American Medical Association (AMA), and Center for Medicare Services (CMS), all practices offering procedures requiring more than just local anesthesia or oral sedation must comply with which of the following accreditation councils?***

   E. Accreditation Association for Ambulatory Health Care (AAAHC).

   ASPS and ASAPS mandated in 1999 that members performing plastic surgery using more than local anesthesia or oral sedation should be in a facility with either:

   - State licensure,
   - Medicare certification, or
   - Accreditation by an organization like the AAAASF, Accreditation Association for Ambulatory Health Care (AAAHC), or Joint Commission on the Accreditation of Health Care Organizations (JCAHO).

   The mandate does not require practices to obtain accreditation or licensure through all of these agencies. Rather, any one of them would offer sufficient accreditation on its own to verify the safety of the practice facility based on the ASPS, ASAPS, AMA, and CMS standards.[1]

REFERENCE

1. American Society of Plastic Surgeons and American Society for Aesthetic Plastic Surgery, Inc. Policy Statement on Accreditation of Office Facilities. Available at www.plasticsurgery.org

LEGAL CONSIDERATIONS

8. *Which of the following statements is true regarding nonphysician aesthetic providers?*

D. They are able to offer nonsurgical aesthetic services when competent, trained, and licensed.

Nonphysician aesthetic providers can be a vital part of any practice's success. From 2012 data as cited in the text, office injectable procedure numbers in the U.S. increase by 20% when those by nonphysician injectors are included. As demand continues to rise faster than the number of board-certified physicians can accommodate, practice productivity and revenue can multiply with surgeries, while qualified nonphysician providers perform nonsurgical cosmetic procedures.[1]

REFERENCE

1. American Society for Aesthetic Plastic Surgery. News releases: cosmetic procedures increase in 2012. Available at www.surgery.org

PATIENT SELECTION AND PATIENT SAFETY

9. *Which of the following aesthetic procedures, when combined with an additional procedure, puts patients at greatest risk of postoperative complication?*

E. Abdominoplasty.

Although abdominoplasty procedures are not associated with a higher risk for overall postoperative morbidity, the data do support that when combined with an additional procedure, abdominoplasty carries a statistically significant higher risk for postoperative complications compared to all other aesthetic procedures. In order to minimize potential complications, the aesthetic surgeon should remain vigilant, avoid hypotensive surgery, and thoroughly evaluate such patients undergoing combined procedures before their discharge from the PACU.[1,2,3]

REFERENCES

1. Soltani AM, Keyes GR, Singer R, et al. Outpatient surgery and sequelae: an analysis of the AAAASF internet-based quality assurance and peer review database. Clin Plast Surg 2013;40:465
2. Iverson RE, Gomez JL. Deep venous thrombosis: prevention and management. Clin Plast Surg 2013;40:389
3. Iverson RE. Patient safety in office-based surgery facilities: I. Procedures in the office-based surgery setting. Plast Reconstr Surg 2002;110:1337

13. Anatomy, Physiology, and Disorders of the Skin

Sammy Sinno, Jeremie Oliver Piña
See *Essentials of Aesthetic Surgery*, pp. 181–190

ANATOMY

1. *Which of the following cell types provides UV protection to the skin?*
A. Keratinocytes.
B. Melanocytes.
C. Merkel cells.
D. Langerhans cells.
E. Squamous cells.

ANATOMY

2. *Which epidermal cell layer is mitotically active, providing stem cells to repopulate the epidermis each month (Fig. 13.1)?*
A. Stratum corneum.
B. Stratum lucidum.
C. Stratum granulosum.
D. Stratum spinosum.
E. Stratum basale.

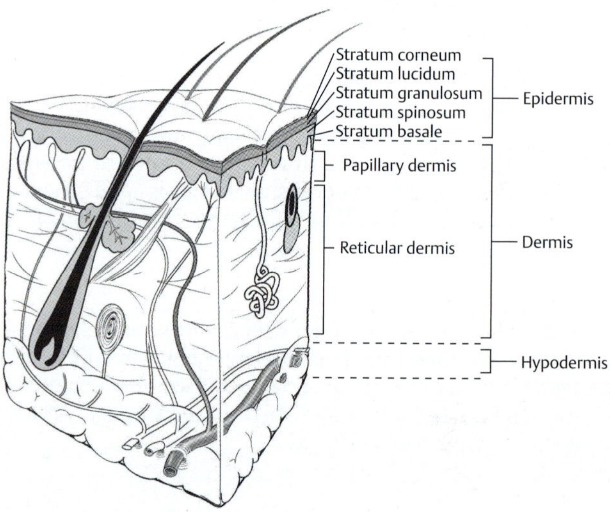

Fig. 13.1 Layers of the skin with adnexal structures. (Source: Anatomy. In: Janis J, ed. Essentials of Aesthetic Surgery. 1st Edition. New York: Thieme; 2018.)

SKIN PHYSIOLOGY

3. *What is the approximate ratio of type I:III collagen in the dermis of a normal adult?*
A. 1:1.
B. 2:1.
C. 4:1.
D. 3:1.
E. 5:1.

SKIN PHYSIOLOGY

4. *Which of the following characteristics of skin is most relevant to surgical planning of scar formation?*

A. Pigmentation.
B. Comedones.
C. Pore size.
D. Gland density.
E. Fitzpatrick type.

SKIN PHYSIOLOGY

5. *Which cell type is the most important in regulating promotion of growth factors and affecting wound healing?*

A. Neutrophils.
B. Basophils.
C. Macrophages.
D. Fibroblasts.
E. Melanocytes.

SKIN PHYSIOLOGY

6. *A patient is told to stop smoking cigarettes 4 to 6 weeks prior to her upcoming breast augmentation surgery. By having her stop cigarette use, what primary negative effect on wound healing are you trying to mitigate?*

A. Epithelial injury.
B. Endothelial injury.
C. DNA strand breaks and helical cross-linking.
D. Increased inflammatory state.
E. Peripheral microvascular vasoconstriction.

SKIN PHYSIOLOGY

7. *Final scar healing strength will reach a maximum of 80% original strength by approximately __ days.*

A. 15.
B. 30.
C. 45.
D. 60.
E. 90.

FACTORS AFFECTING WOUND HEALING

8. *In which of the following skin conditions can surgical correction be beneficial?*

A. Ehlers-Danlos.
B. Elastoderma.
C. Cutis laxa.
D. Progeria.
E. Stevens-Johnson syndrome.

FACTORS AFFECTING WOUND HEALING

9. *Which of the following medications is associated with decreasing collagen synthesis?*

A. Antineoplastic agents.
B. Interferon.
C. Nicotine.
D. Systemic anticoagulants.
E. Anti-inflammatory agents.

SKIN ANALYSIS

10. *How does treatment approach differ for static versus dynamic rhytids of the face?*
A. Static rhytids cannot be treated, dynamic rhytids can.
B. Static rhytids do not respond well to surgery.
C. Dynamic rhytids require excision of muscle.
D. Static rhytids can be treated with laser resurfacing, fillers, or surgery.
E. Dynamic rhytids do not respond well to botulinum toxin injection.

SKIN ANALYSIS

11. *In determining aggressiveness of a melanoma, which of the following characteristics is most predictive of staging and prognosis?*
A. Asymmetric shape/border.
B. Dark pigmentation.
C. Ulceration.
D. Depth >2 mm.
E. Evolution of morphology.

PHYSIOLOGY OF COMMON MEDICAL SKIN THERAPIES

12. *A retired farmer presents with multiple, small, rough and scaly erythematous plaques on his face. Which of the following is an appropriate initial course of action in treating this patient?*
A. Watch and wait.
B. Topical 5-FU.
C. Steroid injection.
D. Standard surgical excision.
E. 2.5% Hydrocortisone cream.

PHYSIOLOGY OF COMMON MEDICAL SKIN THERAPIES

13. *Which of the following potentially predisposing factors contributes most to a patient's increased likelihood of developing malignant melanoma?*
A. Frequent current sun exposure.
B. History of sun burns as a teenager.
C. Family history of melanoma.
D. Multiple actinic keratoses.
E. Fitzpatrick type I skin.

Answers

ANATOMY

1. *Which of the following cell types provides UV protection to the skin?*

B. Melanocytes.

As the pigment-producing (melanin) skin cells, melanocytes provide the skin with UV protection. Melanocytes are located mostly within the basal layer of the epidermis.[1]

REFERENCE

1. Chu DH, Haake AR, Holbrook K, et al. The structure and development of skin. In: Freedberg IM, Eisen AZ, Wolff K, et al, eds. Fitzpatrick's Dermatology in General Medicine. 6th ed. New York: McGraw-Hill; 2003

ANATOMY

2. *Which epidermal cell layer is mitotically active, providing stem cells to repopulate the epidermis each month (Fig. 13.1)?*

E. Stratum basale.

The stratum basale is mitotically active, providing stem cells to the upper layers of the epidermis for differentiation. In regenerative medicine, these epidermal stem cells can be modified in vitro (induced-pluripotent stem cells, iPSCs) and used for stem cell replacement of other tissue types in the body.[1]

REFERENCE

1. Chu DH, Haake AR, Holbrook K, et al. The structure and development of skin. In: Freedberg IM, Eisen AZ, Wolff K, et al, eds. Fitzpatrick's Dermatology in General Medicine. 6th ed. New York: McGraw-Hill; 2003

SKIN PHYSIOLOGY

3. *What is the approximate ratio of type I:III collagen in the dermis of a normal adult?*

C. 4:1.

The dermis is the component making up the majority of the skin tissue. It is divided into a papillary (superficial) and reticular (deep) layers and is composed primarily of elastic fibers and collagen (types I and III in a 4:1 ratio) maintained by fibroblasts.[1,2]

REFERENCES

1. Janis JE, Harrison B. Wound healing: part I. Basic science. Plast Reconst Surg 2014;133:199e
2. Glat P, Longaker M. Wound healing. In: Aston SJ, Beasley RW, Thorne CH, et al, eds. Grabb and Smith's Plastic Surgery. 5th ed. Philadelphia: Lippincott-Raven; 1997

SKIN PHYSIOLOGY

4. *Which of the following characteristics of skin is most relevant to surgical planning of scar formation?*

D. Gland density.

Glands in the skin come in several varieties, including sebaceous, eccrine, and apocrine. Their primary functions involve maintaining skin hydration, assisting with thermal regulation, and providing a regenerative source for the epidermis to repopulate. Increased gland density (particularly in the face) allows for resurfacing procedures to have positive effect; on the other hand, reduced gland density (i.e., below the jawline) delays epidermal regeneration, which can lead to more severe scarring.[1,2]

REFERENCES

1. Janis JE, Harrison B. Wound healing: part I. Basic science. Plast Reconst Surg 2014;133:199e
2. Glat P, Longaker M. Wound healing. In: Aston SJ, Beasley RW, Thorne CH, et al., eds. Grabb and Smith's Plastic Surgery. 5th ed. Philadelphia: Lippincott-Raven; 1997

SKIN PHYSIOLOGY

5. *Which cell type is the most important in regulating promotion of growth factors and affecting wound healing?*

C. Macrophages.

The macrophage is the most important regulator of growth factors in the wound-healing process. They are the second in line to arrive on the scene, following neutrophils, in the acute inflammatory response (days 1–6).[1]

REFERENCE

1. Janis JE, Harrison B. Wound healing: part I. Basic science. Plast Reconst Surg 2014;133:199e

SKIN PHYSIOLOGY

6. *A patient is told to stop smoking cigarettes 4 to 6 weeks prior to her upcoming breast augmentation surgery. By having her stop cigarette use, what primary negative effect on wound healing are you trying to mitigate?*

E. Peripheral microvascular vasoconstriction.

Although cigarette use has been shown to have a host of negative effects on wound healing, the primary mechanism by which it is proposed to affect healing is by having negative effects on the inflammatory phase of wound healing by causing peripheral microvascular vasoconstriction.[1,2,3,4]

REFERENCES

1. Janis JE, Harrison B. Wound healing: part I. Basic science. Plast Reconstr Surg 2016; 138(3, Suppl):9S–17S
2. Coon D, Tuffaha S, Christensen J, et al. Plastic surgery and smoking: a prospective analysis of incidence, compliance, and complications. Plast Reconstr Surg 2013;131(2):385–391
3. Rinker B. The evils of nicotine: an evidence-based guide to smoking and plastic surgery. Ann Plast Surg 2013;70(5):599–605
4. Silverstein P. Smoking and wound healing. Am J Med 1992;93(1A):22S–24S

SKIN PHYSIOLOGY

7. *Final scar healing strength will reach a maximum of 80% original strength by approximately __ days.*

E. 90.

During the maturation phase (week 3 to 1 year) of wound healing, there is equilibrium between collagen formation, deposition, and breakdown. Stronger cross-links are formed through increased collagen organization, as type I collagen replaces type III to revert back to the original 4:1 ratio. Finally, healing tensile strength will begin to plateau, achieving a maximum of 80% of original strength by about 90 days from initiation of wound-healing process.[1,2,3,4,5]

REFERENCES

1. Janis JE, Harrison B. Wound healing: part I. Basic science. Plast Reconst Surg 2014;133:199e
2. Glat P, Longaker M. Wound healing. In: Aston SJ, Beasley RW, Thorne CH, et al, eds. Grabb and Smith's Plastic Surgery. 5th ed. Philadelphia: Lippincott-Raven; 1997
3. Levenson SM, Geever EF, Crowley, Oates JF 3rd, Berard CW, Rosen H. The healing of rat skin wounds. Ann Surg 1965;161(2):293–308
4. Madden JW, Peacock EE Jr. Studies on the biology of collagen during wound healing. I. Rate of collagen synthesis and deposition in cutaneous wounds of the rat. Surgery 1968;64(1):288–294
5. Ireton JE, Unger JG, Rohrich RJ. The role of wound healing and its everyday application in plastic surgery: a practical perspective and systematic review. Plast Reconstr Surg Glob Open 2013;1(1):e10–e19

FACTORS AFFECTING WOUND HEALING

8. *In which of the following skin conditions can surgical correction be beneficial?*

C. Cutis laxa.

Cutis laxa may benefit from surgical correction. This originates from a nonfunctioning elastase inhibitor, which leads to gradual degeneration of elastic fibers in the skin of those affected. The skin develops a coarse texture, drooping all over the body. Although the condition slowly worsens over time, surgical correction may still be indicated and can also be quite beneficial for patients with cutis laxa (unlike A, B, D, and E). The primary treatment of Stevens-Johnson syndrome is stopping nonessential medications that may be the cause, supportive care with fluid management in addition to wound care, and antibiotics to control infection if needed.[1,2]

References

1. Janis JE, Harrison B. Wound healing: part I. Basic science. Plast Reconst Surg 2014;133:199e
2. Glat P, Longaker M. Wound healing. In: Aston SJ, Beasley RW, Thorne CH, et al, eds. Grabb and Smith's Plastic Surgery. 5th ed. Philadelphia: Lippincott-Raven; 1997

FACTORS AFFECTING WOUND HEALING

9. *Which of the following medications is associated with decreasing collagen synthesis?*

E. Anti-inflammatory agents.

A thorough history of medication usage (recent past, present) is vital to understanding a patient's potential for adverse wound healing. Anti-inflammatory drugs in particular have been associated with decreasing the amount of collagen synthesis significantly, by about 45%. This can have a detrimental effect on wound-healing properties of skin following aesthetic procedures. Thus, patients should be counseled well before surgery to abstain for at least 2 weeks prior and after surgery.[1]

Reference

1. Fairweather M, Heit YI, Buie J, Rosenberg LM, Briggs A, Orgill DP, Bertagnolli MM. Celecoxib inhibits early cutaneous wound healing. J Surg Res 2015;194(2):717–724

SKIN ANALYSIS

10. *How does treatment approach differ for* static *versus* dynamic *rhytids of the face?*

D. Static rhytids can be treated with laser resurfacing, fillers, or surgery.

Static rhytids of the face appear at rest, without requiring facial expression muscle movement to accentuate. These are best treated by laser resurfacing, filler injection, or (definitively) with surgery. Dynamic rhytids, on the other hand, *are* accentuated with animation of facial expression musculature, and thus respond well to neurotoxin treatment.[1]

Reference

1. Baker TJ, Stuzin JM, Baker TM, eds. Facial Skin Resurfacing. New York: Thieme Publishers; 1998

SKIN ANALYSIS

11. *In determining aggressiveness of a melanoma, which of the following characteristics is most predictive of staging and prognosis?*

D. Depth >2 mm.

Breslow thickness (measurement of depth of invasion, superficial to deep) is the most important factor in the staging and prognosis of melanoma-type skin cancer. Best prognosis is given for depth of <0.75 mm; the worst is classified by >4 mm of depth. Any depth between these values warrants a sentinel lymph node biopsy. Although the other factors listed are important in the identification of melanoma-type skin cancer, only the depth is used as a prognostic, staging tool.[1]

Reference

1. Langley RG, Barnhi llRL, Mihm MC Jr, et al. Neoplasms: cutaneous melanoma. In: Freedberg IM, Eisen AZ, Wolff K, et al, eds. Fitzpatrick's Dermatology in General Medicine. 6th ed. New York: McGraw-Hill; 2003

PHYSIOLOGY OF COMMON MEDICAL SKIN THERAPIES

12. *A retired farmer presents with multiple, small, rough and scaly erythematous plaques on his face. Which of the following is an appropriate initial course of action in treating this patient?*

B. Topical 5-FU.

Actinic keratoses are rough, scaly, erythematous patches or plaques, often appearing on sun-exposed areas such as the scalp, face, rim of ear, or dorsal upper extremity. They are considered premalignant lesions, as approximately 10% will eventually progress to squamous cell carcinoma, and 60% of squamous cell carcinomas arise within an actinic keratosis. When multiple actinic keratoses are present, it is often not practical to treat each spot individually. Standard of care includes either topical therapy with 5-fluorouracil (5-FU) or topical imiquimod. Standard surgical excision in order to prevent progression to cancer is also an accepted method of treatment. However, this is often reserved for cases where it is difficult to tell if the lesion is an actinic keratosis or an earlycancer.[1]

REFERENCE

1. Marks R, Rennie G, Selwood TS. Malignant transformation of solar keratoses to squamous cell carcinoma. Lancet 1988;1:795

PHYSIOLOGY OF COMMON MEDICAL SKIN THERAPIES

13. *Which of the following potentially predisposing factors contributes most to a patient's increased likelihood of developing malignant melanoma?*

C. Family history of melanoma.

Among the options listed, none of the factors predisposes to melanoma development more strongly than does a positive family history of melanoma. Another notable risk factor is patients with multiple atypical nevi throughout their life.[1]

REFERENCE

1. Langley RG, Barnhi llRL, Mihm MC, Jr, et al. Neoplasms: cutaneous melanoma. In: Freedberg IM, Eisen AZ, Wolff K, et al, eds. Fitzpatrick's Dermatology in General Medicine. 6th ed. New York: McGraw-Hill; 2003

14. Cosmeceuticals and Other Office Products

Sammy Sinno, Michael E. Nissan
See *Essentials of Aesthetic Surgery*, pp. 191–196

CLEANSERS

1. ***Which of the following is true regarding high detergent surfactants?***
   A. They are most appropriate for patients with dry skin.
   B. They may lead to barrier damage and inability of skin to hold water.
   C. Compared with other cleansers, high detergent surfactants remove less skin surface sebum.
   D. Cleansers based on sodium cocoyl isethionate are high detergent.
   E. Synthetic moisturizers, such as *syndets*, are considered high detergent surfactants.

MOISTURIZERS

2. ***Which of the following moisturizers acts by drawing water from deeper skin layers to the dehydrated stratum corneum?***
   A. Petrolatum.
   B. Lanolin.
   C. Mineral oil.
   D. Dimethicone.
   E. Glycerin.

MOISTURIZERS

3. ***A patient is seen in clinic for an itchy, erythematous perioral rash. He says that the rash appeared the day after he began applying a new balm for increasingly chapped lips. Which of the following agents is the most likely cause of this reaction?***
   A. Petrolatum.
   B. Lanolin.
   C. Mineral oil.
   D. Dimethicone.
   E. Glycerin.

ALPHA-HYDROXY ACIDS

4. ***Which of the following is an advantage of alpha-hydroxy acids such as glycolic acid and lactic acid?***
   A. Stimulates collagen synthesis.
   B. Inhibits elastase.
   C. Exerts antioxidant effects by preventing lipid oxidation, protecting the cellular membrane from free radicals.
   D. Enhances exfoliation of the stratum corneum.
   E. Regulates epithelial cell growth and differentiation.

SUNSCREENS

5. ***Which of the following is true regarding sunscreens?***
   A. UVA radiation causes sunburn.
   B. Inorganic filters should be used with organic filters to prevent skin whitening.
   C. Sunscreens prevent photoaging and reverse existing damage.
   D. Paraaminobenzoic acid, salicylates, and cinnamates can be applied to prevent photoaging.
   E. Zinc oxide and titanium dioxide are examples of organic filters.

BOTANICALS

6. *Which of the following compounds acts as a topical antioxidant that can improve photodamaged skin?*

A. Soy.
B. Silymarin.
C. Retinol.
D. Curcumin.
E. Grape seed extract.

TREATMENT OF PIGMENTED SKIN

7. *Regimens to treat pigmented skin should include a cleanser (such as glycolic acid) followed by a serum that inhibits which of the following enzymes?*

A. Tyrosinase.
B. Phenylalanine hydroxylase.
C. Homogentisate oxidase.
D. Tyrosine hydroxylase.
E. DOPA decarboxylase.

Answers

CLEANSERS

1. ***Which of the following is true regarding high detergent surfactants?***

   B. They may lead to barrier damage and inability of skin to hold water.

   The active ingredients of cleansers are surfactants. Compared with low detergent surfactants that remove less skin surface sebum, high detergent surfactants may remove skin surface sebum and intracellular lipids, leading to barrier damage and dry skin. For this reason, patients with dry skin benefit from surfactants that remove less skin surface sebum, such as cleansers based on sodium cocoyl isethionate. Synthetic moisturizers would be considered low detergent surfactants as they remove less sebum; therefore, E is incorrect.[1]

REFERENCE

1. Draelos ZD. Active agents in common skin care products. Plast Reconstr Surg 2010;125:719

MOISTURIZERS

2. ***Which of the following moisturizers acts by drawing water from deeper skin layers to the dehydrated stratum corneum?***

   E. Glycerin.

   Glycerin is a humectant, a class of moisturizer that hydrates the stratum corneum by drawing water from the dermis and epidermis below. Its action is mediated by regulation of aquaporin channels in the skin. Petrolatum, lanolin, oils, and dimethicone are occlusive agents that act as barriers, physically reducing transepidermal water loss.[1,2]

REFERENCES

1. Friberg SE, Ma Z. Stratum corneum lipids, petrolatum and white oils. Cosmet Toilet 1993;107:55
2. Spencer TS. Dry skin and skin moisturizers. Clin Dermatol 1988;6:24

MOISTURIZERS

3. ***A patient is seen in clinic for an itchy, erythematous perioral rash. He says that the rash appeared the day after he began applying a new balm for increasingly chapped lips. Which of the following agents is the most likely cause of this reaction?***

   B. Lanolin.

   Based on the location of the rash and the patient's history of application of a new skin product, allergic contact dermatitis is the most likely diagnosis. The etiology is a delayed-type hypersensitivity reaction to an antigen in the balm the patient applied to the lips. Although any product may potentially cause such a reaction, lanolin, a derivative of sheep sebaceous secretions, is particularly associated with allergic contact dermatitis.[1,2]

REFERENCES

1. Friberg SE, Ma Z. Stratum corneum lipids, petrolatum and white oils. Cosmet Toilet 1993;107:55
2. Spencer TS. Dry skin and skin moisturizers. Clin Dermatol 1988;6:24

ALPHA-HYDROXY ACIDS

4. ***Which of the following is an advantage of alpha-hydroxy acids such as glycolic acid and lactic acid?***

   D. Enhances exfoliation of the stratum corneum.

   Alpha-hydroxy acids comprise a wide variety of products, including glycolic acid, lactic acid, malic acid, citric acid, and tartaric acid. Preparations are available for over-the-counter use or for in-office peel treatments. They exert their effect by enhancing exfoliation of the stratum corneum, the keratinous outermost layer of the epidermis. Common applications include treatment of photodamage, hyperpigmentation, melasma, dry skin, acne, and rosacea.[1]

Reference

1. Sinno S, Lee DS, Khachemoune A. Vitamins and cutaneous wound healing. J Wound Care 2011;20:287

SUNSCREENS

5. *Which of the following is true regarding sunscreens?*

B. Inorganic filters should be used with organic filters to prevent skin whitening.

Sunscreens are designed to absorb or reflect UVA and UVB radiation.[1] UVA radiation is responsible for photoaging, while UVB radiation is responsible for sunburn. Examples of UVB filters include paraaminobenzoic acid, salicylates, and cinnamates—application of these agents aids in preventing UVB-induced sunburn, but not photoaging, which is a sequela of UVA exposure. Although it is true that some sunscreens can prevent photoaging, they cannot reverse existing damage. Zinc oxide and titanium dioxide are examples of inorganic filters, which should be used with organic filters to prevent skin whitening.[1,2,3]

References

1. Chatterjee L, Agarwal R, Mukhtar H. Ultraviolet B radiation-induced DNA lesions in mouse epidermis: an assessment using a novel 32P-postlabeling technique. Biochem Biophys Res Commun 1996;229:590
2. Duell EA, Derguini F, Kang S, et al. Extraction of human epidermis treated with retinol yields retro-retinoids in addition to free retinol and retinyl esters. J Invest Dermatol 1996;107:178
3. Torras H. Retinoids in aging. Clin Dermatol 1996;14:207

BOTANICALS

6. *Which of the following compounds acts as a topical antioxidant that can improve photodamaged skin?*

C. Retinol.

Retinol is the naturally occurring form of vitamin A, and it acts as an antioxidant when applied to the skin. On the skin, it is converted to retinoic acid, which improves photodamage. Soy increases collagen synthesis, silymarin decreases the formation of DNA-damaging pyrimidine dimers, and curcumin acts as a moisturizer. Although grape seed extract does act as a free radical scavenger, it has not been shown to improve photodamaged skin.[1,2]

References

1. Duell EA, Derguini F, Kang S, et al. Extraction of human epidermis treated with retinol yields retro-retinoids in addition to free retinol and retinyl esters. J Invest Dermatol 1996;107:178
2. Torras H. Retinoids in aging. Clin Dermatol 1996;14:207

TREATMENT OF PIGMENTED SKIN

7. *Regimens to treat pigmented skin should include a cleanser (such as glycolic acid) followed by a serum that inhibits which of the following enzymes?*

A. Tyrosinase.

Treatment of pigmented skin is twofold; both a cleanser such as glycolic acid and a tyrosinase-inhibiting serum/moisturizer such as kojic acid or hydroquinone are required. Tyrosinase inhibition hinders pigmentation, as tyrosinase is the rate-limiting enzyme controlling the production of melanin.[1,2,3]

References

1. Friberg SE, Ma Z. Stratum corneum lipids, petrolatum and white oils. Cosmet Toilet 1993;107:55
2. Spencer TS. Dry skin and skin moisturizers. Clin Dermatol 1988;6:24
3. Aston SJ, Steinbrech DS, Walden JL. Aesthetic Plastic Surgery. Philadelphia: Saunders Elsevier; 2010

15. Ethnic Skin Care

Sammy Sinno, Michael E. Nissan
See *Essentials of Aesthetic Surgery*, pp. 197–201

ETHNIC SKIN

1. *Which of the following characteristics is more applicable to ethnic skin rather than white skin?*
A. Ethnic skin contains a higher concentration of melanocytes.
B. Ethnic skin contains more cell layers in the stratum corneum.
C. Ethnic skin has decreased lipid content.
D. Ethnic skin has decreased desquamation.
E. Darker skin provides increased photoprotection and low response to dermal injury.

FITZPATRICK SCALE

2. *A patient is seen in clinic after returning from a tropical vacation. Her sun-exposed skin is visibly sunburnt, and she states that though she is sometimes able to tan, she usually burns when she is exposed to sunlight. Her skin is fair and white without freckles. Which of the following is the patient's Fitzpatrick skin type?*
A. Type I.
B. Type II.
C. Type III.
D. Type IV.
E. Type V.

HYDRATION

3. *Which of the following is characteristic of dry skin in ethnic populations?*
A. Darker skin is associated with higher transepidermal water loss.
B. Dryness of skin layers confers lower predisposition for acne development.
C. Pigmented skin is more likely to camouflage the observable signs of dryness.
D. Pigmented skin has lower rates of stratum corneum shedding.
E. Dry skin is characterized by lower rates of inflammation, irritation, and hyperpigmentation.

HYPOPIGMENTATION

4. *A 28-year-old woman is seen in clinic for a concerning new patch of depigmented skin on the left cheek. The lesion is flat, 5 cm in diameter, and sharply demarcated. Other than autoimmune thyroid disease requiring her to take exogenous thyroid hormone, she is healthy. Which of the following is the most appropriate response to the patient regarding management of this lesion?*
A. Excision with wide margins is necessary.
B. There are no interventions that can be taken at this time.
C. A biopsy of the lesion is necessary.
D. Referral for Mohs surgery.
E. Manage with phototherapy, immunomodulators, and topical steroids.

PIGMENTATION INHIBITORS

5. *Which of the following pigmentation inhibitors acts by suppressing the formation of melanocytes?*
A. Hydroquinone.
B. Kojic acid.
C. Lactic acid.
D. Retinoids.
E. Lanolin.

ACNE

6. *Which of the following is the most effective strategy for preventing postinflammatory hyperpigmentation in darker-skinned individuals?*

A. Topical clindamycin.
B. Topical retinoids.
C. Doxycycline therapy.
D. Initiating combination therapy only if signs of postinflammatory hyperpigmentation are identified.
E. Immediate treatment with topical clindamycin, topical retinoid, and benzoyl peroxide.

SUNSCREEN

7. *A female patient of Northern European heritage who has a history of rosacea would like to know which is the most appropriate sunscreen she should use and why?*

A. An organic sunscreen is most appropriate, as it does not cause skin whitening.
B. An organic sunscreen is most appropriate, as it is less likely to exacerbate preexisting skin conditions such as rosacea.
C. An inorganic sunscreen is most appropriate, as it does not cause skin whitening.
D. An inorganic sunscreen is most appropriate, as it is less likely to exacerbate preexisting skin conditions such as rosacea.
E. Patients with rosacea should avoid using sunscreen.

HAIR REMOVERS

8. *Which of the following is true regarding use of chemical depilatories?*

A. Frequency of use of chemical depilatories is similar across ethnic groups.
B. Chemical depilatories are an alternative to shaving that do not cause irritation or postinflammatory hyperpigmentation.
C. Chemical depilatories work by degrading disulfide bonds in the hair shaft.
D. Any active ingredient can effectively be used regardless of coarseness of hair.
E. Calcium thioglycolate and sodium thioglycolate are the most effective ingredients for removal of coarse hair.

Answers

ETHNIC SKIN

1. *Which of the following characteristics is more applicable to ethnic skin rather than white skin?*

B. Ethnic skin contains more cell layers in the stratum corneum.

Darker pigmentation in ethnic skin is provided by an increased rate of melanin production compared with white skin. However, melanocyte concentration does not differ between skin types. The increased melanin does provide photoprotection; however, darker skin is characterized by increased reaction to tissue injury,[1] particularly hypertrophic scars and keloids. Ethnic skin is further characterized by increased lipid content, more cell layers in the stratum corneum (22 layers in black skin versus 17 in white skin),[2] and a resultant increased rate of desquamation.

REFERENCES

1. Reed JT, Ghadially R, Elias PM. Skin type, but neither race nor gender, influence epidermal permeability barrier function. Arch Dermatol 1995;131:1134
2. Andersen KE, Maibach HI. Black and white human skin differences. J Am Acad Dermatol 1979;1:276

FITZPATRICK SCALE

2. *A patient is seen in clinic after returning from a tropical vacation. Her sun-exposed skin is visibly sunburnt, and she states that though she is sometimes able to tan, she usually burns when she is exposed to sunlight. Her skin is fair and white without freckles. Which of the following is the patient's Fitzpatrick skin type?*

B. Type II.

The Fitzpatrick scale was developed to classify skin by responses to UV light.[1] Given this patient's predisposition to sunburn, limited ability to tan, and lack of freckles, her skin is classified as Fitzpatrick skin type II (**Table 15.1**).

Table 15.1 *Fitzpatrick Skin Type Classification*

Skin Type	Characteristics	Sun Exposure History
I	Pale white, freckles, blue eyes, blond or red hair	Always burns, never tans
II	Fair white, blue/green/hazel eyes, blond or red hair	Usually burns, minimally tans
III	Cream white, any hair or eye color	Sometimes burns, tans uniformly
IV	Moderate brown (Mediterranean)	Rarely burns, always tans well
V	Dark brown (Middle Eastern)	Rarely burns, tans easily
VI	Dark brown to black	Never burns, tans easily

(Source: Data from Fitzpatrick TB. The validity and practicality of sun-reactive skin types I through VI. Arch Dermatol 124:869, 1988.)

REFERENCE

1. Odunze M, Cohn A, Few JW. Restylane and people of color. Plast Reconst Surg 2007;120:2011

HYDRATION

3. *Which of the following is characteristic of dry skin in ethnic populations?*

A. Darker skin is associated with higher transepidermal water loss.

Dryness in ethnic skin is partially attributable to increased transepidermal water loss. The resultant dry skin is prone to cracks, which predispose the patient to develop acne. Another cosmetic concern related to dryness in pigmented skin is stratum corneum shedding, which produces an ashy-appearing scale that is difficult to camouflage on a pigmented backdrop. Additionally, there are higher rates of inflammation, irritation, and hyperpigmentation due to impaired barrier function.[1]

Reference

1. Montagna W, Prota G, Kenney JA Jr, eds. Black Skin Structure and Function. San Diego: Academic Press; 1993

HYPOPIGMENTATION

4. *A 28-year-old woman is seen in clinic for a concerning new patch of depigmented skin on the left cheek. The lesion is flat, 5 cm in diameter, and sharply demarcated. Other than autoimmune thyroid disease requiring her to take exogenous thyroid hormone, she is healthy. Which of the following is the most appropriate response to the patient regarding management of this lesion?*

E. Manage with phototherapy, immunomodulators, and topical steroids.

Although the underlying condition cannot be totally cured, the lesion can be managed with phototherapy, immunomodulators, and topical steroids. Given the characteristics of the lesion (flat, well-demarcated, depigmented) and the patient's previous history of autoimmune disease, a clinical diagnosis of vitiligo can reliably be made without surgical measures such as biopsy or excision. Telling the patient that no interventions can be taken is not appropriate; phototherapy, immunomodulators, and topical steroids can all be used to manage vitiligo lesions.[1]

Reference

1. Baldini E, Odorisio T, Sorrenti S, et al. Vitiligo and autoimmune thyroid disorders. Front Endocrinol (Lausanne) 2017;8:290

PIGMENTATION INHIBITORS

5. *Which of the following pigmentation inhibitors acts by suppressing the formation of melanocytes?*

C. Lactic acid.

Lactic acid acts by suppressing the formation of melanocytes. Hydroquinone inhibits tyrosinase, the enzyme responsible for production of melanin, via inhibition of DNA and RNA synthesis. Kojic acid likewise inhibits tyrosinase, but via a different mechanism: it chelates tyrosinase-bound copper, inactivating the enzyme (**Table 15.2**).[1]

Table 15.2 *Commonly Used Pigmentation Inhibitors*

Inhibitor	Mechanism of Action
Hydroquinone	Inhibits tyrosinase by inhibiting DNA and RNA synthesis
Kojic acid	Chelates copper bound to tyrosinase rendering it inactive
Azelaic acid	Naturally derived from grain products and by oxygenation of oleic acid Cytotoxic to melanocytes
Lactic acid	Suppresses formation of melanocytes
Retinoids	Inhibits tyrosinase activity
Arbutin	Found naturally in cranberries
	Inhibits melanosome maturation
	Less irritating than hydroquinone

Reference

1. Taylor SC. Utilizing combination therapy for ethnic skin. Cutis 2007;80(1 Suppl):15

ACNE

6. *Which of the following is the most effective strategy for preventing postinflammatory hyperpigmentation in darker-skinned individuals?*

E. Immediate treatment with topical clindamycin, topical retinoid, and benzoyl peroxide.

Postinflammatory hyperpigmentation is a major sequela of acne in darker-skinned individuals. For this reason, the primary goal of acne treatment in this population is prevention of this phenomenon. Early intervention is necessary to achieve this goal, rendering watchful waiting an inappropriate course of action. Additionally, monotherapy often proves ineffective. Studies have shown that the most effective therapy involves prompt treatment with clindamycin, topical retinoid, and benzoyl peroxide.[1]

REFERENCE

1. Taylor SC. Utilizing combination therapy for ethnic skin. Cutis 2007;80(1 Suppl):15

SUNSCREEN

7. *A female patient of Northern European heritage who has a history of rosacea would like to know which is the most appropriate sunscreen she should use and why?*

D. An inorganic sunscreen is most appropriate, as it is less likely to exacerbate preexisting skin conditions such as rosacea.

Sunscreen use is important to prevent skin cancer in all patients, including darker-skinned individuals, regardless of skin conditions such as rosacea. The advantage of organic sunscreens is that they do not cause the skin whitening that is seen in inorganic sunscreens such as titanium dioxide and zinc dioxide. The mechanism of action of organic sunscreens involves absorption of solar radiation, which produces heat. Unfortunately, heat can trigger various skin conditions, particularly rosacea. For this reason, an inorganic sunscreen is most appropriate for patients with rosacea.[1]

REFERENCE

1. Draelos ZD. Cosmeceuticals for rosacea. Clin Dermatol 2017;35(2):213–217

HAIR REMOVERS

8. *Which of the following is true regarding use of chemical depilatories?*

C. Chemical depilatories work by degrading disulfide bonds in the hair shaft.

Chemical depilatories are an alternative method of hair removal to shaving, which function by degrading disulfide bonds in the hair shaft, causing swelling within the hair shaft. Importantly, this swelling can cause irritation that can lead to postinflammatory hyperpigmentation. Regardless, the use of chemical depilatories remains higher in the black population due to higher incidence of pseudofolliculitis barbae after shaving. The most common active ingredients in chemical depilatories are calcium thioglycolate and sodium thioglycolate—however, patients with coarser hair find that stronger ingredients are needed to achieve hair removal. Stronger ingredients for use in patients with coarse hair include strontium sulfide, barium sulfide, potassium hydroxide, and sodium hydroxide.[1]

REFERENCE

1. Taylor SC. Utilizing combination therapy for ethnic skin. Cutis 2007;80(1 Suppl):15

Part V

Noninvasive and Minimally Invasive Therapy

16. Basics of Laser Therapy

Ara A. Salibian
See *Essentials of Aesthetic Surgery*, pp. 205–211

PHYSICS OF LASERS

1. *Which of the following characteristics of a laser determines its target chromophore?*
   A. Wavelength.
   B. Spot size.
   C. Pulse duration.
   D. Beam shape.
   E. Fluence.

MAJOR TYPES OF LASERS

2. *What is the target chromophore for ablative CO_2 or erbium:YAG lasers?*
   A. Oxyhemoglobin.
   B. Melanin.
   C. Collagen.
   D. Water.
   E. Fat.

INDICATIONS AND CONTRAINDICATIONS

3. *Which of the following factors is a contraindication to facial laser treatment?*
   A. Moderate perioral rhytides.
   B. Mild acne scarring.
   C. Facial tattoo with iron oxide.
   D. Solar lentigines.
   E. Erythematous hypertrophic scar.

PREOPERATIVE EVALUATION

4. *A patient who sometimes burns but usually tans uniformly is designated as which skin type in Fitzpatrick classification?*
   A. I.
   B. II.
   C. III.
   D. IV.
   E. V.

PREOPERATIVE EVALUATION

5. *Which of the following medications should not be given to patients prior to facial laser resurfacing?*
   A. Hydroquinone.
   B. Vitamin C.
   C. Trenitoin.
   D. Isotretinoin.
   E. Acyclovir.

PREOPERATIVE EVALUATION

6. *Which of the following viral infections is most common after facial laser resurfacing?*
   A. Cytomegalovirus.
   B. Varicella-zoster.

C. Herpes simplex virus.
D. Human immunodeficiency virus.
E. Human papilloma virus.

INFORMED CONSENT

7. *Which of the following is true for facial resurfacing with lasers?*
A. Have low efficacy with poor outcomes.
B. Lower risk for hyperpigmentation in patients with darker skin tone.
C. Multiple treatments are almost always needed.
D. Do not treat tattoos.
E. Are ineffective for vascular lesions.

Answers

PHYSICS OF LASERS

1. *Which of the following characteristics of a laser determines its target chromophore?*

A. Wavelength.

Lasers generate in phase, monochromatic and coherent light that causes tissue injury based on wavelength-specific light absorption by a target chromophore. Each wavelength has an absorption spectrum that identifies the optimal targets. The absorption spectrum of oxyhemoglobin is at lower wavelengths, with melanin and finally water having higher wavelengths of optimal absorption. The principle is used in selective photothermolysis to minimize heat damage to surrounding tissues by targeting specific chromophores.[1]

REFERENCE

1. Atiyeh BS, Dibo SA. Nonsurgical non-ablative treatment of aging skin: radiofrequency technologies between aggressive marketing and evidence-based efficacy. Aesth Plast Surg 2009;33:283

MAJOR TYPES OF LASERS

2. *What is the target chromophore for ablative CO_2 or erbium:YAG lasers?*

D. Water.

High-energy ablative lasers target water in living cells, damaging the epidermis and parts of the dermis. Ablative lasers produce an open wound and have a higher risk of scarring and pigmentation than nonablative lasers depending on the depth of tissue injury.

CO_2 lasers (10,600 nm) and the erbium:YAG laser (2,940 nm) are the most common type of ablative lasers and can effectively treat rhytides, finer acne scars, and sun damage. Erbium lasers are absorbed more readily by water than CO_2 lasers, penetrating less deeply and causing less photomechanical injury. This results in faster healing and less risk of hypopigmentation but also less collagen contraction than CO_2 lasers.[1]

REFERENCE

1. Brightman LA, Brauer JA, Anolik R, et al. Ablative and fractional ablative lasers. Dermatol Clin 2009;27:479

INDICATIONS AND CONTRAINDICATIONS

3. *Which of the following factors is a contraindication to facial laser treatment?*

C. Facial tattoo with iron oxide.

Several types of tattoos are amenable to laser treatment, particularly with different q-switched lasers. These lasers lyse cells that contain tattoo pigments, which are then phagocytosed by surrounding immune cells. Although effective, multiple treatments are often needed, and side effects can include depigmentation. However, laser treatment of tattoos with iron oxide in the ink should be avoided. Lasers will convert the ferrous oxide into ferric oxide and can permanently darken the skin.[1]

REFERENCE

1. Alexiades-Armenakas M. Laser-mediated photodynamic therapy. Clin Dermatol 2006;24:16

PREOPERATIVE EVALUATION

4. *A patient who sometimes burns but usually tans uniformly is designated as which skin type in Fitzpatrick classification?*

C. III.

The Fitzpatrick skin type classification stratifies patients based on their propensity to have pigmentary changes after laser resurfacing (**Table 16.1**). Fitzpatrick I patients have pale white skin and freckles and will always burn and never tan with sun exposure. Fitzpatrick VI patients, on the other hand, have black skin, never burn, and tan very easily. Fitzpatrick III patients have creamy white skin, will sometimes burn, and tan relatively uniformly. Fitzpatrick skin types I–III are the ideal candidates for laser resurfacing, whereas as those with IV–VI skin types are at a higher risk of transient hyperpigmentation and long-term hypopigmentation. Patients with lighter skin, however, have a higher risk of prolonged postoperative erythema. It is important to discuss these risks with patients prior to treatment to set appropriate patient expectations with regards to outcomes and side effects.[1]

Table 16.1 *Fitzpatrick Skin Type Classification*

Skin Type	Characteristics	Sun Exposure History
I	Pale white, freckles, blue eyes, blond or red hair	Always burns, never tans
II	Fair white, blue/green/hazel eyes, blond or red hair	Usually burns, tans minimally
III	Cream white, any hair or eye color	Sometimes burns, tans uniformly
IV	Moderate brown (Mediterranean)	Rarely burns, always tans well
V	Dark brown (Middle Eastern)	Rarely burns, tans easily
VI	Dark brown to black	Never burns, tans easily

(Source: Data from Fitzpatrick TB. The validity and practicality of sun-reactive skin types I through VI. Arch Dermatol 124:869, 1988.)

REFERENCE

1. Fitzpatrick RE, Williams B, Goldman MP. Preoperative anesthesia and postoperative considerations in laser resurfacing. Semin Cutan Med Surg 1996;15:170

PREOPERATIVE EVALUATION

5. *Which of the following medications should not be given to patients prior to facial laser resurfacing?*

D. Isotretinoin.

Laser resurfacing is contraindicated in patients taking isotretinoin (Accutane). This medication should be stopped for at least 12 to 18 months prior to any laser procedures. Isotretinoin is a common medication for cystic acne and impairs re-epithelialization, which is necessary to heal the tissue damage caused by lasers. This impairment can subsequently lead to severe scarring after laser therapy. Hydroquinone is a tyrosine kinase inhibitor and is used as a pretreatment of the skin to prevent hyperpigmentation. Trenitoin (Retin-A) promotes re-epithelialization and is used as a pretreatment to promote healing after laser therapy.[1,2,3]

REFERENCES

1. Saedi N, Hamilton HK, Arndt KA, et al. How to prepare patients for ablative laser procedures. J Am Acad Dermatol 2013;69:e49
2. Mysore V, Mahadevappa OH, Barua S, et al. Standard guidelines of care: performing procedures in patients on or recently administered with isotretinoin. J Cutan Aesthet Surg 2017;10(4):186–194
3. Ward PD, Baker SR. Long term results of carbon dioxide laser resurfacing of the face. Arch Facial Plast Surg 2008;10:238

PREOPERATIVE EVALUATION

6. *Which of the following viral infections is most common after facial laser resurfacing?*

C. Herpes simplex virus.

Patients undergoing facial resurfacing procedures are at a potential risk for herpes simplex virus (HSV) infection. This risk is significantly higher in patients who have a history of HSV infection. All patients should receive antiviral pretreatment for HSV which includes acyclovir 400 mg by mouth three times per day, famciclovir 250 mg by mouth twice per day, or valacyclovir 500 mg by mouth twice per day for 1 to 3 days before treatment until re-epithelialization at 5 to 14 days.[1,2]

REFERENCES

1. Fitzpatrick RE, Williams B, Goldman MP. Preoperative anesthesia and postoperative considerations in laser resurfacing. Semin Cutan Med Surg 1996;15:170

2. Manuskiatti W, Fitzpatrick RE, Goldman MP. Long term effectiveness and side effects of carbon dioxide laser resurfacing for phyotoaged facial skin. J Am Acad Dermatol 1999;40:401

INFORMED CONSENT

7. *Which of the following is true for facial resurfacing with lasers?*

C. Multiple treatments are almost always needed.

Preoperative patient counseling and informed consent are key parts of any procedure, including laser treatments. Lasers can be very effective tools for treating numerous skin lesions and dispigmentations including vascular lesions, melanocytic pigmentations, lymphatic malformations, hair, angiokeratomas, rhytides, scars, and tattoos. Depending on the depth of the lesion and the penetration of the laser, multiple treatments are typically required to achieve the desired result, especially with nonablative lasers.[1,2]

REFERENCES

1. Alexiades Armenakas MR, Dover JS, Arndt KA. The spectrum of laser skin resurfacing: nonablative, fractional, and ablative laser resurfacing. J Am Acad Dermatol 2008;58:719
2. Atiyeh BS, Dibo SA. Nonsurgical non-ablative treatment of aging skin: radiofrequency technologies between aggressive marketing and evidence-based efficacy. Aesth Plast Surg 2009;33:283

17. Ablative Laser Resurfacing

Juan L. Rendon, Simon Moradian
See *Essentials of Aesthetic Surgery*, pp. 212–222

EQUIPMENT

1. *Which of the following lasers provide ablative resurfacing?*

A. Carbon dioxide laser only.
B. Carbon dioxide laser and erbium:yttrium aluminum garnet (ER:YAG) laser.
C. Carbon dioxide laser and neodymium-doped:yttrium aluminum garnet (ND:YAG) laser.
D. Erbium:yttrium aluminum garnet (ER:YAG) laser and neodymium-doped:yttrium aluminum garnet (ND: YAG) laser.
E. Carbon dioxide laser and Q-switched neodymium-doped:yttrium aluminum garnet (ND:YAG) laser.

EQUIPMENT

2. *Compared to the carbon dioxide laser, the erbium:yttrium aluminum garnet (ER:YAG) laser produces which of the following?*

A. More residual thermal damage and less precise tissue vaporization.
B. Less residual thermal damage and more precise tissue vaporization.
C. Equivalent residual thermal damage but more precise tissue vaporization.
D. No residual thermal damage and an increasing depth of tissue penetration with each additional pass.
E. More thermal damage and an increasing depth of tissue penetration with each additional pass.

EQUIPMENT

3. *A 52-year-old woman comes to the office for evaluation of persistent erythema 2 weeks after she underwent ablative carbon dioxide laser treatment. Which of the following topical treatments is most appropriate to decrease this patient's postoperative erythema?*

A. Amoxicillin.
B. Hydroquinone.
C. Ascorbic acid.
D. Valacyclovir.
E. Prednisone.

EQUIPMENT

4. *Which of the following lasers has the greatest affinity for water and therefore greatest dermal ablative potential?*

A. Carbon dioxide.
B. Neodymium-doped:yttrium aluminum garnet (ND:YAG).
C. Q-switched neodymium-doped:yttrium aluminum garnet (ND:YAG).
D. Erbium:yttrium aluminum garnet (ER:YAG).
E. Intense pulse light (IPL).

TECHNIQUE

5. *The use of tumescent local anesthesia for ablative laser is associated with which of the following?*

A. Increased depth of penetration.
B. Decreased depth of penetration.
C. Faster healing times.
D. More predictable treatment area.
E. Increased residual thermal damage.

TECHNIQUE

6. *The addition of hyaluronidase to local anesthetics achieves which of the following?*

A. pH neutralization.
B. Increased tissue diffusion.
C. Increased hemostasis.
D. Increased depth of tissue ablation.
E. Vasoconstriction.

TECHNIQUE

7. *A 45-year-old woman comes to the office because of rhytides caused by photoaging. Treatment using CO_2 laser resurfacing is planned. Laser resurfacing with a carbon dioxide laser should employ which of the following techniques and clinical endpoints?*

A. Multiple overlapping passes until there is a brown coloration of the treated area without skin contracture.
B. Multiple overlapping passes until there is a brown coloration of the treated area with skin contracture.
C. Multiple overlapping passes until there is a yellow coloration of the treated area with skin contracture.
D. Nonoverlapping passes until there is a brown coloration of treated area without skin contracture.
E. Nonoverlapping passes until there is a yellow coloration of treated area with skin contracture.

TECHNIQUE

8. *A 67-year-old woman with Fitzpatrick type I skin comes to the office with concerns over deep rhytides and signs of photoaging. She would like to avoid surgery and has had limited results with prior chemical peels. She is interested in laser therapy and wants recovery to have as little downtime as possible, but with maximal results. She elects for erbium:yttrium aluminum garnet (ER:YAG) laser resurfacing. Resurfacing with an ER:YAG laser should employ which of the following techniques and clinical endpoints?*

A. Overlapping passes until there is eradication of the rhytid and penetration into the papillary dermis as demonstrated by fine fibrillar bleeding.
B. Overlapping passes until there is eradication of the rhytid and penetration into the mid-reticular dermis as demonstrated by large dermal bleeding spots.
C. Nonoverlapping passes until there is eradication of the rhytid and penetration into the papillary dermis as demonstrated by fine fibrillar bleeding.
D. Nonoverlapping passes until there is eradication of the rhytid and penetration into the reticular dermis as demonstrated by large dermal bleeding spots.
E. Nonoverlapping passes until there is eradication of the rhytid and penetration past the reticular dermis with small exposed areas of subcutaneous fat.

POSTOPERATIVE CARE

9. *A 45-year-old female with a history of well-controlled diabetes and a Fitzpatrick type III skin type who underwent ER:YAG laser resurfacing 4 days ago presents to your clinic with worsening blanching erythema over the past 24 hours that is warm to touch and has a grape-like odor over the treated area. She was advised to perform bio-occlusive dressing changes daily and ice water soaks. You suspect a pseudomonas infection and cultures are taken and empiric treatment is started. What do you suspect the primary cause of such an infection to be?*

A. Fitzpatrick type III skin or above.
B. Prolonged use of bio-occlusive dressings for >72 hours.
C. ER:YAG laser use which is associated with a higher risk of infection when compared to other laser types.
D. History of diabetes.
E. Minimal ice water soaks.

POSTOPERATIVE CARE

10. *In open wound care protocols, which of the following topical agents should be used during the reepithelialization healing phase?*

A. Mupirocin.
B. Bacitracin.
C. Polymyxin B.
D. Non-antibiotic petroleum-based ointment.
E. Hydroquinone.

COMPLICATIONS

11. *Which of the following prophylactic measures should be universally continued pre and post ablative resurfacing?*

A. Antifungals, antibiotics, and antivirals.
B. Antifungals and antibiotics.
C. Antibiotics and antivirals.
D. Antibiotics alone.
E. Antivirals alone.

COMPLICATIONS

12. *Hyperpigmentation is most associated with which of the following?*

A. Preoperative use of hydroquinone.
B. Preoperative use of retinoid.
C. Heavy sun exposure.
D. Increased Fitzpatrick score.
E. Decreased Fitzpatrick score.

COMPLICATIONS

13. *A 54-year-old female patient with a Fitzpatrick skin type III is noted to have immediate hypopigmentation after ablative laser resurfacing in the preauricular area directly adjacent to an area of untreated skin. How will you counsel this patient?*

A. This phenomenon occurs more often with erbium:yttrium aluminum garnet (ER:YAG) than with carbon dioxide resurfacing.
B. It is a normal finding related to the transition between treated and untreated areas.
C. It can be addressed with steroid injection.
D. This is likely permanent.
E. This is related to her Fitzpatrick skin type.

Answers

EQUIPMENT

1. *Which of the following lasers provide ablative resurfacing?*

B. Carbon dioxide laser and erbium:yttrium aluminum garnet (ER:YAG) laser.

The CO_2 laser was the first ablative laser of its kind and originally used as a continuous wave in the 1960s. However, newer laser technologies developed to include erbium:yttrium aluminum garnet (ER:YAG) lasers and fractional lasers. The most commonly used ablative lasers to date continue to be **CO_2 laser** (10,600 nm) and the **erbium:YAG laser** (2,940 nm) with their target chromophore being water. The goals of all these devices are to eliminate or reduce sun-damaged collagen and encourage new collagen deposition and remodeling through a combination of tissue vaporization and collagen denaturation.

It should be noted that the absorption coefficient of a (ER:YAG) laser is 10 times greater than that of CO_2 laser (12,000 cm^{-1}). It produces more precise tissue vaporization and less thermal coagulation than CO_2 lasers. Alternatively, other ablative lasers include the yttrium scandium gallium garnet (YSGG) fractional lasers. The neodymium-doped:yttrium aluminum garnet (ND:YAG) and the Q-switched neodymium-doped:yttrium aluminum garnet (ND:YAG) lasers are both nonablative lasers.[1,2,3]

REFERENCES

1. Alexiades Armenakas MR, Dover JS, Arndt KA. The spectrum of laser skin resurfacing: non-ablative, fractional, and ablative laser resurfacing. J Am Acad Dermatol 2008;58:719
2. Brightman LA, Brauer JA, Anolik R, et al. Ablative and fractional ablative lasers. Dermatol Clin 2009;27:479
3. Walsh JT Jr, Flotte TJ, Anderson RR, et al. Pulsed CO_2 laser tissue ablation: effect of tissue type and pulse duration on thermal damage. Lasers Surg Med 1988;8:108

EQUIPMENT

2. *Compared to the carbon dioxide laser, the erbium:yttrium aluminum garnet (ER:YAG) laser produces which of the following?*

B. Less residual thermal damage and more precise tissue vaporization.

Ablative lasers vaporize the epidermis and possibly part of the dermis. Additionally, they cause mild to significant edema and an open wound, all dependent on the depth of injury.

Compared to the carbon dioxide laser, the erbium:yttrium aluminum garnet (ER:YAG) laser produces more precise tissue vaporization and less thermal coagulation, and therefore results in less residual thermal damage and faster healing times.[1,2,3]

REFERENCES

1. Alexiades Armenakas MR, Dover JS, Arndt KA. The spectrum of laser skin resurfacing: non-ablative, fractional, and ablative laser resurfacing. J Am Acad Dermatol 2008;58:719
2. Walsh JT Jr, Flotte TJ, Anderson RR, et al. Pulsed CO_2 laser tissue ablation: effect of tissue type and pulse duration on thermal damage. Lasers Surg Med 1988;8:108
3. Fitzpatrick RE, Williams B, Goldman MP. Preoperative anesthesia and postoperative considerations in laser resurfacing. Semin Cutan Med Surg 1996;15:170

EQUIPMENT

3. *A 52-year-old woman comes to the office for evaluation of persistent erythema 2 weeks after she underwent ablative carbon dioxide laser treatment. Which of the following topical treatments is most appropriate to decrease this patient's postoperative erythema?*

C. Ascorbic acid.

Erythema following laser treatment is an expected consequence of therapy. Postoperative topical application of ascorbic acid has been shown to decrease the duration as well as the severity of erythema by restoring the normal skin pH. Topical therapy with ascorbic acid should be applied following reepithelialization. Antibiotics or antivirals have not been shown to decrease erythema. Hydroquinone is a skin bleaching agent that does not treat erythema. Topical corticosteroids postoperatively may delay reepithelialization and have not been associated with a decrease in erythema.[1,2]

References

1. Alster TS, Lupton JR. Prevention and treatment of side effects and complications of cutaneous laser resurfacing. Plast Reconstr Surg 2002;109(1):308–316
2. Neaman KC, Baca ME, Piazza RC III, et al. Outcomes of fractional CO_2 laser application in aesthetic surgery: a retrospective review. Aesthet Surg J 2010;30(6):845–852

EQUIPMENT

4. *Which of the following lasers has the greatest affinity for water and therefore greatest dermal ablative potential?*

D. Erbium:yttrium aluminum garnet (ER:YAG).

Although both the carbon dioxide and the erbium:yttrium aluminum garnet (ER:YAG) lasers target the chromophore water, the absorption coefficient of the ER:YAG laser is 10 times greater than that of carbon dioxide laser. This produces **more precise tissue vaporization** and **less thermal coagulation** than CO_2 lasers. The ER:YAG laser is quite comprehensive and versatile. It has quicker healing times, or it can be much more aggressive and ablative than CO_2 with less residual thermal damage and an optimal efficacy safety profile (i.e., can be as aggressive or as superficial as needed).[1]

Reference

1. Alexiades, Armenakas MR, Dover JS, Arndt KA. The spectrum of laser skin resurfacing: non-ablative, fractional, and ablative laser resurfacing. J Am Acad Dermatol 2008;58:719

TECHNIQUE

5. *The use of tumescent local anesthesia for ablative laser is associated with which of the following?*

B. Decreased depth of penetration.

Because tumescent anesthesia introduces water into the tissue, it ultimately decreases the depth of penetration, which may not be desired as this would alter your predicted treatment depth and ultimately affect the final outcome. For example, a fractionated laser only treats a fraction of the skin (as the name implies) leaving the intervening skin untouched. These treated areas are known as ablative microthermal treatment zones (MTZs). This is accomplished by the laser emitting numerous narrow microscopic columns. The higher energy within those small spot sizes will increases the depth of the laser per given volume of tissue; however, if this depth is infiltrated with tumescence at varying areas/depths, this may affect your penetration and effect. Kessels etal reported using 0.11% solution of 500 mL lactated Ringer solution, 20 mL 1% ropivacaine, 20 mL 2% xylocaine, and 0.5 mL epinephrine, with a minimum of 6 mL/kg.[1,2,3]

References

1. Kessels JP, Ostertag JU. The use of tumescent local anesthesia in ablative laser treatments. J Eur Acad Dermatol Venereol 2012;26:1456
2. Cartee TV, Wasserman DI. Commentary: Ablative fractionated CO_2 laser treatment of photoaging: a clinical and histologic study. Dermatol Surg 2012;38:1790
3. Hantash BM, Bedi VP, Kapadia B, et al. In vivo histological evaluation of a novel ablative fractional resurfacing device. Lasers Surg Med 2007;39:96

TECHNIQUE

6. *The addition of hyaluronidase to local anesthetics achieves which of the following?*

B. Increased tissue diffusion.

The addition of hyaluronidase increases tissue diffusion. The addition of sodium bicarbonate to the local anesthesia to the lateral face neutralizes the pH. Epinephrine combined with a local anesthetic would provide a hemostatic effect. Hyaluronidase would not affect the depth of tissue ablation.[1,2,3,4]

References

1. Alexiades Armenakas MR, Dover JS, Arndt KA. The spectrum of laser skin resurfacing: non-ablative, fractional, and ablative laser resurfacing. J Am Acad Dermatol 2008;58:719
2. Fitzpatrick RE, Williams B, Goldman MP. Preoperative anesthesia and postoperative considerations in laser resurfacing. Semin Cutan Med Surg 1996;15:170
3. Saedi N, Hamilton HK, Arndt KA, et al. How to prepare patients for ablative laser procedures. J Am Acad Dermatol 2013;69:e49

4. Tierney EP, Hanke CW, Petersen J. Ablative fractionated CO_2 laser treatment of photoaging: a clinical and histologic study. Dermatol Surg 2012;38:1777

TECHNIQUE

7. *A 45-year-old woman comes to the office because of rhytides caused by photoaging. Treatment using CO_2 laser resurfacing is planned. Laser resurfacing with a carbon dioxide laser should employ which of the following techniques and clinical endpoints?*

E. Nonoverlapping passes until there is a yellow coloration of treated area with skin contracture.

With the carbon dioxide laser, ablation in the treatment area is performed in a nonoverlapping manner. After the first pass, debris is removed, and the treatment area will have a pink color as the papillary dermis is exposed. A second pass is then performed, also in a nonoverlapping manner. With the second pass, the treated area will transition to a yellow color, and the dermis will contract. In CO_2 laser resurfacing, the safety endpoint is the appearance of a "**chamois**" yellow skin color, which is seen at the reticular dermis. Most treatment areas will only need two or three passes to achieve optimal results. Clinical endpoints for the carbon dioxide laser include a yellow-brown discoloration, no further skin contraction, and disappearance of the photodamaged area or rhytid. Of note, additional laser treatment may be applied to deep rhytides to soften transition zones. Excessive laser exposure should be avoided as browncolorationindicates thermal necrosis and charring of the skin.[1,2]

REFERENCES

1. Alexiades Armenakas MR, Dover JS, Arndt KA. The spectrum of laser skin resurfacing: non-ablative, fractional, and ablative laser resurfacing. J Am Acad Dermatol 2008;58:719
2. Batra RS, Ort RJ, Jacob C, et al. Evaluation of a silicone occlusive dressing after laser skin resurfacing. Arch Dermatol 2001;137:1317

TECHNIQUE

8. *A 67-year-old woman with Fitzpatrick type I skin comes to the office with concerns over deep rhytides and signs of photoaging. She would like to avoid surgery and has had limited results with prior chemical peels. She is interested in laser therapy and wants recovery to have as little downtime as possible, but with maximal results. She elects for erbium:yttrium aluminum garnet (ER:YAG) laser resurfacing. Resurfacing with an ER:YAG laser should employ which of the following techniques and clinical endpoints?*

B. Overlapping passes until there is eradication of the rhytid and penetration into the mid-reticular dermis as demonstrated by large dermal bleeding spots.

With the erbium:yttrium aluminum garnet (ER:YAG) laser, ablation in the treatment area is performed in an overlapping manner. The amount of overlap depends on the energy distribution profile for each laser. As much as 50% overlap should be used on the most popular erbium laser system. Initially, fine fibrillar bleeding is noted from the papillary dermis. Larger bleeding spots that are less dense imply bleeding from the reticular dermis. Here, endpoints include eradication of the rhytid or penetration to the mid-reticular dermis. A common misconception is that erbium is a more superficial laser. This is unequivocally false. The erbium laser can penetrate deeply if an adequately powered system is used, in addition to providing a faster recovery period which would be ideal for the patient in the above clinical vignette.[1]

REFERENCE

1. Alexiades Armenakas MR, Dover JS, Arndt KA. The spectrum of laser skin resurfacing: non-ablative, fractional, and ablative laser resurfacing. J Am Acad Dermatol 2008;58:719

POSTOPERATIVE CARE

9. *A 45-year-old female with a history of well-controlled diabetes and a Fitzpatrick type III skin type who underwent ER:YAG laser resurfacing 4 days ago presents to your clinic with worsening blanching erythema over the past 24 hours that is warm to touch and has a grape-like odor over the treated area. She was advised to perform bio-occlusive dressing changes daily and ice water soaks. You suspect a pseudomonas infection and cultures are taken and empiric treatment is started. What do you suspect the primary cause of such an infection to be?*

B. Prolonged use of bio-occlusive dressings for >72 hours.

Bio-occlusive dressings have been found to improve patient comfort but require frequent changes. Also, prolonged use (>72 hours) of bio-occlusive dressings is associated with an increased incidence of pseudomonas infection. Fitzpatrick skin type or ER:YAG laser use vs. any other laser use is not associated with an increased risk of infection. This patient has a history of well-controlled diabetes, which also would not be a major contributor in this scenario. Ice water soaks are for minimizing edema and helping with exudate removal. They have not been shown to be a major contributor of infection if not performed.[1,2,3,4]

References

1. Batra RS, Ort RJ, Jacob, C, et al. Evaluation of a silicone occlusive dressing after laser skin resurfacing. Arch Dermatol 2001;137:1317
2. Batra RS. Ablative laser resurfacing—postoperative care. Skin Therapy Lett 2004;9:6
3. Manuskiatti W, Fitzpatrick RE, Goldman MP, et al. Prophylactic antibiotics in patients undergoing laser resurfacing of the skin. J Am Acad Dermatol 1999;40:77
4. Goldman MP, Roberts TL III, Skover G, et al. Optimizing wound healing in the face after laser abrasion. J Am Acad Dermatol 2002;46:399

POSTOPERATIVE CARE

10. *In open wound care protocols, which of the following topical agents should be used during the reepithelialization healing phase?*

D. Non-antibiotic petroleum-based ointment.

In addition to soaks, open wound care protocols require application of petroleum-based healing ointments after each soak. Antibiotic ointments—mupirocin, bacitracin, and bacitracin/polymyxin B—should be avoided to prevent dermatitis. Care should be taken to apply the petroleum-based ointment uniformly over the entire treated area to avoid areas from drying out.[1,2,3]

References

1. Batra RS. Ablative laser resurfacing—postoperative care. Skin Therapy Lett 2004;9:6
2. Manuskiatti W, Fitzpatrick RE, Goldman MP, et al. Prophylactic antibiotics in patients undergoing laser resurfacing of the skin. J Am Acad Dermatol 1999;40:77
3. Goldman MP, Roberts TL III, Skover G, et al. Optimizing wound healing in the face after laser abrasion. J Am Acad Dermatol 2002;46:399

COMPLICATIONS

11. *Which of the following prophylactic measures should be universally continued pre and post ablative resurfacing?*

E. Antivirals alone.

Herpes simplex, candida, and Gram positive/negative bacterial infections can occur with ablative resurfacing. All patients should be treated with antivirals for herpes simplex preoperatively and postoperatively. Conversely, antifungals and antibiotics are reserved for active infections.[1,2]

References

1. Fitzpatrick RE, Williams B, Goldman MP. Preoperative anesthesia and postoperative considerations in laser resurfacing. Semin Cutan Med Surg 1996;15:170
2. Nanni CA, Alster TS. Complications of cutaneous laser surgery. A review. Dermatol Surg 1998;24:209

COMPLICATIONS

12. *Hyperpigmentation is most associated with which of the following?*

D. Increased Fitzpatrick score.

The risk of hyperpigmentation increases with increasing Fitzpatrick score. Treatments include hydroquinone, a retinoid, and sunlight avoidance. Additionally, often times hydroquinone 4% and tretinoin 0.05% are recommended 4 to 6 weeks pretreatment to stimulate faster healing and prevent post-treatment hyperpigmention.[1,2]

References

1. Fabi S, Massaki N, Goldman MP. Efficacy and tolerability of two commercial hyperpigmentation kits in the treatment of facial hyperpigmentation and photo-aging. J Drugs Dermatol 2012;11:964

2. Sriprachya-Anunt S, Marchell NL, Fitzpatrick RE, et al. Facial resurfacing in patients with Fitzpatrick skin type IV. Lasers Surg Med 2002;30:86

COMPLICATIONS

13. *A 54-year-old female patient with a Fitzpatrick skin type III is noted to have immediate hypopigmentation after ablative laser resurfacing in the preauricular area directly adjacent to an area of untreated skin. How will you counsel this patient?*

B. It is a normal finding related to the transition between treated and untreated areas.

Hypopigmentation after ablative resurfacing occurs in 16 to 57% of cases and can be immediate or delayed. Immediate hypopigmentation is likely caused by the transition between treated areas and untreated/photodamaged areas. Delayed hypopigmentation appears 6 to 12 months after resurfacing and can be addressed with UV light, glycolic acid peels, and fractional laser treatments. Hypopigmentation occurs far less often with ER:YAG laser resurfacing when compared with CO_2 laser treatments. Steroid injection is incorrect as this may worsen hypopigmentation. Although her Fitzpatrick skin type III can increase her risk of hyperpigmentation and hypopigmentation, post-inflammatory hyperpigmentation is more likely to occur.[1,2,3]

REFERENCES

1. Alexiades Armenakas MR, Dover JS, Arndt KA. The spectrum of laser skin resurfacing: non-ablative, fractional, and ablative laser resurfacing. J Am Acad Dermatol 2008;58:719
2. Bolognia JL, Jorizzo JL, Schaffer JV, eds. Dermatology. 3rd ed. Philadelphia: Elsevier; 2012
3. Dijkema SJ, van der Lei B. Long-term results of upper lips treated for rhytides with carbon dioxide laser. Plast Reconstr Surg 2005;115:1731

18. Nonablative Laser Resurfacing

Ira L. Savetsky
See *Essentials of Aesthetic Surgery*, pp. 223–230

EQUIPMENT

1. ***Which of the following nonablative lasers is most useful for resurfacing atrophic acne scars?***
   A. ND:YAG 1320 nm.
   B. Q-switched ND:YAG 1064 nm.
   C. Pulsed dye 585–595 nm.
   D. Intense pulsed light.
   E. Radiofrequency.

EQUIPMENT

2. ***Which of the following nonablative lasers is most useful for treating tattoos?***
   A. Erbium-doped 1550 nm.
   B. Pulsed dye 585–595 nm.
   C. Q-switched ND:YAG 1064 nm.
   D. ND:YAG 1320 nm.
   E. Diode 1450 nm.

EQUIPMENT

3. ***A 47-year-old female with Fitzpatrick type II skin is interested in laser resurfacing for her facial rhytids. Which of the following nonablative lasers is most useful for treating her rhytids?***
   A. Erbium-doped 1550 nm.
   B. Pulsed dye 585–595 nm.
   C. Q-switched ND:YAG 1064 nm.
   D. Diode 1450 nm.
   E. ND:YAG 1320 nm.

EQUIPMENT

4. ***What is the main mechanism of action of radiofrequency?***
   A. Target chromophore is water.
   B. Target chromophore is melanin.
   C. Target chromophore is oxyhemoglobin.
   D. Lipolysis.
   E. Collagen denaturation via heat.

ANESTHESIA

5. ***To achieve the maximal effect of topical anesthetic agents such as EMLA (2.5% prilocaine/2.5% lidocaine) or LMX (4% or 5% lidocaine), how long prior to treatment should these agents be applied?***
   A. No minimal time required.
   B. 5 minutes.
   C. 15 minutes.
   D. 30 minutes.
   E. 60 minutes.

SAFETY

6. ***Which of the following steps are taken to ensure the upmost safety when operating a laser?***
   A. All persons in the room must wear wavelength-specific safety goggles.
   B. The laser does not need to be test fired prior to use.
   C. A standard ET tube can be used if treating around the mouth, and the lowest possible FiO_2 should be given.

D. A dry blue or black towel should be placed around the treatment area to absorb heat energy.
E. Masks and special ventilation systems are not required.

TECHNIQUE

7. *What is the clinical end point when using a nonablative laser for tattoo removal?*
A. Skin whitening.
B. Skin darkening.
C. Mild purpura.
D. Severe purpura.
E. Pinpoint bleeding.

TECHNIQUE

8. *What is the recommended overlap between treatment zones when using a pulsed dye laser?*
A. 5–10%.
B. 10–20%.
C. 30–40%.
D. 40–50%.
E. 50–60%.

APPLICATIONS

9. *Which of the following nonablative lasers is most useful for treating scar pliability and texture?*
A. Fractional laser.
B. Q-switched ND:YAG 1064 nm.
C. Pulsed dye laser.
D. Intense pulsed light.
E. Radiofrequency.

APPLICATIONS

10. *A 33-year-old male actor post mole removal from his left cheek 4 weeks ago has some erythema and irritation in his immature scar and is interested in laser treatment. Which of the following nonablative lasers is most useful for treating erythema and irritation of his immature scar?*
A. Fractional laser.
B. Q-switched ND:YAG 1064 nm.
C. Pulsed dye laser.
D. Intense pulsed light.
E. Radiofrequency.

APPLICATIONS

11. *Of the modalities listed, which of the following is most useful for treating scar rosacea?*
A. Fractional laser.
B. Q-switched ND:YAG 1064 nm.
C. Pulsed dye laser.
D. Intense pulsed light.
E. Radiofrequency.

APPLICATIONS

12. *Which of the following nonablative lasers is most useful for removing green pigment in tattoos?*
A. Q-switched ND:YAG 1064 nm.
B. Q-switched ruby 694 nm.
C. Q-switched alexandrite.
D. Intense pulsed light.
E. Radiofrequency.

APPLICATIONS

13. *What is the mechanism of action of using a laser for hair removal?*
A. Target chromophore is water.
B. Target chromophore is melanin.
C. Target chromophore is oxyhemoglobin.
D. Collagen denaturation via heat.
E. Laser must reach the stratum corneum.

APPLICATIONS

14. *Laser hair reduction is most effective in which individuals?*
A. Light hair and fair skin.
B. Dark hair and fair skin.
C. Light hair and dark skin.
D. Dark hair and dark skin.
E. No significant difference among any skin type.

COMPLICATIONS

15. *Which of the following is the most likely complication after nonablative laser therapy?*
A. Hyperpigmentation.
B. Hypopigmentation.
C. Blistering.
D. Scarring.
E. Unsatisfactory result.

COMPLICATIONS

16. *Which of the following is the most likely complication after monopolar radiofrequency therapy?*
A. Hyperpigmentation.
B. Hypopigmentation.
C. Subdermal fat atrophy.
D. Blistering.
E. Scarring.

SIDE EFFECTS

17. *Which of the following is the most likely side effect after nonablative laser therapy?*
A. Erythema.
B. Swelling.
C. Hyperpigmentation.
D. Purpura.
E. Herpes simplex virus outbreak.

SIDE EFFECTS

18. *A patient with Fitzpatrick skin type V is how many times more likely to have hyperpigmentation compared to a patient with Fitzpatrick skin type I after nonablative laser therapy?*
A. 5×.
B. 10×.
C. 20×.
D. 50×.
E. 100×.

Answers

EQUIPMENT

1. *Which of the following nonablative lasers is most useful for resurfacing atrophic acne scars?*

A. ND:YAG 1320 nm.

Of the choices listed, the ND:YAG 1320 nm laser is the most effective in resurfacing atrophic acne scars. The Q-switched ND:YAG 1064 nm laser is very effective in treating tattoos. The pulsed dye 585–595 nm laser is most effective at treating port-wine stains. Intense pulsed light is not a laser but is very effective in treating hypervascularity and dyspigmentation. Radiofrequency is not a laser and is used to improve skin laxity.[1,2,3,4]

REFERENCES

1. Bellew SG, Lee C, Weiss MA, et al. Improvement of atrophic acne scars with a 1,320 nm Nd:YAG laser: retrospective study. Dermatol Surg 2005;31:1218
2. Rogachefsky AS, Hussain M, Goldberg DJ. Atrophic and a mixed pattern of acne scars improved with a 1320-nm Nd:YAG laser. Dermatol Surg 2003;29:904
3. Sadick NS, Schecter AK. A preliminary study of utilization of the 1320-nm Nd:YAG laser for the treatment of acne scarring. Dermatol Surg 2004;30:995
4. Goldberg DJ, Cutler KB. Nonablative treatment of rhytids with intense pulsed light. Lasers Surg Med 2000;26:196

EQUIPMENT

2. *Which of the following nonablative lasers is most useful for treating tattoos?*

C. Q-switched ND:YAG 1064 nm.

Compared with a continuous or shuttered mode of energy delivery by a laser, the energy is not blocked but stored and then released in a super pulse, which greatly exceeds the energy in the on phase of the continuous or shuttered modes. In turn, this allows for a short burst but with a very high energy, known as Q-switching. Of the choices listed, the Q-switched ND:YAG 1064 nm laser is very effective in treating tattoos. The erbium-doped 1550 nm has multiple applications such as dyschromia, fine rhytids, acne scars, and burn scars. The pulsed dye 585–595 nm laser is most effective at treating port-wine stains. The ND: YAG 1320 nm and diode 1450 nm laser are both effective in resurfacing atrophic acne scars.[1,2,3,4,5,6,7,8]

REFERENCES

1. Bellew SG, Lee C, Weiss MA, et al. Improvement of atrophic acne scars with a 1,320 nm Nd:YAG laser: retrospective study. Dermatol Surg 2005;31:1218
2. Rogachefsky AS, Hussain M, Goldberg DJ. Atrophic and a mixed pattern of acne scars improved with a 1320-nm Nd:YAG laser. Dermatol Surg 2003;29:904
3. Zelickson BD, Kilmer SL, Bernstein E, et al. Pulsed dye laser therapy for sun damaged skin. Lasers Surg Med 1999;25:229
4. Sadick NS, Schecter AK. A preliminary study of utilization of the 1320-nm Nd:YAG laser for the treatment of acne scarring. Dermatol Surg 2004;30:995
5. Cohen JL, Ross EV. Combined fractional ablative and nonablative laser resurfacing treatment: a split-face comparative study. J Drugs Dermatol 2013;12:175
6. Collawn SS. Fraxel skin resurfacing. Ann Plast Surg 2007;58:237
7. Ong MW, Bashir SJ. Fractional laser resurfacing for acne scars: a review. Br J Dermatol 2012;166:1160
8. Glaich AS, Rahman Z, Goldberg LH, et al. Fractional resurfacing for the treatment of hypopigmented scars: a pilot study. Dermatol Surg 2007;33:289

EQUIPMENT

3. *A 47-year-old female with Fitzpatrick type II skin is interested in laser resurfacing for her facial rhytids. Which of the following nonablative lasers is most useful for treating her rhytids?*

A. Erbium-doped 1550 nm.

Of the choices listed, the erbium-doped 1550 nm is most effective in treating fine rhytids. The pulsed dye 585–595 nm laser is most effective at treating port-wine stains. The Q-switched ND:YAG 1064 nm laser is very effective in treating tattoos. The ND:YAG 1320 nm and diode 1450 nm laser are both effective in resurfacing atrophic acne scars.[1,2,3,4,5,6,7,8]

References

1. Bellew SG, Lee C, Weiss MA, et al. Improvement of atrophic acne scars with a 1,320 nm Nd:YAG laser: retrospective study. Dermatol Surg 2005;31:1218
2. Rogachefsky AS, Hussain M, Goldberg DJ. Atrophic and a mixed pattern of acne scars improved with a 1320-nm Nd:YAG laser. Dermatol Surg 2003;29:904
3. Zelickson BD, Kilmer SL, Bernstein E, et al. Pulsed dye laser therapy for sun damaged skin. Lasers Surg Med 1999;25:229
4. Sadick NS, Schecter AK. A preliminary study of utilization of the 1320-nm Nd:YAG laser for the treatment of acne scarring. Dermatol Surg 2004;30:995
5. Cohen JL, Ross EV. Combined fractional ablative and nonablative laser resurfacing treatment: a split-face comparative study. J Drugs Dermatol 2013;12:175
6. Collawn SS. Fraxel skin resurfacing. Ann Plast Surg 2007;58:237
7. Ong MW, Bashir SJ. Fractional laser resurfacing for acne scars: a review. Br J Dermatol 2012;166:1160
8. Glaich AS, Rahman Z, Goldberg LH, et al. Fractional resurfacing for the treatment of hypopigmented scars: a pilot study. Dermatol Surg 2007;33:289

EQUIPMENT

4. *What is the main mechanism of action of radiofrequency?*

E. Collagen denaturation via heat.

Radiofrequency waves cause collagen denaturation when heated to 55 to 62° C, and the amount of collagen in the skin increases over time. The amount of tissue heating and the placement of that heating zone can be controlled by modifying the fluence of the radiofrequency waves and the intensity of the cryogenic cooling spray. Although multiple reports have described fat atrophy from heat damage to adipose tissue early in the treatment's evolution, current treatment protocols greatly minimize or eliminate this risk. Radiofrequency is not a laser and does not target any specific chromophores.[1]

Reference

1. Low DW. Lasers in plastic surgery. In: Thorne CH, Bartlett SP, Beasley RW, et al, eds. Grabb and Smith's Plastic Surgery. 6th ed. Philadelphia: Lippincott Williams & Wilkins; 2007

ANESTHESIA

5. *To achieve the maximal effect of topical anesthetic agents such as EMLA (2.5% prilocaine/2.5% lidocaine) or LMX (4% or 5% lidocaine), how long prior to treatment should these agents be applied?*

E. 60 minutes.

Topical anesthesia, typically with EMLA (2.5% prilocaine/2.5% lidocaine) or LMX (4% or 5% lidocaine) must be applied at least 1 hour before treatment, covered with an occlusive dressing, and wiped off just before treatment.[1]

Reference

1. Low DW. Lasers in plastic surgery. In: Thorne CH, Bartlett SP, Beasley RW, et al, eds. Grabb and Smith's Plastic Surgery. 6th ed. Philadelphia: Lippincott Williams & Wilkins; 2007

SAFETY

6. *Which of the following steps are taken to ensure the upmost safety when operating a laser?*

A. All persons in the room must wear wavelength-specific safety goggles.

Medical lasers are all class IV devices. They are hazardous to view directly, under reflection or under scatter. Therefore, all persons in the room must wear wavelength-specific safety goggles. A warning sign must be placed on each entrance, with extra goggles hanging outside the door. Corneal eye shields are placed, with ophthalmic ointment lubrication. The laser must be test fired prior to use. If the patient is under general anesthesia, a laser-safe ET tube must be used if treating around the mouth, and the lowest possible FiO_2 should be given. Wet towels should be applied around the treatment area to absorb heat energy; the color of the towel is irrelevant. If treating viral warts, live viral particles can be transmitted into personnel's airway. Therefore, appropriate masks and ventilation systems must be in place.[1] Additionally, a smoke evacuator is often times used to remove the laser plume.

REFERENCE

1. Low DW. Lasers in plastic surgery. In: Thorne CH, Bartlett SP, Beasley RW, et al, eds. Grabb and Smith's Plastic Surgery. 6th ed. Philadelphia: Lippincott Williams & Wilkins; 2007

TECHNIQUE

7. *What is the clinical end point when using a nonablative laser for tattoo removal?*

A. Skin whitening.

Skin whitening is the clinical end point in tattoo removal. When treating hypervascularity, mild pupura is the clinical end point. Pinpoint bleeding is often the clinical end point in skin resurfacing techniques for rhytids when using ablative lasers.[1]

REFERENCE

1. Low DW. Lasers in plastic surgery. In: Thorne CH, Bartlett SP, Beasley RW, et al, eds. Grabb and Smith's Plastic Surgery. 6th ed. Philadelphia: Lippincott Williams & Wilkins; 2007

TECHNIQUE

8. *What is the recommended overlap between treatment zones when using a pulsed dye laser?*

B. 10–20%.

Most authors recommend a 10 to 20% overlap between treatment zones because of the Gaussian distribution of intensity within each treatment zone if using a pulse dyed laser.[1]

REFERENCE

1. Low DW. Lasers in plastic surgery. In: Thorne CH, Bartlett SP, Beasley RW, et al, eds. Grabb and Smith's Plastic Surgery. 6th ed. Philadelphia: Lippincott Williams & Wilkins; 2007

APPLICATIONS

9. *Which of the following nonablative lasers is most useful for treating scar pliability and texture?*

A. Fractional laser.

Of the choices listed, the fractional laser is the most effective for scar pliability and texture. The pulsed dye laser is very effective in treating erythema and irritation of immature scar. Intense pulsed light is not a laser but is very effective in treating scar dyschromia. Radiofrequency is not a laser and is used to improve skin laxity. The Q-switched ND:YAG 1064 nm laser is very effective in treating tattoos.[1,2,3,4,5,6]

REFERENCES

1. Haedersdal M, Moreau KE, Beyer DM, et al. Fractional nonablative 1540 nm laser resurfacing for thermal burn scars: a randomized controlled trial. Lasers Surg Med 2009;41:189
2. Parrett BM, Donelan MB. Pulsed dye laser in burn scars: current concepts and future directions. Burns 2010;36:443
3. Allison KP, Kiernan MN, Water RA, et al. Pulsed dye laser treatment of burn scars. Alleviation or irritation? Burns 2003;29:207
4. Donelan MB, Parrett BM, Sheridan RL. Pulsed dye laser therapy and z-plasty for facial burn scars: the alternative to excision. Ann Plast Surg 2008;60:480
5. Hultman CS, Edkins RE, Wu C, et al. Prospective, before-after cohort study to assess the efficacy of laser therapy on hypertrophic burn scars. Ann Plast Surg 2013;70:521
6. Erol OO, Gurlek A, Agaoglu G, et al. Treatment of hypertrophic scars and keloids using intense pulsed light (IPL). Aesth Plast Surg 2008;32:902

APPLICATIONS

10. *A 33-year-old male actor post mole removal from his left cheek 4 weeks ago has some erythema and irritation in his immature scar and is interested in laser treatment. Which of the following nonablative lasers is most useful for treating erythema and irritation of his immature scar?*

C. Pulsed dye laser.

Of the choices listed, the pulsed dye laser is very effective in treating erythema and irritation of immature scar. The fractional laser is the most effective for scar pliability and texture. Intense pulsed light is not a laser but is very effective in treating scar dyschromia. Radiofrequency is not a laser and is used to improve skin laxity. The Q-switched ND:YAG 1064 nm laser is very effective in treating tattoos.[1,2,3,4,5,6]

REFERENCES

1. Haedersdal M, Moreau KE, Beyer DM, et al. Fractional nonablative 1540 nm laser resurfacing for thermal burn scars: a randomized controlled trial. Lasers Surg Med 2009;41:189
2. Parrett BM, Donelan MB. Pulsed dye laser in burn scars: current concepts and future directions. Burns 2010;36:443
3. Allison KP, Kiernan MN, Water RA, et al. Pulsed dye laser treatment of burn scars. Alleviation or irritation? Burns 2003;29:207
4. Donelan MB, Parrett BM, Sheridan RL. Pulsed dye laser therapy and z-plasty for facial burn scars: the alternative to excision. Ann Plast Surg 2008;60:480
5. Hultman CS, Edkins RE, Wu C, et al. Prospective, before-after cohort study to assess the efficacy of laser therapy on hypertrophic burn scars. Ann Plast Surg 2013;70:521
6. Erol OO, Gurlek A, Agaoglu G, et al. Treatment of hypertrophic scars and keloids using intense pulsed light (IPL). Aesth Plast Surg 2008;32:902

APPLICATIONS

11. *Of the modalities listed, which of the following is most useful for treating scar rosacea?*

D. Intense pulsed light.

Of the choices listed, intense pulsed light is very effective in treating hypervascularity such as rosacea or telangiectasias. The pulsed dye laser is very effective in treating erythema and irritation of immature scar, or scar dyschromia. The fractional laser is the most effective for scar pliability and texture. Radiofrequency is not a laser and is used to improve skin laxity. The Q-switched ND:YAG 1064 nm laser is very effective in treating tattoos.[1,2,3,4,5,6]

REFERENCES

1. Haedersdal M, Moreau KE, Beyer DM, et al. Fractional nonablative 1540 nm laser resurfacing for thermal burn scars: a randomized controlled trial. Lasers Surg Med 2009;41:189
2. Parrett BM, Donelan MB. Pulsed dye laser in burn scars: current concepts and future directions. Burns 2010;36:443
3. Allison KP, Kiernan MN, Water RA, et al. Pulsed dye laser treatment of burn scars. Alleviation or irritation? Burns 2003;29:207
4. Donelan MB, Parrett BM, Sheridan RL. Pulsed dye laser therapy and z-plasty for facial burn scars: the alternative to excision. Ann Plast Surg 2008;60:480
5. Hultman CS, Edkins RE, Wu C, et al. Prospective, before-after cohort study to assess the efficacy of laser therapy on hypertrophic burn scars. Ann Plast Surg 2013;70:521
6. Erol OO, Gurlek A, Agaoglu G, et al. Treatment of hypertrophic scars and keloids using intense pulsed light (IPL). Aesth Plast Surg 2008;32:902

APPLICATIONS

12. *Which of the following nonablative lasers is most useful for removing green pigment in tattoos?*

C. Q-switched alexandrite.

Q-switching is necessary in order to produce the high energy pulse to break up large particles into smaller particles that can then be phagocytized by macrophages by a photoacoustic effect from the laser. Of the choices listed, Q-switched alexandrite is very effective in removing green pigment in tattoos. The Q-switched ND:YAG 1064 nm and the Q-switched ruby 694 nm are very effective in removing black-blue pigment in tattoos. Radiofrequency is not a laser and is used to improve skin laxity. Intense pulsed light is not a laser but is very effective in treating scar dyschromia.[1]

REFERENCE

1. Alster TS. Q-switched alexandrite laser treatment (755nm) of professional and amateur tattoos. J Am Acad Dermatol 1995;33:69

APPLICATIONS

13. *What is the mechanism of action of using a laser for hair removal?*

B. Target chromophore is melanin.

Lasers that target melanin are effective in hair reduction. The laser needs to reach the dermal papilla to destroy the follicle which is below the stratum basale. Radiofrequency is not a laser and does not target any specific chromophores. It causes collagen denaturation when heated to 55 to 62°C, and the amount of collagen in the skin increases over time.[1]

REFERENCE

1. Lanigan SW. Incidence of side effects after laser hair removal. J Am Acad Dermatol 2003;49:882

APPLICATIONS

14. *Laser hair reduction is most effective in which individuals?*

B. Dark hair and fair skin.

Lasers used for hair removal target the chromophore melanin. Therefore, the lower the concentration of melanin in the skin and the more melanin in the hair will allow the laser to be more effective at targeting the hair follicles.[1]

REFERENCE

1. Lanigan SW. Incidence of side effects after laser hair removal. J Am Acad Dermatol 2003;49:882

COMPLICATIONS

15. *Which of the following is the most likely complication after nonablative laser therapy?*

E. Unsatisfactory result.

Several treatments are often needed to achieve the desired clinical result. Hypopigmentation occurs in 10 to 20% of cases and is usually transient and self-limiting. Rarely, delayed hypopigmentation can develop 6 to 12 months after treatment. Blistering is usually mild and self-limiting. Scarring is very rare.[1]

REFERENCE

1. Guimarães P, Hadad A, Sabino Neto M, et al. Striae distensae after breast augmentation: treatment using the nonablative fractionated 1550-nm erbium glass laser. Plast Reconst Surg 2013;131:636

COMPLICATIONS

16. *Which of the following is the most likely complication after monopolar radiofrequency therapy?*

C. Subdermal fat atrophy.

The frequency of subdermal fat atrophy is unclear but is associated with the use of monopolar radiofrequency devices. Although multiple reports have described fat atrophy from heat damage to adipose tissue early in the treatment's evolution, current treatment protocols greatly minimize or eliminate this risk. The remaining complications are more commonly associated with nonablative lasers.[1]

Reference

1. Guimarães P, Hadad A, Sabino Neto M, et al. Striae distensae after breast augmentation: treatment using the nonablative fractionated 1550-nm erbium glass laser. Plast Reconst Surg 2013;131:636

SIDE EFFECTS

17. *Which of the following is the most likely side effect after nonablative laser therapy?*

A. Erythema.

Erythema occurs very commonly (60%). Swelling occurs commonly (15–20%). Hyperpigmentation is much less common (0.7%). Purpura is more common when using a pulsed dye laser. Herpes simplex virus outbreak occurs most commonly in patients with a history of herpes simplex virus (2–7%).[1,2]

References

1. Fodor L, Peled IJ, Ullmann Y, et al. Using intense pulsed light for cosmetic purposes: our experience. Plast Reconstr Surg 2004;113:1789
2. Graber EM, Tanzi EL, Alster TS. Side effects and complications of fractional laser photo-thermolysis: experience with 961 treatments. Dermatol Surg 2008;34:301

SIDE EFFECTS

18. *A patient with Fitzpatrick skin type V is how many times more likely to have hyperpigmentation compared to a patient with Fitzpatrick skin type I after nonablative laser therapy?*

E. 100×.

Hyperpigmentation is thought to be caused by melanocyte stimulation by heat energy. Patients with dark skin types are at much higher risk. General incidence is 0.3 to 0.7% in Fitzpatrick skin type I and 33% in Fitzpatrick skin type V.[1,2]

References

1. Fodor L, Peled IJ, Ullmann Y, et al. Using intense pulsed light for cosmetic purposes: our experience. Plast Reconstr Surg 2004;113:1789
2. Graber EM, Tanzi EL, Alster TS. Side effects and complications of fractional laser photo-thermolysis: experience with 961 treatments. Dermatol Surg 2008;34:301

19. Chemical Peels

Juan L. Rendon, Simon Moradian
See *Essentials of Aesthetic Surgery*, pp. 231–258

TREATMENT CONSIDERATIONS

1. *Which of the following is an absolute contraindication for a chemical peel?*

A. Recent facelift.
B. Fitzpatrick skin types IV, V, VI.
C. Isotretinoin therapy within the last 6 months.
D. Pigmentary dyschromias.
E. Actinic keratoses.

TREATMENT CONSIDERATIONS

2. *Antiviral prophylaxis before a chemical peel is recommended in which patient population?*

A. All patients.
B. Patients with a history of herpes simplex.
C. Patients with active herpes simplex infection.
D. Antiviral prophylaxis is not recommended prior to chemical peel.
E. Immunosuppressed patients.

TREATMENT CONSIDERATIONS

3. *Which of the following findings would indicate an abnormal result when evaluating a patient under a Wood's lamp?*

A. Under a Wood's lamp, epidermal hyperpigmentation would not be seen or is less pronounced.
B. Under a Wood's lamp, deep dermal hyperpigmentation would be bright and accentuated.
C. The deeper the pigmentation, the worse the patient would look.
D. Under a Wood's lamp, the worse the patient looks the more superficial the pigmentation.
E. The skin will not shine or fluoresce under UV light.

TREATMENT CONSIDERATIONS

4. *Superficial and medium depth chemical peels provide excellent results for which of the following patients?*

A. Fitzpatrick II skin type with seborrheic keratoses.
B. Fitzpatrick II skin type with epidermal melasma.
C. Fitzpatrick VI skin type with epidermal melasma.
D. Fitzpatrick IV skin type with dermal hyperpigmentation.
E. Fitzpatrick II skin type with dermal melasma.

TREATMENT ENDPOINTS

5. *A 42-year-old male with Fitzpatrick skin type II is interested in treating his sunburn freckles on his chest. Which of the following is pertinent to this patient's desired treatment area when discussing chemical peels in nonfacial areas such as the chest?*

A. Usually take 50 to 100% longer to heal than facial areas.
B. Provide excellent results for dermal hyperpigmentation.
C. Achieve optimal results after a single treatment.
D. Dermal peels are less prone to scarring and abnormal textural changes.
E. Carry a lower risk for systemic reaction than facial chemical peels.

TREATMENT CONSIDERATIONS

6. *You are discussing the indications and limitations of a chemical peels with a 37-year-old Fitzpatrick II female patient. Which of the following is an unrealistic expectation of a chemical peel?*
A. Correction of sun damage.
B. Flattening of mild scarring.
C. Correction of rhytids.
D. Improvement of hyperpigmentation.
E. Decreased pore size.

TREATMENT CONSIDERATIONS

7. *A 55-year-old Fitzpatrick skin type II female patient who is being treated for hyperpigmentation is undergoing a chemical peel with two sequential applications of Jessner's solution. Application first causes a faint erythema followed by a more pronounced erythema on second application. What is the expected depth of penetration of Jessner's solution?*
A. Penetration into the epidermis.
B. Penetration into the papillary dermis.
C. Penetration into the mid-reticular dermis.
D. Penetration to the deep reticular dermis.
E. The depth of penetration is limited regardless of the number of applications.

TREATMENT CONSIDERATIONS

8. *You are applying a full facial trichloroacetic acid peel. An appearance of a solid white frost indicates which peel penetration depth?*
A. Removal of the stratum corneum.
B. Intraepidermal peel.
C. Extension into the papillary dermis only.
D. Full-thickness epidermal peel.
E. Extension into the reticular dermis.

TREATMENT CONSIDERATIONS

9. *A 63-year-old female who is Fitzpatrick skin type II is planning to address her deep facial rhytids using a chemical peel. For which of the following chemical peels is cardiac monitoring required?*
A. Glycolic acid.
B. Croton oil.
C. Trichloroacetic acid.
D. Salicylic acid.
E. Beta-lipohydroxy acid.

TREATMENT CONSIDERATIONS

10. *With both phenol-croton and trichloroacetic acid peels, what is the most critical determinant of the depth of the peel?*
A. Degree and nature of the resultant frost.
B. The concentration of the agent used.
C. The number of applications.
D. The wetness of the applicator.
E. The type of applicator used.

TREATMENT CONSIDERATIONS

11. *A 45-year-old Fitzpatrick skin type IV Hispanic female with melasma would like to discuss her options for chemical peels. Which of the following chemical peel formulations is considered not safe to use for ethnic skin?*
A. Trichloroacetic acid: 10 to 20%.
B. Glycolic acid: 20 to 70%.
C. Phenol-Croton.
D. Salicylic acid: 20 to 30%.
E. Jessner's solution.

TREATMENT CONSIDERATIONS

12. *For medium and deep peels, the use of tretinoin prior to performing chemical peel is associated with which of the following?*

A. Increased risk of dyschromias post chemical peel.
B. Attenuated effect of the peel.
C. Slower epidermal healing post chemical peel.
D. Increased dermal layer cell division and remodeling.
E. Faster epidermal healing and enhanced effect of the chemical peel.

TREATMENT CONSIDERATIONS

13. *A patient with dyschromias would like to undergo a chemical peel. She is already taking a tretinoin. Which of the following bleaching agents should she take in combination with her tretinoin prior to the peel?*

A. 2% hydroquinone.
B. 4% hydroquinone.
C. 2% hydroquinone with 20% glycolic acid gel.
D. 4% hydroquinone with 10% glycolic acid gel.
E. 4% hydroquinone with 2% kojic acid and 6% alpha-hydroxy acid gel base.

TREATMENT CONSIDERATIONS

14. *Prior to a trichloroacetic acid facial chemical peel, a patient is treated with topical EMLA cream. Which of the following adjustments should be made?*

A. A higher strength of trichloroacetic acid than originally planned should be used because vasoconstriction will lead to a more superficial peel.
B. A lower strength of trichloroacetic acid than originally planned should be used because vasoconstriction will lead to a deeper peel.
C. A higher strength of trichloroacetic acid than originally planned should be used because vasodilation will lead to a more superficial peel.
D. A lower strength of trichloroacetic acid than originally planned should be used because vasodilation will lead to a deeper peel.
E. No change to the strength of trichloroacetic acid is necessary with the use of topical anesthetics.

TREATMENT CONSIDERATIONS

15. *Strategies for performing an optimal trichloroacetic acid periorbital peel should include which of the following?*

A. Maintaining the head of the bed at 30 to 45 degrees.
B. Applying product below the superior tarsal plate.
C. Protective ophthalmic antibiotic ointment.
D. Avoiding skin tension along the crow's feet during application.
E. Increasing the strength of the TCA in the second coat.

TREATMENT CONSIDERATIONS

16. *After a trichloroacetic acid chemical peel, a patient presents with a sharply demarcated area of bright erythema. The patient denies picking any scabs. On examination, there is premature peeling of the skin. Which of the following is most likely to have contributed to her presentation?*

A. Reactivation of dormant herpes virus.
B. Copious use of petrolatum-containing ointment to keep treated areas moist.
C. Avoiding gentle exfoliation of the treated area.
D. Minimizing facial expressions.
E. Use ice packs or cold compresses to decrease the swelling.

TREATMENT CONSIDERATIONS

17. *A 57-year-old female with Fitzpatrick skin type II is about to undergo a facelift with simultaneous chemical peel. Which of the following peels should not be used on undermined facelift flaps?*

A. Phenol-croton oil.
B. Glycolic acid.
C. Jessner's solution.

D. Trichloroacetic acid.
E. Beta-lipohydroxy acid.

TREATMENT CONSIDERATIONS

18. ***A patient who underwent a chemical peel 3 days ago presents with sudden-onset inflammation and blistering of a chemically peeled area on the face. The patient has a history of gout who takes colchicine regularly. What is the likely diagnosis?***

A. Normal peeling and healing process.
B. Staphylococcus or streptococcus infection.
C. Reactivation of dormant herpetic infection.
D. Fungal infection.
E. Pseudomonas infection.

Answers

TREATMENT CONSIDERATIONS

1. *Which of the following is an absolute contraindication for a chemical peel?*

C. Isotretinoin therapy within the last 6 months.

Absolute contraindications to a chemical peel include isotretinoin therapy within the last 6 months, complete absence of intact pilosebaceous units on the face, active infection or open wounds, poor physician–patient relationship, lack of psychological stability, unrealistic expectations, and/or poor general health and nutritional status. It should be noted that these contraindications are for medium- and deep-depth peels and do not apply to touchups (**Table 19.1**). Some relative contraindications may include recent facial surgery; however, a full-face phenol peel should be avoided whereas Jessner/TCA peels can be performed safely. Pigmentary dyschromias and actinic keratosis would be indications to perform a chemical peel.[1,2,3,4,5]

Table 19.1 *Contraindications for Chemical Peels*

Absolute	• Poor physician–patient relationship • Lack of psychological stability and mental preparedness • Unrealistic expectations • Poor general health and nutritional status • Isotretinoin therapy within the last 6 months* • Complete absence of intact pilosebaceous units on the face • Active infection or open wounds (such as herpes, excoriations, or open acne cysts)
Relative	• Medium-depth or deep resurfacing procedure within the last 3 to 12 months* • Recent facial surgery involving extensive undermining, such as a facelift* • History of abnormal scar formation or delayed wound healing • History of therapeutic radiation exposure • History of particular skin diseases (such as rosacea, seborrheic dermatitis, atopic dermatitis, psoriasis, and vitiligo) or active retinoid dermatitis • Fitzpatrick skin types IV, V, and VI*

*These contraindications are for medium- and deep-depth peels and do not apply to touchups.

REFERENCES

1. Collins PS. Trichloroacetic acid peels revisited. J Dermatol Surg Oncol 1989;15:933
2. Duffy DM. Informed consent for chemical peels and dermabrasion. Dermatol Clin 1989;7:183
3. Clark CP III. Office-based skin care and superficial peels: the scientific rationale. Plast Reconstr Surg 1999;104:854, discussion 865
4. Fulton JE. Simultaneous face lifting and skin resurfacing. Plast Reconstr Surg 1998;102:2480
5. Ozturk CN, Huettner F, Ozturk C, Bartz-Kurycki MA, Zins JE. Outcomes assessment of combination face lift and perioral phenol-croton oil peel. Plast Reconstr Surg 2013;132:743e

TREATMENT CONSIDERATIONS

2. *Antiviral prophylaxis before a chemical peel is recommended in which patient population?*

A. All patients.

All patients should receive antiviral prophylaxis regardless of history. Active herpes simplex infection is a contraindication to chemical peel. Additionally, reactivation of dormant herpetic infections can lead to disastrous long-term sequelae; early detection and prophylactic treatment are always recommended.[1,2,3]

REFERENCES

1. Clark CP III. Office-based skin care and superficial peels: the scientific rationale. Plast Reconstr Surg 1999;104:854, discussion 865
2. Stuzin JM, Baker TJ, Gordon HL. Chemical peel: a change in the routine. Ann Plast Surg 1989;23:166

3. Rubin MG, ed. Manual of Chemical Peels: Superficial and Medium Depth. Philadelphia: Lippincott Williams & Wilkins; 1995

TREATMENT CONSIDERATIONS

3. *Which of the following findings would indicate an abnormal result when evaluating a patient under a Wood's lamp?*

D. Under a Wood's lamp, the worse the patient looks the more superficial the pigmentation.

Under a Wood's lamp, epidermal hyperpigmentation is bright and accentuated while deep dermal hyperpigmentation is not seen or is less pronounced. Additionally, the skin not shining or fluorescing under UV light would also indicate a normal result. Therefore, the worse the patient looks under a Wood's lamp, the more superficial the pigmentation. In order to properly evaluate a patient, individuals should be in a darkest room, if possible, the lamp held 8 to 12 inches from the patient's face, and the wrist is rotated to change angles.[1,2]

REFERENCES

1. Duffy DM. Informed consent for chemical peels and dermabrasion. Dermatol Clin 1989;7:183
2. Clark CP III. Office-based skin care and superficial peels: the scientific rationale. Plast Reconstr Surg 1999;104:854. discussion 865

TREATMENT CONSIDERATIONS

4. *Superficial and medium depth chemical peels provide excellent results for which of the following patients?*

B. Fitzpatrick II skin type with epidermal melasma.

Fitzpatrick skin types IV, V, and VI are relative contraindications to chemical peels. Superficial and medium depth chemical peels are associated with excellent results in the treatment of ephelides, epidermal hyperpigmentation, and epidermal melasma. They are associated with poor results in the treatment of dermal hyperpigmentation, dermal hyperpigmentation, nevi, and seborrheic keratoses (**Table 19.2**).[1,2]

Table 19.2 *Peel Results for Different Dyschromias*

Superficial Peel	***Excellent Results***	Ephelides
		Epidermal hyperpigmentation
		Epidermal melasma
	Variable Results	Lentigines simplex
		Mixed (epidermal and dermal) melisma
		Mixed postinflammatory hyperpigmentation
		Senile lentigines
	Poor Results	Dermal melisma
		Dermal postinflammatory hyperpigmentation
		Junctional nevi
		Seborrheic keratoses
Medium-Depth Peel	***Excellent Results***	Ephelides
		Epidermal melisma
		Epidermal postinflammatory hyperpigmentation
		Lentigines simplex
		Senile lentigines
	Variable Results	Dermal and mixed melisma
		Dermal and mixed postinflammatory hyperpigmentation
		Seborrheic keratoses
	Poor Results	Nevi
		Some exophytic seborrheic keratoses

REFERENCES

1. Duffy DM. Informed consent for chemical peels and dermabrasion. Dermatol Clin 1989;7:183
2. Clark CP III. Office-based skin care and superficial peels: the scientific rationale. Plast Reconstr Surg 1999;104:854. discussion 865

TREATMENT ENDPOINTS

5. *A 42-year-old male with Fitzpatrick skin type II is interested in treating his sunburn freckles on his chest. Which of the following is pertinent to this patient's desired treatment area when discussing chemical peels in nonfacial areas such as the chest?*

A. Usually take 50 to 100% longer to heal than facial areas.

It usually takes nonfacial areas 50 to 100% longer to heal than the face after a chemical peel. Moreover, it is safer to perform epidermal peels in these areas as dermal peels on the arms, hands, neck, and chest are more prone to scarring or abnormal textural changes. Dermal hyperpigmentation and most types of scars on nonfacial areas will not improve significantly with chemical peels. Nonfacial peels are usually repeated several times to achieve the best response. Most nonfacial peels are performed on large areas of skin (a larger surface area than the face). If a peeling agent with potential toxicity is used, there is a greater risk of developing a systemic reaction.[1]

REFERENCE

1. Duffy DM. Informed consent for chemical peels and dermabrasion. Dermatol Clin 1989;7:183

TREATMENT CONSIDERATIONS

6. *You are discussing the indications and limitations of a chemical peels with a 37-year-old Fitzpatrick II female patient. Which of the following is an unrealistic expectation of a chemical peel?*

E. Decreased pore size.

It is imperative to discuss the indications and limitations of a chemical peel with your patient prior to treatment. Chemical peels can improve sun damage, flatten mild scarring, remove rhytids, and improve hyperpigmentation. They cannot decrease pore size; in fact, chemical peels might increase pore size. They also cannot improve skin laxity, improve deep scarring, remove vascular lesions, or remove hyperpigmentation in dark-skinned whites, Asians, and blacks (**Table 19.3**).[1]

Table 19.3 *Things Chemical Peels Can and Cannot Do*

Things Chemical Peels Can Do	Correct sun damage (actinic degeneration) Flatten mild scarring Remove rhytids Improve irregular hyperpigmentation
Things Chemical Peels Cannot Do	Decrease pore size—chemical peels might increase pore size Improve skin laxity Improve deep scarring Totally remove hyperpigmentation in dark-skinned whites, Asians, and blacks Remove vascular lesions

REFERENCE

1. Duffy DM. Informed consent for chemical peels and dermabrasion. Dermatol Clin 1989;7:183

TREATMENT CONSIDERATIONS

7. *A 55-year-old Fitzpatrick skin type II female patient who is being treated for hyperpigmentation is undergoing a chemical peel with two sequential applications of Jessner's solution. Application first causes a faint erythema followed by a more pronounced erythema on second application. What is the expected depth of penetration of Jessner's solution?*

A. Penetration into the epidermis.

Jessner's solution results in a superficial epidermal peel. It is thought to break the intracellular bridges between keratinocytes and has the capacity to remove the epidermis. Application first causes a faint erythema followed by a more pronounced erythema on second application. After further applications, a frost begins to form. Significant exfoliation is seen for 8 to 10 days when a frost is achieved. It does not require neutralization and the depth is controlled by the number of applications.[1]

Reference

1. Clark CP III. Office-based skin care and superficial peels: the scientific rationale. Plast Reconstr Surg 1999;104:854. discussion 865

TREATMENT CONSIDERATIONS

8. ***You are applying a full facial trichloroacetic acid peel. An appearance of a solid white frost indicates which peel penetration depth?***

E. Extension into the reticular dermis.

Trichloroacetic acid can achieve four levels of superficial and intermediate peels. Level 0 has no frost, and the skin looks slick and shiny, which represents removal of the stratum corneum. Level 1 has an irregular, light frost with some erythema; this is an intraepidermal peel that creates 2 to 4 days of light flaking. Level 2 has a pink-white frost, which suggests a full-thickness epidermal peel, and heals in about 5 days. Level 3 has a solid white frost and is thought to extend into the superficial retinacular dermis.[1,2]

References

1. Dolezal J. Trichloroacetic acid solutions and basic pharmacy. In: Rubin MG, ed. Manual of Chemical Peels: Superficial and Medium Depth. Philadelphia: Lippincott Williams & Wilkins; 1995
2. Johnson JB, Ichinose H, Obagi ZE, et al. Obagi's modified trichloroacetic acid (TCA)-controlled variable-depth peel: a study of clinical signs correlating with histological findings. Ann Plast Surg 1996;36:225

TREATMENT CONSIDERATIONS

9. ***A 63-year-old female who is Fitzpatrick skin type II is planning to address her deep facial rhytids using a chemical peel. For which of the following chemical peels is cardiac monitoring required?***

B. Croton oil.

Croton oil peels are rapidly absorbed through the skin, metabolized in the liver, and excreted renally. Croton oil peels are associated with renal failure, hepatotoxicity, and irritation to the myocardium causing arrhythmias. The dysrhythmias can include supraventricular tachycardia, premature ventricular contractions, atrial fibrillation, and ventricular fibrillation. Therefore, cardiac monitoring and testing of kidney, liver, and cardiac function are required prior to treatment. Of note, phenol peels, which is not listed above, is also associated with cardiac dysrhythmias. As a result, it is recommended that patients who undergo phenol peels should also have electrocardiographic monitoring and intravenous access. Glycolic acid, TCA peels, salicylic acid, and beta-lipohydroxy acid peels are not associated with cardiac arrythmias.[1,2]

References

1. Gatti JE. Eyelid phenol peel: an important adjunct to blepharoplasty. Ann Plast Surg 2008;60:14
2. Pathak A, Mohan R, Rohrich RJ. Chemical peels: role of chemical peels in facial rejuvenation today. Plast Reconstr Surg 2020;145(1):58e–66e

TREATMENT CONSIDERATIONS

10. ***With both phenol-croton and trichloroacetic acid peels, what is the most critical determinant of the depth of the peel?***

A. Degree and nature of the resultant frost.

The most critical to the level of the peel is the degree and nature of the frost obtained. A pink-white frost suggests injury to the papillary dermis, dense white frost suggests superficial reticular dermal injury, and gray-white suggests mid-reticular dermal injury. The concentration of the agent used, number of applications, and wetness of the applicator can all affect the depth of penetration but are not as critical as resultant frost. Although multiple applicators exist such as cotton balls, cotton tipped applicators, 4 × 4 gauze, sable brush, and proctology swabs, the proctology swabs have a risk of delivering too much phenol to the skin; however, that is not relevant to this question stem.[1,2]

References

1. Rubin MG, ed. Manual of Chemical Peels: Superficial and Medium Depth. Philadelphia: Lippincott Williams & Wilkins; 1995
2. Monheit GD. The Jessner's-trichloroacetic acid peel. An enhanced medium-depth chemical peel. Dermatol Clin 1995;13:277

TREATMENT CONSIDERATIONS

11. *A 45-year-old Fitzpatrick skin type IV Hispanic female with melasma would like to discuss her options for chemical peels. Which of the following chemical peel formulations is considered not safe to use for ethnic skin?*

B. Glycolic acid: 20 to 70%.

Ethnic skin may respond unpredictably to chemical peels regardless of phenotype. Latino and Hispanic patients are prone to an increased incidence of *melasma* and *postinflammatory hyperpigmentation,* and chemical peels should be approached with caution in this patient population. Prolonged pretreatment suppression with 4% hydroquinone is critical. Often times, spot treating facial lesions is a way to modify the peel technique to minimize potential postinflammatory hyperpigmentation risks. Safe chemical peel formulations for use in ethnic skin include: beta-lipohydroxy acid: 5 to 10%; TCA: 10 to 20%; glycolic acid: 20 to 70%; salicylic acid: 20 to 30%; lactic acid; Jessner's solution.[1,2]

References

1. Fitzpatrick TB. The validity and practicality of sun-reactive skin types I through VI. Arch Der- matol 1988;124:869
2. Salam A, Dadzie OE, Galadari H. Chemical peeling in ethnic skin: an update. Br J Dermatol 2013;169(Suppl 3):82–90

TREATMENT CONSIDERATIONS

12. *For medium and deep peels, the use of tretinoin prior to performing chemical peel is associated with which of the following?*

E. Faster epidermal healing and enhanced effect of the chemical peel.

All-trans-retinoic acid (tretinoin) will speed epidermal healing only and enhance the effect of the peel. Patients should be instructed to start a vitamin A (retinoic acid 0.1% cream daily for a minimum of 2 weeks before the peel) and glycolic acid skin conditioning program for 6 to 8 weeks before the procedure. Preconditioning the skin causes treated skin to heal faster by 3 to 4 days by increasing its metabolism from accelerated cellular division and new collagen formation. Moreover, patients undergoing a peel to improve hyperpigmentation and patients at risk for developing a postinflammatory hyperpigmentation should use tretinoin in combination with a bleaching agent (such as hydroquinone) before a chemical peel.[1,2,3]

References

1. Hevia O, Nemeth AJ, Taylor JR. Tretinoin accelerates healing after trichloroacetic acid chemical peel. Arch Dermatol 1991;127:678
2. Nemeth AJ, Eaglstein WH, Falanga V, et al. Methods to speed healing after skin biopsy or trichloroacetic acid chemical peel. Prog Clin Biol Res 1991;365:267
3. Mandy SH. Tretinoin in the preoperative and postoperative management of dermabrasion. J Am Acad Dermatol 1986;15:878

TREATMENT CONSIDERATIONS

13. *A patient with dyschromias would like to undergo a chemical peel. She is already taking a tretinoin. Which of the following bleaching agents should she take in combination with her tretinoin prior to the peel?*

B. 4% hydroquinone.

Patients undergoing a peel to improve hyperpigmentation and patients at risk for developing a postinflammatory hyperpigmentation should use tretinoin in combination with a bleaching agent before a chemical peel. The bleaching agent should be 4% hydroquinone, not 2%. In addition to tretinoin, two other products are available, hydroquinone and kojic acid, in the following preparations: 2% hydroquinone with 10% glycolic acid gel, 2% hydroquinone with 2% kojic acid and 6% AHA gel base.[1,2]

REFERENCES

1. Peikert JM, Krywonis NA, Rest EB, et al. The efficacy of various degreasing agents used in trichloroacetic acid peels. J Dermatol Surg Oncol 1994;20:724
2. Stuzin JM, Baker TJ, Gordon HL. Chemical peel: a change in the routine. Ann Plast Surg 1989;23:166

TREATMENT CONSIDERATIONS

14. *Prior to a trichloroacetic acid facial chemical peel, a patient is treated with topical EMLA cream. Which of the following adjustments should be made?*

B. A lower strength of trichloroacetic acid than originally planned should be used because vasoconstriction will lead to a deeper peel.

In general, topical anesthetics, including EMLA, will cause vasoconstriction. Therefore, a lower strength of trichloroacetic acid than originally planned should be used because vasoconstriction will lead to a deeper peel.[1,2]

REFERENCES

1. Collins PS. Trichloroacetic acid peels revisited. J Dermatol Surg Oncol 1989;15:933
2. Duffy DM. Informed consent for chemical peels and dermabrasion. Dermatol Clin 1989;7:183

TREATMENT CONSIDERATIONS

15. *Strategies for performing an optimal trichloroacetic acid periorbital peel should include which of the following?*

A. Maintaining the head of the bed at 30 to 45 degrees.

In treating the periorbital region during a chemical peel, the head is elevated to 30 to 45 degrees to prevent pooling of the product around the eyes; the product is applied from lateral to medial; and the product is not applied below the superior tarsal plate to prevent edema. Ophthalmic ointment petrolatum may promote excessive tearing and blinking and is unnecessary if the cotton-tipped applicator is well wrung out. Antibiotic ophthalmic ointment is not necessary. It is safest to decrease the strength of TCA in the second coat by 5 to 10% to prevent too deep a peel.[1,2]

REFERENCES

1. Johnson JB, Ichinose H, Obagi ZE, et al. Obagi's modified trichloroacetic acid (TCA)-controlled variable-depth peel: a study of clinical signs correlating with histological findings. Ann Plast Surg 1996;36:225
2. Rubin MG, ed. Manual of Chemical Peels: Superficial and Medium Depth. Philadelphia: Lippincott Williams & Wilkins; 1995

TREATMENT CONSIDERATIONS

16. *After a trichloroacetic acid chemical peel, a patient presents with a sharply demarcated area of bright erythema. The patient denies picking any scabs. On examination, there is premature peeling of the skin. Which of the following is most likely to have contributed to her presentation?*

E. Use ice packs or cold compresses to decrease the swelling.

Ice packs or cold compresses should NOT be applied to the face to decrease the swelling. The moisture from these may cause the skin to peel prematurely. The face should be washed gently for 20 to 30 seconds twice a day using a mild, quality liquid soap. Then petrolatum-containing ointment should be applied to keep treated areas moist. Patients should avoid any rubbing or picking of scabs. Minimizing facial expressions has been noted to prevent premature skin to crack.[1,2]

REFERENCES

1. Rubin MG, ed. Manual of Chemical Peels: Superficial and Medium Depth. Philadelphia: Lippincott Williams & Wilkins; 1995
2. Brody HJ. Chemical Peeling and Resurfacing. 2nd ed. St Louis: Mosby–Year Book; 1997

TREATMENT CONSIDERATIONS

17. *A 57-year-old female with Fitzpatrick skin type II is about to undergo a facelift with simultaneous chemical peel. Which of the following peels should not be used on undermined facelift flaps?*

A. Phenol-croton oil.

Originally, it was thought that the skin flap from a facelift cannot be safely resurfaced simultaneously with a chemical peel. Fulton and colleagues showed that a Jessner/TCA peel can be safely used on the skin flap from a facelift. A deep, full-face phenol peel should NOT be done simultaneously over undermined facelift flaps to prevent injury to the subdermal plexus and compromise wound healing. More superficial peels—glycolic acid, Jessner, trichloroacetic acid—can safely be performed at the time of facelift surgery. Patients can expect the skin to begin peeling around day 3 or 4 after the peel. The duration of exfoliation is directly related to the depth of the peeling.[1,2,3,4]

REFERENCES

1. Baker TJ. Chemical face peeling and rhytidectomy. A combined approach for facial rejuvenation. Plast Reconstr Surg Transplant Bull 1962;29:199e
2. Litton C. Chemical face lifting. Plast Reconstr Surg Transplant Bull 1962;29:371
3. Fulton JE. Simultaneous face lifting and skin resurfacing. Plast Reconstr Surg 1998;102:2480
4. Ozturk CN, Huettner F, OzturkC, Bartz-Kurycki MA, Zins JE. Outcomes assessment of combination face lift and perioral phenol-croton oil peel. Plast Reconstr Surg 2013;132:743e

TREATMENT CONSIDERATIONS

18. *A patient who underwent a chemical peel 3 days ago presents with sudden-onset inflammation and blistering of a chemically peeled area on the face. The patient has a history of gout who takes colchicine regularly. What is the likely diagnosis?*

C. Reactivation of dormant herpetic infection.

Reactivation of dormant herpetic infection is a serious early complication of chemical peel treatments and warrants early detection and aggressive treatment. All patients should receive prophylactic antiviral therapy. Notably, bacterial and fungal infections are rare in the absence of prolonged occlusive taping methods.[1,2,3]

REFERENCES

1. Brody HJ. Chemical Peeling and Resurfacing. 2nd ed. St Louis: Mosby–Year Book; 1997
2. Duffy DM. Informed consent for chemical peels and dermabrasion. Dermatol Clin 1989;7:183
3. Clark CP III. Office-based skin care and superficial peels: the scientific rationale. Plast Reconstr Surg 1999;104:854. discussion 865

20. Dermabrasion

Stelios C. Wilson
See *Essentials of Aesthetic Surgery*, pp. 259–268

PREOPERATIVE EVALUATION

1. *Which of the following Fitzpatrick skin types should you proceed with caution when considering dermabrasion?*

A. I.
B. II.
C. III.
D. IV.
E. V.

PREOPERATIVE EVALUATION

2. *When performing a "test spot" for a patient who is considering dermabrasion to the face or neck, what is a reasonable anatomic location?*

A. Preauricular.
B. Postauricular.
C. Cheek.
D. Neck.
E. Abdomen.

PREOPERATIVE EVALUATION

3. *A 30-year-old patient comes to you requesting dermabrasion. Her history is notable for occasional cold sores, most recently 2 years prior. Which of the following should be part of your preprocedural instructions?*

A. Acyclovir 1 g once on the day of the procedure.
B. Acyclovir 2 g twice on the day before the procedure.
C. Acyclovir 1 g starting 1 day before the procedure and lasting 5 to 7 days.
D. Acyclovir 1 g, twice per day, starting 1 day before the procedure and lasting 5 to 7 days.
E. No antiviral medication necessary for this patient.

INDICATIONS AND CONTRAINDICATIONS

4. *Which of the following is a contraindication to dermabrasion?*

A. Acne.
B. Basal cell carcinoma (superficial type).
C. Facial rhytids.
D. Traumatic scars.
E. Isotretinoin therapy within 6 to 12 months.

INFORMED CONSENT

5. *As part of the informed consent, the patient should understand that the most likely complication from dermabrasion is which of the following?*

A. Scarring.
B. Prolonged hyperemia.
C. Dyspigmentation.
D. Failure to improve treated area.
E. Milia.

EQUIPMENT AND PREPARATION

6. ***Which of the following combination of abrading tips offers the greatest margin of safety?***
A. Narrow-barrel fraise with coarse-grade diamonds.
B. Wide-barrel fraise with fine-grade diamonds.
C. Wire brush tip with fine-grade diamonds.
D. Wire brush tip.
E. Serrated wheel tip.

PERFORMANCE DETAILS

7. ***When working with tissues with leading (free) edges, which of the following is the correct combination of movements?***
A. Handpiece toward leading edge, drum rotation toward leading edge.
B. Handpiece away from leading edge, drum rotation toward the leading edge.
C. Handpiece toward leading edge, drum rotation away from leading edge.
D. Handpiece perpendicular to the leading edge, drum rotation toward leading edge.
E. Handpiece away from leading edge, drum rotation toward the leading edge.

PERFORMANCE DETAILS

8. ***What is the endpoint for dermabrasion?***
A. Epidermal exfoliation.
B. Bleeding dermis.
C. Superficial papillary dermis.
D. White frost.
E. Uniformly spaced, punctate bleeding.

POSTOPERATIVE CARE

9. ***A patient who had dermabrasion several weeks ago comes in with persistent redness. There is no concern for infection. What treatment adjunct can you offer to this patient?***
A. Finish full course of oral antibiotics.
B. Finish full course of antivirals.
C. Wear sunblock every day.
D. 2 g ascorbic acid (vitamin C) daily.
E. Topical steroid cream.

MICRODERMABRASION

10. ***What is the endpoint for microdermabrasion?***
A. Erythema.
B. Bleeding dermis.
C. Pseudofrost.
D. White frost.
E. Uniformly spaced, punctate bleeding.

COMPLICATIONS

11. ***When does hypopigmentation occur following dermabrasion?***
A. When treatment was too superficial.
B. When treatment was too deep.
C. When performed in patients with darker skin types.
D. In an unpredictable manner.
E. If a steroid cream is used postoperatively.

COMPLICATIONS

12. ***When does hyperpigmentation most likely occur following dermabrasion?***
A. When treatment was too superficial.
B. When treatment was too deep.
C. When performed in patients with darker skin types.
D. In an unpredictable manner.
E. If the patient takes vitamin C supplementation.

Answers

PREOPERATIVE EVALUATION

1. *Which of the following Fitzpatrick skin types should you proceed with caution when considering dermabrasion?*

D. IV.

Fitzpatrick skin types I through III will have a uniform blended skin color postoperatively. Proceed with caution in type IV, and it is best to not dermabrade types V and VI due to hyperpigmentation postoperatively. A review of Fitzpatrick skin type classification can be found below (**Table 20.1**).[1]

Table 20.1 *Fitzpatrick Skin Type Classification*

Skin Type	Characteristics	Sun Exposure History
I	Pale white, freckles, blue eyes, blond or red hair	Always burns, never tans
II	Fair white, blue/green/hazel eyes, blond or red hair	Usually burns, minimally tans
III	Cream white, any hair or eye color	Sometimes burns, tans uniformly
IV	Moderate brown (Mediterranean)	Rarely burns, always tans well
V	Dark brown (Middle Eastern)	Rarely burns, tans easily
VI	Dark brown to black	Never burns, tans easily

(Source: Data from Fitzpatrick TB. The validity and practicality of sun-reactive skin types I through VI. Arch Dermatol 124:869, 1988.)

REFERENCE

1. Baker JL. Dermabrasion. In: Nahai F, ed. The Art of Aesthetic Surgery: Principles & Techniques. New York: Thieme Publishers; 2005

PREOPERATIVE EVALUATION

2. *When performing a "test spot" for a patient who is considering dermabrasion to the face or neck, what is a reasonable anatomic location?*

B. Postauricular.

The test spot should be located close to the area to be treated but in an obscured area that can easily be camouflaged or hidden if further treatment is not performed. For facial or neck candidates, placing the "test spot" behind the ear can give a reasonable assessment of effect. This is usually a 1-cm spot that is abraded with the patient under local anesthesia. It is important to stress that the test spot is *not* predictive of the overall outcome. This point cannot be overstressed.[1]

REFERENCE

1. Baker JL. Dermabrasion. In: Nahai F, ed. The Art of Aesthetic Surgery: Principles & Techniques. New York: Thieme Publishers; 2005

PREOPERATIVE EVALUATION

3. *A 30-year-old patient comes to you requesting dermabrasion. Her history is notable for occasional cold sores, most recently 2 years prior. Which of the following should be part of your preprocedural instructions?*

D. Acyclovir 1 g, twice per day, starting 1 day before the procedure and lasting 5 to 7 days.

Patients are generally given an antibacterial cleanser to wash and shampoo the night before and the morning of surgery. Prescriptions for cephalexin 500 mg twice per day for 5 to 7 days, acyclovir 1 g once per day (twice per day for patients with history of oral herpes, start the day before the procedure) for 5 to 7 days.

For this patient with a history of cold sores, acyclovir 1 g, twice per day, would be the recommendation. Avoidance of reactivation of oral herpes during the healing process is very important.[1,2,3]

References

1. Baker JL. Dermabrasion. In: Nahai F, ed. The Art of Aesthetic Surgery: Principles & Techniques. New York: Thieme Publishers; 2005
2. Duffy DM. Informed consent for chemical peels and dermabrasion. Dermatol Clin 1989;7:183
3. Hruza GJ. Dermabrasion. Facial Plast Surg Clin North Am 2001;9:267

INDICATIONS AND CONTRAINDICATIONS

4. *Which of the following is a contraindication to dermabrasion?*

E. Isotretinoin therapy within 6 to 12 months.

Dermabrasion has been used for numerous traumatic and medical conditions. Please see **Box 20.1** and **Box 20.2** for indications (partial list) and contraindication (partial list). Of the choices listed, only history of isotretinoin therapy within the last 6 to 12 months would be considered a contraindication to dermabrasion.[1,2]

Box 20.1 *Conditions Treatable with Dermabrasion*

Acne rosacea
Actinically damaged skin
Active acne
Adenoma sebaceum
Angiofibromas of tuberous sclerosis
Basal cell carcinoma (superficial type)
Blast tattoos (gunpowder)
Chloasma
Chronic radiation dermatitis (mild)
Congenital pigmented nevi
Darier's disease
Dermatitis papillaris capillitii
Early operative scars
Facial rhytids
Favre-Racouchot syndrome
Fox-Fordyce disease
Freckles
Hair transplantation (elevated recipient sites)
Hemangiomas
Hypertrophic scars
Keratoacanthomas
Lentigines
Lichen amyloidosis
Lichenified dermatoses
Linear epidermal nevus
Discoid lupus erythematosus
Mibelli porokeratosis
Multiple pigmented nevi
Multiple seborrheic keratoses
Multiple trichoepitheliomas
Neurotic excoriations
Postacne scars
Pseudofolliculitis barbae
Rhinophyma
Scleromyxedema
Smallpox or chickenpox scars
Striae distensae
Syringomas
Syringocystadenoma papilliferum
Tattoos (decorative and traumatic)

Telangiectasias
Traumatic scars
Verrucous nevus
Vitiligo
Xanthelasma
Xeroderma pigmentosum

(Source: Data from Hruza GJ. Dermabrasion. Facial Plast Surg Clin North Am 9:267, 2001.)

Box 20.2 *Contraindications to Dermabrasion*

Absolute	Isotretinoin therapy within the last 6 to 12 months* Congenital ectodermal defects Radiodermatitis (only if severe) Pyoderma Psychosis Active herpes labialis
Relative	History of hypertrophic scars History of keloids Burns—deep thermal or chemical Fitzpatrick skin types IV, V, VI (test patch should be tried first) History of hepatitis or HIV†

*Seven patients with atrophic acne scars on the face taking oral isotretinoin to treat facial acne had manual dermabrasion on an area approximately 1 cm^2. At the 6-month follow-up, all patients had normal cicatrization, and the atrophic acne scar revision was deemed excellent. In another study, 10 patients treated with oral isotretinoin for acne had a medium-depth chemical peel applied to the entire face and manual sandpaper dermabrasion (until the appearance of a blood dew) 1 to 3 months after the isotretinoin therapy was concluded. At the 6-month follow-up, all patients had normal cicatrization, and no hypertrophic scars or keloids were observed. Depressed acne scar revision was satisfactory.

†Personal decision of the surgeon.

(Source: Data from Hruza GJ. Dermabrasion. Facial Plast Surg Clin North Am 9:267, 2001.)

References

1. Bagatin E, dos Santos Guadanhim LR, Yarak S, et al. Dermabrasion for acne scars during treatment with oral isotretinoin. Dermatol Surg 2010;36:483
2. Picosse FR, Yarak S, Cabral NC, et al. Early chemabrasion for acne scars after treatment with oral isotretinoin. Dermatol Surg 2012;38:1521

INFORMED CONSENT

5. *As part of the informed consent, the patient should understand that the most likely complication from dermabrasion is which of the following?*

E. Milia.

The most common complication from dermabrasion is milia, which are small white cysts over the surface of the treated area. One-third of patients will develop them. They typically appear within 2 to 4 weeks after treatment and will clear spontaneously in most patients. These small cysts can be unroofed with a buff puff or a mildly abrasive skin cleaner. Other less common complications include scarring, catastrophic intraoperative disaster (avulsion of soft tissue such as lips and eyelids), dyspigmentation, and failure of the procedure to adequately improve the treated area. Additionally, while the surgeon (and the patient) should always be aware of fire risk and minimizing potential for intraoperative fire, this risk is less than from other devices such as cautery and lasers.[1,2]

References

1. Duffy DM. Informed consent for chemical peels and dermabrasion. Dermatol Clin 1989;7:183
2. Dubina M, Tung R. Management of complications of microdermabrasion and dermabrasion. In: Tosti A, Beer K, De Padova MP, eds. Management of Complications of Cosmetic Procedures: Handling Problems and More Uncommon Problems. Berlin, Heidelberg: Springer; 2012

EQUIPMENT AND PREPARATION

6. *Which of the following combination of abrading tips offers the greatest margin of safety?*

B. Wide-barrel fraise with fine-grade diamonds.

For novice surgeons, a wide-barrel fraise with fine-grade diamonds offers the greatest margin of safety. The wider the barrel, the less easily you can gauge through the skin. The coarser the diamond surface, the faster the cutting speed, the greater the penetration into tissue. Wire brush tips should be used with great care because tissue damage can easily occur. Similarly, the serrated wheel should only be employed by experienced surgeons because of its greater potential to cause tissue damage.[1,2]

REFERENCES

1. Baker JL. Dermabrasion. In: Nahai F, ed. The Art of Aesthetic Surgery: Principles & Techniques. New York: Thieme Publishers; 2005
2. Hruza GJ. Dermabrasion. Facial Plast Surg Clin North Am 2001;9:267

PERFORMANCE DETAILS

7. *When working with tissues with leading (free) edges, which of the following is the correct combination of movements?*

A. Handpiece toward leading edge, drum rotation toward leading edge.

The correct way to move the handpiece of a dermabrader is depicted in **Fig. 20.1.** The tissue should be swept away from the rotating drum. The handpiece should be moved toward the leading edge. This will help prevent the free edge from being dragged up over the drum, which could forcefully avulse tissues with free edges (lips and eyelids).[1,2]

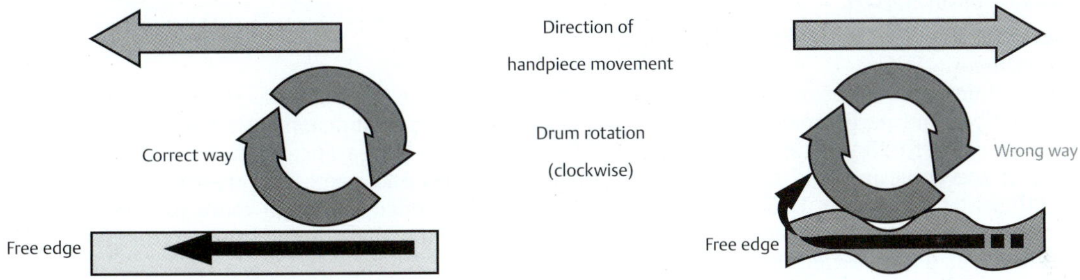

Fig. 20.1 Correct way to move the handpiece of a dermabrader. When the handpiece is moved in the direction of rotation (correct way), the tissue is swept away from the rotating drum. When the handpiece is moved in the direction opposite the drum's rotation, the abrasive tip will clutch the tissue; the rotating drum, in combination with the moving handpiece, will "dig into" the tissue and cause the upcoming tissue to be forcefully and rapidly pulled toward the rotating drum. A free edge would be dragged up and over the drum. This can forcefully avulse tissues with free edges (lips and eyelids). (Source: Performance Details. In: Janis J, ed. Essentials of Aesthetic Surgery. 1st Edition. New York: Thieme; 2018.)

REFERENCES

1. Baker JL. Dermabrasion. In: Nahai F, ed. The Art of Aesthetic Surgery: Principles & Techniques. New York: Thieme Publishers; 2005
2. Hruza GJ. Dermabrasion. Facial Plast Surg Clin North Am 2001;9:267

PERFORMANCE DETAILS

8. *What is the endpoint for dermabrasion?*

E. Uniformly spaced, punctate bleeding.

The abraded surface needs to be wiped frequently with a gauze to observe the bleeding pattern. The endpoint of dermabrasion is uniformly spaced, punctate bleeding. After dermabrasion treatment, the skin is cleaned using a saline solution rinse and a soft bristle brush or rough gauze is used to remove excess skin debris.[1,2]

References

1. Baker JL. Dermabrasion. In: Nahai F, ed. The Art of Aesthetic Surgery: Principles & Techniques. New York: Thieme Publishers; 2005
2. Hruza GJ. Dermabrasion. Facial Plast Surg Clin North Am 2001;9:267

POSTOPERATIVE CARE

9. *A patient who had dermabrasion several weeks ago comes in with persistent redness. There is no concern for infection. What treatment adjunct can you offer to this patient?*

E. Topical steroid cream.

Patients should continue or finish both oral antibiotics and antivirals initially prescribed. The patient in this scenario does not have a bacterial or viral infection. Ascorbic acid (vitamin C) can be recommended for hyperpigmentation, but not persistent redness. Instead, the patient has persistent redness that can be treated with topical steroid cream (Temovate [clobetasol propionate] 0.05%) applied twice per day for 2 weeks. This regimen is repeated until normal skin color returns. Patients should not use this continuously and should not use it on the eyelids. Patients should be wearing sunblock every day—regardless of the season and whether the patient works inside or outside. This must be stressed.[1,2]

References

1. Baker JL. Dermabrasion. In: Nahai F, ed. The Art of Aesthetic Surgery: Principles & Techniques. New York: Thieme Publishers; 2005
2. Hruza GJ. Dermabrasion. Facial Plast Surg Clin North Am 2001;9:267

MICRODERMABRASION

10. *What is the endpoint for microdermabrasion?*

A. Erythema.

With microdermabrasion, longer contact of the abrasive crystals with the skin by slowly moving the handpiece and performing more passes will result in a deeper abrasion. Two passes will exfoliate to a depth of 15 to 25 μm causing epidermal exfoliation in the appearance of erythema. This should only affect the epidermis and is ineffective for deeper wrinkles and scars. Two treatments per session are sufficient for the face. Usually, 5 to 12 treatments are needed, although more may be warranted in heavily scarred/damaged areas. The endpoint for each session is erythema.[1] Pseudofrost only applies to salicylic acid peels when the salicylic acid crystalizes.

Reference

1. Holck DE, Ng JD. Facial skin rejuvenation. Curr Opin Ophthalmol 2003;14:246

COMPLICATIONS

11. *When does hypopigmentation occur following dermabrasion?*

B. When treatment was too deep.

Proper patient selection is the best treatment for hyperpigmentation and hypopigmentation. In general hypopigmentation occurs from dermabrasion that is too deep. Usually this problema corrects with time.[1,2]

References

1. Baker JL. Dermabrasion. In: Nahai F, ed. The Art of Aesthetic Surgery: Principles & Techniques. New York: Thieme Publishers; 2005
2. Hruza GJ. Dermabrasion. Facial Plast Surg Clin North Am 2001;9:267

COMPLICATIONS

12. *When does hyperpigmentation most likely occur following dermabrasion?*

C. When performed in patients with darker skin types.

Hyperpigmentation occurs most commonly in patients with type III or IV skin and in those who have not used sunblock. Hyperpigmentation can sometimes be minimized with 2 g of ascorbic acid (vitamin C) daily. Pigmentation is usually limited to the superficial epidermis and is treatable with topical applications of Retin-A, hydroquinone, and glycolic acids. If pigment persists for several months, a medium-depth peel may be necessary.[1,2]

References

1. Baker JL. Dermabrasion. In: Nahai F, ed. The Art of Aesthetic Surgery: Principles & Techniques. New York: Thieme Publishers; 2005
2. Hruza GJ. Dermabrasion. Facial Plast Surg Clin North Am 2001;9:267

21. Botulinum Toxin

Sammy Sinno, Simon Moradian, Aaron M. Kearney
See *Essentials of Aesthetic Surgery*, pp. 269–279

BOTOX PHYSIOLOGY

1. ***What is the mechanism of action of botulinum toxin?***
   A. Acts at presynaptic nerve terminals to inhibit the release of acetylcholine.
   B. Acts at postsynaptic receptors to prevent binding of acetylcholine.
   C. Prevents production of acetylcholine.
   D. Binds muscarinic receptors.
   E. Stimulation of Rho/Rho kinase pathway.

BOTOX PHYSIOLOGY

2. ***On average, how long is Botox usually effective?***
   A. 1 month.
   B. 3 months.
   C. 6 months.
   D. 9 months.
   E. 1 year.

CLINICAL CONSIDERATIONS

3. ***What muscle forms only vertical glabellar lines?***
   A. Depressor supercilii.
   B. Nasalis.
   C. Procerus.
   D. Corrugator supercilii.
   E. Frontalis.

CLINICAL CONSIDERATIONS

4. ***A 42-year-old male is seeking treatment of his forehead rhytids with Botox. He has a friend who had this done but told him one eyebrow was lower than the other for several months after. He asks what can be done to prevent this from happening to him. What would be the safest way to minimize brow ptosis when injecting for forehead rhytids in this patient?***
   A. Inject in a supraperiosteal plane.
   B. Inject at least 2 cm above the eyebrow.
   C. Do not inject forehead lines.
   D. Inject along the upper border of the eyebrow.
   E. Inject along the superior border of the levator palpebrae superiorus.

CLINICAL CONSIDERATIONS

5. ***Where should perioral rhytids be injected to avoid adverse effects on the lip?***
   A. Deep, at least 5 mm from the vermilion border.
   B. Deep, within 5 mm of the vermilion border.
   C. Superficial, within 5 mm of the vermilion border.
   D. Superficial, 5 mm from the vermilion border.
   E. Superficial, 10 to 15 mm from the vermilion border.

CLINICAL CONSIDERATIONS

6. *What portion of the masseter should be injected to correct masseteric hypertrophy?*
A. The most prominent point of muscle.
B. Along the inferior border of the angle of the mandible only.
C. The superficial layer.
D. The middle layer of muscle.
E. The deep layer of muscle.

CLINICAL CONSIDERATIONS

7. *When is the typical onset of action of botulinum toxin following injection?*
A. 1 hour.
B. 1 day.
C. 3 to 4 days.
D. 14 days.
E. 21 days.

CLINICAL CONSIDERATIONS

8. *What is the most commonly reported adverse effect of botulinum toxin?*
A. Hypersensitivity.
B. Dysphagia.
C. Headache.
D. Ecchymosis.
E. Transient eyelid ptosis.

Answers

BOTOX PHYSIOLOGY

1. *What is the mechanism of action of botulinum toxin?*

A. Acts at presynaptic nerve terminals to inhibit the release of acetylcholine.

The neurotoxin acts at presynaptic nerve terminals to inhibit the release of acetylcholine, producing chemodenervation. The protein consists of a heavy chain and a light chain. The heavy chain irreversibly binds to the nerve terminal, and the toxin is internalized through endocytosis, where it renders the nerve terminal nonfunctional and blocks the release of acetylcholine into the neuromuscular junction. Botox inhibits Rho kinase which inhibits smooth muscle cell constriction directly through interference with the Ca^{2+} sensitivity of vascular smooth muscle cells and the NO system.[1]

REFERENCE

1. Rohrich RJ, Janis JE, Fagien S, et al. The cosmetic use of botulinum toxin. Plast Reconstr Surg 2003;112(5 Suppl): S117

BOTOX PHYSIOLOGY

2. *On average, how long is Botox usually effective?*

B. 3 months.

Botox is usually effective for approximately 3 months with the upper end of extreme being closer to 6 months. This varies depending on the preparation (Botox, Dysport, and Xeomin) as well as the number of units injected into a given area.[1,2]

REFERENCES

1. Rohrich RJ, Janis JE, Fagien S, et al. The cosmetic use of botulinum toxin. Plast Reconstr Surg 2003;112(5 Suppl): S117
2. Kim EJ, Ramirez AL, Reeck JB, et al. The role of botulinum toxin type B (Myobloc) in the treatment of hyperkinetic facial lines. Plast Reconstr Surg 2003;112(5 Suppl):S88

CLINICAL CONSIDERATIONS

3. *What muscle forms only vertical glabellar lines?*

D. Corrugator supercilii.

The corrugator supercilii, procerus, and depressor supercili (medial orbicularis oculi) are the muscles responsible for brow depression and make up the glabellar muscle units. The corrugator supercilii muscles are the only paired muscles that contribute to a dynamic vertical line. The procerus is a flat, pyramidal muscle on the bridge of the nose which contributes to form a transverse rhytid. The depressor supercilii muscle is a portion of the medial orbicularis oculi muscle which contributes to both vertical and transverse glabellar lines and a lower static medial brow position. The nasalis forms bunny lines and is not involved in the glabellar muscle unit.[1,2]

REFERENCES

1. Carruthers JD, Carruthers JA. Treatment of glabellar frown lines with C. botulinum-Aexotoxin. J Dermatol Surg Oncol 1992;18:17
2. Carruthers J, Fagien S, Matarasso SL; Botox Consensus Group. Consensus recommendations on the use of botulinum toxin type a in facial aesthetics. Plast Reconstr Surg 2004;114(Suppl 6):S1

CLINICAL CONSIDERATIONS

4. *A 42-year-old male is seeking treatment of his forehead rhytids with Botox. He has a friend who had this done but told him one eyebrow was lower than the other for several months after. He asks what can be done to prevent this from happening to him. What would be the safest way to minimize brow ptosis when injecting for forehead rhytids in this patient?*

B. Inject at least 2 cm above the eyebrow.

Brow ptosis can be avoided by staying at least 2 cm above the eyebrow when injecting. Especially in a male patient, who likely will have lower set eyebrows compared to a female, this may be an unreliable landmark to use. Therefore, staying at least 2 cm above the upper brow should lower the risk of brow ptosis. In general, one should inject above the superior orbital rim in order to prevent the neurotoxin from diffusing inferiorly and paralyzing the levator palpebrae superioris, which is innervated by a branch of the oculomotor nerve leading to ptosis. Injecting supraperiosteal or within the forehead lines will not make a difference in relation to brow ptosis.[1,2,3]

REFERENCES

1. Rohrich RJ, Janis JE, Fagien S, et al. The cosmetic use of botulinum toxin. Plast Reconstr Surg 2003;112(5 Suppl): S117
2. Kim EJ, Ramirez AL, Reeck JB, et al. The role of botulinum toxin type B (Myobloc) in the treatment of hyperkinetic facial lines. Plast Reconstr Surg 2003;112(5 Suppl):S88
3. Carruthers J, Fagien S, Matarasso SL; Botox Consensus Group. Consensus recommendations on the use of botulinum toxin type a in facial aesthetics. Plast Reconstr Surg 2004;114(Suppl 6):S1

CLINICAL CONSIDERATIONS

5. *Where should perioral rhytids be injected to avoid adverse effects on the lip?*

C. Superficial, within 5 mm of the vermilion border.

Injecting in a deep plane or further than 5 mm from the vermilion can affect the function of the lips. This should be considered especially in patients such as musicians. The perioral region should generally not be injected in patients who are dependent on their lips for their professions. Additionally, perioral region is often more sensitive, and topical anesthesia is often beneficial in this location (**Fig. 21.1**).[1,2,3,4]

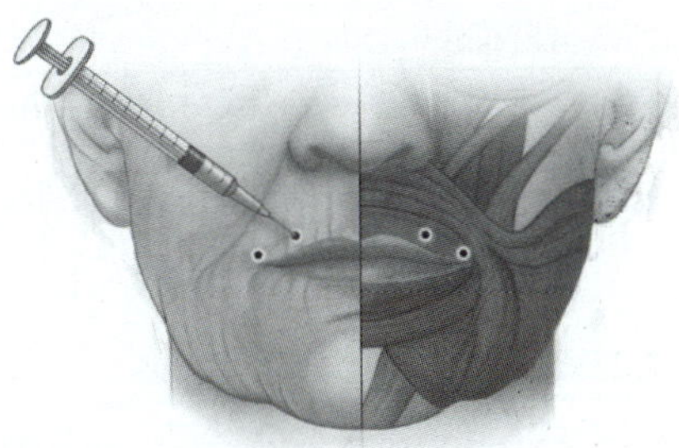

Fig. 21.1 Injection points for perioral rhytids. (Source: Injection. In: Janis J, ed. Essentials of Aesthetic Surgery. 1st Edition. New York: Thieme; 2018.)

REFERENCES

1. Carruthers J, Fagien S, Matarasso SL; Botox Consensus Group. Consensus recommendations on the use of botulinum toxin type a in facial aesthetics. Plast Reconstr Surg 2004;114(Suppl 6):S1
2. Rohrich RJ, Janis JE, Fagien S, et al. The cosmetic use of botulinum toxin. Plast Reconstr Surg 2003;112(5 Suppl):S117
3. Kim EJ, Ramirez AL, Reeck JB, et al. The role of botulinum toxin type B (Myobloc) in the treatment of hyperkinetic facial lines. Plast Reconstr Surg 2003;112(5 Suppl):S88
4. Kwiat DM, Bersani TA, Bersani A. Increased patient comfort utilizing botulinum toxin type a reconstituted with preserved versus nonpreserved saline. Ophthal Plast Reconstr Surg 2004;20:186

CLINICAL CONSIDERATIONS

6. *What portion of the masseter should be injected to correct masseteric hypertrophy?*

A. The most prominent point of muscle.

The most prominent portion of the masseter should be injected to correct hypertrophy. Masseter hypertrophy can lead to a wide contour of the lower face. In 1994, Moore and Wood first used botulinum toxin for functional reasons. Rijsdijk et al later used the toxin for aesthetic wrinkle reduction. The masseter consists of three layers of skeletal muscle: superficial, middle, and deep layers. The myofibers within these layers are arranged in different directions. Superficial layer arises from the anterior zygomatic arch and passes posteriorly and inferiorly, inserting onto the masseter tuberosity. The thinner middle layer arisesfrom the posterior arch and travels downward to the front and inserts into the masseter tuberosity. The deep layer arises from the posterior arch as well and passes back and downward to insert on the masseter tuberosity. These three layers fuse together in the lower third of the muscle. The effective minimal dosage is 20 units and the dosageis increased depending on the strength of the muscle. Results have shown a decrease in masseter thickness and improved contour of the lower face.[1,2]

Reference

1. Xie Y, Zhou J, Li H, et al. Classification of masseter hypertrophy for tailored botulinum toxin type a treatment. Plast Reconstr Surg 2014;134:209e
2. Rijsdijk BA, van ES RJ, Zonneveld FW, Steenks MH, Koole R. De toepassing van botuline A toxine bij cosmetisch storende M.-masseterhypertrofie [Botulinum toxin type A treatment of cosmetically disturbing masseteric hypertrophy]. Ned Tijdschr Geneeskd 1998;142(10):529-532

CLINICAL CONSIDERATIONS

7. *When is the typical onset of action of botulinum toxin following injection?*

C. 3 to 4 days.

Botulinum toxin usually takes effect within 3 to 4 days and the effect plateaus at 14 days after injection. Thus, reassessments and touch-ups can be performed at 14 days. Generally, patients are instructed not to massage the injection sites and to briefly limit activity. Refraining from strenuous activity may be beneficial by limiting ecchymosis and edema.[1,2]

References

1. Botox® Cosmetic Package Insert. Allergan, Inc., Irvine, CA. Available at http://www.allergan.com/assets/pdf/botox_cosmetic_pi.pdf
2. Rohrich RJ, Janis JE, Fagien S, et al. The cosmetic use of botulinum toxin. Plast Reconstr Surg 2003;112(5 Suppl):S117

CLINICAL CONSIDERATIONS

8. *What is the most commonly reported adverse effect of botulinum toxin?*

E. Transient eyelid ptosis.

Transient lid ptosis is reported in 5% of patients. Injection only above the orbital rim is recommended to prevent diffusion resulting in eyelid ptosis. In regard to the glabellar complex, five to seven injection sites are recommended (**Fig. 21.2**). Starting doses are approximately 20 to 30 U for women and 30 to 40 U for men. Midline injection should be at the nasal root to treat the procerus muscle. Injection of the depressor supercilii can raise the static position of the medial brow, if desired. In regard to the frontalis, injection varies depending on gender. Men generally require larger doses because they have thicker muscles. The female brow is arched, whereas the male brow is usually more horizontal. Injection patterns should be tailored with this in mind. Complete paralysis should be avoided because it can lead to brow ptosis and significantly limits facial expression. This is best prevented by injecting 2 cm above the eyebrow.Lateralinjections should be high (especially in women) to prevent drooping of the lateral brow. Starting doses are approximately 10 to 20 U for women and 20 to 30 U for men.[1,2,3]

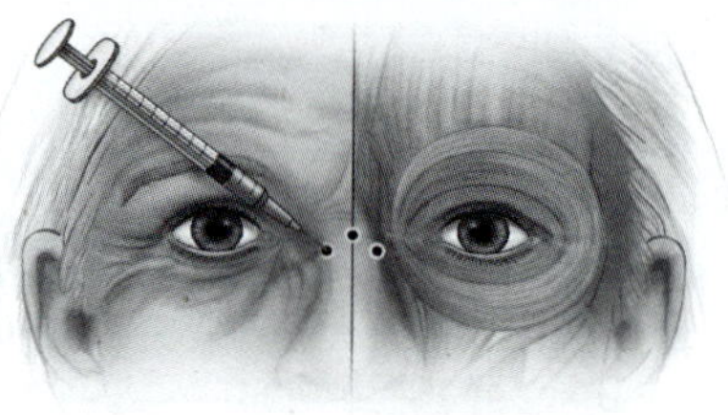

Fig. 21.2 Injection points for bunny lines. (Source: Injection. In: Janis J, ed. Essentials of Aesthetic Surgery. 1st Edition. New York: Thieme; 2018.)

References

1. Rohrich RJ, Janis JE, Fagien S, et al. The cosmetic use of botulinum toxin. Plast Reconstr Surg 2003;112(5 Suppl): S117
2. Kim EJ, Ramirez AL, Reeck JB, et al. The role of botulinum toxin type B (Myobloc) in the treatment of hyperkinetic facial lines. Plast Reconstr Surg 2003;112(5 Suppl):S88
3. Carruthers J, Fagien S, Matarasso SL; Botox Consensus Group. Consensus recommendations on the use of botulinum toxin type a in facial aesthetics. Plast Reconstr Surg 2004;114(Suppl 6):S1

22. Soft Tissue Fillers

Nima Khosravani, Anup Patel, Simon Moradian
See *Essentials of Aesthetic Surgery*, pp. 280–296

ANATOMICAL PRINCIPLES

1. *Which of the following is an important consideration with regards to the fat compartments in the malar region from the lateral zygomaticomaxillary junction to the nasomaxillary region below the tear trough?*

A. These fat compartments consist of only a superficial region requiring only superficial volume rejuvenation.
B. These fat compartments consist of both deep and superficial regions requiring multilevel filling.
C. These fat compartments consist of only a deep region requiring only deep volume rejuvenation.
D. Injection should proceed in the deep and superficial fat compartments as well as the lower eyelid region.
E. Injection to these fat compartments is not indicated for large molecule HA fillers and/or hydroxyapatite.

ANATOMICAL PRINCIPLES

2. *Youthful characteristics of lips include:*

A. Upper lip/lower lip height ratio of 1/3:2/3.
B. Upper lip/lower lip height ratio of 1:1.
C. Flat philtral columns.
D. Poorly defined cupid's bow.
E. Gentle convex sloping lines from nasal base and labiomental groove.

TREATMENT

3. *What is considered to be the most effective treatment for crow's feet?*

A. Chemodenervation.
B. Fat grafting.
C. Large molecule HA fillers.
D. Hydroxyapatite.
E. Laser.

ANATOMICAL PRINCIPLES/TREATMENT

4. *Which of the following should not be injected in the lower lid–cheek junction and tear trough area?*

A. Botox.
B. Calcium hydroxyapatite.
C. Small-molecule HA fillers.
D. Poly-L-lactic acid.
E. Fat.

PREOPERATIVE PLANNING

5. *A 27-year-old female body builder is interested in lip augmentation and would like a dramatic increase in her lip size. What strategy should be used for a patient who demands overcorrection of the lips?*

A. Soft tissue fillers should be avoided in patients who desire overcorrection of lips.
B. Over-enhanced lips should be achieved by using 2× standard aliquot.
C. Advise the patient that the filler will last between 12 and 18 months.
D. Use a dermal fat graft in addition to filler.
E. An incremental approach should be used, with reevaluation from multiple views during the injection.

PREOPERATIVE PLANNING

6. ***Which of the following may interfere with healing at the injection site?***
   A. Family history of smoking, diabetes, or lung cancer.
   B. Presence of a collagen–vascular disease process.
   C. A skin or soft tissue inflammatory process that completely subsided 1 week before injection.
   D. Use of a topical tretinoin.
   E. Active viral upper respiratory infection.

PREOPERATIVE PLANNING

7. ***Which of the following would contraindicate 54-year-old patients from receiving mid face injections with calcium hydroxyapatite?***
   A. History of smoking.
   B. Takes an 81 mg aspirin but stopped taking it 1 week prior to injection.
   C. Presence of facial contour irregularities.
   D. Received filler 2 weeks ago.
   E. Presence of impetigo in the malar region.

PREOPERATIVE PLANNING

8. ***Which of the following should be discussed with patients during informed consent?***
   A. Cosmetic outcomes such as lumpiness, overcorrection/undercorrection, and contour irregularities.
   B. Hypersensitivity and hyposensitivity are common adverse events.
   C. About 12 to 15% of negative skin test patients can produce an allergic reaction to facial injection.
   D. Skin necrosis/ulceration can occur in healthy patients.
   E. Antibiotics are prescribed prophylactically to reduce chance of cellulitis at injection site.

PREOPERATIVE PLANNING

9. ***When counseling a patient on the effects of hyaluronic fillers, which of the following are accurate considerations?***
   A. They are animal based and less likely to cause inflammatory reaction.
   B. Skin testing is required as these fillers have immunologic activity.
   C. They are hydrophilic in nature accounting for initial swollen/overcorrected appearance.
   D. Contraindicated in lower lid–cheek junction and tear trough area.
   E. Degree of cross linking and weight is consistent between products.

OPERATIVE TECHNIQUE

10. ***Which injection technique is most appropriate for the white roll of the vermilion?***
    A. Serial puncture.
    B. Linear threading.
    C. Fanning technique.
    D. Cross radial technique.
    E. Intradermal microdroplet techniques.

OPERATIVE TECHNIQUE

11. ***Which injection technique is most appropriate for the commissures?***
    A. Serial puncture.
    B. Linear threading.
    C. Lip tenting technique.
    D. Fanning technique.
    E. Cross radial technique.

OPERATIVE TECHNIQUE

12. ***Which injection technique is most appropriate when using calcium hydroxyapatite?***
    A. Serial puncture.
    B. Linear threading.
    C. Lip tenting technique.
    D. Fanning technique.
    E. Cross radial technique.

PREOPERATIVE PLANNING

13. *Which of the following would be a reason to consider the use of calcium hydroxyapatite fillers?*

A. Maximum volume effect seen immediately.
B. FDA approved for HIV lipoatrophy of the face.
C. Excellent filler for malar and nasolabial fold augmentation.
D. Meticulous product placement is not crucial as massaging of product is extremely effective.
E. Results commonly seen up to 3 to 6 months.

OPERATIVE TECHNIQUE

14. *Which of the following must be avoided during malar augmentation with calcium hydroxyapatite?*

A. Fanning technique from lateral submalar point and/or medially at upper nasolabial fold.
B. Starting deep in subcutaneous or preperiosteal level and layer.
C. Injecting in region of lower eyelid.
D. Extending inferiorly along medial zygoma.
E. Serial puncture technique from lateral submalar point and/or medially at upper nasolabial fold.

OPERATIVE TECHNIQUE

15. *Which technique must be used when injecting prejowl sulcus?*

A. It is important to remain superficial to avoid neurovascular structures.
B. Start from lateral to medial and use the fanning technique.
C. Start from lateral to medial and use serial puncture technique.
D. Start from medial to lateral and use a combination of serial puncture and linear threading technique.
E. It is important to overcorrect in this region.

PERIOPERATIVE CONSIDERATIONS

16. *Which of the following applies to the use of poly-L-lactic Acid (PLLA)?*

A. May require 3 to 6 treatments that may last up to 2 years.
B. Glycosaminoglycan biopolymer of repeating disaccharide units of N-acetylglucosamine and glucuronic acid.
C. Reconstitution with 3 to 5 mL of sterile water is not necessary as with other injectables.
D. It is not FDA approved for correction of HIV-associated lipoatrophy of the face.
E. The initial, robust appearance of PLLA is from edema and inflammation, which will diminish and return at approximately 8 to 12 weeks as collagen replacement is under way.

PERIOPERATIVE CONSIDERATIONS

17. *Which of the following products is FDA approved for HIV lipoatrophy of the face?*

A. Calcium hydroxyapatite.
B. Poly-L-lactic acid.
C. Large particle hyaluronic acid fillers.
D. Small particle hyaluronic acid fillers.
E. Autologous fat injections.

PREOPERATIVE PLANNING

18. *Which of the following applies to the use of polymethylmethacrylate (PMMA)?*

A. Skin testing is required.
B. Indicated for superficial rhytids and other locations prone to skin ulceration/atrophy.
C. It is considered a temporary filler.
D. Postinjection irregularities are uncommon; however, they should be treated with gentle massage.
E. For depressed scars, large aliquot is injected into scar and defect is corrected during one session.

PREOPERATIVE PLANNING

19. *Which scenario would make injectables an inappropriate treatment in a 31-year-old female patient?*

A. She is getting married in 2 days and desires dermal fillers to enhance her nasolabial folds.
B. She is getting married in 2 months and desires dermal fillers to enhance her nasolabial folds.
C. She is an actress who takes a daily aspirin and desires augmentation of her malar region.
D. She has lipoatrophy of the face due to extreme body fat loss secondary to body building and dieting.
E. She has lipoatrophy of the face and is HIV/AIDS positive.

POSTOPERATIVE CARE

20. ***Which of the following is the most appropriate postinjection care for fillers?***

A. At home manipulation or "shaping" of product when injected properly should be performed every 6 hours for the first 72 hours post injection.
B. Initial ice application may help to reduce facial edema and can be applied for 20 minutes on and 20 minutes off during the first 12 to 24 hours.
C. Initial application of warm packs to help with dispersion of the filler.
D. Patients can resume normal activity that increases heart rate immediately.
E. Patients are encouraged to increase salt intake as this may help decrease edema and erythema.

PERIOPERATIVE CONSIDERATIONS

21. ***Which of the following applies to the appearance of lumpiness following injection of fillers?***

A. It is more likely with malleable products.
B. Should be treated within 48 to 72 hours of being seen, with massage to smooth out the lump.
C. This is a normal immediate effect of filler and will resolve on its own within 2 to 3 days.
D. It is often related to improper technique, fast injection, and placement of disproportionate filler material in one spot.
E. Gentle massage is usually ineffective in smoothing out lumps immediately following injection.

Answers

ANATOMICAL PRINCIPLES

1. ***Which of the following is an important consideration with regards to the fat compartments in the malar region from the lateral zygomaticomaxillary junction to the nasomaxillary region below the tear trough?***

   B. These fat compartments consist of both deep and superficial regions requiring multilevel filling.

   Fat compartments in the malar region from lateral zygomaticomaxillary junction to the nasomaxillary region below the tear trough consist of both deep and superficial compartments requiring multilevel filling. This is an excellent indication for large-molecule HA fillers and/or hydroxyapatite. Injection should be AVOIDED in the lower eyelid region, and one finger should be held at infraorbital rim to block inadvertent needle passes. Malar augmentation is important and complementary to lower lid–tear trough treatments with HA agents. This allows comprehensive and natural blending of the periorbital with malar subcutaneous compartments.[1,2] **Fig. 22.1** depicts the injection of the nasolabial folds and malar mounds with Radiesse.

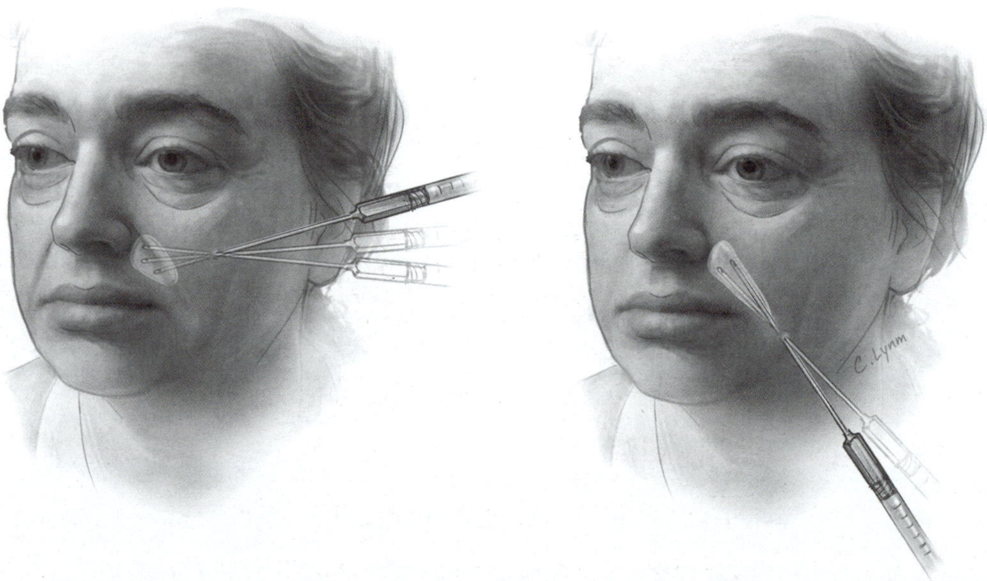

Fig. 22.1 Injection technique. Injection of the nasolabial folds and malar mounds with Radiesse. (Source: From Tonnard PL, Verpaele AM, Bensimon RH, eds. Centrofacial Rejuvenation. New York: Thieme Publishers, 2018.)

REFERENCES

1. Marmur ES, Phelps R, Goldberg DJ. Clinical, histologic, and electron microscopic findings after injection of a calcium hydroxylapatite filler. J Cosmet Laser Ther 2004;6:223
2. Graivier MH, Bass, Lawrence S, et al. Calcium hydroxylapatite (Radiesse) for correction of the mid- and lower face: consensus recommendations. Plast Reconstr Surg 2007;120(6 Suppl):S55

ANATOMICAL PRINCIPLES

2. *Youthful characteristics of lips include:*

A. Upper lip/lower lip height ratio of 1/3:2/3.

Youthful characteristics of lips include upper lip/lower lip height ratio of 1/3:2/3. Cupid's bow should be sharp and well defined. Philtral columns are full. There is a gentle concave sloping from nasal base and labiomental groove. Oral commissures should be slightly upward in orientation with full medial tubercle accompanied by sharp white rolls (vermilion–cutaneous junction) (**Fig. 22.2**).[1,2]

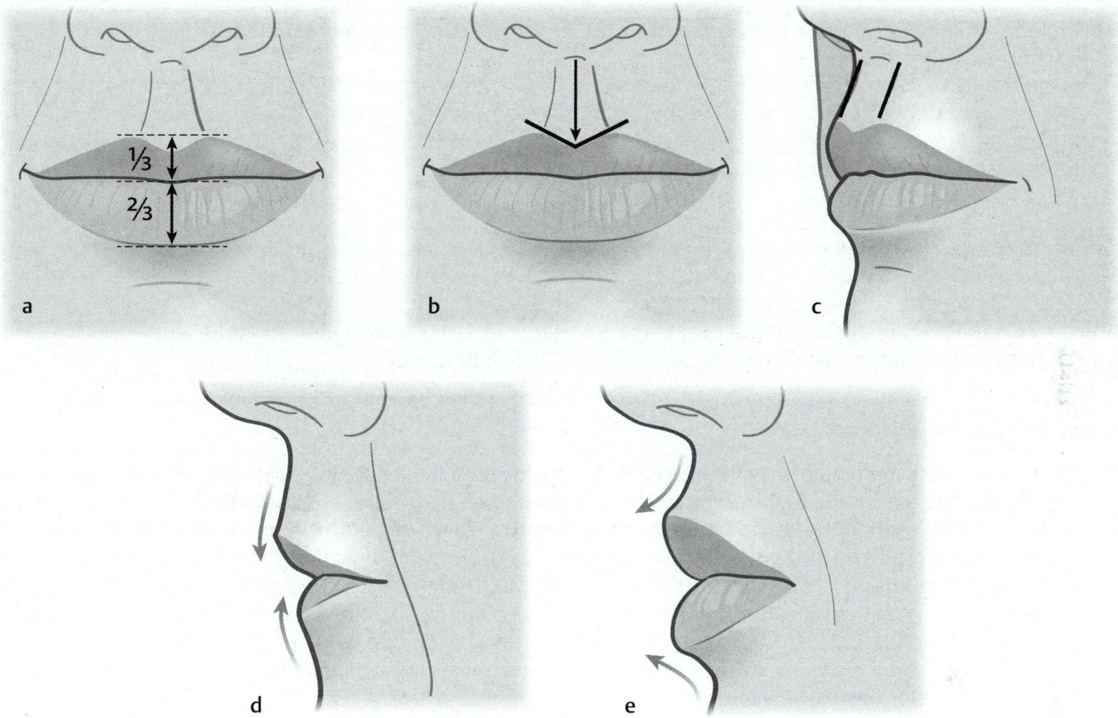

Fig. 22.2 (a–e) Youthful lip characteristics. (Source: Lips. In: Janis J, ed. Essentials of Aesthetic Surgery. 1st Edition. New York: Thieme; 2018.)

REFERENCES

1. Born TM. Soft tissue fillers in aesthetic facial surgery. In: Nahai F, ed. The Art of Aesthetic Surgery: Principles & Techniques. New York: Thieme Publishers; 2007
2. Fagien S, Klein AW. A brief overview and history of temporary fillers: evolution, advantages, and limitations. Plast Reconstr Surg 2007;120(6 Suppl):S8

TREATMENT

3. *What is considered to be the most effective treatment for crow's feet?*

A. Chemodenervation.

Chemodenervation is considered the best treatment for crow's feet. Fat and fillers are rarely effective in this area where the skin is thick and well adherent to the underlying orbicularis. Laser treatment is somewhat unpredictable in the periorbital area given the thinness of the skin and therefore caution should be taken.[1,2,3]

REFERENCES

1. Rohrich RJ, Ghavami A, Crosby MA. The role of hyaluronic acid fillers (Restylane) in facial cosmetic surgery: review and technical considerations. Plast Reconstr Surg 2007;120(6 Suppl):S41
2. Born TM. Soft tissue fillers in aesthetic facial surgery. In: Nahai F, ed. The Art of Aesthetic Surgery: Principles & Techniques. New York: Thieme Publishers; 2007
3. Fagien S, Klein AW. A brief overview and history of temporary fillers: evolution, advantages, and limitations. Plast Reconstr Surg 2007;120(6 Suppl):S8

ANATOMICAL PRINCIPLES/TREATMENT

4. *Which of the following should not be injected in the lower lid–cheek junction and tear trough area?*

B. Calcium hydroxyapatite.

Calcium hydroxyapatite should not be injected in the lower lid–cheek junction and tear trough area. Ideal sites are generally in regions with overlying thicker skin: nasolabial folds, malar augmentation, submalar augmentation, oral commissures, marionette lines, labiomental crease, jawline, prejowl/premental depression, and chin augmentation.[1,2]

REFERENCES

1. Marmur ES, Phelps R, Goldberg DJ. Clinical, histologic, and electron microscopic findings after injection of a calcium hydroxylapatite filler. J Cosmet Laser Ther 2004;6:223
2. Graivier MH, Bass LS, et al. Calcium hydroxylapatite (Radiesse) for correction of the mid- and lower face: consensus recommendations. Plast Reconstr Surg 2007;120(6 Suppl):S55

PREOPERATIVE PLANNING

5. *A 27-year-old female body builder is interested in lip augmentation and would like a dramatic increase in her lip size. What strategy should be used for a patient who demands overcorrection of the lips?*

E. An incremental approach should be used, with reevaluation from multiple views during the injection.

The lips are a vital and central portion of the face that evoke emotion, sensuality, youth, and vitality. An incremental approach should always be used with reevaluation from multiple views during injection. Hyaluronic acid–based fillers are absorbed by the body over time and generally will last between 6 and 12 months. Although a dermal fat graft could be considered, it may not be the best option for patients if they have an extremely low body fat, as in this body builder. Additionally, the concomitant use of a dermal fat graft in addition to filler should be avoided and would be unpredictable.[1,2,3]

REFERENCES

1. Born TM. Soft tissue fillers in aesthetic facial surgery. In: Nahai F, ed. The Art of Aesthetic Surgery: Principles & Techniques. New York: Thieme Publishers; 2007
2. Sundaram H, Cassuto D. Biophysical characteristics of hylauronic acid soft-tissue fillers and their relevance to aesthetic applications. Plast Reconstr Surg 2013;132(4 Suppl):S5
3. Fagien S, Klein AW. A brief overview and history of temporary fillers: evolution, advantages, and limitations. Plast Reconstr Surg 2007;120(6 Suppl):S8

PREOPERATIVE PLANNING

6. *Which of the following may interfere with healing at the injection site?*

B. Presence of a collagen–vascular disease process.

The presence of collagen–vascular disease process may interfere with healing at the injection site and compromise skin blood supply. Any active skin or soft tissue inflammatory infectious process should completely subside before injections. Smoking may delay or interfere with healing and longevity of the product, especially if a collagen response is necessary for results. The use of a topical tretinoin will not affect the use of filler as the filler is used for augmentation in tissues deep to the dermis/epidermis.[1]

REFERENCE

1. Alam M, Dover JS. Management of complications and sequelae with temporary injectable fillers. Plast Reconstr Surg 2007;120(6 Suppl):S98

PREOPERATIVE PLANNING

7. *Which of the following would contraindicate 54-year-old patients from receiving mid face injections with calcium hydroxyapatite?*

E. Presence of impetigo in the malar region.

Any active skin or soft tissue inflammatory process should completely subside before injections. Patients should not take aspirin, NSAIDs, and other blood thinning medications for at least 1 week prior to injection. Patients should understand that smoking may delay or interfere with healing and longevity of the product. Maximum volume effect is seen at 4 to 6 weeks post injection; therefore, it would not be advisable to inject at 2 weeks after a prior injection as the final aesthetic outcome would be overcorrected.[1,2]

REFERENCES

1. Alam M, Dover JS. Management of complications and sequelae with temporary injectable fillers. Plast Reconstr Surg 2007;120(6 Suppl):S98
2. Fagien S, Klein AW. A brief overview and history of temporary fillers: evolution, advantages, and limitations. Plast Reconstr Surg 2007;120(6 Suppl):S8

PREOPERATIVE PLANNING

8. *Which of the following should be discussed with patients during informed consent?*

A. Cosmetic outcomes such as lumpiness, overcorrection/undercorrection, and contour irregularities.

Cosmetic outcomes such as lumpiness, overcorrection and undercorrection, and contour irregularities should be explained during informed consent. Rarely hypersensitivity/hyposensitivity has been reported with all types of fillers. In fact, 1 to 5% of negative skin test patients can produce an allergic reaction to facial injection. Skin necrosis ulcerations are rare but are more likely in poorly selected patients.[1]

REFERENCE

1. Alam M, Dover JS. Management of complications and sequelae with temporary injectable fillers. Plast Reconstr Surg 2007;120(6 Suppl):S98

PREOPERATIVE PLANNING

9. *When counseling a patient on the effects of hyaluronic fillers, which of the following are accurate considerations?*

C. They are hydrophilic in nature accounting for initial swollen/overcorrected appearance.

Hyaluronic acid fillers are not animal based. They do not require skin testing, and do not have immunologic activity. They are hydrophilic which accounts for the initial swollen/overcorrected appearance. Calcium hydroxyapatite is contraindicated in lower lid–cheek junction and tear trough area. Hyaluronic acid is a normal ground substance that is found in many tissues such as bone, skin, cartilage, and synovial fluid which decreases with age. The degree of cross linking and weight differs between products.[1,2,3]

REFERENCES

1. Rohrich RJ, Ghavami A, Crosby MA. The role of hyaluronic acid fillers (Restylane) in facial cosmetic surgery: review and technical considerations. Plast Reconstr Surg 2007;120(6 Suppl):S41
2. Sundaram H, Cassuto D. Biophysical characteristics of hyaluronic acid soft-tissue fillers and their relevance to aesthetic applications. Plast Reconstr Surg 2013;132(4 Suppl):S5
3. Flynn TC, Thompson DH, Hyun SH. Molecular weight analysis and enzymatic degradation profiles of the soft-tissue fillers Belotero Balance, Restylane, and Juvéderm Ultra. Plast Reconstr Surg 2013;132(4 Suppl):S22

OPERATIVE TECHNIQUE

10. *Which injection technique is most appropriate for the white roll of the vermilion?*

B. Linear threading.

Different locations are best served with different injection techniques. The white roll of the vermilion necessitates linear threading. **Fig. 22.3** shows the following: (a) serial puncture; (b) linear threading; (c) fanning technique; (d) cross-radial technique or cross-hatching.[1,2]

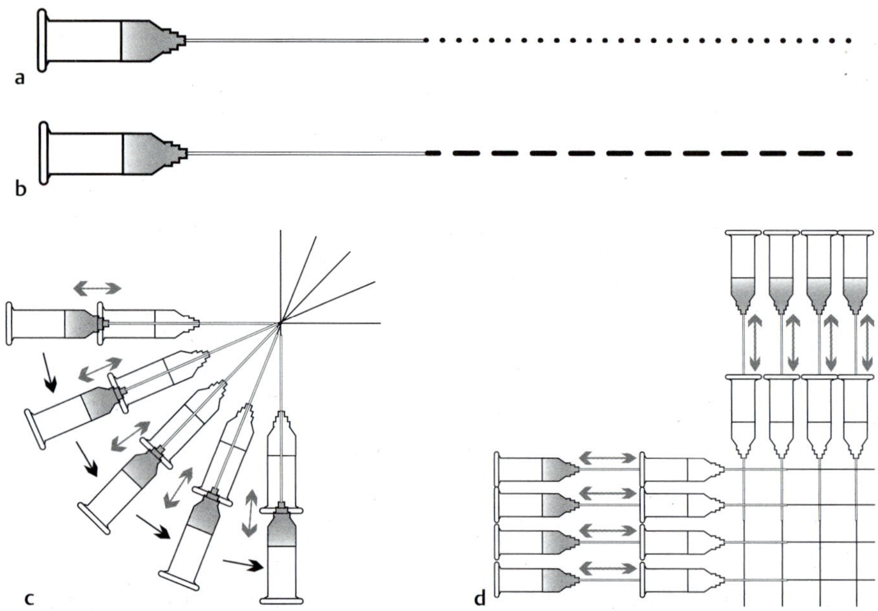

Fig. 22.3 **(a)** Serial puncture. **(b)** Linear threading. **(c)** Fanning technique. **(d)** Cross-radial technique or cross-hatching. (Source: Injection Techniques. In: Pu L, ed. Aesthetic Plastic Surgery in Asians: Principles & Techniques. 1st Edition. New York: Thieme; 2015.)

References

1. Born TM. Soft tissue fillers in aesthetic facial surgery. In: Nahai F, ed. The Art of Aesthetic Surgery: Principles & Techniques. New York: Thieme Publishers; 2007
2. Sundaram H, Cassuto D. Biophysical characteristics of hyaluronic acid soft-tissue fillers and their relevance to aesthetic applications. Plast Reconstr Surg 2013;132(4 Suppl):S5

OPERATIVE TECHNIQUE

11. ***Which injection technique is most appropriate for the commissures?***

E. Cross radial technique.

Different locations are best served with different injection techniques. The commissures are best treated with cross-radial injections. **Fig. 22.4** shows the following: (a) serial puncture; (b) linear threading; (c) fanning technique; (d) cross-radial technique or cross-hatching.[1,2]

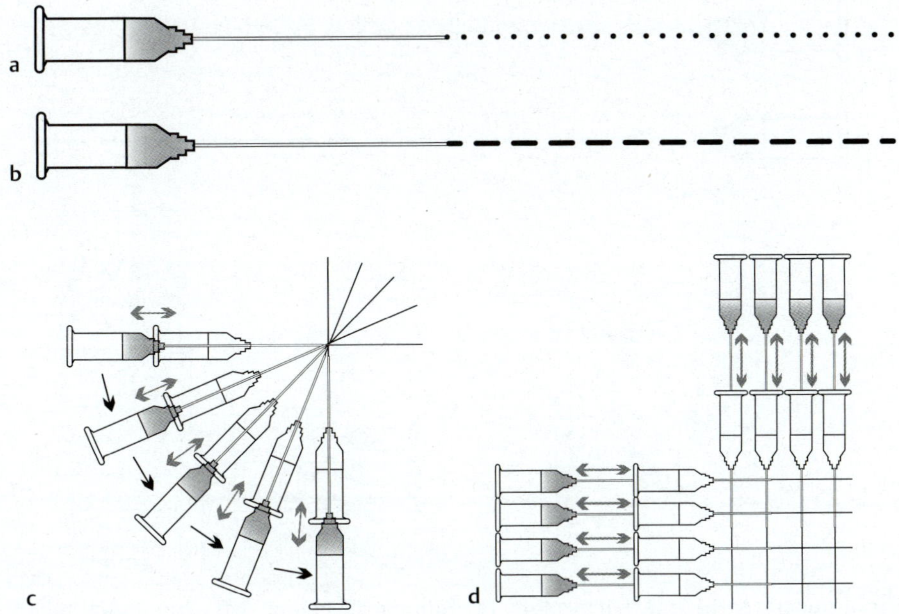

Fig. 22.4 **(a)** Serial puncture. **(b)** Linear threading. **(c)** Fanning technique. **(d)** Cross-radial technique or cross-hatching. (Source: Injection Techniques. In: Pu L, ed. Aesthetic Plastic Surgery in Asians: Principles & Techniques. 1st Edition. New York: Thieme; 2015.)

REFERENCES

1. Born TM. Soft tissue fillers in aesthetic facial surgery. In: Nahai F, ed. The Art of Aesthetic Surgery: Principles & Techniques. New York: Thieme Publishers; 2007
2. Sundaram H, Cassuto D. Biophysical characteristics of hyaluronic acid soft-tissue fillers and their relevance to aesthetic applications. Plast Reconstr Surg 2013;132(4 Suppl):S5

OPERATIVE TECHNIQUE

12. ***Which injection technique is most appropriate when using calcium hydroxyapatite?***

D. Fanning technique.

Fanning technique is most useful when using calcium hydroxyapatite because the product is placed during needle withdrawal. Mindfulness of skin entry and exit sites is essential to prevent inadvertent superficial deposition of product. **Fig. 22.5** shows the following: (a) serial puncture; (b) linear threading; (c) fanning technique; (d) cross-radial technique or cross-hatching.[1,2]

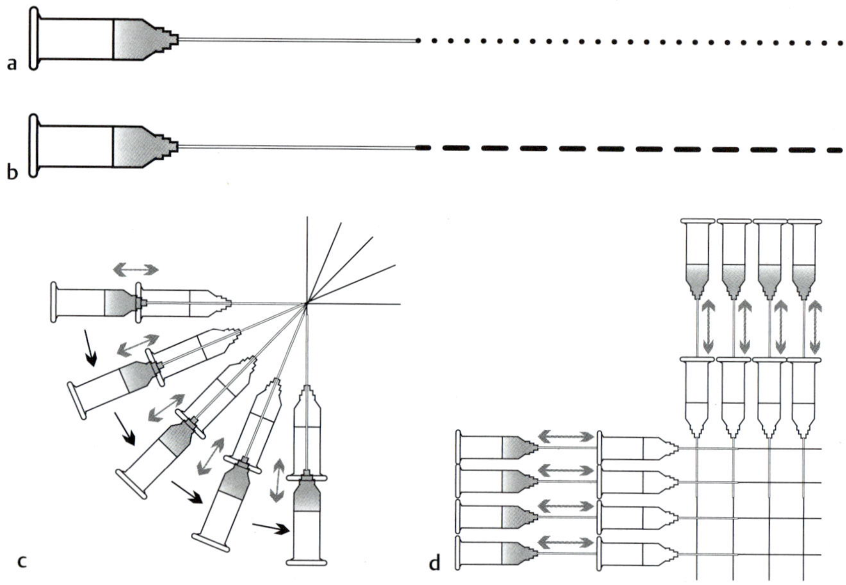

Fig. 22.5 **(a)** Serial puncture. **(b)** Linear threading. **(c)** Fanning technique. **(d)** Cross-radial technique or cross-hatching. (Source: Injection Techniques. In: Pu L, ed. Aesthetic Plastic Surgery in Asians: Principles & Techniques. 1st Edition. New York: Thieme; 2015.)

REFERENCES

1. Born TM. Soft tissue fillers in aesthetic facial surgery. In: Nahai F, ed. The Art of Aesthetic Surgery: Principles & Techniques. New York: Thieme Publishers; 2007
2. Sundaram H, Cassuto D. Biophysical characteristics of hyaluronic acid soft-tissue fillers and their relevance to aesthetic applications. Plast Reconstr Surg 2013;132(4 Suppl):S5

PREOPERATIVE PLANNING

13. ***Which of the following would be a reason to consider the use of calcium hydroxyapatite fillers?***

C. Excellent filler for malar and nasolabial fold augmentation.

Maximum volume effect is seen at 4 to 6 weeks, with results clinically lasting up to 9 to 12 months. Ideal sites are generally in regions with overlying thicker skin (nasolabial folds, malar augmentation, submalar augmentation, oral commissures, etc.). Meticulous placement of product is most critical with the fanning technique most useful because product is placed during needle withdrawal. Results are commonly seen up to 6 to 9 months (**Fig. 22.6**).[1,2]

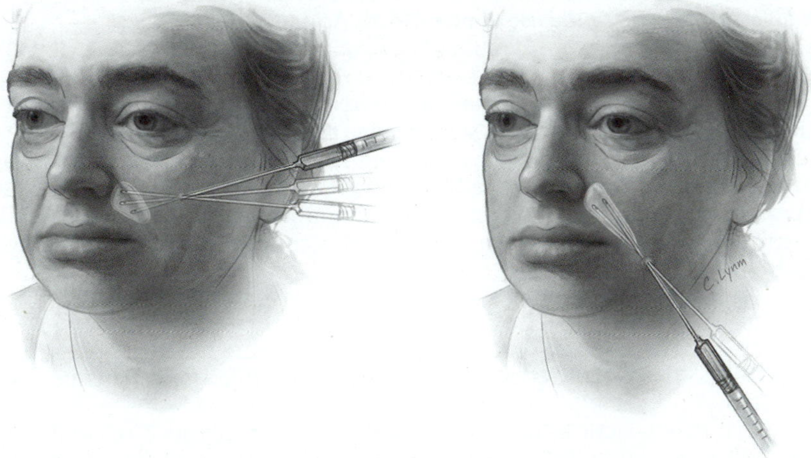

Fig. 22.6 Injection technique. Injection of the nasolabial folds and malar mounds with Radiesse. (Source: From Tonnard PL, Verpaele AM, Bensimon RH, eds. Centrofacial Rejuvenation. New York: Thieme Publishers, 2018.)

REFERENCES

1. Marmur ES, Phelps R, Goldberg DJ. Clinical, histologic, and electron microscopic findings after injection of a calcium hydroxylapatite filler. J Cosmet Laser Ther 2004;6:223
2. Graivier MH, Bass, Lawrence S, et al. Calcium hydroxylapatite (Radiesse) for correction of the mid- and lower face: consensus recommendations. Plast Reconstr Surg 2007;120(6 Suppl):S55

OPERATIVE TECHNIQUE

14. *Which of the following must be avoided during malar augmentation with calcium hydroxyapatite?*

C. Injecting in region of lower eyelid.

Injection in the region of lower eyelid should be avoided. The injector should hold one finger at the infraorbital rim to block inadvertent needle passes. The use of the fanning technique from lateral submalar point and/or medially at upper nasolabial fold, starting deep in the subcutaneous or preperiosteal level and layer, extension inferiorly along the medial zygoma, and HIV-associated malar lipoatrophy are all appropriate principles and reasons to use calcium hydroxyapatite filler when injecting along the malar region.[1]

REFERENCE

1. Graivier MH, Bass, Lawrence S, et al. Calcium hydroxylapatite (Radiesse) for correction of the mid- and lower face: consensus recommendations. Plast Reconstr Surg 2007;120(6 Suppl):S55

OPERATIVE TECHNIQUE

15. *Which technique must be used when injecting prejowl sulcus?*

B. Start from lateral to medial and use the fanning technique.

It is important to stay deep, and to start from lateral to medial while using the fanning technique when correcting the prejowl sulcus. In general, fanning technique is the safest method to use for injections of the lower third of the face as well as staying deep to not injure superficial neurovascular structures.[1]

REFERENCE

1. Born TM. Soft tissue fillers in aesthetic facial surgery. In Nahai F, ed. The Art of Aesthetic Surgery: Principles & Techniques. New York: Thieme Publishers; 2007

PERIOPERATIVE CONSIDERATIONS

16. ***Which of the following applies to the use of poly-L-lactic Acid (PLLA)?***

E. The initial, robust appearance of PLLA is from edema and inflammation, which will diminish and return at approximately 8 to 12 weeks as collagen replacement is under way.

PLLA may last up to 2 years and may require 3 to 6 treatments. It must be reconstituted prior to injection with sterile water, which will allow for easier injection as viscosity is lowered. Initial effects results from an inflammatory process between the soft tissue and PLLA. Macrophages and fibroblasts form a capsule around the microspheres. PLLA is eventually all degraded and replaced with collagen; therefore, the initial robust appearance of the product is from edema and inflammation, which will diminish and return at approximately 8 to 12 weeks as collagen replacement occurs. It is FDA approved for the use of HIV-associated lipoatrophy of the face.[1,2,3]

REFERENCES

1. Woerle B, Hanke CW, Sattler G. Poly-L-lactic acid: a temporary filler for soft tissue augmentation. J Drugs Dermatol 2004;3:385
2. Sterling JB, Hanke CW. Poly-L-lactic acid as a facial filler. Skin Therapy Lett 2005;10:9
3. Borelli C, Kunte C, Weisenseel P, et al. Deep subcutaneous application of poly-L-lactic acid as a filler for facial lipoatrophy in HIV-infected patients. Skin Pharmacol Physiol 2005;18:273

PERIOPERATIVE CONSIDERATIONS

17. ***Which of the following products is FDA approved for HIV lipoatrophy of the face?***

B. Poly-L-lactic acid.

Poly-L-lactic acid (PLLA) is FDA approved for HIV lipoatrophy of the face. PLLA is a synthetic polymer. It is biodegradable, biocompatible, immunologically inert, and no skin test required. PLLA is delivered as microparticles that are broken down by nonenzymatic hydrolysis into lactic acid monomers. Lactic acid polymers are then broken down to CO_2 or glucose.

The initial effect results from an inflammatory process between the soft tissue and PLLA whereby macrophages and fibroblasts form a capsule around the microspheres and PLLA is eventually all degraded and replaced with collagen.[1]

REFERENCE

1. Borelli C, Kunte C, Weisenseel P, et al. Deep subcutaneous application of poly-L-lactic acid as a filler for facial lipoatrophy in HIV-infected patients. Skin Pharmacol Physiol 2005;18:273

PREOPERATIVE PLANNING

18. ***Which of the following applies to the use of polymethylmethacrylate (PMMA)?***

A. Skin testing is required.

Skin testing is required when using PMMA. PMMA is considered a permanent filler; however, more filler may be required at 1.5 years, and initial results may not be seen for 6 to 8 months. PMMA is not safe for superficial rhytids or locations prone to skin ulceration/atrophy as product becomes more visible with time as soft tissue and skin atrophy with age. For depressed scars, release scar first (18 gauge or pickle fork instrument), and fill the scar gradually using serial injection over several weeks to months.[1,2]

REFERENCES

1. Lemperle G, Romano JJ, Busso M. Soft tissue augmentation with Artecoll: 10-year history, indications, techniques, and complications. Dermatol Surg 2003;29:573
2. Alcalay J, Alkalay R, Gat A, et al. Late onset granuloma to reaction to Artecoll. Dermatol Surg 2003;29:859

PREOPERATIVE PLANNING

19. ***Which scenario would make injectables an inappropriate treatment in a 31-year-old female patient?***

A. She is getting married in 2 days and desires dermal fillers to enhance her nasolabial folds.

There will be edema, erythema, and bruising for up to 2 weeks, and therefore a patient getting married in 2 days should be aware of the presence of edema and erythema. The remaining scenarios would all be considered appropriate patients to augment using filler.[1]

REFERENCE

1. Born TM. Soft tissue fillers in aesthetic facial surgery. In: Nahai F, ed. The Art of Aesthetic Surgery: Principles & Techniques. New York: Thieme Publishers; 2007

POSTOPERATIVE CARE

20. *Which of the following is the most appropriate postinjection care for fillers?*

B. Initial ice application may help to reduce facial edema and can be applied for 20 minutes on and 20 minutes off during the first 12 to 24 hours.

Initial ice application may help to reduce facial edema and can be applied for 20 minutes on and 20 minutes off during the first 12 to 24 hours. Application of heat packs would not be beneficial after filler injection, nor would it assist in filler dispersion. Additionally, manipulation of the filler would not be recommended to be performed by the patient. Filler volume and shape should be optimal before the patient leaves the office precluding the need for manipulation or shaping of the product at home. Patients are instructed to limit activity that increases heart rate for 3 to 7 days. Patients can resume previous diet as tolerated but limiting salt intake may help decrease edema slightly.[1,2]

REFERENCES

1. Born TM. Soft tissue fillers in aesthetic facial surgery. In: Nahai F, ed. The Art of Aesthetic Surgery: Principles & Techniques. New York: Thieme Publishers; 2007
2. Alam M, Dover JS. Management of complications and sequelae with temporary injectable fillers. Plast Reconstr Surg 2007;120(6 Suppl):S98

PERIOPERATIVE CONSIDERATIONS

21. *Which of the following applies to the appearance of lumpiness following injection of fillers?*

D. It is often related to improper technique, fast injection, and placement of disproportionate filler material in one spot.

#Lumps are often related to improper technique, fast injection, and placement of disproportionate filler material in one spot. Injection is performed with an even flow to prevent lumpiness and irregularities. If lumpiness is seen or felt, the area needs to be massaged immediately to smooth the product, not days later. Lumpiness is more likely with less malleable products or semipermanent compared to fully permanent products.[1,2,3]

REFERENCES

1. Born TM. Soft tissue fillers in aesthetic facial surgery. In: Nahai F, ed. The Art of Aesthetic Surgery: Principles & Techniques. New York: Thieme Publishers; 2007
2. Alam M, Dover JS. Management of complications and sequelae with temporary injectable fillers. Plast Reconstr Surg 2007;120(6 Suppl):S98
3. Lombardi T, Samson J, Plantier F, et al. Orofacial granulomas after injection of cosmetic fillers. Histopathological and clinical study of 11 cases. J Oral Pathol Med 2004;33:115

23. Fat Grafting

Stelios C. Wilson
See *Essentials of Aesthetic Surgery*, first edition, pp. 297–312

HARVEST SITE

1. ***Which harvest site has been shown to have the best fat longevity?***
   A. Abdomen.
   B. Flanks.
   C. Medial thigh.
   D. Lateral thigh.
   E. There is no difference based on donor site.

FAT PROCESSING

2. ***According to the Coleman technique of fat preparation, how long the fat should be centrifuged?***
   A. 3 minutes at 3000 rpm.
   B. 5 minutes at 5000 rpm.
   C. 8 minutes at 8000 rpm.
   D. 10 minutes at 10,000 rpm.
   E. 12 minutes at 15,000 rpm.

FAT PROCESSING

3. ***Following centrifugation, the lipoaspirate separates into three layers. Which layer contains potentially viable parcels of fat?***
   A. Upper level.
   B. Middle level.
   C. Lower level.
   D. Upper and middle layers only.
   E. All three layers.

FAT PLACEMENT

4. ***To strengthen soft tissue projection over bony prominences, fat should be placed in which of the following levels?***
   A. Subperiosteal.
   B. Supraperiosteal.
   C. In the subcutaneous fat.
   D. Immediately subdermal.
   E. Intradermal.

EDEMA

5. ***According to the Coleman technique description, when is the patient allowed to start massaging the recipient site after the procedure?***
   A. Immediately after surgery.
   B. 1 week after surgery.
   C. 2 weeks after surgery.
   D. 4 weeks after surgery.
   E. 6 weeks after surgery.

EDEMA

6. *According to the Coleman technique, when is the patient allowed to start massaging the donor site after the procedure?*
A. Immediately after surgery.
B. 1 week after surgery.
C. 2 weeks after surgery.
D. 4 weeks after surgery.
E. 6 weeks after surgery.

EDEMA

7. *How long should you tell a patient to expect postoperative edema of the face following fat grafting?*
A. 1 week after surgery.
B. 1 month after surgery.
C. 2 months after surgery.
D. Greater than 4 months after surgery.
E. Up to 8 to 12 months after surgery.

TREATMENT OF SELECT AREAS

8. *When treating the lips, what layer is the preferred layer for fat injection?*
A. Into the vermilion and white roll.
B. Immediately deep to the mucosa or vermilion.
C. Immediately deep to the mucosa only.
D. Intramuscular.
E. Deep to the muscle.

COMPLICATIONS

9. *Which of the following is the most common potential complication in fat grafting to the face?*
A. Hematoma.
B. Infection.
C. Blindness.
D. Skin necrosis.
E. Inaccurate volume.

COMPLICATIONS

10. *Although rare, blindness is the most feared potential complication in fat grafting to the face. This complication generally occurs from induction of fat (or filler) around which artery?*
A. Lateral nasal artery.
B. Infraorbital artery.
C. Supratrochlear artery.
D. Superior labial artery.
E. Transverse facial artery.

COMPLICATIONS

11. *Which of the following potential complications is more likely to be associated with direct trauma rather than intraarterial fat injection?*
A. Severe pain.
B. Skin loss.
C. Blindness.
D. Petechia.
E. Numbness.

FATE OF TRANSPLANTED ADIPOCYTES

12. *How long can adipose-derived stromal cells remain viable in vitro?*
A. 4 hours.
B. 1 day.
C. 3 days.
D. 7 days.
E. 12 days.

Answers

HARVEST SITE

1. *Which harvest site has been shown to have the best fat longevity?*

E. There is no difference based on donor site.

There is no difference of grafted fat longevity based on donor site. Thus, fat should be harvested from sites that enhance body contour and are easily accessible in the supine position. The most common sites used are the abdomen and medial thigh. Other sites include the flanks, knees, lateral thighs, and anterior thighs.[1,2,3]

REFERENCES

1. Coleman SR. Structural Fat Grafting. New York: Thieme Publishers; 2004
2. Coleman SR. Facial recontouring with lipostructure. Clin Plast Surg 1997;24:347
3. Coleman SR. Long-term survival of fat transplants: controlled demonstrations. Aesthetic Plast Surg 1995;19:421

FAT PROCESSING

2. *According to the Coleman technique of fat preparation, how long the fat should be centrifuged?*

A. 3 minutes at 3000 rpm.

Using the Coleman technique of fat preparation, a syringe is filled, the cannula is removed, and a dual-function Luer-Lok plug is used to cap the syringe. This is then tightly capped, the plunger is removed, and the syringe is placed in a centrifuge for 3 minutes at 3000 rpm. After centrifugation, the harvested fat will separate into three layers.[1,2,3,4]

REFERENCES

1. Coleman SR. Structural Fat Grafting. New York: Thieme Publishers; 2004
2. Coleman SR. Facial recontouring with lipostructure. Clin Plast Surg 1997;24:347
3. Coleman SR. Long-term survival of fat transplants: controlled demonstrations. Aesthetic Plast Surg 1995;19:421
4. Coleman SR. Structural fat grafts: the ideal filler? Clin Plast Surg 2001;28:111

FAT PROCESSING

3. *Following centrifugation, the lipoaspirate separates into three layers. Which layer contains potentially viable parcels of fat?*

B. Middle level.

After centrifugation, the harvested fat will separate into three layers (**Fig. 23.1**). The upper level contains oil from ruptured fat cells, the middle level contains potentially viable parcels of tissue, and the lowest level contacts blood, water, and lidocaine.[1,2,3,4]

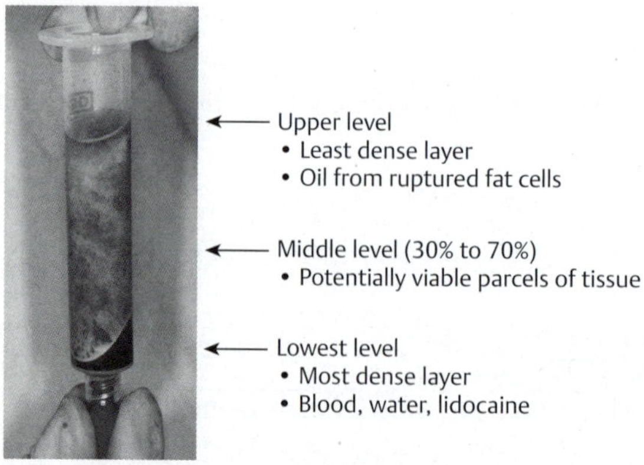

Fig. 23.1 Three different layers of harvested fat after centrifugation. (Source: Centrifugation. In: Coleman S, Mazzola R, Pu L, ed. Fat Injection: From Filling to Regeneration. 2nd Edition. New York: Thieme; 2017.)

REFERENCES

1. Coleman SR. Structural Fat Grafting. New York: Thieme Publishers; 2004
2. Coleman SR. Facial recontouring with lipostructure. Clin Plast Surg 1997;24:347
3. Coleman SR. Long-term survival of fat transplants: controlled demonstrations. Aesthetic Plast Surg 1995;19:421
4. Coleman SR. Structural fat grafts: the ideal filler? Clin Plast Surg 2001;28:111

FAT PLACEMENT

4. *To strengthen soft tissue projection over bony prominences, fat should be placed in which of the following levels?*

B. Supraperiosteal.

The level of fat placement is important and dictated by the goal. To strengthen soft tissue projection over bony prominences, fat should be injected deep against the bone or cartilage in a supraperiosteal location.[1,2,3]

REFERENCES

1. Coleman SR. Structural Fat Grafting. New York: Thieme Publishers; 2004
2. Coleman SR. Long-term survival of fat transplants: controlled demonstrations. Aesthetic Plast Surg 1995;19:421
3. Coleman SR. Structural fat grafts: the ideal filler? Clin Plast Surg 2001;28:111

EDEMA

5. *According to the Coleman technique description, when is the patient allowed to start massaging the recipient site after the procedure?*

C. 2 weeks after surgery.

Edema is one of the most common problems after fat grafting to the face. In addition to elevation and cold therapy that should be performed in the first 48 hours, patients are encouraged to massage the recipient site. That being said, this is not recommended until 2 weeks after the procedure. Further, fat placed in folds or grooves should not be massaged.[1]

REFERENCE

1. Coleman SR. Structural Fat Grafting. New York: Thieme Publishers; 2004

EDEMA

6. *According to the Coleman technique, when is the patient allowed to start massaging the donor site after the procedure?*

A. Immediately after surgery.

In comparison to the recipient site, which should not be massaged until 2 weeks after surgery, Dr. Coleman encourages massage of the donor site as soon as tenderness in the area permits it. Thus, the patients can start immediately after surgery to help with edema.[1]

REFERENCE

1. Coleman SR. Structural Fat Grafting. New York: Thieme Publishers; 2004

EDEMA

7. *How long should you tell a patient to expect postoperative edema of the face following fat grafting?*

D. Greater than 4 months after surgery.

As previously mentioned, edema is one of the most common problems. Patients should be informed preoperatively about what to expect. Patients will have the worst swelling on postoperative day 3 but will continue to have some varying degrees of swelling even at the 4-month period. Thus, patients should be prepared for prolonged swelling following fat grafting to the face.[1]

REFERENCE

1. Coleman SR. Structural Fat Grafting. New York: Thieme Publishers; 2004

TREATMENT OF SELECT AREAS

8. *When treating the lips, what layer is the preferred layer for fat injection?*

B. Immediately deep to the mucosa or vermilion.

When fat grafting to the lips, fat needs to be precisely placed to achieve a favorable result. Specifically, the fat needs be injected in the plane immediately deep to the mucosa or vermilion. Placement of fat within the muscle only creates a fat lip. Fat should not be placed deep to the muscle given the location of the blood supply of the orbicularis oris (**Fig. 23.2**).[1,2]

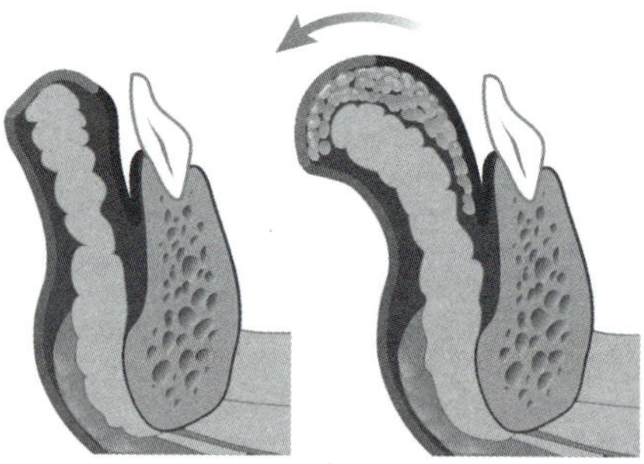

Fig. 23.2 Fat used for lip augmentation should be placed with precise accuracy in the plane immediately deep to the mucosa or vermilion and should not be infiltrated into the muscle. (Source: Coleman SR, Mazzola RF, Pu LL, eds. Fat Injection: From Filling to Regeneration, 2nd ed. New York, NY: Thieme; 2018.)

REFERENCES

1. Coleman SR. Structural Fat Grafting. New York: Thieme Publishers; 2004
2. Coleman SR. Facial recontouring with lipostructure. Clin Plast Surg 1997;24:347

COMPLICATIONS

9. *Which of the following is the most common potential complication in fat grafting to the face?*

E. Inaccurate volume.

The most common potential complication in fat grafting to the face is inaccurate volume causing undercorrection or overcorrection. Some surgeons will slightly overfill with the idea that not all of the fat will be viable postoperatively while others would rather undercorrect and fat graft again than manage an overcorrected face.[1,2,3,4,5]

REFERENCES

1. Coleman SR. Structural Fat Grafting. New York: Thieme Publishers; 2004
2. Coleman SR. Facial recontouring with lipostructure. Clin Plast Surg 1997;24:347
3. Coleman SR. Long-term survival of fat transplants: controlled demonstrations. Aesthetic Plast Surg 1995;19:421
4. Coleman SR. Structural fat grafts: the ideal filler? Clin Plast Surg 2001;28:111
5. Coleman SR. Hand rejuvenation with structural fat grafting. Plast Reconstr Surg 2002;110:1731; discussion 1745

COMPLICATIONS

10. *Although rare, blindness is the most feared potential complication in fat grafting to the face. This complication generally occurs from induction of fat (or filler) around which artery?*

C. Supratrochlear artery.

Although rare, arterial occlusion is the most feared potential complication of fat grafting to the face. This will result in excruciating pain followed by skin loss. More importantly, this complication is even more devastating in the periorbita as central arterial injection can cause blindness. This complication generally occurs from induction of fat (or filler) around the supratrochlear, supraorbital, and dorsal nasal arteries.[1,2,3,4,5]

REFERENCES

1. Coleman SR. Structural Fat Grafting. New York: Thieme Publishers; 2004
2. Coleman SR. Facial recontouring with lipostructure. Clin Plast Surg 1997;24:347
3. Coleman SR. Long-term survival of fat transplants: controlled demonstrations. Aesthetic Plast Surg 1995;19:421
4. Coleman SR. Structural fat grafts: the ideal filler? Clin Plast Surg 2001;28:111
5. Coleman SR. Hand rejuvenation with structural fat grafting. Plast Reconstr Surg 2002;110:1731; discussion 1745

COMPLICATIONS

11. ***Which of the following potential complications is more likely to be associated with direct trauma rather than intraarterial fat injection?***

E. Numbness.

Intra-arterial injection is a feared complication of surgeons who perform fat grafting to the face. Severe pain, skin/soft tissue loss, and blindness are all documented complications from arterial occlusion. Intra-arterial injection of fat will not affect the sensory nervous distribution; this would only occur through direct trauma to a sensory nerve. A strong understanding of vascular anatomy should be obtained prior to performing these procedures and great caution should be taken prior to injecting in the periorbita.[1,2,3,4,5]

REFERENCES

1. Coleman SR. Structural Fat Grafting. New York: Thieme Publishers; 2004
2. Coleman SR. Facial recontouring with lipostructure. Clin Plast Surg 1997;24:347
3. Coleman SR. Long-term survival of fat transplants: controlled demonstrations. Aesthetic Plast Surg 1995;19:421
4. Coleman SR. Structural fat grafts: the ideal filler? Clin Plast Surg 2001;28:111
5. Coleman SR. Hand rejuvenation with structural fat grafting. Plast Reconstr Surg 2002;110:1731; discussion 1745

FATE OF TRANSPLANTED ADIPOCYTES

12. ***How long can adipose-derived stromal cells remain viable in vitro?***

C. 3 days.

In vitro studies have shown that transplanted adipocytes are susceptible to an ischemic death, whereas adipose-derived stromal cells can remain viable for 3 days. It has been shown that most adipocytes die on day 1, with some survivors. After 7 days of grafting, there is an increase in viable adipocytes, suggesting that repair and regeneration of adipocytes occurs during this time period.[1,2,3,4,5,6,7]

REFERENCES

1. Eto H, Kato H, Suga H, et al. The fate of adipocytes after nonvascularized fat grafting: evidence of early death and replacement of adipocytes. Plast Reconstr Surg 2012;129:1081
2. Coleman SR. Structural Fat Grafting. New York: Thieme Publishers; 2004
3. Coleman SR. Facial recontouring with lipostructure. Clin Plast Surg 1997;24:347
4. Coleman SR. Long-term survival of fat transplants: controlled demonstrations. Aesthetic Plast Surg 1995;19:421
5. Coleman SR. Structural fat grafts: the ideal filler? Clin Plast Surg 2001;28:111
6. Coleman SR. Hand rejuvenation with structural fat grafting. Plast Reconstr Surg 2002;110:1731; discussion 1745
7. Eto H, Kato H, Suga H, et al. The fate of adipocytes after nonvascularized fat grafting: evidence of early death and replacement of adipocytes. Plast Reconstr Surg 2012;129:1081–1092

24. Treatment of Prominent Veins

Sammy Sinno, Jeremie Oliver Piña
See *Essentials of Aesthetic Surgery*, pp. 313–320

TREATMENT OPTIONS

1. *What is the standard preoperative workup for an asymptomatic patient desiring sclerotherapy of varicose veins?*

A. Ultrasound.
B. D-dimer blood test.
C. CT scan.
D. Venous duplex imaging.
E. Physical examination only.

TREATMENT OPTIONS

2. *For symptomatic patients, why is it necessary to obtain venous duplex imaging prior to treatment?*

A. Decrease risk of pulmonary embolism.
B. Identify superficial or deep venous insufficiency.
C. Identify vascular calcification or plaque.
D. To measure vessel patency.
E. Symptomatic patients do not require preoperative venous duplex imaging.

TREATMENT OPTIONS

3. *When both superficial and deep veins are affected, in which order should you treat them?*

A. Superficial first, then deep.
B. Deep first, then superficial.
C. Treat simultaneously with multiple injectors.
D. Does not matter.
E. Treatment of superficial veins may obviate the need for deep vein treatment.

TREATMENT OPTIONS

4. *How should the surgeon counsel a patient about expectations of sclerotherapy treatment for varicose veins and telangiectasias?*

A. It is reasonable to expect 100% clearance of treated varicose veins and telangiectasias after 4 to 6 treatment sessions.
B. Sun exposure after sclerotherapy will complement treatment and enhance results.
C. Compressive stockings are recommended for the morbidly obese.
D. New telangiectasias will tend to occur over time, thus annual maintenance treatments are recommended.
E. Exercise immediately after treatment sessions will help maintain results.

TREATMENT OPTIONS

5. *Which of the following sclerosing agents carries the lowest risk of telangiectatic matting?*

A. Sodium tetradecyl sulfate.
B. Polidocanol.
C. Hypertonic saline.
D. Normal saline.
E. Glycerin.

TREATMENT OPTIONS

6. ***Which of the following potential complications of sclerotherapy treatment for prominent veins has the highest relative risk of occurrence?***
   A. Ulceration.
   B. Telangiectatic matting.
   C. Hyperpigmentation.
   D. Skin necrosis.
   E. Thrombophlebitis.

TREATMENT OPTIONS

7. ***In which of the following scenarios should you consider laser therapy for telangiectatic veins rather than sclerotherapy?***
   A. Telangiectasias are too small or superficial for needle cannula diameter.
   B. Patient has a history of a deep vein thrombosis.
   C. Patients who have a Fitzpatrick score of III to VI.
   D. Patient has a history of phlebitis.
   E. Deep telangiectatic veins.

TREATMENT OPTIONS

8. ***When treating prominent veins with laser therapy, what is the maximum number of attempts over the same area that can be safely made before risking burns?***
   A. Single pass.
   B. Two.
   C. Three.
   D. Five.
   E. There is no maximum.

TREATMENT OPTIONS

9. ***How does the postoperative care differ in patients who undergo laser therapy compared to sclerotherapy for prominent veins?***
   A. No differences exist.
   B. Avoidance of sun exposure to treatment areas is heavily advised.
   C. Repeat therapy is typically needed.
   D. Immediate return to normal daily activities.
   E. Bed rest for 1 to 2 days.

TREATMENT OPTIONS

10. ***Before proceeding with laser treatment of varicose veins in a patient with Fitzpatrick skin type IV, what preoperative assessment should be documented?***
    A. Complete blood count (CBC).
    B. Skin biopsy.
    C. Wood's lamp test.
    D. Test spot.
    E. Proceed without preoperative evaluation.

TREATMENT OPTIONS

11. ***Which of the following varicose vein treatment options yields the highest reported recurrence rates?***
    A. Sclerotherapy.
    B. Laser.
    C. Surgery.
    D. Nonendothermal endovenous ablation.
    E. Radiofrequency ablation (RFA).

Answers

TREATMENT OPTIONS

1. ***What is the standard preoperative workup for an asymptomatic patient desiring sclerotherapy of varicose veins?***

   E. Physical examination only.

   Asymptomatic patients presenting for cosmetic sclerotherapy treatment of varicose veins do not require further preoperative workup beyond a standard physical examination prior to administering treatment.[1,2]

REFERENCES

1. Schwartz L, Maxwell H. Sclerotherapy for lower limb telangiectasias. Cochrane Database Syst Rev 2011;18: CD008826
2. Tisi PV, Beverley C, Rees A. Injection sclerotherapy for varicose veins. Cochrane Database Syst Rev 2006;(4): CD001732

TREATMENT OPTIONS

2. ***For symptomatic patients, why is it necessary to obtain venous duplex imaging prior to treatment?***

   C. Identify vascular calcification or plaque.

   While asymptomatic patients do not require preoperative diagnostic workup beyond a standard physical examination, *symptomatic* patients should undergo venous duplex imaging to identify potential presence of superficial or deep venous insufficiency.[1,2]

REFERENCES

1. Callam MJ. Epidemiology of varicose veins. Br J Surg 1994;81:167
2. Chiesa R, Marone EM, Limoni C, et al. Chronic venous disorders: correlation between visible signs, symptoms, and presence of functional disease. J Vasc Surg 2007;46:322

TREATMENT OPTIONS

3. ***When both superficial and deep veins are affected, in which order should you treat them?***

   B. Deep first, then superficial.

   Larger underlying reticular varicose veins should first be treated with sclerotherapy before more superficial, telangiectatic vessels are addressed.[1,2,3]

REFERENCES

1. Callam MJ. Epidemiology of varicose veins. Br J Surg 1994;81:167
2. Chiesa R, Marone EM, Limoni C, et al. Chronic venous disorders: correlation between visible signs, symptoms, and presence of functional disease. J Vasc Surg 2007;46:322
3. Langer RD, Ho E, Denenberg JO, et al. Relationships between symptoms and venous disease: the San Diego population study. Arch Intern Med 2005;165:1420

TREATMENT OPTIONS

4. ***How should the surgeon counsel a patient about expectations of sclerotherapy treatment for varicose veins and telangiectasias?***

   D. New telangiectasias will tend to occur over time, thus annual maintenance treatments are recommended.

   In the sclerotherapy consultation, it is important to inform patients that new spider veins will tend to recur over time and annual maintenance treatments are encouraged.[1,2,3,4]

REFERENCES

1. Chiesa R, Marone EM, Limoni C, et al. Chronic venous disorders: correlation between visible signs, symptoms, and presence of functional disease. J Vasc Surg 2007;46:322
2. Langer RD, Ho E, Denenberg JO, et al. Relationships between symptoms and venous disease: the San Diego population study. Arch Intern Med 2005;165:1420
3. Chang CJ, Chua JJ. Endovenous laser photocoagulation (EVLP) for varicose veins. Lasers Surg Med 2002;31:257
4. Schwartz L, Maxwell H. Sclerotherapy for lower limb telangiectasias. Cochrane Database Syst Rev 2011;18: CD008826

TREATMENT OPTIONS

5. *Which of the following sclerosing agents carries the lowest risk of telangiectatic matting?*

E. Glycerin.

Among those listed, glycerin (ideally 72%) carries the lowest risk of associated telangiectatic matting, as well as ulceration and necrosis. However, the disadvantages of glycerin include potential contact sensitivity, urethral colic, hematuria (although rare), as well as the fact that it is off-label for treatment of prominent veins (**Table 24.1**).[1,2,3]

Table 24.1 *Common Sclerosing Agents for the Treatment of Prominent Veins*

Agent	Vessel Size (mm)	Concentration (%)	Volume (mL)	Maximum Dose	Advantages	Disadvantages
Sodium tetradecyl sulfate	0.3–1 1–3 3–5 >5	0.1–0.25 0.25–0.5 0.5–1 1–3	0.25 0.5 0.5–1 1–2	10 mL of 3%	Less telangiectatic matting	Allergy Hyperpigmentation at high concentrations Ulceration/ necrosis
Polidocanol	**<0.5** 0.5–1 **1–3**	0.25 0.5 1	0.1–0.3 0.1–0.3 0.1–0.3	2 mg/kg	Painless Nontoxic Rare ulceration No necrosis	Allergy Telangiectatic matting Hyperpigmentation
Hypertonic saline	**<0.5** 0.5–1 1–3	11.7 11.7 23.4	0.25 0.5 0.5–1	None	No allergy	Pain Muscle cramping Ulceration/ necrosis Hyperpigmentation
Glycerin	<1	25–72	0.25	10 mL of 72%	No matting No ulceration No necrosis	Contact sensitivity Urethral colic Hematuria (rare) Off-label, not FDA approved

REFERENCES

1. Schwartz L, Maxwell H. Sclerotherapy for lower limb telangiectasias. Cochrane Database Syst Rev 2011;18: CD008826
2. Tisi PV, Beverley C, Rees A. Injection sclerotherapy for varicose veins. Cochrane Database Syst Rev 2006; CD001732
3. Leach BC, Goldman MP. Comparative trial between sodium tetradecyl sulfate and glycerin in the treatment of telangiectatic leg veins. Dermatol Surg 2003;29:612; discussion 615

TREATMENT OPTIONS

6. *Which of the following potential complications of sclerotherapy treatment for prominent veins has the highest relative risk of occurrence?*

C. Hyperpigmentation.

Hyperpigmentation, caused by deposition of hemosiderin within the treated skin areas, has a relative occurrence rate of 30% in patients undergoing sclerotherapy; however, this tends to be transient, resolving spontaneously in 80% of patients within 2 years of final treatment. Comparatively, the risk of ulceration is between 1 and 5% (usually small, heals with home wound care within 4–6 weeks), and the risk of telangiectatic matting is about 15 to 24% (also transient, resolving within 3–12 months).[1]

REFERENCE

1. Gillet JL, Guedes JM, Guex JJ, et al. Side-effects and complications of foam sclerotherapy of the great and small saphenous veins: a controlled multicentre prospective study including 1,025 patients. Phlebology 2009;24:131

TREATMENT OPTIONS

7. *In which of the following scenarios should you consider laser therapy for telangiectatic veins rather than sclerotherapy?*

A. Telangiectasias are too small or superficial for needle cannula diameter.

There are certain circumstances under which the surgeon should treat telangiectatic veins with laser therapy rather than sclerosing agents. These include the following: the patient does not tolerate sclerotherapy well or has already tried and failed to respond to treatment; superficial telangiectatic veins are too small in diameter for sclerotherapy needle; the patient is too afraid of the needle to undergo treatment; history of acute venous thrombosis or phlebitis; and pregnancy. Other relative contraindications include diabetes mellitus, peripheral arterial disease, as well as Fitzpatrick skin types III to VI.[1]

REFERENCE

1. McCoppin HH, Hovenic WW, Wheeland RG. Laser treatment of superficial leg veins: a review. Dermatol Surg 2011;37:729

TREATMENT OPTIONS

8. *When treating prominent veins with laser therapy, what is the maximum number of attempts over the same area that can be safely made before risking burns?*

C. Three.

As a preventative technique to avoid risk of burning the skin, the surgeon should avoid exceeding a maximum of three attempts passing over the same area with laser therapy of prominent veins.[1,2,3,4]

REFERENCES

1. Munavalli GS,Weiss RA. Complications of sclerotherapy. Semin Cutan Med Surg 2007;26:22
2. Gillet JL, Guedes JM, Guex JJ, et al. Side-effects and complications off sclerotherapy of the great and small saphenous veins: a controlled multicentre prospective study including 1,025 patients. Phlebology 2009;24:131
3. McCoppin HH, Hovenic WW, Wheel and RG. Laser treatment of superficial leg veins: a review. Dermatol Surg 2011;37:729
4. Eremia S, Li C, Umar SH. Aside-by side comparative study of 1064 nm Nd:YAG, 810 nm diode and 755 nm alexandrite lasers for treatment of 0.3–3 mm leg veins. Dermatol Surg 2002;28:224

TREATMENT OPTIONS

9. *How does the postoperative care differ in patients who undergo laser therapy compared to sclerotherapy for prominent veins?*

D. Immediate return to normal daily activities.

Unlike in postoperative care for sclerotherapy (which requires compressive stockings and avoidance of exercise for 2–4 weeks), laser therapy allows patients to resume daily activities immediately.[1,2,3,4]

References

1. Hamahata A, Yamaki T, Sakurai H. Outcomes of ultrasound-guided foam sclerotherapy for varicose veins of the lower extremities: a single center experience. Dermatol Surg 2001;37:804
2. Eremia S, Li C,Umar SH.A side-by-side comparative study of 1064 nmNd:YAG, 810 nm diode and 755 nm alexandrite lasers for treatment of 0.3–3 mm leg veins. Dermatol Surg 2002;28:224
3. Chen JZ, Alexiades-Armenakas MR, Bernstein LJ, et al.Two randomized, double-blind, placebo-controlled studies evaluating the S-Caine Peel for induction of local anesthesia before long- pulsed Nd:YAG laser therapy for leg veins. Dermatol Surg 2003;29:1012
4. Desmyttère J, Grard C, Wassmer B, et al. Endovenous 980-nm laser treatment of saphenous veins in a series of 500 patients. J Vasc Surg 2007;46:1242

TREATMENT OPTIONS

10. ***Before proceeding with laser treatment of varicose veins in a patient with Fitzpatrick skin type IV, what preoperative assessment should be documented?***

D. Test spot.

Given the heightened risk of hyperpigmentation (can be transient) and hypopigmentation (more typically permanent), a test spot should be performed before proceeding with laser therapy on patients with Fitzpatrick skin types III to VI.[1]

Reference

1. McCoppin HH, Hovenic WW, Wheeland RG. Laser treatment of superficial leg veins: a review. Dermatol Surg 2011;37:729

TREATMENT OPTIONS

11. ***Which of the following varicose vein treatment options yields the highest reported recurrence rates?***

C. Surgery.

Of the options listed, surgical management of varicose veins has largely been replaced by less-invasive methods of treatment (for varicose veins <1.5 cm diameter), as surgical techniques are associated with a 20 to 28% recurrence rate of varicose veins.[1,2]

References

1. Ravi R, Trayler EA, Barrett DA, et al. Endovenous thermal ablation of superficial venous insufficiency of the lower extremity: single-center experience with 3000 limbs treated in a 7-year period. J Endovasc Ther 2009;16:500
2. Merchant RF, Pichot O; Closure Study Group. Long-term outcomes of endovenous radiofrequency obliteration of saphenous reflux as a treatment for superficial venous insufficiency. J Vasc Surg 2005;42:502; discussion 509

Part VI

Adjuncts to Aesthetic Surgery

25. Tissue Glues

Sammy Sinno, Jeremie Oliver Piña
See *Essentials of Aesthetic Surgery*, pp. 323–328

FIBRIN SEALANT

1. *In addition to being a tissue sealant, fibrin is also used in aesthetic surgery as a ____ and ____.*

A. Anticoagulant and adhesive.
B. Hemostat and adhesive.
C. Lubricant and hemostat.
D. Emollient and adhesive.
E. Hemostat and synthetic capsule.

FIBRIN SEALANT

2. *Which of the following is a proven advantage (through multiple double-blind, randomized, controlled trials) of the use of fibrin sealant in rhytidectomy?*

A. Significantly reduced drainage output on fibrin sealant side compared to control.
B. Significantly reduced hematoma rates.
C. Significantly less postoperative edema.
D. Significantly less postoperative ecchymosis.
E. Significantly reduced seroma rates.

FIBRIN SEALANT

3. *Which of the following is true regarding fibrin sealants in abdominoplasty?*

A. Fibrin sealant is more effective at achieving closure than quilting sutures alone.
B. Seroma formation is significantly lower when fibrin sealant is applied compared to either drains or quilting sutures.
C. Seroma formation is significantly greater with fibrin sealant compared to both drain and quilting sutures.
D. Fibrin sealant is only helpful when achieving closure of a fleur-de-lis abdominoplasty technique.
E. There is no evidence to support its efficacy.

FIBRIN SEALANT

4. *What is a potential disadvantage of using a fibrin sealant–only technique in upper blepharoplasty?*

A. Higher likelihood of milia formation.
B. Slightly higher risk of conjunctivitis.
C. Irritation/allergic reaction.
D. Potential for wound separation.
E. More swelling postoperatively.

CYANOACRYLATES

5. *What is a relative disadvantage of using cyanoacrylate glue for wound closure compared to fibrin sealant?*

A. Cyanoacrylate is less effective for larger wounds.
B. Cyanoacrylate takes more time to polymerize compared to fibrin sealant.
C. Cyanoacrylates have been associated with foreign body reactions.
D. Cyanoacrylates have not been associated with carcinogenicity.
E. Cyanoacrylates have not been associated with tissue necrosis.

CYANOACRYLATES

6. *When cyanoacrylates are applied to clean, well-approximated, tension-free wound closures, how do they compare to standard monofilament suture closure?*

A. Significantly lower cosmetic score.
B. Higher cost.
C. Lower physician and assistant satisfaction with use.
D. More cost-effective.
E. Significantly slower closure time.

CYANOACRYLATES

7. *Which of the following is a major potential complication of utilizing bovine tissue sealant products?*

A. Infection.
B. Wound dehiscence.
C. Bloodborne pathogen risk (i.e., viral, prion).
D. Greater risk of edema.
E. Increased operative time.

Answers

FIBRIN SEALANT

1. *In addition to being a tissue sealant, fibrin is also used in aesthetic surgery as a ____ and ____.*

B. Hemostat and adhesive.

Fibrin tissue sealant, also known by the trade name Artiss (Baxter), is approved by the FDA as a hemostat, adhesive, and sealant. Its mechanism of action as a hemostat involves polymerization through reacting with fibrinogen and thrombin, which eventually forms a clot that degrades within 10 to 14 days.[1,2]

REFERENCES

1. Spotnitz WD. Fibrin sealant: past, present, and future: a brief review. World J Surg 2010;34:632
2. Buchta C, Hedrich HC, Macher M, et al. Biochemical characterization of autologous fibrin sealants produced by CryoSeal and Vivostat in comparison to the homologous fibrin sealant product Tissucol/Tisseel. Biomaterials 2005;26:6233

FIBRIN SEALANT

2. *Which of the following is a proven advantage (through multiple double-blind, randomized, controlled trials) of the use of fibrin sealant in rhytidectomy?*

A. Significantly reduced drainage output on fibrin sealant side compared to control.

The only example from those listed which has been repeatedly shown in high-powered studies[1,2,3] is the association between fibrin sealant use and a significantly reduced drainage output volume compared to control side of rhytidectomy (which did not use any tissue glue). All of the other choices are anecdotally supported by some, but have not been substantiated to the extent as choice A.[1,2,3]

REFERENCES

1. Hester TR Jr, Shire JR, Nguyen DB, et al. Randomized, controlled, phase 3 study to evaluate the safety and efficacy of fibrin sealant VH S/D 4 s-apr (Artiss) to improve tissue adherence in subjects undergoing rhytidectomy. Aesthet Surg J 2013;33:487
2. Oliver DW, Hamilton SA, Figle AA, et al. A prospective, randomized, double-blind trial of the use of fibrin sealant for face lifts. Plast Reconstr Surg 2001;108:2101
3. Marchac D, Greensmith AL. Early postoperative efficacy of fibrin glue in face lifts: a prospective randomized trial. Plast Reconstr Surg 2005;115:911

FIBRIN SEALANT

3. *Which of the following is true regarding fibrin sealants in abdominoplasty?*

C. Seroma formation is significantly greater with fibrin sealant compared to both drain and quilting sutures.

Although data seems to be contradictory depending on the study, one prospective analysis demonstrated fibrin sealant to possibly be inferior to surgical drains or quilting sutures.[1] This study observed a significantly lower rate of seroma formation in association with drain (13.9 mL) and quilting suture (16.1 mL) groups compared with the fibrin sealant (53.6 mL) group ($p < 0.05$).[1]

REFERENCE

1. Bercial ME, Sabino Neto M, Calil JA, et al. Suction drains, quilting sutures, and fibrin sealant in the prevention of seroma formation in abdominoplasty: which is the best strategy? Aesthetic Plast Surg 2012;36:370

FIBRIN SEALANT

4. *What is a potential disadvantage of using a fibrin sealant–only technique in upper blepharoplasty?*

D. Potential for wound separation.

Although there is a small risk of wound separation in the "glue only" technique for upper blepharoplasty, when compared with standard suture techniques, the incidence of minor problems such as milia formation was lower.[1] This was shown to be an acceptable alternative or adjunct to sutures for closure in upper blepharoplasty.

REFERENCE

1. Mandel MA. Minimal suture blepharoplasty: closure of incisions with autologous fibrin glue. Aesthetic Plast Surg 1992;16:269

CYANOACRYLATES

5. *What is a relative disadvantage of using cyanoacrylate glue for wound closure compared to fibrin sealant?*

C. Cyanoacrylates have been associated with foreign body reactions.

Although fibrin sealant can safely be used internally within the wound bed, cyanoacrylates are *not* for internal use, as they have been associated with foreign body reactions, carcinogenicity, and tissue necrosis.[1]

REFERENCE

1. Toriumi DM, Raslan WF, Friedman M, Tardy ME. Histotoxicity of cyanoacrylate tissue adhesives. A comparative study. Arch Otolaryngol Head Neck Surg 1990;116:546

CYANOACRYLATES

6. *When cyanoacrylates are applied to clean, well-approximated, tension-free wound closures, how do they compare to standard monofilament suture closure?*

D. More cost-effective.

Given the clean, well-approximated, tension-free application of cyanoacrylates, they have been validated by multiple prospective randomized trials in plastic surgery procedures to have equivalent rates of wound infection, dehiscence, and cosmesis compared to standard suture closure methods, with an additional advantage of greater cost-effectiveness through decreased operative times and elimination of suture removal or secondary dressing requirements.[1,2,3,4]

REFERENCES

1. Gennari R, Rotmensz N, Ballardini B, et al. A prospective, randomized, controlled clinical trial of tissue adhesive (2-octylcyanoacrylate) versus standard wound closure in breast surgery. Surgery 2004;136:593
2. Scott GR, Carson CL, Borah GL. Dermabond skin closures for bilateral reduction mammaplasties: a review of 255 consecutive cases. Plast Reconstr Surg 2007;120:1460
3. Greene D, Koch RJ, Goode, RL. Efficacy of octyl-2-cyanoacrylate tissue glue in blepharoplasty. A prospective controlled study of wound-healing characteristics. Arch Facial Plast Surg 1999;1:292
4. Nipshagen MD, Hage JJ, Beckman WH. Use of 2-octyl-cyanoacrylate skin adhesive (Dermabond) for wound closure following reduction mammaplasty: a prospective, randomized intervention study. Plast Reconstr Surg 2008;122:10

CYANOACRYLATES

7. *Which of the following is a major potential complication of utilizing bovine tissue sealant products?*

C. Bloodborne pathogen risk (i.e., viral, prion).

Commercial preparations of tissue sealants carry the risk of spreading bloodborne pathogens (i.e., viral, prions) upon application.[1] All standard precautions for patient and staff safety must be followed.

REFERENCE

1. O'Grady KM, Agrawal A, Bhattacharyya TK, et al. An evaluation of fibrin tissue adhesive concentration and application thickness on skin graft survival. Laryngoscope 2000;110:1931

26. Fixation Devices

Sammy Sinno, Jeremie Oliver Piña
See *Essentials of Aesthetic Surgery*, pp. 329–334

FIXATION OF BROWLIFTS, MIDFACE LIFTS, AND NECKLIFTS

1. *After placement of a polylactic acid/polyglycolic acid (Endotine) tack in browlift surgery, how long will it take for the tack to be completely absorbed?*
A. 3 months.
B. 6 months.
C. 12 months.
D. 18 months.
E. 24 months.

FIXATION OF BROWLIFTS, MIDFACE LIFTS, AND NECKLIFTS

2. *Which of the following is a relative disadvantage of the polylactic acid/polyglycolic acid tack technique in browlift surgery?*
A. Steep learning curve for surgeons to adapt.
B. Device remains palpable and tender prior to absorption.
C. Cannot be used in conjunction with endoscope.
D. Adds substantially to operative time.
E. Very high infection rate.

FIXATION OF BROWLIFTS, MIDFACE LIFTS, AND NECKLIFTS

3. *The Ultratine tack has been shown to be more rapidly absorbed compared to the Endotine tack. Which of the following potential implications of this modification could impact surgical outcomes?*
A. Decreased infection risk.
B. Potential loss of fixation.
C. Less inflammation.
D. Decreased need for revision surgery.
E. Decreased cost of procedure.

FIXATION OF BROWLIFTS, MIDFACE LIFTS, AND NECKLIFTS

4. *When considering the use of Endotine ribbon as an adjunct for ptosis correction at the cervicomental junction of a patient with thin soft tissue in the face and neck, which of the following is an important potential long-term result of placement of this device?*
A. Wound dehiscence.
B. Tenderness/pain at placement site after 12 months postoperatively.
C. Potential for palpability of ribbon.
D. Reversal of cervicomental ptosis.
E. Overcorrection of ptosis.

FIXATION OF BROWLIFTS, MIDFACE LIFTS, AND NECKLIFTS

5. *Which of the following differentiates the Mini-Mitek soft tissue anchor (Ethicon) from Endotine fixation devices?*
A. It is less applicable to facial aesthetic surgery.
B. Potential for the device to be palpable through thin soft tissue areas.
C. Much more expensive.
D. Does not absorb.
E. Low learning curve for surgeons to adapt to practice.

FIXATION OF BROWLIFTS, MIDFACE LIFTS, AND NECKLIFTS

6. ***Which of the following pertains to the use of the V-Loc barbed suture (Covidien)[1] compared to traditional suture in wound closure?***
   A. Decreased operative time.
   B. 10 to 15% longer scars through the "accordion effect."
   C. Increased risk of suture extrusion.
   D. Increased cost of the procedure.
   E. V-Loc 180 (Polyglyconate) has a shorter time to absorption.

FIXATION OF BROWLIFTS, MIDFACE LIFTS, AND NECKLIFTS

7. ***How does the Quill suture (Angiotech Pharmaceuticals)[1,2] differ from the V-Loc suture?***
   A. Quill suture is used in the closure of body contouring procedures.
   B. Quill suture is composed of both bioabsorbable and permanent material.
   C. Quill suture is a barbed suture.
   D. Quill suture is bidirectional.
   E. These two suture types do not differ functionally.

OUTCOMES

8. ***Despite its significant association with retention cysts, when comparing Ultratine vs. Endotine tacks in browlift surgery, the Ultratine tack has shown higher patient satisfaction scores compared to Endotine tack in browlift surgery. Which of the following is a potential reason for this finding?***
   A. Decreased cost with the Ultratine tack.
   B. Ultratine tack is 50% bioabsorbed by 4 months.
   C. Ultratine tack is 75% bioabsorbed by 18 months.
   D. Ultratine tack is 90% bioabsorbed by 24 months.
   E. Increased palpability.

Answers

FIXATION OF BROWLIFTS, MIDFACE LIFTS, AND NECKLIFTS

1. ***After placement of a polylactic acid/polyglycolic acid (Endotine) tack in browlift surgery, how long will it take for the tack to be completely absorbed?***

   C. 12 months.

   Endotine tacks (COAPT Systems)[1,2] are made of 82:18 ratio of polylactic acid/polyglycolic acid and are secured through the outer cortex of the cranium for fixation in browlift surgery. These materials are bioabsorbable; thus, they do not need to be removed. The degradation process is achieved through hydrolysis and enzymatic breakdown of (first) polyglycolic component and (second) polylactic acid component over a period of 12 months.

REFERENCES

1. Saltz R, Ohana B. Thirteen years of experience with the endoscopic midface lift. Aesthet Surg J 2012;32:927
2. Holzapfel AM, Mangat DS. Endoscopic forehead-lift using a bioabsorbable fixation device. Arch Facial Plast Surg 2004;6:389

FIXATION OF BROWLIFTS, MIDFACE LIFTS, AND NECKLIFTS

2. ***Which of the following is a relative disadvantage of the polylactic acid/polyglycolic acid tack technique in browlift surgery?***

   B. Device remains palpable and tender prior to absorption.

   Several advantages to utilizing Endotine tack technology in browlift surgery include the ability to achieve timely, direct fixation to the cranium and soft tissue through digital pressure, low learning curve for surgeons to apply the technique to their practice, capability to be used in conjunction with an endoscope, and bioabsorption of the device within 12 months of placement. However, the relative disadvantages include the added costs to the procedure for the device itself (not for extra time in the OR), *postoperative tenderness over the device and palpability until the device begins to absorb*, and the difficulty in application for temporal laxity and/or more severe cases of brow ptosis.[1]

REFERENCE

1. Cervelli V. An original application of the Endotine Ribbon device for brow lift. Plast Reconstr Surg 2009;124:1652

FIXATION OF BROWLIFTS, MIDFACE LIFTS, AND NECKLIFTS

3. ***The Ultratine tack has been shown to be more rapidly absorbed compared to the Endotine tack. Which of the following potential implications of this modification could impact surgical outcomes?***

   B. Potential loss of fixation.

   Although the Ultratine tack (COAPT Systems)[1,2,3] undergoes 50% absorption by 4 months, and 70% by 10 months postoperatively, the reported disadvantages compared to Endotine tack include the potential for loss of fixation point (likely given the faster absorptive action, allowing less time for soft tissue adhesion to device on outer cortex of cranium), as well as reports of inflammatory retention cysts requiring surgical correction and increasing costs of the procedure.

REFERENCES

1. Servat JJ, Black EH. A comparison of surgical outcomes with the use of 2 different biodegradable multipoint fixation devices for endoscopic forehead rejuvenation. Ophthal Plast Reconstr Surg 2012;28:401
2. Savar A, Shore J. Ultratine retention: report of a case. Ophthal Plast Reconstr Surg 2009;25:501
3. Apfelberg DB, Newman J, Graivier M, et al. Multispecialty contralateral study of clinical experience with the Ultratine forehead fixation device: evolution of the original Endotine device. Arch Facial Plast Surg 2008;10:280

FIXATION OF BROWLIFTS, MIDFACE LIFTS, AND NECKLIFTS

4. *When considering the use of Endotine ribbon as an adjunct for ptosis correction at the cervicomental junction of a patient with thin soft tissue in the face and neck, which of the following is an important potential long-term result of placement of this device?*

C. Potential for palpability of ribbon.

Although a useful adjunct for correction of cervicomental ptosis, in a patient with thin soft tissue the placement of an Endotine ribbon can potentially result in chronic palpability of the ribbon beneath the skin.[1,2,3]

REFERENCES

1. Knott PD, Newman J, Keller GS, et al. A novel bioabsorbable device for facial suspension and rejuvenation. Arch Facial Plast Surg 2009;11:129
2. Cervelli V. An original application of the Endotine ribbon device for brow lift. Plast Reconstr Surg 2009;124:1652
3. Bartsich S, Swartz KA, Spinelli HM. Lateral canthoplasty using the Mitek Anchor system. Aesthetic Plast Surg 2012;36:3

FIXATION OF BROWLIFTS, MIDFACE LIFTS, AND NECKLIFTS

5. *Which of the following differentiates the Mini-Mitek soft tissue anchor (Ethicon) from Endotine fixation devices?*

D. Does not absorb.

The Mini-Mitek anchor device, in contrast to Endotine fixation devices described previously, is a *permanent* implantable device. Otherwise, it is very applicable to facial aesthetic surgery, is relatively easy to use, and has a similar cost to other implantable fixation devices.[1,2]

REFERENCES

1. Cervelli V. An original application of the Endotine ribbon device for brow lift. Plast Reconstr Surg 2009;124:1652
2. Bartsich S, Swartz KA, Spinelli HM. Lateral canthoplasty using the Mitek Anchor system. Aesthetic Plast Surg 2012;36:3

FIXATION OF BROWLIFTS, MIDFACE LIFTS, AND NECKLIFTS

6. *Which of the following pertains to the use of the V-Loc barbed suture (Covidien)[1] compared to traditional suture in wound closure?*

A. Decreased operative time.

The V-Loc barbed suture has shown superior results in wound closure compared to traditional buried suture closure in that it shortens the operative time (and may reduce operative costs as a result), potentially shortens scar length from the "accordion effect" of barbed suture placement, evenly distributes tension along the wound closure, and has shown decreased numbers of suture extrusion during wound healing given the fewer number of buried knots in subcutaneous and dermal planes.[1] V-Loc 90 has an approximate time to absorption of 90 days whereas V-Loc 180 has an approximate time to absorption of 180 days.[1]

REFERENCE

1. Nguyen AT, Ritz M. Body contouring surgery with the V-loc suture. Plast Reconstr Surg 2011;128:332

FIXATION OF BROWLIFTS, MIDFACE LIFTS, AND NECKLIFTS

7. *How does the Quill suture (Angiotech Pharmaceuticals)[1,2] differ from the V-Loc suture?*

D. Quill suture is bidirectional.

While the V-Loc barbed suture is unidirectional and uses a loop at the end for fixation, the Quill barbed suture is bidirectional with a tapered needle at both ends of the suture. This differs functionally from other barbed suture in that suture is run starting in the mid-portion of the wound and running in both directions away from the mid-point, and finally either run back toward the midline or cut at the wound endpoint.[1,2]

REFERENCES

1. Hurwitz DJ, Reuben B. Quill barbed sutures in body contouring surgery: a 6-year comparison with running absorbable braided sutures. Aesthet Surg J 2013;33(3 Suppl):S44
2. Moya AP. Barbed sutures in body surgery. Aesthet Surg J 2013;33(3 Suppl):S57

OUTCOMES

8. *Despite its significant association with retention cysts, when comparing Ultratine vs. Endotine tacks in browlift surgery, the Ultratine tack has shown higher patient satisfaction scores compared to Endotine tack in browlift surgery. Which of the following is a potential reason for this finding?*

B. Ultratine tack is 50% bioabsorbed by 4 months.

Ultratine undergoes hydrolysis at a faster rate than Endotine. About 50% of the device is absorbed in 4 months, and 70% is absorbed in 10 months. This in turn makes it less palpable due to a faster absorption. Ultratine tack does show greater patient satisfaction outcomes in browlift surgery compared to Endotine, despite the significant association of required surgical correction of postoperative retention cysts.[1]

REFERENCE

1. Servat JJ, Black EH. A comparison of surgical outcomes with the use of 2 different biodegradable multipoint fixation devices for endoscopic forehead rejuvenation. Ophthal Plast Reconstr Surg 2012;28:401

27. Implants and Alloplasts (Nonbreast)

Nima Khosravani, Sammy Sinno, Jeremie Oliver Piña
See *Essentials of Aesthetic Surgery*, pp. 335–343

BIOMETRICAL IMPLANTS

1. ***What is the most important clinical aspect of any implanted biomaterial?***

A. Ability to visualize on radiographic imaging studies.
B. Cost-effectiveness.
C. Size.
D. Permanence.
E. Weight.

AUTOGRAFTS

2. ***Which of the following describes a methodology to help reduce inevitable free bone graft resorption and remodeling?***

A. Use of cancellous rather than cortical bone in free bone graft.
B. Placement of greater amounts of graft in recipient site.
C. Fixation of graft under mobile tissue recipient site.
D. Extensive dicing of graft material prior to implantation.
E. Addition of platelet-rich plasma to bone graft.

AUTOGRAFTS

3. ***What is a relative advantage of using cartilage as an autograft compared to free autologous bone graft?***

A. Easier to mold.
B. Does not warp over time.
C. Resorption is rare.
D. More potential donor sources.
E. Lower infection rate.

AUTOGRAFTS

4. ***What is the most worrisome potential complication of allogeneic graft material placement?***

A. Delayed hypersensitivity reaction.
B. Hypercoagulability.
C. Infection.
D. Graft failure.
E. Infectious disease transmission.

ALLOGENEIC MATERIALS

5. ***Which of the following is a considerable disadvantage of utilizing bi-layered acellular dermal regenerative templates (Integra)?***

A. Cannot be used on wounds greater than 20 cm.
B. Lacks matrix strength.
C. Cost.
D. Difficult to apply.
E. Cause congestion/fluid build-up behind graft.

ALLOGENEIC MATERIALS

6. *Which of the following has become the most commonly placed alloplastic material in aesthetic surgery (nonbreast)?*

A. Stainless steel.
B. High-density porous polyethylene.
C. Vitallium alloy.
D. Titanium alloy.
E. Hydroxyapatite.

ALLOGENEIC MATERIALS

7. *Which of the following is an important consideration pertaining to high-density porous polyethylene (Medpor) implants?*

A. Has a low fatigue tolerance compared to other implants.
B. Difficult to stabilize.
C. High propensity to resorb.
D. Is very radiodense.
E. Must soak in antibiotic solution prior to placement.

ALLOGENEIC MATERIALS

8. *Particularly with regard to aesthetic surgery, which of the following is a substantial disadvantage of using hydroxyapatite in the facial skeleton?*

A. Reports of high inflammatory burden on surrounding soft tissue.
B. High rate of infection.
C. Very difficult to remove.
D. High resorption rate.
E. Does not allow ingrowth of host tissue.

ALLOGENEIC MATERIALS

9. *Which of the following is considered a potential advantage of silicone facial implants compared to other alloplastic material types?*

A. Implant infections easily managed nonsurgically.
B. Allows in-growth of host tissue.
C. Becomes incorporated into facial skeleton.
D. Easily removed.
E. Hydrophilic nature.

Answers

BIOMETRICAL IMPLANTS

1. *What is the most important clinical aspect of any implanted biomaterial?*

D. Permanence.

Although there are a number of important ideal properties to consider of any implanted biomaterial (**Box 27.1**), the most important clinical aspect of an implanted biomaterial is its permanence, as this will determine the functional long-term relationship between the host and the implant.[1]

Box 27.1 Ideal Properties for Generic Biomaterial

Chemically inert
Biocompatible
Nonallergenic
Noncarcinogenic
Cost-effective
Sterilizable
Easy to handle
Radiopaque
Ability to stabilize

Reference

1. Rubin PJ, Yaremchuck MJ. Complications and toxicities of implantable biomaterials used in facial reconstructive and aesthetic surgery: a comprehensive review of the literature. Plast Reconstr Surg 1997;100:1336

AUTOGRAFTS

2. *Which of the following describes a methodology to help reduce inevitable free bone graft resorption and remodeling?*

C. Fixation of graft under mobile tissue recipient site.

Although all free bone grafts do inevitably undergo variable degrees of resorption and remodeling, there are a couple of techniques which can help maintain the volume of grafted material after placement. Cortical grafts have been shown to maintain their volume significantly better than their cancellous bone graft equivalents[1] and fixation of bone grafts under mobile recipient tissues reduces resorption rates.[1]

Reference

1. Ozaki W, Buchman SR. Volume maintenance of onlay grafts in the craniofacial skeleton: microarchitecture versus embryologic origin. Plast Reconstr Surg 1998;102:291

AUTOGRAFTS

3. *What is a relative advantage of using cartilage as an autograft compared to free autologous bone graft?*

C. Resorption is rare.

Compared to autologous free bone graft, cartilage graft has significantly lower rate of resorption.[1] Chondrocytes are capable of surviving within normal matrix without fibrous ingrowth or resorption risk,[2,3,4,5,6] which allows for great fidelity of graft take and permanence. However, cartilage does tend to warp[3,7,8] and can be difficult to mold given its flexibility compared to bone graft.

References

1. Vuyk HD, Adamson PA. Biomaterials in rhinoplasty. Clin Otolaryngol 1998;23:209
2. Lin KY, Bartlett SP, Yaremchuck MJ, et al. The effect of rigid fixation on the survival of onlay bone grafts: an experimental study. Plast Reconstr Surg 1990;86:449
3. Peer LA. Diced cartilage grafts. Arch Otolaryngol 1943;38:156
4. Peer LA. Cartilage grafting. Br J Plast Surg 1954;7:250

5. Ballantyne DL, Rees TD, Seidman I. Silicone fluid: response to massive subcutaneous injections of dimethylpolysiloxane fluid in animals. Plast Reconstr Surg 1965;36:330
6. Werther JR. Not seeing eye to eye about septal grafts for orbital fractures. J Oral Maxillofac Surg 1998;56:906
7. Antonyshyn O, Gruss JS, Galbraith DJ, et al. Complex orbital fractures: a critical analysis of immediate bone graft reconstruction. Ann Plast Surg 1989;22:220
8. Waite PD, Clantons JT. Orbital floor reconstruction with lyophilized dura. J Oral Maxillofac Surg 1988;46:727

AUTOGRAFTS

4. *What is the most worrisome potential complication of allogeneic graft material placement?*

E. Infectious disease transmission.

Although the other options are certainly potential complications of allogeneic graft material placement, the most worrisome is that of infectious disease (i.e., blood-borne pathogens) transmission. Careful sterilization techniques have evolved over time, but the risk still remains.[1]

REFERENCE

1. Vuyk HD, Adamson PA. Biomaterials in rhinoplasty. Clin Otolaryngol 1998;23:209

ALLOGENEIC MATERIALS

5. *Which of the following is a considerable disadvantage of utilizing bi-layered acellular dermal regenerative templates (Integra)?*

C. Cost.

Although there is certainly a role of the existing products, the Integra bi-layered acellular dermal matrix comes with a very high financial burden. Also, it has limited application in aesthetic surgery; products such as autologous acellular dermal matrix may be of more use, as these can be used for fascial replacement, soft tissue volume increase, and breast implant encapsulation.[1,2,3]

REFERENCES

1. Liu DZ, Mathes DW, Neligan PC, et al. Comparison of outcomes using AlloDerm versus FlexHD for implant-based breast reconstruction. Ann Plast Surg 2014;72:503
2. Ho G, Nguyen DJ, Shahabi A, et al. A systematic review and meta-analysis of complications associated with acellular dermal matrix-assisted breast reconstruction. Ann Plast Surg 2012;68:346
3. Yeong EK, Chen SH, Tang YB. The treatment of bone exposure in burns by using artificial dermis. Ann Plast Surg 2012;69:607

ALLOGENEIC MATERIALS

6. *Which of the following has become the most commonly placed alloplastic material in aesthetic surgery (nonbreast)?*

D. Titanium alloy.

Given its high tolerability, strength, and malleability, titanium alloy alloplasts have become the most commonly used material in aesthetic surgery (nonbreast).[1]

REFERENCE

1. Haug RH, Kimberly D, Bradick JP. A comparison of microscrew and suture fixation of porous high density polyethylene orbital floor implants. J Oral Maxillofac Surg 1993;51:1217

ALLOGENEIC MATERIALS

7. *Which of the following is an important consideration pertaining to high-density porous polyethylene (Medpor) implants?*

E. Must soak in antibiotic solution prior to placement.

Medpor implants are very easily fixated and stabilized through use of screws,[1] are not resorbed by the body, and are not radiodense; however, they must be thoroughly soaked in an antibiotic solution prior to implant placement to avoid infection complications.

Reference

1. Holmes R, Hagler H. Porous hydroxyapatite as a bone graft substitute on cranial reconstruction: a histometric study. Plast Reconstr Surg 1988;81:662

ALLOGENEIC MATERIALS

8. *Particularly with regard to aesthetic surgery, which of the following is a substantial disadvantage of using hydroxyapatite in the facial skeleton?*

C. Very difficult to remove.

In the event that the removal of a hydroxyapatite implant is aesthetically indicated or desired, the removal process is extremely difficult to the point that its removal can potentially endanger the mental nerve or infraorbital nerve, cause excessive bleeding, hematoma, seroma, and undesirable scar tissue.[1,2]

References

1. Ellis E III, Sinn DP. Use of homologous bone in maxillofacial surgery. J Oral Maxillofac Surg 1993;51:1181
2. Holmes R, Hagler H. Porous hydroxyapatite as a bone graft substitute on cranial reconstruction: a histometric study. Plast Reconstr Surg 1988;81:662

ALLOGENEIC MATERIALS

9. *Which of the following is considered a potential advantage of silicone facial implants compared to other alloplastic material types?*

A. Implant infections easily managed nonsurgically.

One substantial advantage of silicone facial implants in aesthetic surgery is the capability to manage a potential postoperative infection with (often) antibiotics alone, or (sometimes) needle aspiration for fluid drainage from the implant pocket. Other alloplastic materials would not lend as well to nonoperative management of suspected infection.[1,2,3]

References

1. Terino EO, Flowers RS. The Art of Alloplastic Facial Contouring. St Louis: Mosby–Year Book; 2000
2. Ridwan-Pramana A, Wolff J, Raziei A, et al. Porous polyethylene implants in facial reconstruction: outcome and complications. J Craniomaxillofac Surg 2015;43:1330
3. Rubin PJ, Yarem chuck MJ. Complications and toxicities of implantable biomaterials used in facial reconstructive and aesthetic surgery: a comprehensive review of the literature. Plast Reconstr Surg 1997;100:1336

28. Progressive Tension Sutures

Stelios C. Wilson, Simon Moradian
See *Essentials of Aesthetic Surgery*, first edition, pp. 344–352

DEFINITION

1. *Progressive tension suturing refers to the technique of which of the following?*
A. Anchor flaps over multiple points of fixation in an advanced position.
B. Bringing together rectus abdominis muscles to the midline.
C. High lateral tension closure to improve contour.
D. Closure of the abdominoplasty incision in three layers.
E. Closure of the Scarpa's fascia in an abdominoplasty.

DEFINITION

2. *Which of the following applies to the use of progressive tension suturing?*
A. Extremely costly.
B. Technically difficult.
C. Takes an extra 60 minutes of operating time, on average.
D. Increases hematoma rates.
E. Decreases seroma rates.

INDICATIONS AND CONTRAINDICATIONS

3. *In which of the following reconstructions would progressive tension sutures be inappropriate?*
A. Abdominoplasty.
B. Facelift.
C. Subcutaneous brow lift.
D. Reconstructive advancement flaps.
E. Skin grafting.

INFORMED CONSENT

4. *When discussing progressive tension suturing (PTSs) with your patients, what should you mention?*
A. PTSs eliminate the risk of seroma.
B. Dimpling will not occur.
C. Revision rates are no greater than with traditional techniques.
D. Higher rates of venous thromboembolism.
E. They decrease infection rates.

TECHNIQUE

5. *Excessive or obvious dimpling once the next suture is tied may result from which of the following in a patient with a BMI of 35?*
A. Too superficial suture placement.
B. Little to no advancement of the flap.
C. Placement of the sutures in the opposing direction of the flap advancement.
D. Placement of sutures by taking bites of Scarpa's fascia during an abdominoplasty.
E. More likely to occur if using a braided suture.

TECHNIQUE

6. *Once a surgeon–assistant coordination is achieved, placement of progressive tension sutures for an abdominoplasty should take approximately how many additional minutes?*

A. Less than 5 minutes.
B. 15 minutes.
C. 25 minutes.
D. 40 minutes.
E. 60 minutes.

EQUIPMENT AND PREPARATION

7. *What is the preferred suturing technique for placement of progressive tension sutures?*

A. Suturing in an interrupted fashion only.
B. Suturing in a continuous fashion only.
C. There is no difference in technique used.
D. Primarily using absorbable sutures in a continuous running fashion.
E. Primarily using nonabsorbable sutures in an interrupted fashion.

OUTCOMES

8. *What is the approximate percentage of seroma formation with the use of progressive tension sutures in abdominoplasties with no drains versus traditional abdominoplasties with drains?*

A. 2%.
B. 5%.
C. 10%.
D. 15%.
E. 22%.

OUTCOMES

9. *When counseling a patient on risks/benefits of the use of progressive tension sutures (PTSs) during an abdominoplasty, which of the following is associated with the use of PTSs?*

A. Decreased hematoma rate.
B. Increased hematoma rate.
C. No significant increased risk of hematomas.
D. Decreased chance of infection.
E. Increased risk of superficial wound dehiscence.

OUTCOMES

10. *Which of the following is associated with the use of using progressive tension sutures and forgoing drains in abdominoplasty?*

A. Increased hematoma rates.
B. Increased long-term skin dimpling.
C. Increased seroma rates.
D. Low levels of patient satisfaction.
E. High levels of patient satisfaction.

Answers

DEFINITION

1. *Progressive tension suturing refers to the technique of which of the following?*

A. Anchor flaps over multiple points of fixation in an advanced position.

Progressive tension suturing is intended to securely anchor flaps over multiple points of fixation in an advanced position. There are several benefits including eliminating dead space and minimizing tension on the flap closure. Rectus plication brings the rectus muscles together in the midline. High lateral tension closure to improve contour is a principle popularized by Lockwood.[1,2,3]

REFERENCES

1. Pollock H, Pollock T. Progressive tensions sutures: a technique to reduce local complications in abdominoplasty. Plast Reconstr Surg 2000;105:2583
2. Andrades P, Prado A. Composition of postabdominoplasty seromas. Aesthetic Plast Surg 2007;31:514
3. Lockwood T. High-lateral-tension abdominoplasty with superficial fascial system suspension. Plast Reconstr Surg 1995;96:603–615

DEFINITION

2. *Which of the following applies to the use of progressive tension suturing?*

E. Decreases seroma rates.

Progressive tension suturing helps to reduce or eliminate dead space. This can help eliminate the need for drains. Also, progressive tension suturing can improve wound healing through limiting motion, minimizing tension on advancement flaps, and distributing tension over multiple points of fixation. Although fluid accumulation is generally compartmentalized to smaller-volume areas that are easily absorbed, thus limiting seroma, there is no advantage related to infection.[1,2]

REFERENCES

1. Pollock H, Pollock T. Progressive tensions sutures: a technique to reduce local complications in abdominoplasty. Plast Reconstr Surg 2000;105:2583
2. Andrades P, Prado A. Composition of postabdominoplasty seromas. Aesthetic Plast Surg 2007;31:514

INDICATIONS AND CONTRAINDICATIONS

3. *In which of the following reconstructions would progressive tension sutures be inappropriate?*

E. Skin grafting.

Progressive tension sutures are based on a simple surgical concept that can be applied to any procedure involving an advancement flap. Therefore, they have no specific indications or contraindications.[1,2,3,4,5] The placement and healing process of skin grafts would not be an appropriate situation to use progression tension sutures.

REFERENCES

1. Pollock H, Pollock T. Progressive tensions sutures: a technique to reduce local complications in abdominoplasty. Plast Reconstr Surg 2000;105:2583
2. Andrades P, Prado A. Composition of postabdominoplasty seromas. Aesthetic Plast Surg 2007;31:514
3. Pollock H, Pollock T. Management of face lifts with progressive tension sutures. Aesthet Surg J 2003;23:28
4. Pollock H, Pollock T. Subcutaneous brow lift with progressive tension suture fixation and advancement. Aesthet Surg J 2007;27:388
5. Rios JL, Pollock T, Adams WP. Progressive tension sutures to prevent seroma formation after latissimus dorsi harvest. Plast Reconstr Surg 2003;112:1779

INFORMED CONSENT

4. *When discussing progressive tension suturing (PTSs) with your patients, what should you mention?*

C. Revision rates are no greater than with traditional techniques.

Progressive tension sutures (PTSs) have similar revision rates to operations without the use of PTSs. However, the use of PTSs significantly reduces the risk of seroma but does not eliminate it. Dimpling can occur but is almost always temporary. In cases where the dermis rather than the superficial fascial system is being sutured, such as in a subcutaneous facelift flap, temporary dimpling is more common. There is no evidence to suggest that the use of PTSs decrease infection rates. It is believed that using PTSs allows for early ambulation in an upright position for abdominoplasty patients, improving venous circulation and reducing the risk of venous thromboembolism.[1,2,3]

REFERENCES

1. Pollock H, Pollock T. Progressive tensions sutures: a technique to reduce local complications in abdominoplasty. Plast Reconstr Surg 2000;105:2583
2. Antonetti JW, Antonetti AR. Reducing seroma in outpatient abdominoplasty: analysis of 516 consecutive cases. Aesthet Surg J 2010;30:418
3. Pollock H, Pollock T. Progressive tension sutures in abdominoplasty: a review of 597 consecutive cases. Aesthet Surg J 2012;32:729

TECHNIQUE

5. *Excessive or obvious dimpling once the next suture is tied may result from which of the following in a patient with a BMI of 35?*

A. Too superficial suture placement.

When placing progressive tension sutures (PTSs), it is not uncommon to have dimpling that is temporary in your last suture. Once the next suture is placed, the dimpling should resolve. Excessive or obvious dimpling can occur with bites that are too superficial, on placing excessive advancement of the flap, and on placing the sutures in the opposing direction. Of note, you can use a slight dimpling to your advantage. There is no evidence to suggest that using a braided suture will result in more or less dimpling. For instance, midline PTSs during abdominoplasty with slight dimpling can mimic a natural aesthetic contour.[1,2]

REFERENCES

1. Pollock H, Pollock T. Progressive tensions sutures: a technique to reduce local complications in abdominoplasty. Plast Reconstr Surg 2000;105:2583
2. Pollock H, Pollock T. Progressive tension sutures in abdominoplasty: a review of 597 consecutive cases. Aesthet Surg J 2012;32:729

TECHNIQUE

6. *Once a surgeon–assistant coordination is achieved, placement of progressive tension sutures for an abdominoplasty should take approximately how many additional minutes?*

C. 25 minutes.

For trained surgeons, no special skills are required to perform this technique and the learning curve is short. Once a surgeon–assistant coordination is achieved, placement of the sutures takes 20 to 30 minutes, including the in-continuity inset of the umbilicus. In a meta-analysis performed by Jabbour and colleagues, the mean difference in surgical time was 23 minutes.[1]

REFERENCE

1. Jabbour S, Awaida C, Mhawej R, et al. Does the addition of progressive tension sutures to drains reduce seroma incidence after abdominoplasty? A systematic review and meta-analysis. Aesthet Surg J 2017;37:440–447

EQUIPMENT AND PREPARATION

7. *What is the preferred suturing technique for placement of progressive tension sutures?*

C. There is no difference in technique used.

When placing progressive tension sutures (PTSs), the surgeon can use either an interrupted or a continuous suture. For both techniques, absorbable sutures are generally employed. The use of both smooth and barbed sutures has been described. Smooth sutures are thought to be equally as effective and less expensive (**Fig. 28.1**, **Fig. 28.2**).[1,2,3,4]

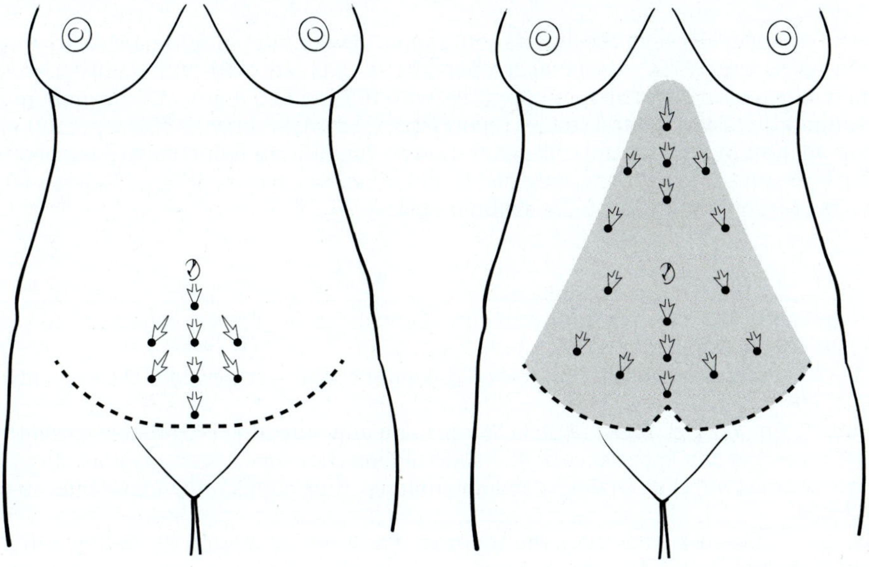

Fig. 28.1 Progressive tension sutures. (Source: Reprinted with permission from Pollock H, Pollock T. Progressive tension sutures: a technique to reduce local complications in abdominoplasty. Plast Reconstr Surg 105:2583; discussion 2587, 2000.)

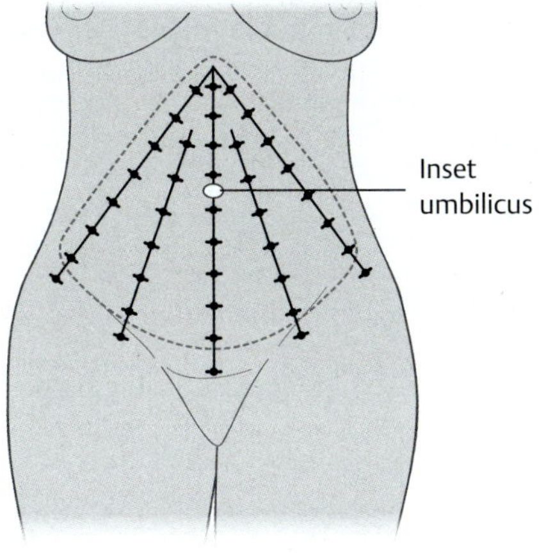

Fig. 28.2 Continuous sutures. (Source: Technique for Progressive Tension Sutures. In: Janis J, ed. Essentials of Aesthetic Surgery. 1st Edition. New York: Thieme; 2018.)

References

1. Pollock H, Pollock T. Progressive tensions sutures: a technique to reduce local complications in abdominoplasty. Plast Reconstr Surg 2000;105:2583
2. Pollock H, Pollock T. Progressive tension sutures in abdominoplasty: a review of 597 consecutive cases. Aesthet Surg J 2012;32:729
3. Gutowski KA, Warner JP. Incorporating barbed sutures in abdominoplasty. Aesthet Surg J 2013;33(3 Suppl):S76
4. Warner JP, Gutowski KA. Abdominoplasty with progressive tension closure using a barbed suture technique. Aesthet Surg J 2009;29:221

OUTCOMES

8. *What is the approximate percentage of seroma formation with the use of progressive tension sutures in abdominoplasties with no drains versus traditional abdominoplasties with drains?*

A. 2%.

True, there is strong evidence in the literature to support lower rates of seroma formation when using progressive tension sutures (PTSs). Macias et al reported a seroma rate of 9% with traditional abdominoplasties with drains compared to 2% for abdominoplasties with PTSs and no drains. Although there is no level I evidence to support this claim, several studies report large case series showing efficacy in this practice. In addition, a meta-analysis by Jabbour and colleagues showed a significant reduction in postoperative seroma rate when using PTSs compared to drains alone and no difference when comparing individuals who had PTSs and drains to PTSs without drains following abdominoplasty.[1,2,3,4,5]

REFERENCES

1. Antonetti JW, Antonetti AR. Reducing seroma in outpatient abdominoplasty: analysis of 516 consecutive cases. Aesthet Surg J 2010;30:418
2. Pollock H, Pollock T. Progressive tension sutures in abdominoplasty: a review of 597 consecutive cases. Aesthet Surg J 2012;32:729
3. Macias LH, Kwon E, Gould DJ, et al. Decrease in seroma rate after adopting progressive tension sutures without drains: a single surgery center experience of 451 abdominoplasties over 7 years. Aesthet Surg J 2016;36:1029
4. Isaac KV, Lista F, McIsaac MP, et al. Drainless abdominoplasty using barbed progressive tension sutures. Aesthet Surg J 2017;37:428
5. Jabbour S, Awaida C, Mhawej R, et al. Does the addition of progressive tension sutures to drains reduce seroma incidence after abdominoplasty? A systematic review and meta-analysis. Aesthet Surg J 2017;37:440–447

OUTCOMES

9. *When counseling a patient on risks/benefits of the use of progressive tension sutures (PTSs) during an abdominoplasty, which of the following is associated with the use of PTSs?*

C. No significant increased risk of hematomas.

There is no significant increased risk of hematoma in individuals who undergo abdominoplasty with progressive tension sutures (PTSs). The rate of hematoma for both groups is between 1 and 2%. This has not been shown to be significantly different between individuals who underwent PTSs and those who did not.[1] There is no evidence to suggest that the use of PTSs is associated with any significant change in infection rates or wound healing complications.[2]

REFERENCES

1. Antonetti JW, Antonetti AR. Reducing seroma in outpatient abdominoplasty: analysis of 516 consecutive cases. Aesthet Surg J 2010;30:418
2. Isaac KV, Lista F, McIsaac MP, et al. Drainless abdominoplasty using barbed progressive tension sutures. Aesthet Surg J 2017;37:428

OUTCOMES

10. *Which of the following is associated with the use of using progressive tension sutures and forgoing drains in abdominoplasty?*

E. High levels of patient satisfaction.

Anecdotally, high levels of patient satisfaction are noted when drains are not used with abdominoplasties. Patients may find drain care daunting and cumbersome. True, forgoing drains with the use of progressive tension suturing (PTSs) has been shown in many high-volume studies to be both safe and reliable. Specifically, proponents of this technique show no higher incidence of complications including seroma, hematoma, and infection. This data may support that drains are unnecessary; however, the use of drains is still based on surgeon's discretion.[1,2,3,4,5] Additionally, skin dimpling is temporary and resolves with time.

References

1. Antonetti JW, Antonetti AR. Reducing seroma in outpatient abdominoplasty: analysis of 516 consecutive cases. Aesthet Surg J 2010;30:418
2. Pollock H, Pollock T. Progressive tension sutures in abdominoplasty: a review of 597 consecutive cases. Aesthet Surg J 2012;32:729
3. Macias LH, Kwon E, Gould DJ, et al. Decrease in seroma rate after adopting progressive tension sutures without drains: a single surgery center experience of 451 abdominoplasties over 7 years. Aesthet Surg J 2016;36:1029
4. Isaac KV, Lista F, McIsaac MP, et al. Drainless abdominoplasty using barbed progressive tension sutures. Aesthet Surg J 2017;37:428
5. Jabbour S, Awaida C, Mhawej R, et al. Does the addition of progressive tension sutures to drains reduce seroma incidence after abdominoplasty? A systematic review and meta-analysis. Aesthet Surg J 2017;37:440–447.

PART VII

Facial Surgery

29. Periorbital Anatomy

Anmol Chattha, Elbert E. Vaca
See *Essentials of Aesthetic Surgery*, first edition, pp. 355–371

ANATOMY

1. ***Which deep fat compartment is bordered by the inferior orbital rim superiorly and the zygomatic cutaneous ligaments inferiorly?***
   A. Deep medial cheek fat.
   B. Central lower orbital fat.
   C. Suborbicularis oculi fat (SOOF).
   D. Retroorbicularis oculi fat (ROOF).
   E. Deep lateral cheek fat.

COMPLICATIONS

2. ***After 3 months of transconjunctival lower blepharoplasty with orbital fat excision, a patient complains of persistent double vision exacerbated by head tilt and downward gaze. Examination confirms the presence of strabismus. Visual acuity is intact in both eyes. These findings are most likely explained by damage to which of the following structures?***
   A. Scar contracture of orbital septum.
   B. Retroorbital hematoma.
   C. Scar contracture of the inferior oblique muscle.
   D. Dehiscence of the levator palpebrae muscle.
   E. Palsy of the left inferior rectus muscle.

SURGICAL TECHNIQUE

3. ***A patient underwent hyaluronic acid filler injection to the tear trough and reports decreasing visual acuity immediately after injection. Which of the following injection techniques increases the risk of retrograde occlusion of the ophthalmic artery?***
   A. Supraperiosteal injection.
   B. Use of a blunt canula.
   C. Use of firm pressure on the plunger during injection.
   D. Injection while the needle or canula is in motion.
   E. Using larger gauge needle or cannula.

ANATOMY

4. ***The levator palpebrae muscle is innervated by which of the following cranial nerve?***
   A. II.
   B. III.
   C. IV.
   D. V.
   E. VI.

ANATOMY

5. ***Which of the following best describes the relationship of the corrugator supercilii muscles to the frontalis and orbicularis oculi?***
   A. Deep to both the frontalis and orbicularis oculi.
   B. Superficial to both the frontalis and orbicularis oculi.
   C. Deep to the frontalis, superficial to the orbicularis oculi.
   D. Deep to the orbicularis oculi, superficial to the frontalis.
   E. Within the same plane as orbicularis oculi and deep to frontalis.

COMPLICATIONS

6. *A 27-year-old patient sustains a laceration to the right cheek. Physical examination demonstrates difficulty with voluntary right eyelid closure. Which of the following facial nerve branches is most likely injured?*

A. Frontal.
B. Zygomatic.
C. Buccal.
D. Marginal mandibular.
E. Cervical.

ANATOMY

7. *A 74-year-old female presents with an ulcerated squamous cell carcinoma of the lower eyelid at the level of the medial limbus. Lymph node involvement is confirmed. Which lymph nodes are most likely positive for malignant cells?*

A. Preauricular.
B. Submandibular.
C. Submental.
D. Parotid.
E. Supraclavicular.

ANATOMY

8. *Which of the following most accurately describes the location and insertion of Mueller's muscle?*

A. Superficial to the levator palpebrae muscle, inserts onto posterior surface of upper tarsal plate.
B. Superficial to the levator palpebrae muscle, inserts onto superior edge of upper tarsal plate.
C. Deep to the levator palpebrae muscle, inserts onto the posterior edge of upper tarsal plate.
D. Deep to the levator palpebrae muscle, inserts onto superior edge of upper tarsal plate.
E. In the same plane as levator palpebrae and inserts onto the inferior edge of upper tarsal plate.

ANATOMY

9. *Which component of the orbicularis oculi muscle inserts into the lacrimal sac to aid in lacrimal drainage?*

A. Posterior reflection of the preseptal orbicularis (Jones muscle).
B. Posterior reflection of the pretarsal orbicularis (Horner muscle).
C. Orbital portion of the orbicularis oculi.
D. Lateral palpebral raphae.
E. Entire portion of orbicularis.

ANATOMY

10. *A 54-year-old female presents with complains of dry eye symptoms. Rheumatologic workup is negative. Schirmer's test is normal bilaterally, confirming adequate tear production volume. Which of the following components of the tear film is most likely affected?*

A. The amount of lipid in the tear film.
B. The amount of mucin in the tear film.
C. The antimicrobial properties of the tear film.
D. The dispersion of the tear film.
E. The drainage of the tear film.

ANATOMY

11. *A 25-year-old male reports numbness of the left cheek and lower eyelid after blunt trauma to the left midface. Physical examination reveals crepitus and bruising along the left midface. The described sensory disturbance is a result from trauma to which of the following nerves?*

A. Supraorbital nerve.
B. Supratrochlear nerve.
C. Infratrochlear nerve.
D. Infraorbital nerve.
E. Anterior ethmoid nerve.

Answers

ANATOMY

1. ***Which deep fat compartment is bordered by the inferior orbital rim superiorly and the zygomatic cutaneous ligaments inferiorly?***

C. Suborbicularis oculi fat (SOOF).

The suborbicularis oculi fat (SOOF) pads lie deep to the orbicularis oculi muscle and are bordered by the inferior orbital rim superiorly and zygomatic retaining ligaments inferiorly. The SOOF is composed of two distinct fat pads: the lateral SOOF and medial SOOF divided by the infraorbital foramen. With aging, descent and volumetric deflation of the SOOF along with overlying orbital orbicularis oculi laxity contribute to the formation of malar bags (i.e., festoons).

The deep medial cheek fat pad lies caudal to the zygomatic retaining ligaments and deep to the zygomaticus major muscle. The central lower orbital fat is an orbital fat compartment and lies deep to the orbital septum. The SOOF lies on the midface. The ROOF lies deep to the orbicularis oculi along the superolateral orbital rim.[1]

REFERENCE

1. Rohrich RJ, Pessa JE. The fat compartments of the face: anatomy and clinical implications for cosmetic surgery. Plast Reconstr Surg 2007;119(7):2219–2227

COMPLICATIONS

2. ***After 3 months of transconjunctival lower blepharoplasty with orbital fat excision, a patient complains of persistent double vision exacerbated by head tilt and downward gaze. Examination confirms the presence of strabismus. Visual acuity is intact in both eyes. These findings are most likely explained by damage to which of the following structures?***

C. Scar contracture of the inferior oblique muscle.

The inferior oblique muscle is susceptible to damage during orbital fat excision and is located between the nasal (i.e., central) and middle orbital fat compartments. The inferior oblique muscle is responsible for eye elevation, external rotation, and abduction. The inferior oblique muscle is susceptible to damage during orbital fat excision, which can result in scarring and contracture of the muscle leading to strabismus. Scar contracture of the inferior oblique muscle (a globe elevator) will result in ipsilateral restriction in downward gaze. In contrast, palsy of the inferior oblique muscle would result in ipsilateral globe hypotropia.

Scar contracture of the orbital septum would result in lower eyelid retraction, a common complication after lower blepharoplasty. This would not result in strabismus.

A retroorbital hematoma is a clinical emergency and can occur after lower blepharoplasty. Increasing orbital pressure can result in palsy due to compression of cranial nerves 3, 4, and 6 and blindness due to compression of cranial nerve 2. The patient is 3 months status post blepharoplasty and visual acuity is intact.

Dehiscence of the levator palpebrae muscle can occur after upper blepharoplasty and would result in upper lid ptosis. This would not result in strabismus and double vision.

Palsy of the left interior rectus would result in similar symptoms as left inferior oblique scar contracture, with both causing left eye hypertropia. However, the inferior oblique muscle lies between the nasal and middle fat compartments and is more susceptible to injury than the inferior rectus muscle, which lies deeper and is not typically encountered when dissecting orbital fat during lower blepharoplasty.[1]

REFERENCE

1. Jelks GW, Jelks EB. The influence of orbital and eyelid anatomy on the palpebral aperture. Clin Plast Surg 1991;18:183

SURGICAL TECHNIQUE

3. *A patient underwent hyaluronic acid filler injection to the tear trough and reports decreasing visual acuity immediately after injection. Which of the following injection techniques increases the risk of retrograde occlusion of the ophthalmic artery?*

C. Use of firm pressure on the plunger during injection.

Filler injection under high pressure increases the risk of retrograde filling into the ophthalmic artery if a periorbital artery is cannulated. It is possible that use of a blunt canula may decrease the risk of intravascular injection. Injection in the supraperiosteal plane decreases the risk of vascular cannulation as the arteries and veins course in a more superficial plane. Injecting only while moving the needle or canula may decrease the risk of injecting large aliquots of filler in one location; therefore, a smaller volume of filler will be injected intravascularly if a blood vessel is inadvertently cannulated. Smaller gauge cannulas or needles are more likely to penetrate into smaller vessels.[1]

REFERENCE

1. Mortada H, Seraj H, Barasain O, Bamakhrama B, Alhindi NI, Arab K. Ocular complications post-cosmetic periocular hyaluronic acid injections: a systematic review. Aesthetic Plast Surg 2022;46(2):760–773

ANATOMY

4. *The levator palpebrae muscle is innervated by which of the following cranial nerve?*

B. III.

The levator palpebrae muscle is the main elevator of the upper eyelid and is voluntarily innervated by the oculomotor nerve (CN III). The optic nerve (CN II) is responsible for the transmission of visual information from the retina to the brain. CN II does not have motor function. The abducens nerve (CN IV) innervates the lateral rectus muscle. It does not innervate the levator palpebrae muscle. The trigeminal nerve (CN V) provides sensation to the upper face (V1), middle face (V2), lower face (V3), and anterior two-thirds of the tongue. It also provides motor innervation to the muscles of mastication and the tensor veli palatini muscle. The trochlear nerve (CV VI) provides innervation to the superior oblique muscle.[1]

REFERENCE

1. Jelks GW, Jelks EB. The influence of orbital and eyelid anatomy on the palpebral aperture. Clin Plast Surg 1991;18:183

ANATOMY

5. *Which of the following best describes the relationship of the corrugator supercilii muscles to the frontalis and orbicularis oculi?*

A. Deep to both the frontalis and orbicularis oculi.

The corrugator supercilii muscle lies deep to both the frontalis and orbicularis oculi muscles.[1]

REFERENCE

1. Jelks GW, Jelks EB. The influence of orbital and eyelid anatomy on the palpebral aperture. Clin Plast Surg 1991;18:183

COMPLICATIONS

6. *A 27-year-old patient sustains a laceration to the right cheek. Physical examination demonstrates difficulty with voluntary right eyelid closure. Which of the following facial nerve branches is most likely injured?*

B. Zygomatic.

The orbicularis oculi muscle receives innervation from the zygomatic and buccal branches of the facial nerve. The medial canthal orbicularis is innervated by the buccal branch of the facial nerve and is responsible for involuntary blink and the pumping mechanism of the lacrimal system. Zygomatic branches control voluntary eyelid closure and squinting.[1]

REFERENCE

1. Jelks GW, Jelks EB. The influence of orbital and eyelid anatomy on the palpebral aperture. Clin Plast Surg 1991;18:183

ANATOMY

7. *A 74-year-old female presents with an ulcerated squamous cell carcinoma of the lower eyelid at the level of the medial limbus. Lymph node involvement is confirmed. Which lymph nodes are most likely positive for malignant cells?*

B. Submandibular.

The submandibular lymph nodes drain the medial upper and lower eyelids, while the lateral upper and lower eyelids drain into the preauricular lymph nodes.

The submental lymph nodes drain the apex of the tongue and the central lower lip.[1]

REFERENCE

1. Nijhawan N, Marriott C, Harvey JT. Lymphatic drainage patterns of the human eyelid: assessed by lymphoscintigraphy. Ophthal Plast Reconstr Surg 2010;26:281

ANATOMY

8. *Which of the following most accurately describes the location and insertion of Mueller's muscle?*

D. Deep to the levator palpebrae muscle, inserts onto superior edge of upper tarsal plate.

Mueller's muscle is sympathetically innervated and loss of function results in 2 to 3 mm of ptosis. Muller's muscle lies deep to the levator palpebrae muscle and it inserts into the upper border of the tarsal plate. The levator palpebrae muscle insterts onto the anterosuperior surface of the superior tarsal plate.[1]

REFERENCE

1. Jelks GW, Jelks EB. The influence of orbital and eyelid anatomy on the palpebral aperture. Clin Plast Surg 1991;18:183

ANATOMY

9. *Which component of the orbicularis oculi muscle inserts into the lacrimal sac to aid in lacrimal drainage?*

A. Posterior reflection of the preseptal orbicularis (Jones muscle).

Jones muscle, derived from the medial preseptal orbicularis, inserts onto the lacrimal sac.

Horner's muscle forms part of the posterior reflection of the medial canthal tendon and inserts deep to the lacrimal sac.

The orbital portion of the orbicularis oculi muscle does not insert into the lacrimal sac.

The lateral palpebral raphe is the fascial condensation of the upper and lower orbicularis oculi muscle at the lateral commissure. The lacrimal sac lies medially, not laterally.[1]

REFERENCE

1. Jelks GW, Jelks EB. The influence of orbital and eyelid anatomy on the palpebral aperture. Clin Plast Surg 1991;18:183

ANATOMY

10. *A 54-year-old female presents with complains of dry eye symptoms. Rheumatologic workup is negative. Schirmer's test is normal bilaterally, confirming adequate tear production volume. Which of the following components of the tear film is most likely affected?*

A. The amount of lipid in the tear film.

The tear film is composed of a trilaminar fluid. The deep layer is formed by mucin-secreting goblet cells in the conjunctiva. The mucin layer acts as a surfactant promoting dispersion of the tear film. The middle layer is aqueous and secreted by the lacrimal gland. The aqueous layer produces the majority of the tear film volume and possesses antimicrobial properties. The meibomian glands secrete the outer lipid layer which helps prevent tear film evaporation. Dysfunction of the meibomian glands results in dry eye symptoms due to rapid tear film evaporation.[1]

REFERENCE

1. Tiffany JM. The normal tear film. In: Geerling G, Brewitt H, eds. Surgery for the Dry Eye: Scientific Evidence and Guidelines for the Clinical Management of Dry Eye Associated Ocular Surface Disease (Developments in Ophthalmology, Book 41). 1st ed. Basel, Switzerland: Karger; 2008:1–20

ANATOMY

11. ***A 25-year-old male reports numbness of the left cheek and lower eyelid after blunt trauma to the left midface. Physical examination reveals crepitus and bruising along the left midface. The described sensory disturbance is a result from trauma to which of the following nerves?***

D. Infraorbital nerve.

The clinical vignette describes a fracture of the left maxilla. The infraorbital nerve (V2) courses along the roof of the maxillary sinus and exits through the infraorbital foramen at approximately the level of the medial limbus. Maxillary fractures often traverse the infraorbital foramen resulting in hypoesthesia of the midface and lower eyelid.

The supraorbital and supratrochlear nerves originate from the ophthalmic division of the trigeminal nerve (V1) and provide sensation to the anterior scalp and mid forehead, respectively.

The infratrochlear nerve is a division of the ophthalmic division of the trigeminal nerve (V1) and provides sensation to the upper third of the nose and medial upper eyelid.

The anterior ethmoid nerve is a division of the ophthalmic division of the trigeminal nerve (V1) and provides sensation to the nasal cavity.[1]

REFERENCE

1. Jelks GW, Jelks EB. The influence of orbital and eyelid anatomy on the palpebral aperture. Clin Plast Surg 1991;18:183

30. Face and Neck Anatomy

Jacob Nathaniel Grow, Christopher C. Surek
See *Essentials of Aesthetic Surgery*, pp. 372–389

SOFT TISSUE LAYERS OF THE FACE

1. ***Which of the following represents the most appropriate arrangement of facial layers from most superficial to deep?***
   A. Skin, subcutaneous fat, mimetic muscles, superficial musculoaponeurotic system, parotidomasseteric fascia.
   B. Skin, superficial musculoaponeurotic system, subcutaneous fat, mimetic muscles, parotidomasseteric fascia.
   C. Skin, subcutaneous fat, superficial musculoaponeurotic system, parotidomasseteric fascia, mimetic muscles.
   D. Skin, subcutaneous fat, superficial musculoaponeurotic system, mimetic muscles, parotidomasseteric fascia.
   E. Skin, parotidomasseteric fascia, subcutaneous fat, superficial musculoaponeurotic system, mimetic muscles.

SOFT TISSUE LAYERS OF THE FACE

2. ***A patient consults for complaints primarily related to prominent nasolabial folds. This feature of facial aging may be attributed to pseudoptosis of the nasolabial fat pad secondary to volume loss of which of the following?***
   A. Malar bone.
   B. Deep medial cheek compartment.
   C. Prezygomatic space.
   D. Suborbicularis oculi fat (SOOF).
   E. Nasal ala.

SOFT TISSUE LAYERS OF THE FACE

3. ***While performing a rhytidectomy, you appreciate improvement of jowling. The anatomical basis for this phenomenon of aging is associated with which of the following structures?***
   A. Orbicularis oculi muscle.
   B. Modiolus.
   C. Mentalis muscle.
   D. Nasolabial fat pad.
   E. Depressor anguli oris muscle.

SOFT TISSUE LAYERS OF THE FACE

4. ***Which of the following structures is not continuous with the superficial musculoaponeurotic system (SMAS)?***
   A. Galea.
   B. Platysmal fascia.
   C. Temporoparietal fascia.
   D. Orbicularis fascia.
   E. Parotidomasseteric fascia.

SOFT TISSUE LAYERS OF THE FACE

5. ***Which of the following muscles receives innervation from the facial nerve on its superficial surface?***
   A. Mentalis.
   B. Levator labii superioris.
   C. Depressor anguli oris.
   D. Risorius.
   E. Zygomaticus minor.

SOFT TISSUE LAYERS OF THE FACE

6. *During open neck rejuvenation with platysmal plication in the midline, remaining just superficial to which layer ensures the safest plane for dissection?*

A. Infrahyoid muscle fascia.
B. Prevertebral fascia.
C. Investing deep fascia.
D. Pretracheal fascia.
E. Subcutaneous tissue.

NERVES

7. *Following rhytidectomy, a patient complains of numbness at the ear lobule. Injury to which of the following is the most likely explanation for this complication?*

A. Auriculotemporal nerve.
B. Lesser occipital nerve.
C. Greater occipital nerve.
D. Great auricular nerve.
E. Arnold's nerve.

NERVES

8. *Which of the following is true with regards to Pitanguy's line?*

A. Anterior point is 1.5 cm lateral to tail of the brow.
B. Posterior point is 2 cm below the tragus.
C. Identifies the location of the zygomatic branch of the facial nerve.
D. Courses over the zygomatic arch at its posterior 1/3.
E. Runs parallel with the parotid duct.

NERVES

9. *Following an open neck lift, a patient returns to clinic with complaints of facial asymmetry. On examination, the patient has an elevated right commissure compared to the left on active smile. Lower lip eversion is present and symmetric. Which of the following nerves is most likely injured?*

A. Right facial nerve cervical branch.
B. Left facial nerve cervical branch.
C. Right facial nerve marginal mandibular branch.
D. Left facial nerve marginal mandibular branch.
E. Bilateral facial nerve buccal branches.

FACIAL DANGER ZONES

10. *A patient undergoes a deep plane facelift with undermining to the modiolus. The next day, the patient has inability to elevate the commissure on active smile. Which of the following nerves is likely injured?*

A. Supraorbital nerve.
B. Mental nerve.
C. Zygomatic branch of the facial nerve.
D. Marginal mandibular nerve.
E. Infraorbital nerve.

FACIAL DANGER ZONES

11. *A patient has inability to evert the lower lip 3 days after a deep neck lift surgery. Which nerve is likely injured?*

A. Supraorbital nerve.
B. Mental nerve.
C. Buccal branch of the facial nerve.
D. Marginal mandibular nerve.
E. Infraorbital nerve.

FACIAL DANGER ZONES

12. *A 22-year-old female who is not healing postoperatively from an augmentation genioplasty has chin numbness. Which nerve is likely injured?*

A. Supraorbital nerve.
B. Mental nerve.
C. Buccal branch of the facial nerve.
D. Marginal mandibular nerve.
E. Infraorbital nerve.

FACIAL DANGER ZONES

13. *A patient has residual numbness of the central forehead 2 months after an endoscopic browlift procedure. Which nerve is likely affected?*

A. Supraorbital nerve.
B. Mental nerve.
C. Buccal branch of the facial nerve.
D. Marginal mandibular nerve.
E. Infraorbital nerve.

VASCULAR SUPPLY

14. *Which of the following is derived from the internal carotid arterial system?*

A. Superficial temporal artery.
B. Facial artery.
C. Maxillary artery.
D. Supratrochlear artery.
E. Superior thyroid artery.

VASCULAR SUPPLY

15. *Which of the following is true regarding the sentinel vein?*

A. Located below the zygoma.
B. Found above the temporal crest.
C. Associated with the zygomatic branch of the facial nerve.
D. Branch of the zygomaticotemporal vein.
E. Remains above the inferior temporal septum.

RETAINING LIGAMENTS OF THE FACE AND NECK

16. *A patient presents for improvement of periorbital facial aging. Release of which of the following is essential to blend the lid–cheek junction?*

A. Temporal ligamentous adhesion.
B. Supraorbital ligamentous adhesion.
C. Zygomatic osteocutaneous ligament.
D. Lateral canthal tendon.
E. Orbicularis retaining ligament.

ANTERIOR TRIANGLE OF THE NECK

17. *The borders of the anterior triangle of the neck include which of the following?*

A. Anterior and posterior bellies of digastric muscle, inferior border of the mandible.
B. Anterior bellies of the digastric muscles, hyoid bone.
C. Anterior border of sternocleidomastoid, inferior border of the mandible, median line of the neck.
D. Anterior border of sternocleidomastoid, anterior belly of digastric, median line of the neck.
E. Posterior border of sternocleidomastoid, anterior border of trapezius muscle, clavicle.

Answers

SOFT TISSUE LAYERS OF THE FACE

1. ***Which of the following represents the most appropriate arrangement of facial layers from most superficial to deep?***

   D. Skin, subcutaneous fat, superficial musculoaponeurotic system, mimetic muscles, parotidomasseteric fascia.

   The face is arranged in well-defined, concentric layers that come to define the facial architecture in concert with underlying bone. This consistent arrangement provides not only form, but also function through the complexities of facial movement. Most superficial is the skin, whose mobility and susceptibility to aging varies with dermal thickness. Next, the subcutaneous tissue includes volumizing compartmentalized fat, in addition to the retinacular cutis responsible for bridging the skin to the underlying superficial musculoaponeurotic system (SMAS) which allows for synchronized facial movement. Following this layer is the SMAS, continuous throughout the head and neck as it invests the mimetic muscles and therefore lies superficial to branches of the facial nerve. Just deep to the SMAS are the layered mimetic muscles, providing the motor for facial expression in addition to oral (speech and feeding) and periocular (protective blink) movement. Deep facialfascia,also known as the parotidomasseteric fascia, follows as a continuation of the superficial layer of the deep cervical fascia. Named according to the overlying structure, it includes the parotid capsule, masseteric fascia, and deep temporal fascia. Finally, the deepest plane includes the buccal fat pad, parotid duct, facial artery/facial vein, and zygomatic and buccal branches of the facial nerve.[1]

REFERENCE

1. Nahai F, Mejia JD, Nahai FR. Applied anatomy of the face and neck. In: Nahai F, ed. The Art of Aesthetic Surgery: Principles and Techniques. 2nd ed. New York: Thieme Publishers; 2010

SOFT TISSUE LAYERS OF THE FACE

2. ***A patient consults for complaints primarily related to prominent nasolabial folds. This feature of facial aging may be attributed to pseudoptosis of the nasolabial fat pad secondary to volume loss of which of the following?***

   B. Deep medial cheek compartment.

   The subcutaneous layer of the face is composed primarily of fat, which has been shown through cadaver dissection to be divided into multiple, well-defined compartments (**Fig. 30.1**). Of these superficial compartments, the nasolabial fat pad lies the most medial. With time, this fat pad tends to resist deflation. However, the deep medial cheek compartment is more susceptible to volume loss with aging. As a result, there is gravitationally dependent descent and pseudoptosis of the more superficial nasolabial fat compartment, which accentuates the nasolabial fold.[1]

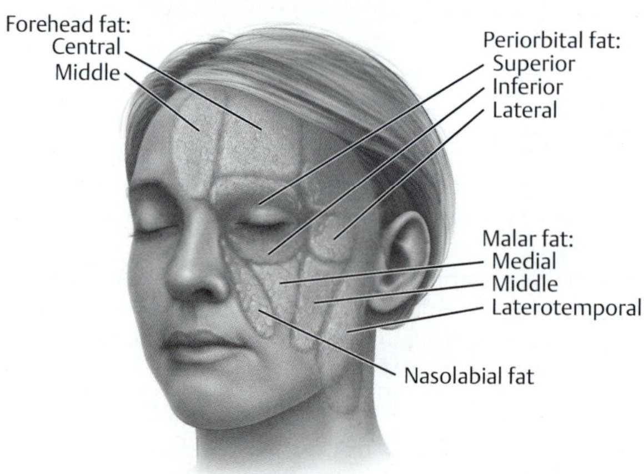

Fig. 30.1 Superficial facial fat compartments. (Source: Soft Tissue Layers of the Face. In: Janis J, ed. Essentials of Aesthetic Surgery. 1st Edition. New York: Thieme; 2018.)

Reference

1. Rohrich RJ, Pessa JE. The fat compartments of the face: anatomy and clinical implications for cosmetic surgery. Plast Reconstr Surg 2007;119:2219

SOFT TISSUE LAYERS OF THE FACE

3. *While performing a rhytidectomy, you appreciate improvement of jowling. The anatomical basis for this phenomenon of aging is associated with which of the following structures?*

E. Depressor anguli oris muscle.

Effacement of the jowls is a common goal when performing rhytidectomy. Anatomically, jowling occurs as descending tissue adherent to the overlying depressor anguli oris muscle is tethered to the mandibulocutaneous ligament, creating the appearance of hanging, deflated tissue. As a result, release of the mandibulocutaneous ligament can be an effective method of correcting this hallmark sign of facial aging during rhytidectomy or isolated neck lift (**Fig. 30.2**).[1]

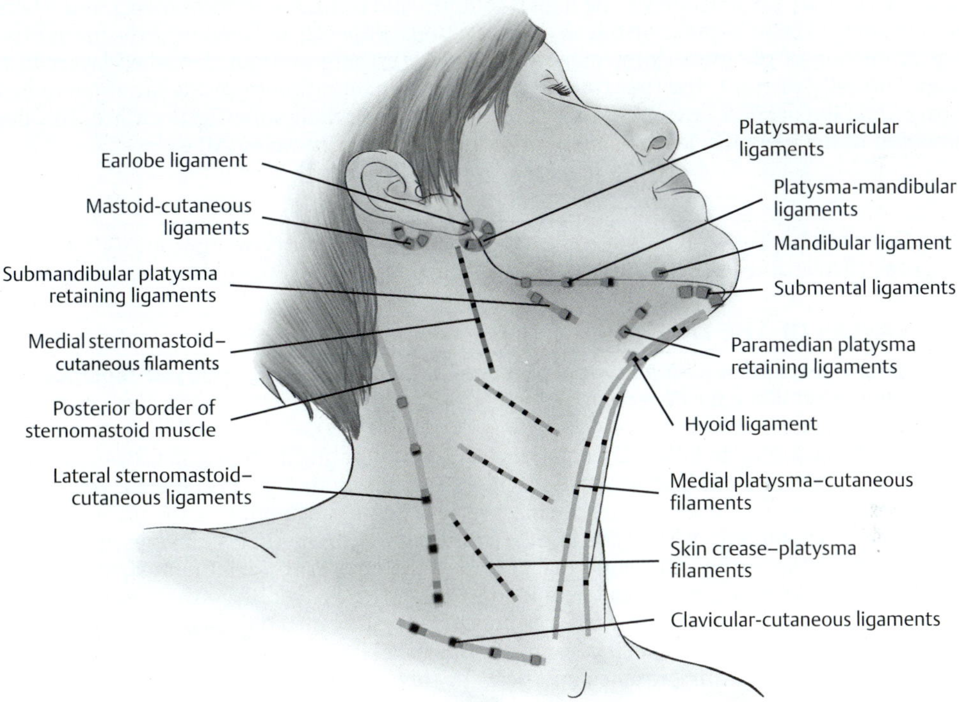

Fig. 30.2 Retaining ligaments and filaments of the neck. (Source: Retaining Ligaments of the Neck. In: Feldman J, ed. Neck Lift. 1st Edition. New York: Thieme; 2006.)

Reference

1. Stuzin JM, Baker TJ, Gordon HL. The relationship of the superficial and deep facial fascias: relevance to rhytidectomy and aging. Plast Reconstr Surg 1992;89:441

SOFT TISSUE LAYERS OF THE FACE

4. *Which of the following structures is not continuous with the superficial musculoaponeurotic system (SMAS)?*

E. Parotidomasseteric fascia.

The superficial musculoaponeurotic system (SMAS) is a continuous layer throughout the face and neck and a vital component to facial aesthetic anatomy. An upward extension of the cervical fascia, the SMAS is continuous with the galea in the scalp, temporoparietal fascia in the temple, and the platysma in the neck. It may be further divided into a fixed portion located more laterally over the parotid gland and a mobile portion anteriorly over the mimetic muscles that allows surgical manipulation during rhytidectomy. Of note, the neurovascular structures, particularly the branches of the facial nerve, lie deep to the SMAS, making it an important layer to identify when performing any procedures on the face. The parotidomasseteric fascia is located deeper to the SMAS as part of the deep facial fascia, including the deep temporal fascia, deep cervical fascia, and parotid fascia.[1]

REFERENCE

1. Mitz V, Peyronie M. The superficial musculo-aponeurotic system (SMAS) in the parotid and cheek area. Plast Reconstr Surg 1976;58:80

SOFT TISSUE LAYERS OF THE FACE

5. *Which of the following muscles receives innervation from the facial nerve on its superficial surface?*

A. Mentalis.

Mimetic muscles are responsible for the highly complex and coordinated movements of the face. This contributes not only to facial expression but also the functions of speech and feeding (orbicularis oris muscle) as well as protection of the globe (orbicularis oculi muscle). There are four described layers of these facial muscles. Clinically relevant, the first three layers receive innervation from the facial nerve on their deep surfaces, while the deepest layer of muscles are innervated on their superficial surface. This deepest layer is composed of the mentalis, levator anguli oris, and buccinator muscles (MLB).[1]

REFERENCE

1. Freilinger G, Gruber H, Happal W, et al. Surgical anatomy of the mimic muscle system and the facial nerve: importance for reconstructive and aesthetic surgery. Plast Reconstr Surg 1987;80:686

SOFT TISSUE LAYERS OF THE FACE

6. *During open neck rejuvenation with platysmal plication in the midline, remaining just superficial to which layer ensures the safest plane for dissection?*

C. Investing deep fascia.

The layers of the neck tend to be a challenging topic. When operating in this region, awareness of the various layers is critical to avoid damage to vital structures that are abundant in the area. Following dissection through the subcutaneous tissue, which can have various degrees of adiposity, the platysma and superficial neck fascia are encountered. Of note, this layer is continuous with the superficial muscular aponeurotic system (SMAS) above the jawline. The superficial fascia of the neck is also continuous with the deep thoracic fascia covering the pectoralis major and deltoid muscles and fuses laterally with investing deep fascia of the sternocleidomastoid and trapezius muscles. Next is the investing deep fascia, also known as the superficial layer of the deep cervical fascia, which is the most superficial layer of the deep cervical fascia. Clinically relevant, no vital structures are present superficial to this layer in the midline, allowing for a safeplane ofdissection deep to the platysma muscle. The infrahyoid muscle fascia is located deeper, investing the sternohyoid, omohyoid, sternothyroid, and thyrohyoid muscles. Visceral fascia includes the pretracheal fascia covering the larynx and trachea, which also invests the thyroid gland. The deepest layer, the prevertebral fascia, invests the vertebral column and forms the floor of the posterior triangle of the neck.[1]

REFERENCE

1. Feldman JJ. Surgical anatomy of the neck. In: Feldman JJ, ed. Neck Lift. New York: Thieme Publishers; 2006

NERVES

7. *Following rhytidectomy, a patient complains of numbness at the ear lobule. Injury to which of the following is the most likely explanation for this complication?*

D. Great auricular nerve.

Innervation of the ear is well defined and derived primarily from the cervical plexus. The great auricular nerve (C2–C3) is responsible for innervation of the lobule and majority of the helix, consistently identified at McKinney's point 6.5 cm inferior to the external auditory canal overlying the sternocleidomastoid muscle running with the external jugular vein. Ozturk et al describe an additional topographic landmark where the nerve is consistently found.[1] This consists of a vertical line perpendicular to the Frankfort's horizontal plane bisecting the lobule of the ear and another line extending from the mid-lobule posteriorly at a 30-degree angle. Given its location and superficial course, it is prone to injury during surgical rejuvenation of the face and-neck. The auriculotemporal nerve, a branch of the mandibular division of the trigeminal nerve (V3), runs just anterior to the ear with the superficial temporal vessels and is responsible for sensationof the helical root and tragus primarily. The lesser occipital and greater occipital nerves (C2) provide sensation more posteriorly with the lesser providing some innervation at the postauricular fold. Arnold's nerve, a branch of CN X, is responsible for sensation within the ear at the external auditory canal lining.

REFERENCE

1. Ozturk CN, Ozturk C, Huettner F, Drake RL, Zins JE. A failsafe method to avoid injury to the great auricular nerve. Aesthetic Surg Journal 2014;34:16–21

NERVES

8. *Which of the following is true with regards to Pitanguy's line?*

A. Anterior point is 1.5 cm lateral to tail of the brow.

One of the long-standing topographic landmarks for the frontal branch of the facial nerve is Pitanguy's line (**Fig. 30.3**). The line is formed by connecting a point 1.5 cm lateral to the tail of the brow to a point 0.5 cm below the tragus. This intersects with the middle third of the zygomatic arch, at which point the frontal branch of the facial nerve also crosses over the arch. In the temple region, the frontal branch is located just deep to or within temporoparietal fascia and continues to course superoanteriorly to innervate the frontalis muscle. Be cognizant that there are typically three to five rami of the frontal branch of the facial nerve.[1]

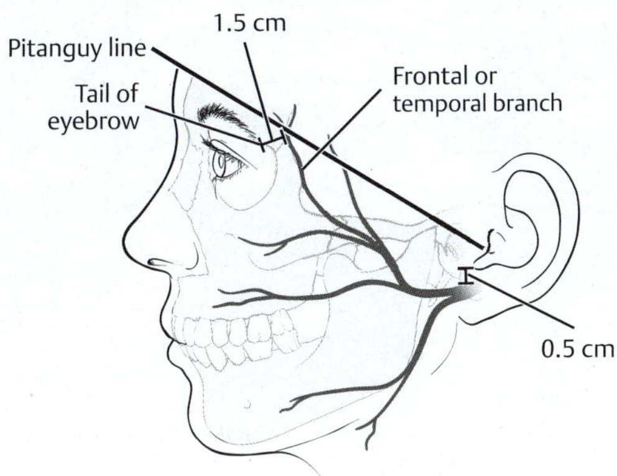

Fig. 30.3 Frontal branch course. (Source: Motor Innervation: Facial Nerve. In: Janis J, ed. Essentials of Aesthetic Surgery. 1st Edition. New York: Thieme; 2018.)

REFERENCE

1. Daane SP, Owsley JQ. Incidence of cervical branch injury with "marginal mandibular nerve pseudo-paralysis" in patients undergoing face lift. Plast Reconstr Surg 2003;111:2414

NERVES

9. *Following an open neck lift, a patient returns to clinic with complaints of facial asymmetry. On examination, the patient has an elevated right commissure compared to the left on active smile. Lower lip eversion is present and symmetric. Which of the following nerves is most likely injured?*

A. Right facial nerve cervical branch.

In this clinical scenario, the right commissure appears higher than the left while smiling due to weakened active lip depression from an injury to the right facial nerve cervical branch. As a result, there is more unopposed lip elevation on the right compared to the left, giving the illusion that the lower side is the injured side. In addition, active lip eversion is solely dependent upon the marginal mandibular nerve, which is intact in this case which eliminates this as a possibility. Of note, avoiding dissection within 2 cm of the lower mandibular border helps protect against injury to the marginal mandibular nerve. Although unilateral injury to the buccal branch may result in impaired elevation of the commissure on the affected side, bilateral involvement is rare and would not manifest with asymmetry. Injuries to the cervical branch of the facial nerve tend to recover over time with conservative management.[1]

REFERENCE

1. Daane SP, Owsley JQ. Incidence of cervical branch injury with "marginal mandibular nerve pseudo-paralysis" in patients undergoing face lift. Plast Reconstr Surg 2003;111:2414

FACIAL DANGER ZONES

10. *A patient undergoes a deep plane facelift with undermining to the modiolus. The next day, the patient has inability to elevate the commissure on active smile. Which of the following nerves is likely injured?*

C. Zygomatic branch of the facial nerve.

The zygomatic branch of the facial nerve innervates the muscles that control the movement of the upper lip, including the muscles responsible for elevating the corner of the mouth (commissure) during smiling. Injury to this nerve can result in difficulty elevating the commissure and lead to a drooping or asymmetric smile on the affected side (**Fig. 30.4**).[1]

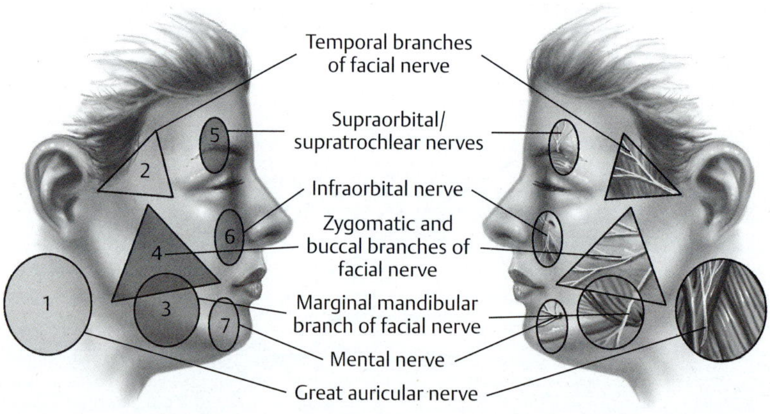

Fig. 30.4 Facial danger zones: motor and sensory nerves. (Source: Facial Danger Zones. In: Janis J, ed. Essentials of Aesthetic Surgery. 1st Edition. New York: Thieme; 2018.)

REFERENCE

1. Nahai F, Mejia JD, Nahai FR. Applied anatomy of the face and neck. In: Nahai F, ed. The Art of Aesthetic Surgery: Principles and Techniques. 2nd ed. New York: Thieme Publishers; 2010

FACIAL DANGER ZONES

11. *A patient has inability to evert the lower lip 3 days after a deep neck lift surgery. Which nerve is likely injured?*

D. Marginal mandibular nerve.

The marginal mandibular nerve is a branch of the facial nerve (cranial nerve VII) that provides innervation to the muscles responsible for controlling the movement of the lower lip, including the depressor anguli oris muscle. Inability to evert the lower lip indicates dysfunction of this nerve, which can occur due to injury during surgery or as a result of swelling and inflammation in the surgical area (**Fig. 30.5**).[1]

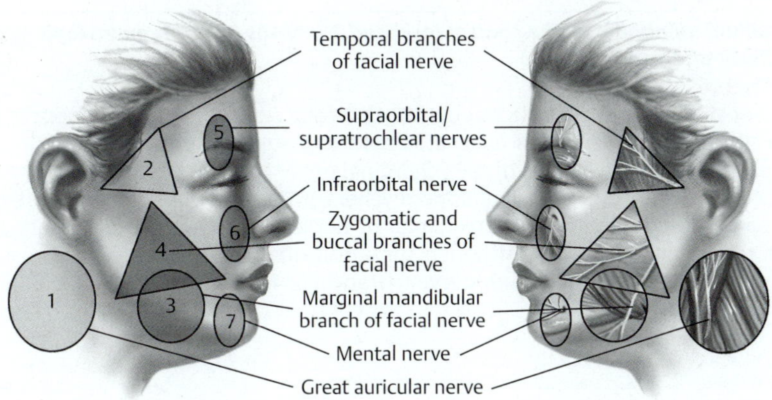

Fig. 30.5 Facial danger zones: motor and sensory nerves. (Source: Facial Danger Zones. In: Janis J, ed. Essentials of Aesthetic Surgery. 1st Edition. New York: Thieme; 2018.)

REFERENCE

1. Nahai F, Mejia JD, Nahai FR. Applied anatomy of the face and neck. In: Nahai F, ed. The Art of Aesthetic Surgery: Principles and Techniques. 2nd ed. New York: Thieme Publishers; 2010

FACIAL DANGER ZONES

12. *A 22-year-old female who is not healing postoperatively from an augmentation genioplasty has chin numbness. Which nerve is likely injured?*

B. Mental nerve.

The mental nerve is a branch of the trigeminal nerve (cranial nerve V) that provides sensory innervation to the chin and lower lip. It runs along the lower jaw and can be affected during genioplasty surgery, leading to numbness and altered sensation in the area. Nerve injury can result from the surgical procedure itself, pressure, stretching, or other factors that may have affected the nerve during surgery (**Fig. 30.6**).[1]

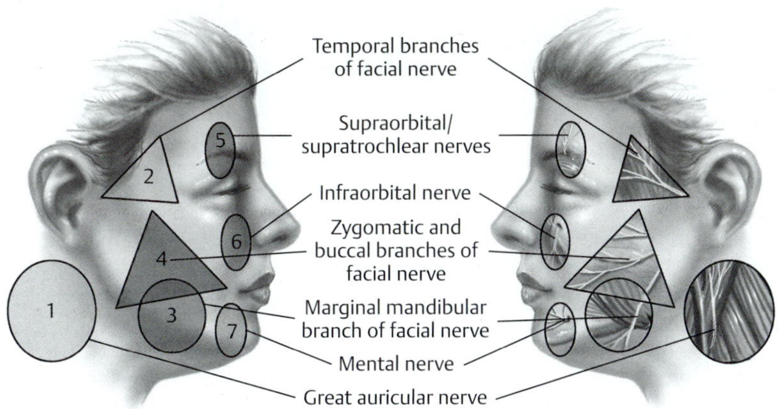

Fig. 30.6 Facial danger zones: motor and sensory nerves. (Source: Facial Danger Zones. In: Janis J, ed. Essentials of Aesthetic Surgery. 1st Edition. New York: Thieme; 2018.)

REFERENCE

1. Nahai F, Mejia JD, Nahai FR. Applied anatomy of the face and neck. In: Nahai F, ed. The Art of Aesthetic Surgery: Principles and Techniques. 2nd ed. New York: Thieme Publishers; 2010

FACIAL DANGER ZONES

13. *A patient has residual numbness of the central forehead 2 months after an endoscopic browlift procedure. Which nerve is likely affected?*

A. Supraorbital nerve.

In case a patient still experiences residual numbness of the central forehead 2 months after an endoscopic browlift procedure, the nerve that is likely affected is the supraorbital nerve.

The supraorbital nerve is a branch of the trigeminal nerve (cranial nerve V) that provides sensory innervation to the central forehead, scalp, and upper eyelid. During an endoscopic browlift, the manipulation of tissues and potential compression or stretching of nerves can result in temporary or even permanent numbness in the innervated areas. Although sensation often improves over time, some patients might experience prolonged numbness due to nerve irritation or injury (**Fig. 30.7**).[1]

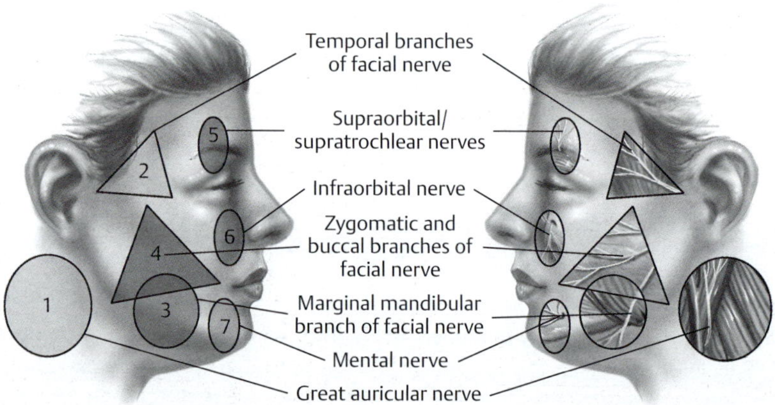

Fig. 30.7 Facial danger zones: motor and sensory nerves. (Source: Facial Danger Zones. In: Janis J, ed. Essentials of Aesthetic Surgery. 1st Edition. New York: Thieme; 2018.)

REFERENCE

1. Nahai F, Mejia JD, Nahai FR. Applied anatomy of the face and neck. In: Nahai F, ed. The Art of Aesthetic Surgery: Principles and Techniques. 2nd ed. New York: Thieme Publishers; 2010

VASCULAR SUPPLY

14. *Which of the following is derived from the internal carotid arterial system?*

D. Supratrochlear artery.

The main vascular supply of the face is provided by the external carotid system, whose branches include the following, from most caudal to cephalad: superior thyroid, ascending pharyngeal, lingual, facial, occipital, posterior auricular, maxillary, and superficial temporal (remembered by the pneumonic SALFOP MS). The internal carotid does contribute a small portion to the facial blood supply, namely, from the ophthalmic artery whose branches include the supraorbital and supratrochlear arteries at the forehead.[1]

REFERENCE

1. Whetzel TP, Mathes SJ. Arterial anatomy of the face: an analysis of vascular territories and perforating cutaneous vessels. Plast Reconstr Surg 1992;89:591

VASCULAR SUPPLY

15. *Which of the following is true regarding the sentinel vein?*

D. Branch of the zygomaticotemporal vein.

The sentinel vein is an important anatomic landmark that is commonly encountered when performing a temporal brow lift. A branch of the zygomaticotemporal vein, it is located above the zygomatic arch and lateral to the lateral canthus, but below the temporal crest in the temporal hollow, classically below the inferior temporal septum (**Fig. 30.8**). Identification and avoidance of the sentinel vein not only assist with decreasing postoperative edema and ecchymosis, but also serve to prevent injury to the frontal branch of the facial nerve, which is found in close proximity.[1]

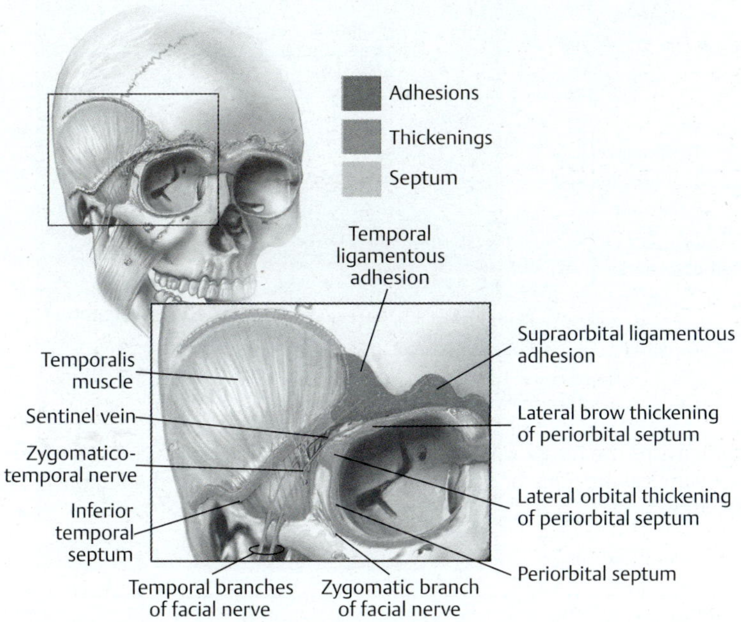

Fig. 30.8 Retaining ligaments of the temporal and orbital regions. (Source: Reprinted with permission from Moss JC, Mendelson BC, Taylor GI. Surgical anatomy of the ligamentous attachments in the temple & periorbital regions. Plast Reconstr Surg 105:1475, 2000.)

REFERENCE

1. Whetzel TP, Mathes SJ. Arterial anatomy of the face: an analysis of vascular territories and perforating cutaneous vessels. Plast Reconstr Surg 1992;89:591

RETAINING LIGAMENTS OF THE FACE AND NECK

16. *A patient presents for improvement of periorbital facial aging. Release of which of the following is essential to blend the lid–cheek junction?*

E. Orbicularis retaining ligament.

The orbicularis retaining ligament (ORL), also known as the orbitomalar ligament, is an important component of lower eyelid rejuvenation surgery. Originating from the periosteum, the ORL passes through the orbicularis oculi muscle and inserts onto the skin at the lid–cheek junction. The ORL includes a lateral extension, which connects to the superficial lateral canthal tendon at the lateral orbital thickening. Medially, the ORL is continuous with the tear trough ligament at the medial origin of the orbicularis oculi muscle (**Fig. 30.9**). Full inferior release of this ligamentous construct allows for a youthful contour transition from the lower eyelid to the midface. The temporal ligamentous adhesion is located at the superolateral orbit at the temple, holding the tail of the brow in position. The zygomatic osteocutaneous ligament originates from inferior border of the zygomatic arch, coursing anteriorly through the malar fat pad and insertingdirectlyonto dermis.[1]

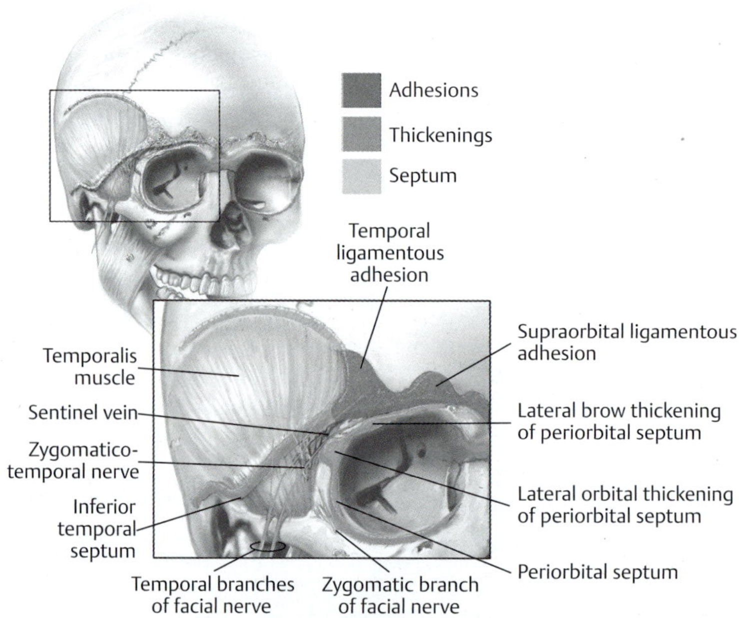

Fig. 30.9 Retaining ligaments of the temporal and orbital regions. (Source: Reprinted with permission from Moss JC, Mendelson BC, Taylor GI. Surgical anatomy of the ligamentous attachments in the temple & periorbital regions. Plast Reconstr Surg 105:1475, 2000.)

Reference

1. Ghavami A, Pessa JE, Janis J, et al. The orbicularis retaining ligament of the medial orbit: closing the circle. Plast Reconstr Surg 2008;121:994

ANTERIOR TRIANGLE OF THE NECK

17. *The borders of the anterior triangle of the neck include which of the following?*

C. Anterior border of sternocleidomastoid, inferior border of the mandible, median line of the neck.

The anterior triangle of the neck is bordered posteriorly by the anterior border of the sternocleidomastoid muscle, anteriorly by the median line of the neck, and superiorly by the inferior border of the mandible. Within the anterior triangle of the neck, the submandibular and submental triangles may be found. Their boundaries include both the anterior and posterior bellies of the digastric muscle and inferior border of the mandible, and the anterior bellies of the digastric muscles and hyoid bone, respectively. The posterior neck triangle is bound anteriorly by the posterior border of sternocleidomastoid, posteriorly by the anterior border of trapezius muscle, and inferiorly by the clavicle.[1]

Reference

1. Nahai F, Mejia JD, Nahai FR. Applied anatomy of the face and neck. In: Nahai F, ed. The Art of Aesthetic Surgery: Principles and Techniques. 2nd ed. New York: Thieme Publishers; 2010

31. Facial Analysis

Ira L. Savetsky, Anmol Chattha
See *Essentials of Aesthetic Surgery*, pp. 390–401

SKIN QUALITY

1. ***Which of the following Fitzpatrick skin types tans moderately and easily, burns minimally?***
   A. I.
   B. II.
   C. III.
   D. IV.
   E. V.

SKIN QUALITY

2. ***By what percentage does dermal thickness decrease per decade?***
   A. 2%.
   B. 6%.
   C. 12%.
   D. 20%.
   E. 30%.

SKIN QUALITY

3. ***According to the Glogau classification, which of the following best describes "Group III, Advanced"?***
   A. Early wrinkling, mild scarring; sallow color with early actinic keratosis; requires little makeup.
   B. Persistent wrinkling; discoloration with telangiectasias and actinic keratosis; wears makeup always.
   C. Little wrinkling or scarring; no keratosis; requires little or no makeup.
   D. Wrinkling; photoaging: gravitational, dynamic; actinic keratosis with or without skin cancer; wears makeup with poor coverage.
   E. No wrinkling or photoaging, however with some keratosis.

FACIAL CANONS OF DIVINE PROPORTION

4. ***What is the golden ratio of Fibonacci?***
   A. 1:1.
   B. 1:1.3.
   C. 1:1.6.
   D. 1:1.9.
   E. 1:2.

FACIAL CANONS OF DIVINE PROPORTION

5. ***On frontal view, how is the face classically divided into?***
   A. Vertical thirds, horizontal halves.
   B. Vertical halves, horizontal thirds.
   C. Vertical thirds, horizontal fifths.
   D. Vertical fifths, horizontal thirds.
   E. Vertical halves, horizontal fifths.

FACIAL CANONS OF DIVINE PROPORTION

6. *The desired lip–chin complex relationship in a female patient is an upper lip that projects approximately how many millimeters more than the lower lip?*

A. 1 mm.
B. 2 mm.
C. 3 mm.
D. 4 mm.
E. 5 mm.

REGION-SPECIFIC ANALYSIS

PERIORBITAL

7. *With the lid closed, the brow should be how many centimeters above the upper lid margin?*

A. 0.5 cm.
B. 1 cm.
C. 2 cm.
D. 3 cm.
E. 4 cm.

REGION-SPECIFIC ANALYSIS

PERIORBITAL

8. *In Caucasian females, what is considered to be the most attractive intercanthal distance?*

A. 20–25 mm.
B. 25–30 mm.
C. 30–35 mm.
D. 35–40 mm.
E. 40–45 mm.

REGION-SPECIFIC ANALYSIS

PERIORBITAL

9. *What is the minimum distance the upper eyelid should extend below the upper limbus?*

A. 0.5 mm.
B. 1 mm.
C. 1.5 mm.
D. 2 mm.
E. 2.5 mm.

REGION-SPECIFIC ANALYSIS

PERIORBITAL

10. *Which of the following is an indicator of levator dehiscence?*

A. High supratarsal fold, thinning of the lid above the tarsal plate.
B. High supratarsal fold, thickening of the lid above the tarsal plate.
C. Low supratarsal fold, thinning of the lid above the tarsal plate.
D. Low supratarsal fold, thickening of the lid above the tarsal plate.
E. Low supratarsal fold, no change to the lid above the tarsal plate.

REGION-SPECIFIC ANALYSIS

NOSE

11. ***The width of the body of the nose at the nasal–cheek junction should equal what percentage of the alar base width?***
A. 20%.
B. 40%.
C. 60%.
D. 80%.
E. 100%.

REGION-SPECIFIC ANALYSIS

NOSE

12. ***How many millimeters is considered normal alar flaring in white females?***
A. 0.5 mm.
B. 1 mm.
C. 2 mm.
D. 3 mm.
E. 4 mm.

REGION-SPECIFIC ANALYSIS

NOSE

13. ***When evaluating the nose from the basal view, what is the ideal ratio of columella to lobular portion?***
A. 1:2.
B. 1:1.
C. 2:1.
D. 3:1.
E. 4:1.

REGION-SPECIFIC ANALYSIS

NOSE

14. ***When evaluating the nasal dorsum in women, how many millimeters should the nasal dorsum lie behind and parallel to a line connecting the nasofrontal angle with the desired tip projection?***
A. 0.5 mm.
B. 1 mm.
C. 2 mm.
D. 3 mm.
E. 4 mm.

REGION-SPECIFIC ANALYSIS

NOSE

15. ***What is the preferred nasolabial angle in women?***
A. 85–90 degrees.
B. 90–95 degrees.
C. 95–100 degrees.
D. 100–105 degrees.
E. 105–120 degrees.

REGION-SPECIFIC ANALYSIS

NOSE

16. *What is the preferred nasolabial angle in men?*
A. 85–90 degrees.
B. 90–95 degrees.
C. 95–100 degrees.
D. 100–105 degrees.
E. 105–120 degrees.

REGION-SPECIFIC ANALYSIS

NOSE

17. *What is the preferred columellar–lobular angle?*
A. 15–30 degrees.
B. 30–45 degrees.
C. 45–60 degrees.
D. 60–75 degrees.

REGION-SPECIFIC ANALYSIS

NOSE

18. *Compared with nasal ideals for white patients, the noses of black patients have which of the following characteristics?*
A. Increased nasal length and tip projection.
B. Strong nasal tip definition.
C. Obtuse columellar–labial angle.
D. Alar flaring.
E. High radix.

REGION-SPECIFIC ANALYSIS

EAR

19. *When considering ideal ear aesthetics, approximately how many degrees should the long vertical axis incline posteriorly from the scalp?*
A. 10.
B. 20.
C. 30.
D. 40.
E. 50.

REGION-SPECIFIC ANALYSIS

NECK

20. *What is the ideal cervicomental angle?*
A. 90–100 degrees.
B. 100–105 degrees.
C. 105–120 degrees.
D. 120–130 degrees.
E. 130–135 degrees.

Answers

SKIN QUALITY

1. ***Which of the following Fitzpatrick skin types tans moderately and easily, burns minimally?***

D. IV.

The Fitzpatrick skin scale, developed by dermatologist Thomas B. Fitzpatrick in 1975, categorizes human skin into six different types based on their response to sun exposure. It takes into account factors such as skin color, reaction to UV radiation, and tendency to tan or burn. This classification system helps determine the appropriate treatments for various skin concerns, such as sun protection recommendations, laser therapies, and chemical peels, taking into consideration the differing characteristics and sensitivities of each skin type.

Fitzpatrick skin type IV refers to a specific category in the Fitzpatrick skin scale, which is a classification system used to categorize human skin based on its response to sun exposure. Skin type IV represents individuals with moderately pigmented skin that typically tans easily and rarely burns. Fitzpatrick skin type III burns "moderately" compared to type IV which burns minimally. Both tan moderately. Fitzpatrick skin type I burns easily and can be severe. Fitzpatrick II usually burns and tans minimally. Fitzpatrick V rarely burns and patients have dark brown skin (**Table 31.1**).[1,2]

Table 31.1 *Fitzpatrick Skin Type Classification*

Skin Type	Sun Exposure History/Skin Color
I	Never tans; burns easily and severely; extremely fair skin
II	Usually burns; tans minimally
III	Burns moderately; tans moderately
IV	Tans moderately and easily; burns minimally
V	Rarely burns; dark brown skin
VI	Never burns; dark brown or black skin

(Source: Data from Fitzpatrick TB. The validity and practicality of sun-reactive skin types I through VI. Arch Dermatol 124:869, 1988.)

REFERENCES

1. Barton FE Jr, ed. Facial Rejuvenation. New York: Thieme Publishers; 2008
2. Nahai F, ed. The Art of Aesthetic Surgery: Principles & Techniques. New York: Thieme Publishers; 2005

SKIN QUALITY

2. ***By what percentage does dermal thickness decrease per decade?***

B. 6%.

Total dermal thickness decreases approximately 6% per decade. Actinic exposure and smoking increase the rate of dermal deterioration.[1,2]

REFERENCES

1. Barton FE Jr, ed. Facial Rejuvenation. New York: Thieme Publishers; 2008
2. Nahai F, ed. The Art of Aesthetic Surgery: Principles & Techniques. New York: Thieme Publishers; 2005

SKIN QUALITY

3. ***According to the Glogau classification, which of the following best describes "Group III, Advanced"?***

B. Persistent wrinkling; discoloration with telangiectasias and actinic keratosis; wears makeup always.

The Glogau classification is a system used to categorize the severity of facial aging and sun damage based on visible signs such as wrinkles, pigmentation changes, and skin texture. It was developed by Dr. Richard Glogau, a dermatologist, as a way to help clinicians and researchers communicate more effectively about the degree of facial aging in patients. Group III is defined as wrinkles visible both at rest and with facial expressions. This category represents more significant photoaging, characterized by moderate to severe wrinkles, age spots (also known as sunspots or liver spots), and noticeable texture changes.[1,2]

References

1. Barton FE Jr, ed. Facial Rejuvenation. New York: Thieme Publishers; 2008
2. Nahai F, ed. The Art of Aesthetic Surgery: Principles & Techniques. New York: Thieme Publishers; 2005

FACIAL CANONS OF DIVINE PROPORTION

4. *What is the golden ratio of Fibonacci?*

C. 1:1.6.

In aesthetic surgery, the golden ratio is a concept derived from the mathematical proportion of approximately 1.618. It is thought to define a pleasing and harmonious symmetry in facial or bodily proportions. Surgeons sometimes utilize this ratio as a tool to guide their surgical approach, aiming to achieve outcomes that align with this aesthetically acclaimed ratio.[1]

Reference

1. Bashour M. History and current concepts in the analysis of facial attractiveness. Plast Reconstr Surg 2006;118:741

FACIAL CANONS OF DIVINE PROPORTION

5. *On frontal view, how is the face classically divided into?*

D. Vertical fifths, horizontal thirds.

Vertical fifths are divided by lines drawn adjacent to the most lateral projection of the head, the lateral canthi, and the medial canthi (**Fig. 31.1a**). Horizontal thirds are divided by lines drawn adjacent to the menton, nasal base, brows at the supraorbital notch level, and hairline (**Fig. 31.1b**).[1,2]

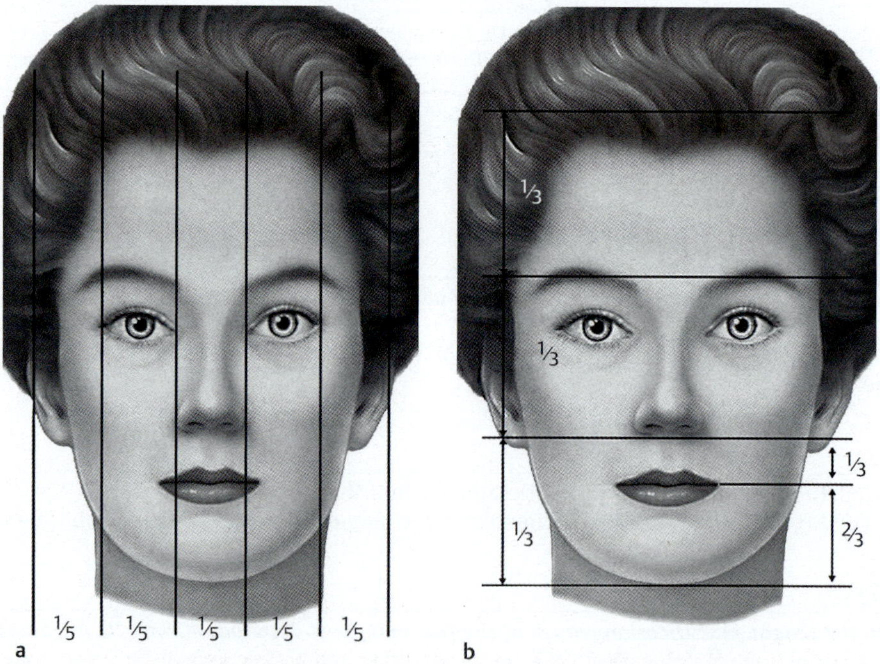

Fig. 31.1 (a) Vertical fifths. **(b)** Horizontal thirds. (Source: Proportions of the Face. In: Rohrich R, Adams W, Ahmad J, Gunter J, ed. Dallas Rhinoplasty: Nasal Surgery by the Masters. 3rd Edition. New York: Thieme; 2014.)

REFERENCES

1. Bashour M. History and current concepts in the analysis of facial attractiveness. Plast Reconstr Surg 2006;118:741
2. Gunter JP, Rohrich RJ, Adams WP Jr, eds. Dallas Rhinoplasty: Nasal Surgery by the Masters. New York: Thieme Publishers; 2002

FACIAL CANONS OF DIVINE PROPORTION

6. *The desired lip–chin complex relationship in a female patient is an upper lip that projects approximately how many millimeters more than the lower lip?*

B. 2 mm.

The desired lip–chin complex relationship is an upper lip that projects approximately 2 mm more than the lower lip. In women the chin lies slightly posterior to the lower lip. In men the chin is slightly stronger (**Fig. 31.2**).[1]

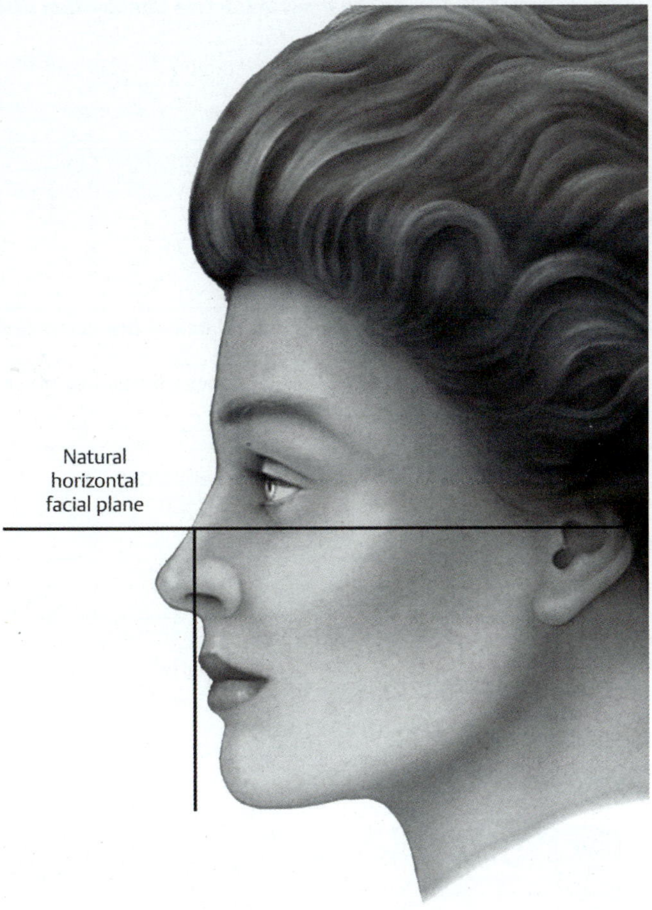

Fig. 31.2 Desired lip-chin complex relationship. (Source: Proportions of the Face. In: Rohrich R, Adams W, Ahmad J, Gunter J, ed. Dallas Rhinoplasty: Nasal Surgery by the Masters. 3rd Edition. New York: Thieme; 2014.)

REFERENCE

1. Gunter JP, Rohrich RJ, Adams WP Jr, eds. Dallas Rhinoplasty: Nasal Surgery by the Masters. New York: Thieme Publishers; 2002

REGION-SPECIFIC ANALYSIS

PERIORBITAL

7. *With the lid closed, the brow should be how many centimeters above the upper lid margin?*

C. 2 cm.

With the lid closed, the brow should be 2 to 2.5 cm above the upper lid margin.[1]

REFERENCE

1. Barton FE Jr, ed. Facial Rejuvenation. New York: Thieme Publishers; 2008

REGION-SPECIFIC ANALYSIS

PERIORBITAL

8. *In Caucasian females, what is considered to be the most attractive intercanthal distance?*

C. 30–35 mm.

The ideal intercanthal distance is 31 to 33 mm; however, 33 to 36 mm can be considered attractive.[1]

REFERENCE

1. Barton FE Jr, ed. Facial Rejuvenation. New York: Thieme Publishers; 2008

REGION-SPECIFIC ANALYSIS

PERIORBITAL

9. *What is the minimum distance the upper eyelid should extend below the upper limbus?*

C. 1.5 mm.

The upper lid extends down at least 1.5 mm below the upper limbus but no more than 3 mm.[1]

REFERENCE

1. Barton FE Jr, ed. Facial Rejuvenation. New York: Thieme Publishers; 2008

REGION-SPECIFIC ANALYSIS

PERIORBITAL

10. *Which of the following is an indicator of levator dehiscence?*

A. High supratarsal fold, thinning of the lid above the tarsal plate.

Indicators of levator dehiscence include elevation of supratarsal fold and an accentuated supratarsal hollow (**Fig. 31.3**).[1]

This woman in the photo shows classic signs of left levator dehiscence with ptosis, a high lid crease, and thinning of the lid above the tarsal plate.

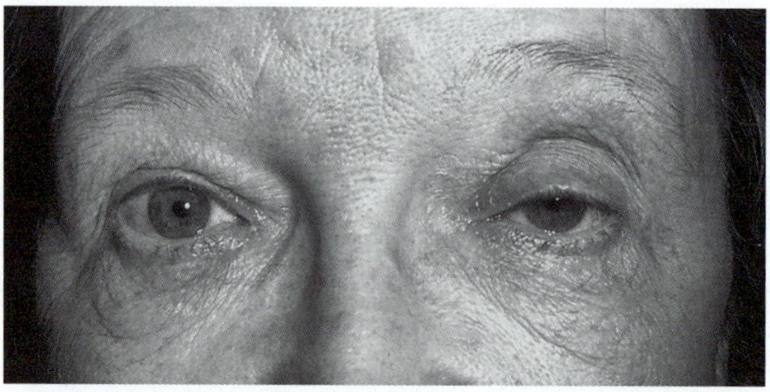

Fig. 31.3 This woman shows classic signs of left levator dehiscence with ptosis, a high lid crease, and thinning of the lid above the tarsal plate. (Source: Is Levator Dehiscence Present?. In: Codner M, McCord C, ed. Eyelid & Periorbital Surgery. 2nd Edition. New York: Thieme; 2016.)

Reference

1. McCord CD Jr, Codner MA, eds. Eyelid & Periorbital Surgery. New York: Thieme Publishers; 2008

REGION-SPECIFIC ANALYSIS

NOSE

11. *The width of the body of the nose at the nasal–cheek junction should equal what percentage of the alar base width?*

D. 80%.

The width of the body of the nose at the nasal–cheek junction should equal 80% of the alar base width (**Fig. 31.4**).[1,2]

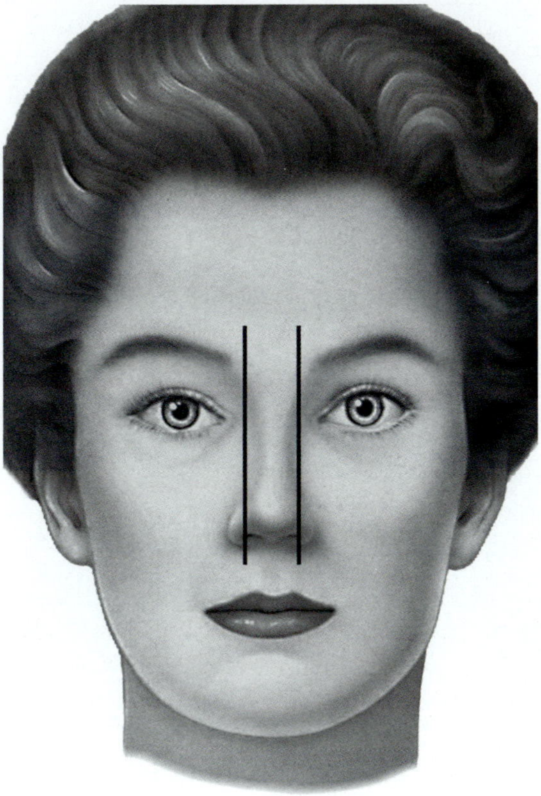

Fig. 31.4 The body of the nose at the nasal-cheek junction should equal 80% of the alar base width. (Source: Proportions of the Face. In: Rohrich R, Adams W, Ahmad J, Gunter J, ed. Dallas Rhinoplasty: Nasal Surgery by the Masters. 3rd Edition. New York: Thieme; 2014.)

References

1. Gunter JP, Rohrich RJ, Adams WP Jr, eds. Dallas Rhinoplasty: Nasal Surgery by the Masters. New York: Thieme Publishers; 2002
2. Byrd HS, Hobar PC. Rhinoplasty: a practical guide for surgical planning. Plast Reconstr Surg 1993;91:642; discussion 655

REGION-SPECIFIC ANALYSIS

NOSE

12. *How many millimeters is considered normal alar flaring in white females?*

C. 2 mm.

Normal alar flaring in white females is 2 mm wider than alar base; if it is greater than this, alar base resection should be considered.[1,2]

REFERENCES

1. Gunter JP, Rohrich RJ, Adams WP Jr, eds. Dallas Rhinoplasty: Nasal Surgery by the Masters. New York: Thieme Publishers; 2002
2. Byrd HS, Hobar PC. Rhinoplasty: a practical guide for surgical planning. Plast Reconstr Surg 1993;91:642; discussion 655

REGION-SPECIFIC ANALYSIS

NOSE

13. *When evaluating the nose from the basal view, what is the ideal ratio of columella to lobular portion?*

C. 2:1.

On basal view, an equilateral triangle is visualized with a 2:1 ratio of columella to lobular portion; the nostrils should be teardrop shaped (**Fig. 31.5**).[1,2]

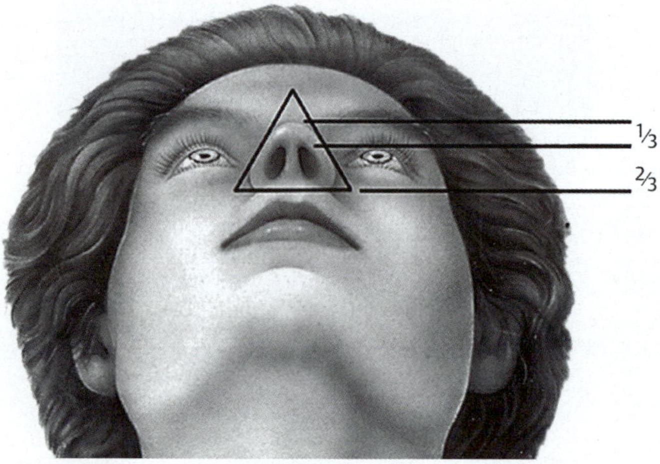

Fig. 31.5 Basal view. (Source: Proportions of the Face. In: Rohrich R, Adams W, Ahmad J, Gunter J, ed. Dallas Rhinoplasty: Nasal Surgery by the Masters. 3rd Edition. New York: Thieme; 2014.)

REFERENCES

1. Gunter JP, Rohrich RJ, Adams WP Jr, eds. Dallas Rhinoplasty: Nasal Surgery by the Masters. New York: Thieme Publishers; 2002
2. Byrd HS, Hobar PC. Rhinoplasty: a practical guide for surgical planning. Plast Reconstr Surg 1993;91:642; discussion 655

REGION-SPECIFIC ANALYSIS

NOSE

14. *When evaluating the nasal dorsum in women, how many millimeters should the nasal dorsum lie behind and parallel to a line connecting the nasofrontal angle with the desired tip projection?*

C. 2 mm.

In women it lies 2 mm behind and parallel to a line connecting the nasofrontal angle with the desired tip projection; a slight supratip break is preferred (**Fig. 31.6**). In men it lies slightly more anteriorly. If it is too far posterior to this line, augmentation will be required. If it is too far anterior to this line, reduction is indicated.[1,2]

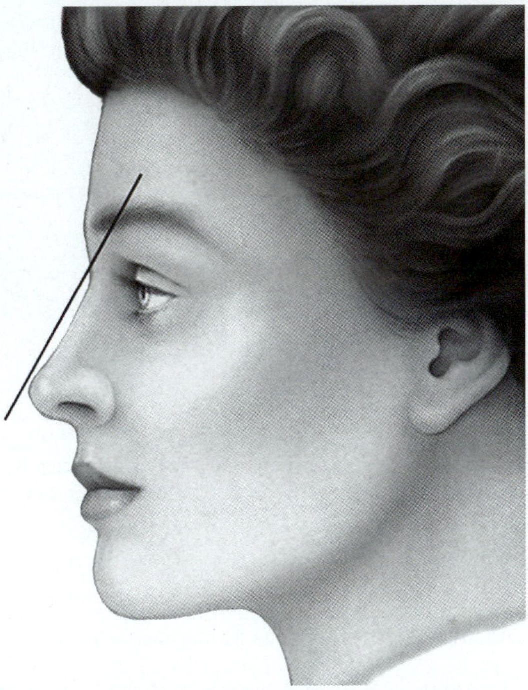

Fig. 31.6 Nasal dorsum evaluation. (Source: Proportions of the Face. In: Rohrich R, Adams W, Ahmad J, Gunter J, ed. Dallas Rhinoplasty: Nasal Surgery by the Masters. 3rd Edition. New York: Thieme; 2014.)

REFERENCES

1. Gunter JP, Rohrich RJ, Adams WP Jr, eds. Dallas Rhinoplasty: Nasal Surgery by the Masters. New York: Thieme Publishers; 2002
2. Byrd HS, Hobar PC. Rhinoplasty: a practical guide for surgical planning. Plast Reconstr Surg 1993;91:642; discussion 655

REGION-SPECIFIC ANALYSIS

NOSE

15. *What is the preferred nasolabial angle in women?*

C. 95–100 degrees.

Tip rotation is determined by the degree of the nasolabial angle. Draw a straight line through the most anterior and posterior points of the nostrils on lateral view. The angle formed when this line bisects a perpendicular line to the natural horizontal facial plane is the nasolabial angle. In women 95- to 100-degree angle is preferred. In men 90- to 95-degree angle is preferred (**Fig. 31.7**).[1,2]

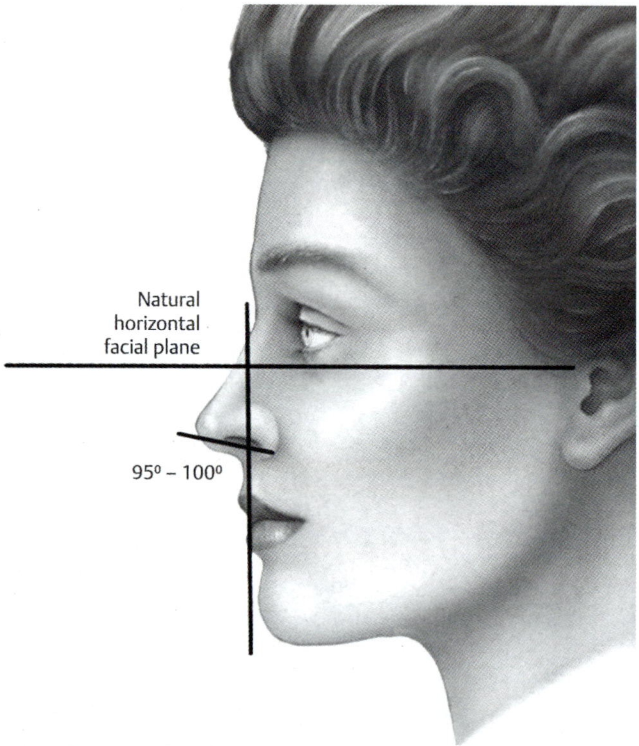

Fig. 31.7 Nasolabial angle. (Source: Proportions of the Face. In: Rohrich R, Adams W, Ahmad J, Gunter J, ed. Dallas Rhinoplasty: Nasal Surgery by the Masters. 3rd Edition. New York: Thieme; 2014.)

References

1. Gunter JP, Rohrich RJ, Adams WP Jr, eds. Dallas Rhinoplasty: Nasal Surgery by the Masters. New York: Thieme Publishers; 2002
2. Byrd HS, Hobar PC. Rhinoplasty: a practical guide for surgical planning. Plast Reconstr Surg 1993;91:642; discussion 655

REGION-SPECIFIC ANALYSIS

NOSE

16. *What is the preferred nasolabial angle in men?*

B. 90–95 degrees.

Tip rotation is determined by the degree of the nasolabial angle. Draw a straight line through the most anterior and posterior points of the nostrils on lateral view. The angle formed when this line bisects a perpendicular line to the natural horizontal facial plane is the nasolabial angle. In women 95- to 100-degree angle is preferred. In men 90- to 95-degree angle is preferred (**Fig. 31.8**).[1,2]

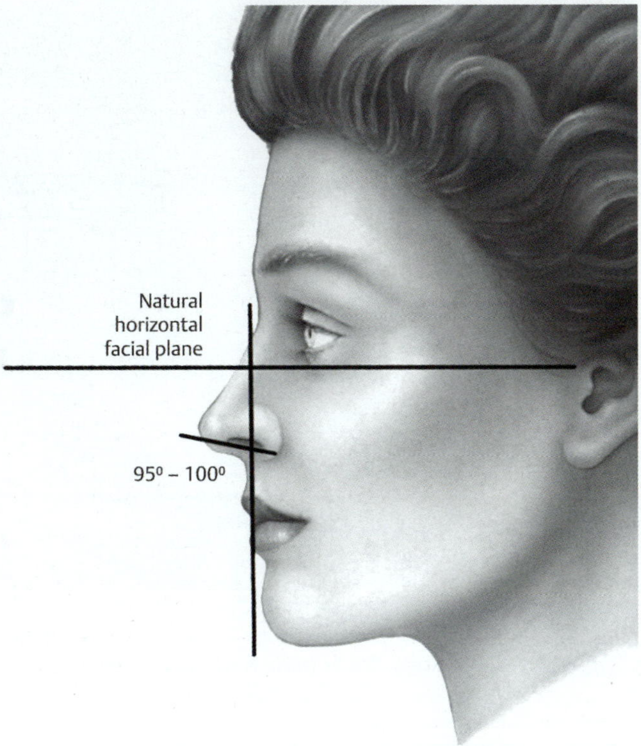

Fig. 31.8 Nasolabial angle. (Source: Proportions of the Face. In: Rohrich R, Adams W, Ahmad J, Gunter J, ed. Dallas Rhinoplasty: Nasal Surgery by the Masters. 3rd Edition. New York: Thieme; 2014.)

REFERENCES

1. Gunter JP, Rohrich RJ, Adams WP Jr, eds. Dallas Rhinoplasty: Nasal Surgery by the Masters. New York: Thieme Publishers; 2002
2. Byrd HS, Hobar PC. Rhinoplasty: a practical guide for surgical planning. Plast Reconstr Surg 1993;91:642; discussion 655

REGION-SPECIFIC ANALYSIS

NOSE

17. *What is the preferred columellar–lobular angle?*

B. 30–45 degrees.

The columellar–lobular angle is formed by the junction of the columella with the infratip lobule. It is usually 30 to 45 degrees. Increased fullness in this area (usually caused by prominent caudal septum) will give the appearance of increased tip rotation even though the angle of rotation (nasolabial angle) is within normal limits (**Fig. 31.9**).[1,2]

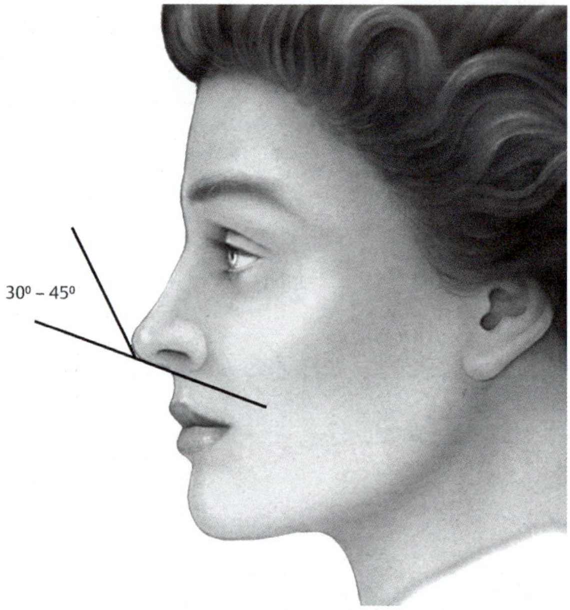

Fig. 31.9 Columellar-lobular angle. (Source: Proportions of the Face. In: Rohrich R, Adams W, Ahmad J, Gunter J, ed. Dallas Rhinoplasty: Nasal Surgery by the Masters. 3rd Edition. New York: Thieme; 2014.)

REFERENCES

1. Gunter JP, Rohrich RJ, Adams WP Jr, eds. Dallas Rhinoplasty: Nasal Surgery by the Masters. New York: Thieme Publishers; 2002
2. Byrd HS, Hobar PC. Rhinoplasty: a practical guide for surgical planning. Plast Reconstr Surg 1993;91:642; discussion 655

REGION-SPECIFIC ANALYSIS

NOSE

18. ***Compared with nasal ideals for white patients, the noses of black patients have which of the following characteristics?***

D. Alar flaring.

Compared with nasal ideals for whites, the nose of black patients has the following characteristics: wide, low nasal dorsum, decreased nasal length and tip projection, poor nasal tip definition, acute columellar-labial angle, and alar flaring (**Fig. 31.10**).[1,2]

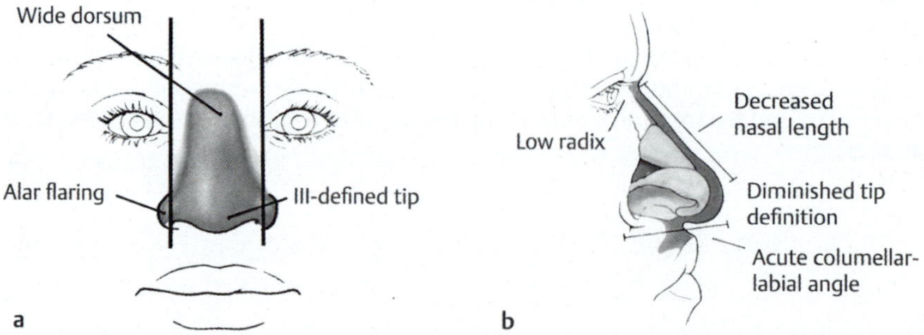

Fig. 31.10 (a,b) Typical characteristics of the noses of black patients. (Source: Proportions of the Face. In: Rohrich R, Adams W, Ahmad J, Gunter J, ed. Dallas Rhinoplasty: Nasal Surgery by the Masters. 3rd Edition. New York: Thieme; 2014.)

References

1. Gunter JP, Rohrich RJ, Adams WP Jr, eds. Dallas Rhinoplasty: Nasal Surgery by the Masters. New York: Thieme Publishers; 2002
2. Byrd HS, Hobar PC. Rhinoplasty: a practical guide for surgical planning. Plast Reconstr Surg 1993;91:642; discussion 655

REGION-SPECIFIC ANALYSIS

EAR

19. *When considering ideal ear aesthetics, approximately how many degrees should the long vertical axis incline posteriorly from the scalp?*

B. 20.

In normal ear aesthetics, the ear is positioned approximately one ear length posterior to the lateral orbital rim and centered in the middle third horizontal plane. The long axis inclines posteriorly approximately 20 degrees from the vertical plane. The ideal width is approximately 55 to 60% of the height. The anterolateral aspect of the helix protrudes 21 to 30 degrees (1.5–2 cm) from the scalp. The helix should project 2 to 5 mm more laterally than the antihelix in frontal view (**Fig. 31.11**).[1,2]

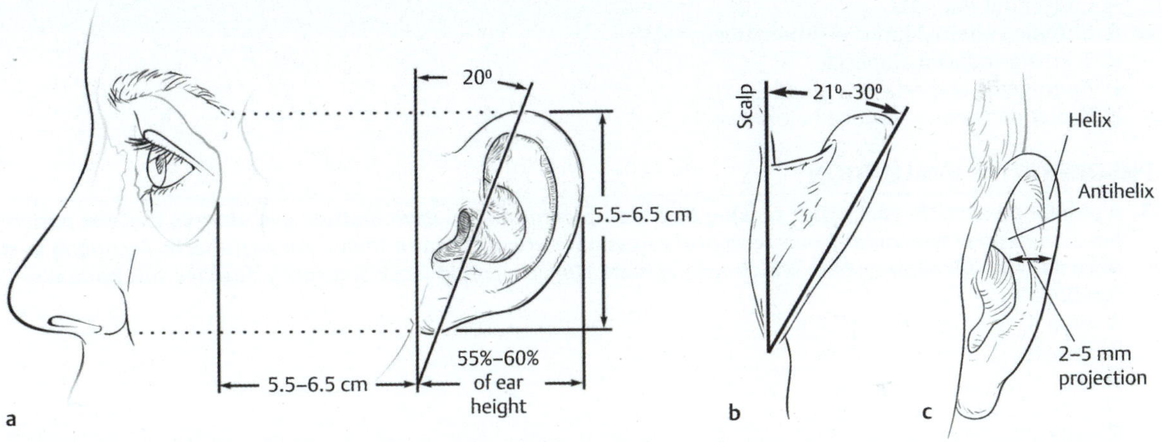

Fig. 31.11 (a–c) Normal ear aesthetics. (Source: Ears. In: Janis J, ed. Essentials of Aesthetic Surgery. 1st Edition. New York: Thieme; 2018.)

References

1. Janis JE, Rohrich RJ, Gutowski KA. Otoplasty. Plast Reconstr Surg 2005;115:60e
2. Ha RY, Trovato MJ. Plastic surgery of the ear. Sel Read Plast Surg 2011;11:1

REGION-SPECIFIC ANALYSIS

NECK

20. *What is the ideal cervicomental angle?*

C. 105–120 degrees.

The qualities of a youthful neck are: a distinct inferior mandibular border, subhyoid depression, a visible thyroid cartilage bulge, a visible anterior border of the sternocleidomastoid, and a cervicomental angle of 105 to 120 degrees.[1]

Reference

1. Ellenbogen R, Karlin JV. Visual criteria for success in restoring the youthful neck. Plast Reconstr Surg 1980;66:826

32. Hair Transplantation

Sammy Sinno, Jeremie Oliver Piña
See *Essentials of Aesthetic Surgery*, pp. 402–410

DEFINITION OF PROBLEM

1. *Which phase of hair growth is prolonged during the thinning and balding process?*

A. Anagen.
B. Catagen.
C. Telogen.
D. Club phase.
E. Papillary.

CONTRAINDICATIONS

2. *Which of the following is a contraindication to pursuing hair transplantation treatment?*

A. Congenital hair loss.
B. Chronic systemic lupus erythematosus (SLE).
C. Scarring-induced alopecia.
D. Androgenic alopecia in a female.
E. Radiation therapy–induced alopecia.

PREOPERATIVE EVALUATION

3. *A patient presents to your office seeking hair transplantation. On examination, you observe that the patient has symmetrical triangular frontotemporal recessions extending more than 2 cm posteriorly. According to the Norwood classification system, which type of male alopecia would most accurately describe this patient's condition?*

A. Type II.
B. Type III.
C. Type V.
D. Type VI.
E. Type VII.

PREOPERATIVE EVALUATION

4. *What is the minimum range of hair follicles per square centimeter that is classified as appearing normal?*

A. 0–30.
B. 30–70.
C. 70–110.
D. 140–220.
E. 240–400.

PREOPERATIVE EVALUATION

5. *Which of the following are the two most ideal donor sites for hair transplantation harvest?*

A. Occipital and frontal.
B. Temporal and frontal.
C. Postauricular and temporal.
D. Temporal and occipital.
E. None of the above.

TECHNIQUE

6. *In a mature patient, which of the following landmarks would be most appropriate for donor site selection?*
A. Two-thirds of the way down from the posterior fringe to the lower hairline.
B. One-third of the way down from upper border of baldness to the lower hairline.
C. One-half the distance down from the upper border of baldness to the lower hairline.
D. 2 inches above the lower hairline.
E. 2 inches below the posterior fringe.

TECHNIQUE

7. *What is the maximum number of hairs acceptable in a mini-graft?*
A. 1.
B. 2.
C. 3.
D. 4.
E. 5.

TECHNIQUE

8. *Which graft placement technique in relation to the scalp epidermis will best prevent cyst and ingrown hair formation?*
A. Graft placed just above scalp epidermis.
B. Graft placed evenly with scalp epidermis.
C. Graft placed just below scalp epidermis.
D. Cysts and ingrown hairs are inevitable.
E. By grasping the bulb of the follicle prior to graft placement, you can reduce potential cyst formation.

TECHNIQUE

9. *In a patient under the age of 23 requesting hair transplantation, what is the appropriate route of initial therapy?*
A. Follicular unit extraction.
B. Strip technique.
C. Combined follicular unit extraction and transplantation.
D. Trial of medical treatment (e.g., minoxidil [Rogaine] or finasteride [Propecia]).
E. Deny treatment until the patient is at least 25 years of age.

Answers

DEFINITION OF PROBLEM

1. ***Which phase of hair growth is prolonged during the thinning and balding process?***

   C. Telogen.

   Normal hair growth includes an active (anagen), degradation (catagen), and resting (telogen) phase. Most of the cycle (90%) is spent in the anagen phase during normal active hair growth. During the process of thinning and balding, the hair growth cycle switches from predominantly anagen phase to a more prolonged telogen phase.[1]

REFERENCE

1. Janis JE, ed. Essentials of Plastic Surgery. 2nd ed. New York: Thieme Publishers; 2014

CONTRAINDICATIONS

2. ***Which of the following is a contraindication to pursuing hair transplantation treatment?***

   B. Chronic systemic lupus erythematosus (SLE).

   All of the choices above are appropriate indications to pursue hair transplantation, except for chronic SLE, as the chronicity of the autoimmune condition would likely lead to a less-than-optimal surgical outcome.

PREOPERATIVE EVALUATION

3. ***A patient presents to your office seeking hair transplantation. On examination, you observe that the patient has symmetrical triangular frontotemporal recessions extending more than 2 cm posteriorly. According to the Norwood classification system, which type of male alopecia would most accurately describe this patient's condition?***

   B. Type III.

   According to the Norwood classification system for male pattern baldness,[1,2] this patient is presenting with Type III alopecia, described as symmetrical triangular frontotemporal recessions extending posteriorly more than 2 cm.

REFERENCES

1. Norwood OT. Male pattern baldness: classification and incidence. South Med J 1975;68:1359
2. Norwood OT, Shiell RC, eds. Hair Transplant Surgery. 2nd ed. Springfield, IL: Charles C Thomas; 1984

PREOPERATIVE EVALUATION

4. ***What is the minimum range of hair follicles per square centimeter that is classified as appearing normal?***

   C. 70–110.

   Although 140 to 220 hairs/cm^2 is the defined range of normal-appearing hair, the accepted lower limit of normal appearance is in the range of 70 to 110 hairs/cm^2.[1,2,3,4]

REFERENCES

1. Barrera A, Oscar Uebel C. Hair Transplantation: The Art of Follicular Unit Micrografting and Minigrafting. 2nd ed. New York: Thieme Publishers; 2014
2. Janis JE, ed. Essentials of Plastic Surgery. 2nd ed. New York: Thieme Publishers; 2014
3. Limmer B. The density issue in hair transplantation. Dermatol Surg 1997;23:747
4. Marritt E. The death of the density debate. Dermatol Surg 1999;25:654

PREOPERATIVE EVALUATION

5. ***Which of the following are the two most ideal donor sites for hair transplantation harvest?***

   D. Temporal and occipital.

   Donor site dominance is a concept that hair will retain growth characteristic of the donor site upon transplantation; the most favorable regions for donor hair harvest are the temporal and occipital scalp.

TECHNIQUE

6. *In a mature patient, which of the following landmarks would be most appropriate for donor site selection?*

C. One-half the distance down from the upper border of baldness to the lower hairline.

An elliptical donor site is mapped approximately 1 cm in thickness, as wide as the number of required follicular units for the transplantation. A reliable landmark for mapping the occipital donor site in a more mature male patient is one-half the distance from upper border of baldness to the lower hairline (**Fig. 32.1**).

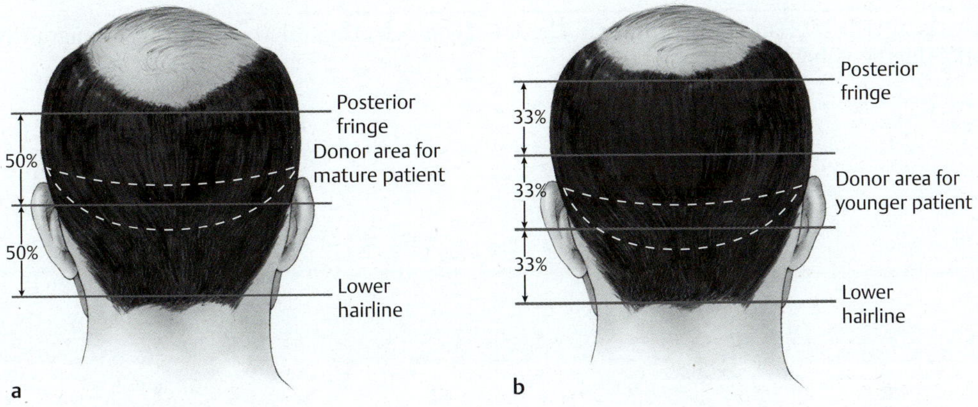

Fig. 32.1 (a,b) The donor strip is harvested from the area with the thickest healthier, most durable hair, generally halfway between the upper border of baldness (or thinning) and the lower neck hairline. (Source: Donor Site Harvesting. In: Barrera A, Uebel C, ed. Hair Transplantation: The Art of Follicular Unit Micrografting and Minigrafting. 2nd Edition. New York: Thieme; 2013.)

TECHNIQUE

7. *What is the maximum number of hairs acceptable in a mini-graft?*

D. 4.

In donor hair harvest, natural grouping of hair follicular units is maintained. A micro-graft is considered 1 to 2 hairs per graft, whereas mini-grafts contain 3 to 4. As grafts should ultimately end up 1 to 2 mm apart, the maximum number of hairs allowable in a mini-graft is 4. Micro-grafts contain 1 or 2 hairs per graft.[1]

REFERENCE

1. Barrera A, Oscar Uebel C. Hair Transplantation: The Art of Follicular Unit Micrografting and Minigrafting. 2nd ed. New York: Thieme Publishers; 2014

TECHNIQUE

8. *Which graft placement technique in relation to the scalp epidermis will best prevent cyst and ingrown hair formation?*

A. Graft placed just above scalp epidermis.

Epidermis of the *graft* should be slightly superficial to scalp epidermis at the time of placement to prevent the formation of cysts and/or ingrown hairs. NEVER GRIP THE BULB.[1]

REFERENCE

1. Barrera A, Oscar Uebel C. Hair Transplantation: The Art of Follicular Unit Micrografting and Minigrafting. 2nd ed. New York: Thieme Publishers; 2014

TECHNIQUE

9. *In a patient under the age of 23 requesting hair transplantation, what is the appropriate route of initial therapy?*

D. Trial of medical treatment (e.g., minoxidil [Rogaine] or finasteride [Propecia]).

As a precaution for incipient baldness, all patients under the age of 23 seeking treatment should first trial medical pharmacotherapy options such as minoxidil (Rogaine) or finasteride (Propecia).[1] Should these trials be unsuccessful, hair transplantation options may be discussed.

REFERENCE

1. Barrera A, Oscar Uebel C. Hair Transplantation: The Art of Follicular Unit Micrografting and Minigrafting. 2nd ed. New York: Thieme Publishers; 2014

33. Browlift

Cameron R. Erickson, Michael R. Lee
See *Essentials of Aesthetic Surgery*, pp. 411–428

IDEAL FACIAL AESTHETICS

1. ***Which statement is true regarding eyebrow position and aesthetics?***
   A. The ideal female eyebrow level is typically 3 to 5 mm above the supratarsal crease.
   B. The medial end of the eyebrow should be tapered, while the lateral end is more club shaped.
   C. The eyebrow peaks just above the lateral limbus of the eye.
   D. Male eyebrow level is approximately 1 cm above the supraorbital ridge.
   E. Anterior hairline is normally 3 to 4 cm above the eyebrow level.

IDEAL FACIAL AESTHETICS

2. ***What eyebrow positioning gives the patient a sad and tired appearance?***
   A. Medial eyebrow is depressed.
   B. Medial eyebrow is elevated.
   C. Lateral eyebrow is elevated.
   D. Lateral eyebrow is depressed.
   E. Both the medial and lateral eyebrow are elevated.

ANATOMY

3. ***What is the correct anatomical relationship of the forehead from superficial to deep?***
   A. Skin and subcutaneous, frontalis, superficial plane of galea, loose areolar tissue.
   B. Skin and subcutaneous, superficial plane of galea, frontalis, deep plane of galea, loose areolar tissue, periosteum.
   C. Skin and subcutaneous, loose areolar tissue, superficial plane of the galea, periosteum.
   D. Superficial plane of galea, loose areolar tissue, subcutaneous tissue, periosteum.
   E. Skin and subcutaneous tissue, frontalis, deep plane of galea, periosteum.

ANATOMY

4. ***The orbital ligament is a fibrous band that secures what structures?***
   A. Deep temporal fascia to periosteum.
   B. Superficial temporal fascia to the superolateral orbital rim.
   C. Superficial temporal fascia to the medial orbital rim.
   D. Skin to the superficial temporal fascia.
   E. Temporalis muscle to the periosteum.

ANATOMY

5. ***Choose the correctly matched muscle with its action.***
   A. Frontalis–movement of the medial brow medially and downward.
   B. Corrugator supercilii–primary eyelid closure.
   C. Procerus–eyebrow elevation.
   D. Orbicularis oculi–lateral brow depression.
   E. Depressor supercilii–medial brow elevation.

ANATOMY

6. ***A 58-year-old male presents to your clinic and is interested in a browlift. You examine the patient and find that the distance between his brow and hairline is approximately 5 cm. Which incisional approach would be recommended for this patient?***
   A. Anterior hairline incision.
   B. Endoscopic assisted incision.
   C. Coronal incision.
   D. Occipital incision.
   E. Direct at brow.

ANATOMY

7. ***Which of the following choices is an advantage of a limited incision temporal scalp hairline approach for brow elevation?***
   A. No risk of alopecia.
   B. Sensory innervation to the forehead is spared.
   C. Optimal medial eyebrow elevation.
   D. Ability to address deep transverse rhytids.
   E. Minimal soft tissue undermining.

ANATOMY

8. ***Regarding the dissection planes for forehead elevation, choose the correctly matched plane and why that plane is advantageous.***
   A. Subcutaneous–relatively avascular plane.
   B. Subcutaneous–allows for a rapid dissection sequence.
   C. Subgaleal–no requirement to release the soft tissues from the bone.
   D. Subgaleal–“natural cleft” and relatively avascular.
   E. Subperiosteal–allows excellent exposure of the deep surface of the frontalis.

ANATOMY

9. ***You are performing a direct skin excision immediately superior to the brow and your presurgical goal is to raise the brow approximately 1.0 cm. You plan your elliptical incision in a transverse fashion above the eyebrow with a marking pen. What should be the distance of the width (cranial to caudal) of the ellipse measured with a caliper?***
   A. 10 mm.
   B. 12 mm.
   C. 15 mm.
   D. 20 mm.
   E. 25 mm.

ANATOMY

10. ***When discussing risks and complications of a browlift procedure with a patient, which of the following statements is accurate?***
    A. Thinning or loss of scalp hair results from loose wound closure and decreased wound edge opposition.
    B. The frontal (temporal) branch of the facial nerve is vulnerable to injury from excessive traction or transection during midline dissection after a coronal incision.
    C. Excessive elevation of the eyebrow produces a “surprised” appearance; this is easily corrected by an in-office procedure.
    D. Skin surface deformities can result from aggressive scoring or excision of the frontalis muscle.
    E. The supraorbital nerve is protected in most dissection planes and does not get injured.

Answers

IDEAL FACIAL AESTHETICS

1. ***Which statement is true regarding eyebrow position and aesthetics?***

   C. The eyebrow peaks just above the lateral limbus of the eye.

   The ideal female eyebrow is typically 3 to 5 mm above the supraorbital ridge, not the supratarsal crease. The medial end of the eyebrow is shaped more like a club and the lateral end is more tapered. Male eyebrow level is aesthetically positioned at the level of the supraorbital ridge. Anterior hairline is 5 to 6 cm from the eyebrow level (**Fig. 33.1**).[1]

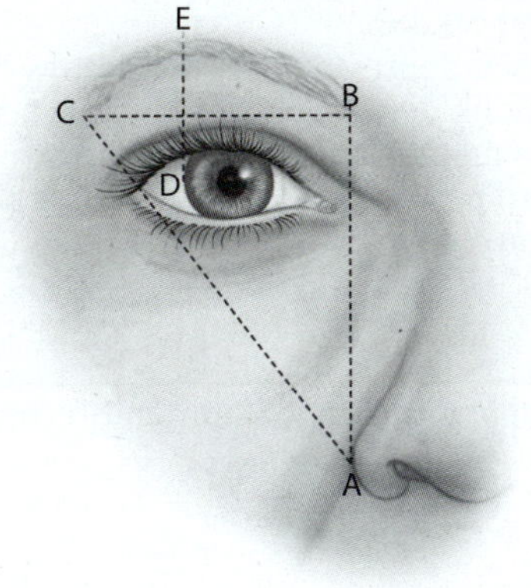

Fig. 33.1 Spatial relationships of the ideal eyebrow. (A, Nasal ala; B, medial bow; C, lateral tail of brow; D, lateral limbus; E, brow apex.) (Source: Ideal Eyebrow Shape & Position will Vary by Gender. In: Janis J, ed. Essentials of Aesthetic Surgery. 1st Edition. New York: Thieme; 2018.)

Reference

1. Gunter JP, Antrobus SD. Aesthetic analysis of the eyebrows. Plast Reconstr Surg 1997;99:1807

IDEAL FACIAL AESTHETICS

2. ***What eyebrow positioning gives the patient a sad and tired appearance?***

   D. Lateral eyebrow is depressed.

   A person looks angry when the medial eyebrow is depressed and surprised when the medial eyebrow is elevated. When the lateral brow is elevated, the person appears quizzical and when it is depressed, the person appears sad or tired.[1]

Reference

1. Freund RM, Nolan WB. Correlation between brow lift outcomes and aesthetic ideals for eyebrow height and shape in females. Plast Reconstr Surg 1996;97:1343

ANATOMY

3. ***What is the correct anatomical relationship of the forehead from superficial to deep?***

   B. Skin and subcutaneous, superficial plane of galea, frontalis, deep plane of galea, loose areolar tissue, periosteum.

   The correct layers of the forehead are arranged from superficial to deep as follows: skin and subcutaneous tissue, superficial plane of galea, frontalis, deep plane of galea, loose areolar tissue, and then periosteum.[1]

Reference

1. Codner MA, Kikkawa DO, Korn BS, et al. Blepharoplasty and brow lift. Plast Reconstr Surg 2010;126:1e

ANATOMY

4. *The orbital ligament is a fibrous band that secures what structures?*

B. Superficial temporal fascia to the superolateral orbital rim.

The orbital ligament is a fibrous band that attaches the superficial temporal fascia to the superolateral orbital rim.[1]

REFERENCE

1. Codner MA, Kikkawa DO, Korn BS, et al. Blepharoplasty and brow lift. Plast Reconstr Surg 2010;126:1e

ANATOMY

5. *Choose the correctly matched muscle with its action.*

D. Orbicularis oculi–lateral brow depression.

The orbicularis oculi lateral portion depresses the lateral brow and creates radial and lateral periorbital rhytids with contraction. Frontalis elevates eyebrow and creates transverse forehead skin lines. Corrugator supercilii causes movement of the medial eyebrow medially and downward. Procerus causes medial eyebrow depression, which produces transverse rhytids at the nasal root. Depressor supercilii also causes medial eyebrow depression.[1]

REFERENCE

1. Knize DM, ed. The Forehead and Temporal Fossa: Anatomy and Technique. Philadelphia: Lippincott Williams & Wilkins; 2001

ANATOMY

6. *A 58-year-old male presents to your clinic and is interested in a browlift. You examine the patient and find that the distance between his brow and hairline is approximately 5 cm. Which incisional approach would be recommended for this patient?*

C. Coronal incision.

This patient has a low hairline, given the distance of his eyebrow to hairline is <6 cm, and therefore would be better served by a coronal incision to lengthen his hairline. This technique is often recommended for individuals with a higher degree of brow sagging or a larger amount of excess skin to address.

The coronal browlift involves a longer incision along the hairline, typically from ear to ear or slightly beyond. The incision is placed within the scalp to hide any scarring. This approach allows for significant lifting and reshaping of the brow and forehead tissues. It is well suited for individuals with more advanced signs of aging in the brow area.[1,2]

REFERENCES

1. Janis JE, Potter JK, Rohrich RJ. Brow lift techniques. In: Fagien S, ed. Putterman's Cosmetic Oculoplastic Surgery. 4th ed. Philadelphia: Elsevier; 2007
2. Guyuron B, Lee M. A reappraisal of surgical techniques and efficacy in forehead rejuvenation. Plast Reconstr Surg 2014;134:426

ANATOMY

7. *Which of the following choices is an advantage of a limited incision temporal scalp hairline approach for brow elevation?*

B. Sensory innervation to the forehead is spared.

The limited incision lateral hairline approach is a minimally invasive approach, with limited scarring, and sensory innervation to the forehead is spared. The approach is skill dependent. It does not elevate the medial eyebrows, is unable to address the deep transverse rhytids, and unfortunately requires a good amount of soft tissue undermining with ligament release in order to obtain a desirable aesthetic outcome. There is also a risk of alopecia.[1,2]

REFERENCES

1. Janis JE, Potter JK, Rohrich RJ. Brow lift techniques. In: Fagien S, ed. Putterman's Cosmetic Oculoplastic Surgery. 4th ed. Philadelphia: Elsevier; 2007
2. Guyuron B, Lee M. A reappraisal of surgical techniques and efficacy in forehead rejuvenation. Plast Reconstr Surg 2014;134:426

ANATOMY

8. *Regarding the dissection planes for forehead elevation, choose the correctly matched plane and why that plane is advantageous.*

D. Subgaleal–"natural cleft" and relatively avascular.

Dissection in subcutaneous plane is considered a simple anatomic dissection and preserves scalp sensation. The subgaleal dissection allows access to the "natural cleft" (surgical plane) in the forehead and is considered relatively avascular. This plane also allows for excellent exposure of the deep surface of the frontalis for scoring and excision. The subperiosteal plane is also relatively avascular and avoids deep division of the supraorbital nerve.[1,2]

REFERENCES

1. Janis JE, Potter JK, Rohrich RJ. Brow lift techniques. In: Fagien S, ed. Putterman's Cosmetic Oculoplastic Surgery. 4th ed. Philadelphia: Elsevier; 2007
2. Guyuron B, Lee M. A reappraisal of surgical techniques and efficacy in forehead rejuvenation. Plast Reconstr Surg 2014;134:426

ANATOMY

9. *You are performing a direct skin excision immediately superior to the brow and your presurgical goal is to raise the brow approximately 1.0 cm. You plan your elliptical incision in a transverse fashion above the eyebrow with a marking pen. What should be the distance of the width (cranial to caudal) of the ellipse measured with a caliper?*

A. 10 mm.

When performing a direct skin excision directly above the brow, the amount of eyebrow elevation is usually equal to the width of the elliptical skin excision at a 1:1 ratio. This is in contrast to the coronal technique where the scalp tissue must be advanced approximately 1.5 cm to obtain 1 mm of eyebrow elevation because of the greater distance of the fixation point from the eyebrow. The "elastic band principle" states that the effectiveness of any fixation method to suspend a forehead flap decreases as the suspension point is placed farther from the eyebrow level.[1,2]

REFERENCES

1. Janis JE, Potter JK, Rohrich RJ. Brow lift techniques. In: Fagien S, ed. Putterman's Cosmetic Oculoplastic Surgery. 4th ed. Philadelphia: Elsevier; 2007
2. Guyuron B, Lee M. A reappraisal of surgical techniques and efficacy in forehead rejuvenation. Plast Reconstr Surg 2014;134:426

ANATOMY

10. *When discussing risks and complications of a browlift procedure with a patient, which of the following statements is accurate?*

D. Skin surface deformities can result from aggressive scoring or excision of the frontalis muscle.

Thinning or loss of scalp hair is due to tight wound closure and wound edge ischemia. The frontal branch is at risk during dissection in the temporal fossa area. Excessive eyebrow elevation is difficult to correct.[1]

REFERENCE

1. Byun S, Mukovozov I, Farrokhyar F, et al. Complications in brow lift techniques: a systematic review. Plast Reconstr Surg 2012;130(5S-1):S90

34. Upper Blepharoplasty

Elbert E. Vaca, Anmol Chattha
See *Essentials of Aesthetic Surgery*, pp. 429–450

ANATOMY

1. ***A patient is asked to tightly close the eyes against resistance. Which muscle is mainly responsible for this action?***
   A. Pretarsal orbicularis.
   B. Corrugator supercilii.
   C. Preseptal orbicularis.
   D. Procerus muscle.
   E. Orbital orbicularis.

ANATOMY

2. ***The levator palpebrae superioris muscle originates from which of the following bones?***
   A. Greater wing of the sphenoid.
   B. Lesser wing of the sphenoid.
   C. Zygoma.
   D. Ethmoid bone.
   E. Lacrimal bone.

SURGICAL JUDGMENT

3. ***A patient presents to clinic 6 days after botulinum toxin A injection to the glabella complaining of left upper lid ptosis. Which of the following best describes the mechanism of action of apraclonidine, which is used to help address this issue?***
   A. Cleavage of SNAP-25 protein, preventing release of acetylcholine from the presynaptic vesicle.
   B. Stimulates levator palpebrae superioris muscle via alpha-2 adrenergic agonist effects.
   C. Stimulates Müller's muscle via alpha-2 adrenergic agonist effects.
   D. Stimulates levator palpebrae superioris via binding of sodium ion channels.
   E. Stimulates Müller's muscle via binding of sodium ion channels.

ANATOMY

4. ***Which of the following correctly describes the function of Whitnall's ligament?***
   A. It redirects the vector of pull of the levator palpebrae muscle on the superior tarsal plate.
   B. It forms an anatomic barrier between the orbital fat pads and the orbicularis oculi muscle.
   C. It redirects the vector of pull of the capsulopalpebral fascia on the inferior tarsal plate.
   D. It redirects the vector of pull of the superior oblique muscle.
   E. It prevents inferior displacement of the levator palpebrae.

SURGICAL JUDGMENT

5. ***A 65-year-old female returns to clinic 2 months after upper blepharoplasty complaining of a "tired" appearance of her left upper lid. There is no evidence of lagophthalmos. Examination reveals 10 mm of levator excursion bilaterally, with an MRD-1 of 2 mm on the left and 4 mm on the right. Which of the following is the most likely reason for this patient's postoperative complaint?***
   A. Greater care in not disrupting levator aponeurosis attachments to the superior tarsus.
   B. Failure to recognize preoperative eyelid ptosis.
   C. A browlift should have been concomitantly performed.
   D. Insufficient resection of excess upper eyelid skin.
   E. Over-resection of skin causing lagophthalmos.

SURGICAL MANAGEMENT

6. *A 58-year-old female is 9 months post bilateral upper blepharoplasty and complains of right eye irritation and dryness. Examination reveals 2 mm of right eye lagophthalmos and conjunctival injection without evidence of ulceration. Which of the following is the most appropriate management?*

A. Reassurance.
B. Instruct the patient to perform downward scar massage on the upper eyelid and re-examine the patient serially until resolution.
C. Corticosteroid injection into the upper eyelid scar line.
D. Full-thickness skin graft.
E. Excise more skin from the upper lid.

ANATOMY

7. *A 61-year-old woman with significant herniation of upper eyelid orbital fat is to undergo bilateral upper blepharoplasty with partial excision of orbital fat. The superior oblique muscle is most susceptible to injury between which of the following structures?*

A. Medial and central fat compartments.
B. Central fat compartment and lacrimal gland.
C. Medial fat compartment and lacrimal gland.
D. Medial fat compartment and medial canthal tendon.
E. Lacrimal gland and lateral canthal tendon.

ANATOMY

8. *During blinking (i.e., eyelid closure), which of the following best describes the action of the lacrimal sac?*

A. It contracts independently.
B. It relaxes.
C. It is compressed by contraction of the orbicularis oculi muscle.
D. It expands due to contraction of the orbicularis oculi muscle.
E. It does not change in size.

PREOPERATIVE EVALUATION

9. *Which of the following is an absolute contraindication to upper blepharoplasty?*

A. Coumadin use for a prosthetic heart valve.
B. History of Lasik procedure 14 months prior.
C. Hypothyroidism.
D. Contact lens use.
E. Controlled hypertension.

PREOPERATIVE EVALUATION

10. *A 72-year-old female presents to your office requesting a skin-only upper blepharoplasty complaining of "extra skin" partially occluding her visual fields bilaterally. Physical examination reveals deep transverse forehead rhytids and pronounced lateral hooding bilaterally. Levator excursion and MRD-1 are 11 and 5 mm bilaterally, respectively. You counsel the patient and recommend which of the following surgical interventions?*

A. Proceed with upper blepharoplasty only.
B. Counsel the patient that she is not a candidate for surgery.
C. Upper blepharoplasty and neurotoxin injection to treat her transverse forehead rhytids.
D. Bilateral upper blepharoplasty and levator advancement.
E. Browlift and upper blepharoplasty.

SURGICAL JUDGMENT

11. *The nurse pages you to evaluate a 60-year-old patient who underwent bilateral upper blepharoplasty 2 hours ago. On examination, the patient complains of severe pain, and proptosis of the left globe is noted along with decreased visual acuity. Which of the following is the correct next step in management?*

A. Emergent ophthalmology consultation.
B. Infusion of IV acetazolamide.
C. Start mannitol infusion and dexamethasone.
D. Apply manual pressure to the globe.
E. Emergent lateral canthotomy and cantholysis.

Answers

ANATOMY

1. *A patient is asked to tightly close the eyes against resistance. Which muscle is mainly responsible for this action?*

E. Orbital orbicularis.

The orbicularis oculi muscle forms a sphincter responsible for eyelid closure. The orbicularis has three parts: pretarsal, preseptal, and orbital. The orbital orbicularis is under voluntary control and is activated during forceful closure of the eyelids and is innervated by frontal and zygomatic branches of the facial nerve. The preseptal orbicularis has both voluntary and involuntary functions and is involved in blinking. The pretarsal orbicularis is also involved in blinking and is involuntary.

The corrugator muscles draw the medial brow downward and medially. The procerus muscle lies primarily over the upper third of the nose and its contraction results in transverse rhytids over the nasion.[1,2,3]

REFERENCES

1. Nahai F. Aesthetic plastic surgery. In: Nahai F, ed. The Art of Aesthetic Surgery: Principles and Techniques. 2nd ed. New York: Thieme Publishers; 2007
2. Zide B, Jelks GW, eds. Surgical Anatomy Around the Orbit. New York: Lippincott Williams & Wilkins; 2007
3. Siegel RJ. Surgical anatomy of the upper eyelid fascia. Ann Plast Surg 1984;13:263

ANATOMY

2. *The levator palpebrae superioris muscle originates from which of the following bones?*

B. Lesser wing of the sphenoid.

The levator palpebrae superioris is innervated by cranial nerve III and originates from the lesser wing of the sphenoid in the bony orbit.[1,2,3]

REFERENCES

1. Nahai F. Aesthetic plastic surgery. In Nahai F, ed. The Art of Aesthetic Surgery: Principles and Techniques. 2nd ed. New York: Thieme Publishers; 2007
2. Zide B, Jelks GW, eds. Surgical Anatomy Around the Orbit. New York: Lippincott Williams & Wilkins; 2007
3. Siegel RJ. Surgical anatomy of the upper eyelid fascia. Ann Plast Surg 1984;13:263

SURGICAL JUDGMENT

3. *A patient presents to clinic 6 days after botulinum toxin A injection to the glabella complaining of left upper lid ptosis. Which of the following best describes the mechanism of action of apraclonidine, which is used to help address this issue?*

C. Stimulates Müller's muscle via alpha-2 adrenergic agonist effects.

Botulinum toxin A inhibits release of acetylcholine from the pre-synaptic terminal; therefore, answer choice A is incorrect as this describes the mechanism of action of botulinum toxin A. Apraclonidine is an alpha-2 adrenergic agonist and stimulates sympathetically innervated muscle. Müller's muscle is a sympathetically innervated involuntary muscle which contributes to 2 to 3 mm of upper eyelid excursion. Apraclonidine, therefore, stimulates Müller's muscle and can be used to ameliorate lid ptosis due to inadvertent botulinum toxin effect on the levator palpebrae superioris muscle. Local anesthetics (i.e., lidocaine) are categorized as class 1 antiarrhythmics and bind/block sodium channel receptors, preventing sodium ion flow and membrane depolarization. Therefore, answer choices D and E are incorrect.[1,2,3]

REFERENCES

1. Nahai F. Aesthetic plastic surgery. In Nahai F, ed. The Art of Aesthetic Surgery: Principles and Techniques. 2nd ed. New York: Thieme Publishers; 2007
2. Zide B, Jelks GW, eds. Surgical Anatomy Around the Orbit. New York: Lippincott Williams & Wilkins; 2007
3. Siegel RJ. Surgical anatomy of the upper eyelid fascia. Ann Plast Surg 1984;13:263

ANATOMY

4. ***Which of the following correctly describes the function of Whitnall's ligament?***

   A. It redirects the vector of pull of the levator palpebrae muscle on the superior tarsal plate.

   Whitnall's ligament functions as a fulcrum, helping to redirect the vector of pull of the levator palpebrae superioris muscle on the superior tarsal plate. Whitnall's ligament also contributes fibers to the medial and lateral canthal tendons. The orbital septum, not Whitnall's ligament, forms the middle lamella of the eyelid and lies between the orbicularis muscle and orbital fat. In the inferior lid, Lockwood's ligament functions as a fulcrum to redirect the vector of pull of the capsulopalpebral fascia.[1,2,3]

REFERENCES

1. Moss CJ, Mendelson BC, Taylor GI. Surgical anatomy of the ligamentous attachments in the temple and periorbital regions. Plast Reconstr Surg 2000;105:1475
2. Muzaffar A, Mendelson BC, Adams WP. Surgical anatomy of the ligamentous attachments of the lower lid and lateral canthus. Plast Reconstr Surg 2002;110:873
3. Ghavami A, Pessa JE, Janis JE, et al. The orbicularis retaining ligament of the medial orbit: closing the circle. Plast Reconstr Surg 2008;121:994

SURGICAL JUDGMENT

5. ***A 65-year-old female returns to clinic 2 months after upper blepharoplasty complaining of a "tired" appearance of her left upper lid. There is no evidence of lagophthalmos. Examination reveals 10 mm of levator excursion bilaterally, with an MRD-1 of 2 mm on the left and 4 mm on the right. Which of the following is the most likely reason for this patient's postoperative complaint?***

   B. Failure to recognize preoperative eyelid ptosis.

   The vignette describes a patient with normal levator excursion (normal 10–15 mm) but left eyelid ptosis. Although iatrogenic disruption of levator aponeurosis attachment to the superior tarsal plate can result in ptosis, it is much more common for postoperative upper lid ptosis to be due to unrecognized preoperative eyelid ptosis. A browlift would have not addressed this patient's ptosis. Insufficient skin resection would result in persistent postoperative dermatochalasis. Over-resection of the skin causing lagophthalmos would have presented differently in a patient who has difficulty closing eyelids due to over-resection.[1,2]

REFERENCES

1. Lisman RD, Hyde K, Smith B. Complications of blepharoplasty. Clin Plast Surg 1988;15:309
2. Rohrich RJ, Coberly DM, Fagien S, et al. Current concepts in aesthetic upper blepharoplasty. Plast Reconstr Surg 2004;113:32e

SURGICAL MANAGEMENT

6. ***A 58-year-old female is 9 months post bilateral upper blepharoplasty and complains of right eye irritation and dryness. Examination reveals 2 mm of right eye lagophthalmos and conjunctival injection without evidence of ulceration. Which of the following is the most appropriate management?***

   D. Full-thickness skin graft.

   Lagophthalmos is a relatively common complication after upper blepharoplasty and can result from excessive resection of skin. If present in the acute postoperative period, conservative management is appropriate including hydrating ocular ointment application and downward scar massage on the upper eyelid, as many cases will resolve over time. However, this patient is 9 months status post upper blepharoplasty with persistent lagophthalmos. A full-thickness skin graft from the contralateral eyelid, cervical, preauricular, or postauricular area is appropriate. A full-thickness skin graft will add additional tissue to the anterior lamella and is an effective treatment of persistent iatrogenic lagophthalmos. Excising more skin from the upper lid would cause worsening of her lagophthalmos.[1,2]

REFERENCES

1. Lisman RD, Hyde K, Smith B. Complications of blepharoplasty. Clin Plast Surg 1988;15:309
2. Rohrich RJ, Coberly DM, Fagien S, et al. Current concepts in aesthetic upper blepharoplasty. Plast Reconstr Surg 2004;113:32e

ANATOMY

7. *A 61-year-old woman with significant herniation of upper eyelid orbital fat is to undergo bilateral upper blepharoplasty with partial excision of orbital fat. The superior oblique muscle is most susceptible to injury between which of the following structures?*

A. Medial and central fat compartments.

The trochlea of the superior oblique muscle separates the medial and central fat compartments of the upper orbit. Therefore, the superior oblique muscle is most susceptible to injury in this location and can result in strabismus (i.e., misalignment of the affected eye).[1,2,3]

REFERENCES

1. Nahai F. Aesthetic plastic surgery. In Nahai F, ed. The Art of Aesthetic Surgery: Principles and Techniques. 2nd ed. New York: Thieme Publishers; 2007
2. Zide B, Jelks GW, eds. Surgical Anatomy Around the Orbit. New York: Lippincott Williams & Wilkins; 2007
3. Siegel RJ. Surgical anatomy of the upper eyelid fascia. Ann Plast Surg 1984;13:263

ANATOMY

8. *During blinking (i.e., eyelid closure), which of the following best describes the action of the lacrimal sac?*

D. It expands due to contraction of the orbicularis oculi muscle.

The lacrimal apparatus is a complex drainage system. The tear film first drains into the punctum, which then drains into the lacrimal sac via the canaliculus. The lacrimal sac then drains into the nasolacrimal duct, which drains into the nasal cavity at the inferior turbinate. Jones's muscle (deep head of the preseptal orbicularis) inserts onto the lacrimal sac. During eyelid closure and orbicularis muscle contraction, Jones's muscle expands the lacrimal sac. Expansion of the lacrimal sac results in negative pressure, which draws the tear film into the lacrimal sac. During eyelid opening, the lacrimal sac recoils (i.e., relaxes) down to its resting size and projects the tear down the nasolacrimal duct.

The lacrimal sac does not contract independently. Expansion and recoil (i.e., relaxation) of the lacrimal gland is secondary to the action of the orbicularis oculi muscle. Furthermore, the lacrimal sac expands during eyelid closure. The lacrimal sac does not "relax" in the same sense as muscles do. Instead, it participates in the ongoing drainage process as tears are produced and the eye blinks and moves. The lacrimal sac does change in size due a variety of factors previously mentioned.[1,2,3]

REFERENCES

1. Nahai F. Aesthetic plastic surgery. In Nahai F, ed. The Art of Aesthetic Surgery: Principles and Techniques. 2nd ed. New York: Thieme Publishers; 2007
2. Zide B, Jelks GW, eds. Surgical Anatomy Around the Orbit. New York: Lippincott Williams & Wilkins; 2007
3. Siegel RJ. Surgical anatomy of the upper eyelid fascia. Ann Plast Surg 1984;13:263

PREOPERATIVE EVALUATION

9. *Which of the following is an absolute contraindication to upper blepharoplasty?*

A. Coumadin use for a prosthetic heart valve.

Retrobulbar hematoma is a rare, but severe, complication after blepharoplasty which can result in blindness due to compression of the optic nerve. Patients on therapeutic anticoagulation are not candidates for upper blepharoplasty due to an increased risk of bleeding.

It is recommended that blepharoplasty should not be performed earlier than 12 months after Lasik procedure. The patient in the above vignette is 14 months after Lasik surgery and therefore blepharoplasty is not contraindicated. Hypothyroidism, contact lens use, and controlled hypertension are not contraindications to blepharoplasty.[1]

REFERENCE

1. Lisman RD, Hyde K, Smith B. Complications of blepharoplasty. Clin Plast Surg 1988;15:309

PREOPERATIVE EVALUATION

10. *A 72-year-old female presents to your office requesting a skin-only upper blepharoplasty complaining of "extra skin" partially occluding her visual fields bilaterally. Physical examination reveals deep transverse forehead rhytids and pronounced lateral hooding bilaterally. Levator excursion and MRD-1 are 11 and 5 mm bilaterally, respectively. You counsel the patient and recommend which of the following surgical interventions?*

E. Browlift and upper blepharoplasty.

The clinical vignette describes a patient with concomitant brow ptosis. Deep transverse forehead rhytids are due to increased frontalis muscle tone. Unconscious frontalis muscle activation can occur to compensate for brow ptosis and/or blepharoptosis. However, the patient has 11 mm (normal) of levator excursion and an appropriate distance between her corneal light reflex and upper lid margin (i.e., MRD-1 5 mm). Therefore, this patient is best served by first treating her brow ptosis and a concomitant upper blepharoplasty.

Isolated upper blepharoplasty is incorrect and would produce a suboptimal aesthetic result. In a patient with concomitant brow ptosis, isolated blepharoplasty also risks excision of excess tissue.

There is no indication that this patient is not a surgical candidate.

Neurotoxin injection of the frontalis would exacerbate the patient's brow ptosis, and potentially result in occlusion of her visual fields.[1]

REFERENCE

1. Guyuron B. Endoscopic forehead rejuvenation: limitations, flaws, and rewards. Plast Reconstr Surg 2006;117:1121

SURGICAL JUDGMENT

11. *The nurse pages you to evaluate a 60-year-old patient who underwent bilateral upper blepharoplasty 2 hours ago. On examination, the patient complains of severe pain, and proptosis of the left globe is noted along with decreased visual acuity. Which of the following is the correct next step in management?*

E. Emergent lateral canthotomy and cantholysis.

The clinical vignette describes a patient with a retrobulbar hematoma. A retrobulbar hematoma can result from a bleeding vessel after orbital fat excision. Although emergent ophthalmology consultation and pharmacologic interventions are indicated, visual compromise is an indication for emergent decompression to prevent permanent blindness. Therefore, a bedside lateral canthotomy and cantholysis under local anesthesia is first indicated, followed by return to the operating room to obtain hemostasis along with ophthalmology consultation and pharmacotherapy.[1]

REFERENCE

1. Lisman RD, Hyde K, Smith B. Complications of blepharoplasty. Clin Plast Surg 1988;15:309

35. Lower Blepharoplasty

Joseph A. Kelling, Michael R. Lee

See *Essentials of Aesthetic Surgery*, pp. 451–460

ANATOMY

1. *An outward turning of the eyelid margin defines which of the following terms?*

A. Entropion.
B. Retraction.
C. Ectropion.
D. Steatoblepharon.
E. Blepharochalasis.

ANATOMY

2. *Which of the following options best describes a youthful aesthetic appearance of the lower eyelid?*

A. Resting position of the lower eyelid is 2 mm below the level of the limbus with scleral show, fullness of the pretarsal orbicularis oculi, and a clear transition from the lower eyelid to cheek with a visible inferior orbital rim.
B. Resting position of the lower eyelid at the level of the limbus without scleral show, fullness of the pretarsal orbicularis oculi, and a smooth, convex transition from the lower eyelid to cheek.
C. Resting position of the lower eyelid is 1 mm below the level of the limbus with scleral show, lack of fullness of the pretarsal orbicularis oculi, and a smooth, convex transition from the lower eyelid to cheek.
D. Resting position of the lower eyelid at the level of the limbus without scleral show, fullness of the pretarsal orbicularis oculi, and concave appearance of the lower eyelid to cheek junction with a defined nasojugal groove.
E. Resting position of the lower eyelid is 2 mm above the level of the limbus, fullness of the pretarsal orbicularis oculi, and a smooth concave transition from the lower eyelid to cheek.

ANATOMY

3. *Understanding the position of the globe relative to the inferior orbital rim is important for predicting which postoperative outcome?*

A. Entropion.
B. Retrobulbar hematoma.
C. Chemosis.
D. Ectropion.
E. Dry eye syndrome.

ANATOMY

4. *What is the definition of an abnormal pull-away test and what procedure is indicated to correct the abnormality?*

A. Delayed return of the lid margin to native position when retracted downward with finger traction indicates that a supplemental canthal anchoring procedure should be performed.
B. Greater than 10 mm of laxity of the lid margin when pulled away from the globe indicates that a supplemental canthal anchoring procedure should be performed.
C. Greater than 6 mm of laxity of the lid margin when pulled away from the globe indicates that skin excision from the lower eyelid should be performed.
D. Forced closure of the eyelid does not improve the redundant, ptotic appearance of the orbicularis oculi muscle, indicating that a septal reset procedure should be performed.
E. Greater than 8 mm of laxity of the lid margin when pulled away from the globe indicates that a transconjunctival fat removal should be performed.

ANATOMY

5. ***A 52-year-old man has come to the plastic surgeon's office seeking improvement in the appearance of his lower eyelids. He expresses concerns about the persistent bags under his eyes that make him look tired and aged. On examination he has a negative vector, skin elasticity, and poor snap-back test. What is the patient at risk for and what maneuver may help decrease the possibility of that complication from arising?***

A. Entropion–canthopexy.
B. Dry eyes–skin pinch.
C. Dry eyes–fat grafting.
D. Ectropion–canthopexy.
E. Ectropion–skin pinch.

SURGICAL TECHNIQUES

6. ***A patient with isolated fine lines would best benefit from which type of procedure?***

A. Skin resurfacing with a chemical peel or laser resurfacing.
B. Transconjunctival fat removal.
C. Skin-only blepharoplasty.
D. External lower blepharoplasty with orbicularis suspension.
E. External lower blepharoplasty with orbicularis suspension and septal reset.

SURGICAL TECHNIQUES

7. ***What is the best indication for a skin-only blepharoplasty?***

A. Patients with excess fat and no excess skin or orbicularis ptosis.
B. Patients with minimal redundant skin or fullness, the presence of pretarsal and preseptal orbicularis hypertrophy, and minimal fat herniation.
C. Patients with minimal redundant skin or fullness, usually isolated to the pretarsal region, and not associated with fat herniation, lid laxity, or orbicularis ptosis.
D. Patients with the presence of skin excess and orbicularis ptosis, but minimal fat herniation.
E. Patients with significant lid laxity, but minimal redundant skin isolated to the pretarsal region.

SURGICAL TECHNIQUES

8. ***A patient presents with apparent skin excess of the lower eyelid and a ptotic orbicularis muscle. What is the key surgical step to address the ptotic orbicularis muscle?***

A. Excision of a strip of the orbicularis oculi muscle.
B. Removal of fat from the postseptal compartment.
C. Performing a canthal anchoring procedure.
D. Suspension of a preseptal orbicularis oculi flap to lateral orbital rim.
E. Release of the arcus marginalis to allow extrusion of the lower eyelid fat.

SURGICAL TECHNIQUES

9. ***Which of the following is an indication to perform a septal reset procedure?***

A. Ptosis of the orbicularis oculi muscle.
B. Redundant lower eyelid skin.
C. Ectropion.
D. Isolated fine lines of the periorbital area.
E. Visible nasojugal groove and fat herniation.

SURGICAL TECHNIQUES

10. ***Which of the following must be considered when determining whether to perform a canthal anchoring procedure (canthopexy or canthoplasty)?***

A. Amount of horizontal lid laxity present.
B. Amount of vertical lid laxity present.
C. Amount of fat resection planned.
D. Presence of a positive vector globe.
E. Past surgical history that includes laser in situ keratomileusis.

COMPLICATIONS

11. ***You are called about a patient in the postanesthesia care unit who has undergone a lower blepharoplasty. The patient is complaining of severe pain in the right eye that is not controlled with intravenous pain medication and reports decreased vision in the eye. What is the most appropriate next step in treatment?***

A. Recommend head of bed elevation.
B. Recommend applying firm pressure to the right eye.
C. Continued administration of pain medication.
D. Prompt return to the operating room for exploration.
E. Administration of mannitol.

COMPLICATIONS

12. ***Prevention of dry eye syndrome is largely related to which component of lower blepharoplasty surgery?***

A. Performing an appropriate preoperative assessment.
B. Manipulation of the conjunctiva.
C. Performing a canthal anchoring procedure.
D. Removal of fat from the postseptal compartment.
E. Excision of excess lower lid skin.

Answers

ANATOMY

1. *An outward turning of the eyelid margin defines which of the following terms?*

C. Ectropion.

An ectropion is defined as an outward turning of the eyelid margin and can be further classified as *senile* or *cicatricial*. Senile ectropion results from age-related laxity of the lower eyelid. Cicatricial ectropion results from scar-induced retraction of the lower eyelid.

An entropion is a rolling in of the eyelid margin toward the sclera. This can result in irritation of the cornea or sclera by the individual's eyelashes. Retraction is a downward displacement of the lower eyelid resulting in inferior scleral show. Steatoblepharon is excess or protruding fat through a lax septum. Blepharochalasis is thin, excessive eyelid skin secondary to recurrent bouts of painless eyelid edema.[1]

REFERENCE

1. Flowers RS, Du Val C. Blepharoplasty and periorbital aesthetic surgery. In: Aston SJ, Beasley RW, Thorne HM, et al, eds. Grabb and Smith's Plastic Surgery. 6th ed. Philadelphia: Lippincott Williams & Wilkins; 2007

ANATOMY

2. *Which of the following options best describes a youthful aesthetic appearance of the lower eyelid?*

B. Resting position of the lower eyelid at the level of the limbus without scleral show, fullness of the pretarsal orbicularis oculi, and a smooth, convex transition from the lower eyelid to cheek.

The lower eyelid should rest at the level of the limbus without scleral show between the limbus and the eyelid margin. The presence of a *pretarsal bulge*, or pretarsal orbicularis hypertrophy, is considered by many to be an aesthetic component of the youthful eye. The eyelid–cheek junction should be a smooth, convex, essentially imperceptible, transition from eyelid to cheek in youthful patients.[1]

REFERENCE

1. Flowers RS, Du Val C. Blepharoplasty and periorbital aesthetic surgery. In: Aston SJ, Beasley RW, Thorne HM, et al, eds. Grabb and Smith's Plastic Surgery. 6th ed. Philadelphia: Lippincott Williams & Wilkins; 2007

ANATOMY

3. *Understanding the position of the globe relative to the inferior orbital rim is important for predicting which postoperative outcome?*

D. Ectropion.

The orbital vector or position of the globe relative to the inferior orbital rim is useful for predicting postoperative tendencies of lid position. Negative vector orbits have poor lower lid suspension and are at risk for postoperative ectropion and retraction.[1]

REFERENCE

1. Flowers RS, Du Val C. Blepharoplasty and periorbital aesthetic surgery. In: Aston SJ, Beasley RW, Thorne HM, et al, eds. Grabb and Smith's Plastic Surgery. 6th ed. Philadelphia: Lippincott Williams & Wilkins; 2007

ANATOMY

4. *What is the definition of an abnormal pull-away test and what procedure is indicated to correct the abnormality?*

B. Greater than 10 mm of laxity of the lid margin when pulled away from the globe indicates that a supplemental canthal anchoring procedure should be performed.

Both the pull-away test and snap-back test are ways to examine for horizontal lid laxity. The pull-away test is abnormal when there is greater than 10 mm of lid laxity when the examiner grabs the lid margin with his or her index finger and thumb and pulls it away from the globe. A snap-back test is abnormal when there is delayed return of the lid margin to native positive when retracted downward with finger traction. A squinch (or squint) test can tell you if festoons are caused by ptosis of the orbicularis oculi muscle. The festoon will improve with forced closure of the eyelids. If either the snap-back or pull-away test is abnormal then the patient would benefit from a supplemental canthal anchoring procedure if undergoing lower blepharoplasty.[1]

REFERENCE

1. Codner MA, Kikkawa DO, Korn BS, et al. Blepharoplasty and brow lift. Plast Reconstr Surg 2010;126:1e

ANATOMY

5. *A 52-year-old man has come to the plastic surgeon's office seeking improvement in the appearance of his lower eyelids. He expresses concerns about the persistent bags under his eyes that make him look tired and aged. On examination he has a negative vector, skin elasticity, and poor snap-back test. What is the patient at risk for and what maneuver may help decrease the possibility of that complication from arising?*

D. Ectropion–canthopexy.

Given the patient's description and examination findings, he is at risk for developing lower eyelid malposition after undergoing lower blepharoplasty surgery. The combination of a negative vector (where the lower eyelid is positioned below the level of the eyeball), poor skin elasticity, and a positive snap-back test (indicating reduced elasticity and poor tissue recoil) can contribute to potential complications involving the position and contour of the lower eyelid post-surgery.

One possible complication that can arise due to these factors is ectropion. Ectropion is a condition in which the lower eyelid turns outward, exposing the inner surface of the eyelid and causing discomfort, irritation, and an unnatural appearance. Given the patient's existing risk factors, there is an increased chance that the lower eyelid might not heal properly and could become pulled downward or have an abnormal position.

To decrease the possibility of ectropion and ensure a successful outcome, the plastic surgeon may employ a surgical maneuver known as a canthopexy or canthoplasty. These procedures involve tightening and stabilizing the lateral canthal tendon, which is the tissue that holds the outer corner of the eyelid in place. By reinforcing this structure, the surgeon can help prevent lower eyelid malposition, mitigate the risk of ectropion, and ensure a more natural and comfortable appearance after the surgery.[1]

REFERENCE

1. Trussler AP, Rohrich RJ. MOC-PSSM CME article: blepharoplasty. Plast Reconstr Surg 2008;121(1 Suppl):S1

SURGICAL TECHNIQUES

6. *A patient with isolated fine lines would best benefit from which type of procedure?*

A. Skin resurfacing with a chemical peel or laser resurfacing.

Patients with isolated fine lines would benefit from an attempt at nonsurgical rejuvenation prior to a surgical procedure. Both nonsurgical and surgical procedures carry risks, but isolated fine lines are not an indication for lower blepharoplasty.[1]

REFERENCE

1. Trussler AP, Rohrich RJ. MOC-PSSM CME article: blepharoplasty. Plast Reconstr Surg 2008;121(1 Suppl):S1

SURGICAL TECHNIQUES

7. *What is the best indication for a skin-only blepharoplasty?*

C. Patients with minimal redundant skin or fullness, usually isolated to the pretarsal region, and not associated with fat herniation, lid laxity, or orbicularis ptosis.

Skin-only or pinch blepharoplasty is indicated in patients with minimal redundant skin or fullness, usually isolated to the pretarsal region, and not associated with fat herniation, lid laxity, or orbicularis ptosis. If pretarsal orbicularis hypertrophy is present and contributing to excessive fullness, a strip of pretarsal muscle may be excised as well. The pinch technique can be combined with other blepharoplasty techniques if indicated.[1]

REFERENCE

1. Kim EM, Bucky LP. Power of the pinch: pinch lower lid blepharoplasty. Ann Plast Surg 2008;60:532

SURGICAL TECHNIQUES

8. *A patient presents with apparent skin excess of the lower eyelid and a ptotic orbicularis muscle. What is the key surgical step to address the ptotic orbicularis muscle?*

D. Suspension of a preseptal orbicularis oculi flap to lateral orbital rim.

External skin-only techniques do not adequately address orbicularis ptosis even if a strip of orbicularis oculi muscle is removed. Along with elevating a pennant flap of the preseptal orbicularis muscle, the surgeon must also release the orbital retaining ligament and lateral orbital thickening in order to adequately suspend the flap to the lateral orbital rim.[1]

REFERENCE

1. Trussler AP, Rohrich RJ. MOC-PSSM CME article: blepharoplasty. Plast Reconstr Surg 2008;121(1 Suppl):S1

SURGICAL TECHNIQUES

9. *Which of the following is an indication to perform a septal reset procedure?*

E. Visible nasojugal groove and fat herniation.

A visible nasojugal groove and fat herniation along with the presence of the tear trough triad (herniation of orbital fat, tight attachment of the orbicular along the arcus marginalis, and malar retrusion) are indications to perform a septal release to allow herniation of the postseptal fat over the inferior orbital rim, or septal reset. Septal reset procedures should be performed with the eyelid under tension (by temporary Frost suture) to prevent excessive tightening of the septum and predisposing patients to ectropion.[1]

REFERENCE

1. Barton FE, Ha R, Awada M. Fat extrusion and septal reset in patients with the tear trough triad: a critical appraisal. Plast Reconstr Surg 2004;13:2115

SURGICAL TECHNIQUES

10. *Which of the following must be considered when determining whether to perform a canthal anchoring procedure (canthopexy or canthoplasty)?*

A. Amount of horizontal lid laxity present.

The decision to perform canthal anchoring is based upon the amount of horizontal lid laxity (preoperatively determined by the "snap-back test" and "pull-away test"), the prominence of the globe (a negative vector globe is at considerably higher risk of developing ectropion), the amount of skin/muscle resection planned, and other ancillary procedures performed (facial rhytidectomy, laser facial resurfacing, chemical peel, etc.). Whether orbicularis oculi muscle incision leads to paralytic ectropion after blepharoplasty is controversial. Pretarsal innervation is maintained through medial branches if the incision is only through the lateral aspect of the muscle. When muscle-splitting techniques are performed it is important to perform proper preoperative risk assessment and routine lateral canthal anchoring procedures for a successful outcome.[1]

REFERENCE

1. Hester RT, Codner MA, McCord CD, et al. Evolution of technique of the direct transblepharoplasty approach for the correction of lower lid and midfacial aging: maximizing results and minimizing complications in a 5-year experience. Plast Reconstr Surg 2000;105:393

COMPLICATIONS

11. *You are called about a patient in the postanesthesia care unit who has undergone a lower blepharoplasty. The patient is complaining of severe pain in the right eye that is not controlled with intravenous pain medication and reports decreased vision in the eye. What is the most appropriate next step in treatment?*

D. Prompt return to the operating room for exploration.

Retrobulbar hematoma is a rare but serious complication with an incidence of 0.04%. A retrobulbar hematoma can compress the neurovascular structures and cause retinal ischemia and optic nerve compression. Symptoms include severe pain, visual changes, proptosis, and ecchymosis. Any indication of retrobulbar hematoma should result in prompt return to the operating room for reexploration. If there is any delay, a bedside lateral canthotomy should be performed as well as release of sutures. The medical treatment of retrobulbar hematoma includes mannitol, acetazolamide, and systemic and topical steroids, but this is not the most appropriate treatment in this scenario.[1]

REFERENCE

1. Wolfort FG, Vaughan TE, Wolfort SF, et al. Retrobulbar hematoma and blepharoplasty. Plast Reconstr Surg 1999;104:2154

COMPLICATIONS

12. ***Prevention of dry eye syndrome is largely related to which component of lower blepharoplasty surgery?***

A. Performing an appropriate preoperative assessment.

Documented dry eyes, history of dry eyes, and abnormal orbital and periorbital anatomy such as lower lid laxity are predictors of postoperative dry eye complications. Blepharoplasty should be delayed at least 6 months in patients who have undergone laser in situ keratomileusis (LASIK). Prevention of this complication is largely due to proper patient screening. Symptoms include itching, foreign body sensation, burning, secretions, and frequent blinking. Patients who wear contact lenses without difficulty have adequate tear production to proceed with blepharoplasty. Treatment includes lubricating drops and ointment. Eye patch or Frost suture can also be used if lubricating measures do not improve symptoms. In prolonged cases (>3 months), ophthalmic cyclosporine can be used to increase tear production.[1,2]

REFERENCES

1. Pacella SJ, Codner MA. Minor complications after blepharoplasty: dry eyes, chemosis, granulomas, ptosis, and scleral show. Plast Reconstr Surg 2010;125:709
2. Lelli GJ Jr, Lisman RD. Blepharoplasty complications. Plast Reconstr Surg 2010;125:1007

36. Asian Blepharoplasty

Sammy Sinno, Michael E. Nissan
See *Essentials of Aesthetic Surgery*, pp. 462–481

PALPEBRAL FOLD

1. *Which of the following explains why Asians lack a palpebral fold?*
A. The levator aponeurosis in the Asian eyelid does not penetrate the orbital septum.
B. There is decreased preseptal fat in the Asian eyelid.
C. The Asian eyelid is characterized by a high insertion of the levator aponeurosis.
D. Tarsal height is longer in the Asian eyelid.
E. The Asian eyelid is characterized by the presence of a medial epicanthal fold.

EYELID ANATOMY

2. *In the upper eyelid, the conjoined fascia is formed by which of the following?*
A. The orbicularis oculi and the orbital septum.
B. The preseptal fat and the orbital septum.
C. The orbital septum and the levator aponeurosis.
D. The levator aponeurosis and the superior tarsus.
E. The orbital septum and the superior tarsus.

SOFT TISSUE CHARACTERISTICS

3. *Which of the following is a characteristic of the Asian eyelid but not the Caucasian eyelid?*
A. Thinner dermis with lower collagen content.
B. More prominent preseptal fibroadipose tissue.
C. Thinner pretarsal subcutaneous tissue.
D. Thinner orbicularis oculi muscle.
E. Well defined palpebral crease.

PRETARSAL SHOW

4. *When evaluating the Asian eyelid for aesthetic characteristics, what is the ideal amount of pretarsal show?*
A. 0–1 mm.
B. 1–4 mm.
C. 4–6 mm.
D. 6–8 mm.
E. 8–10 mm.

INCISIONAL VERSUS NONINCISIONAL

5. *Which of the following patients is best suited for a nonincisional (also known as suture, minimal incision, or closed) blepharoplasty?*
A. A patient with an excessive amount of subcutaneous fat.
B. A patient with dermatochalasis.
C. A patient with thick eyelids that require debulking.
D. A young patient with ptosis.
E. A young patient with thin upper eyelids who does not want a visible scar.

INCISIONAL TECHNIQUE WITH LEVATOR RELEASE

6. *When reapproximating fascial attachments in the incisional technique with levator release, to which structures is the levator aponeurosis sutured?*

A. Orbital septum only.
B. Dermis only.
C. Preseptal fat and orbital septum.
D. Anterior tarsus and dermal margin of lower incision.
E. Orbital septum and orbicularis oculi.

TRAPEZOIDAL DEBULKING TECHNIQUE

7. *Which of the following regarding trapezoidal debulking of preaponeurotic tissues in Asian blepharoplasty is true?*

A. The technique allows precise, physiologic, on-plane debulking.
B. Compared with other upper blepharoplasty techniques, trapezoidal debulking requires more steps.
C. When skin excision is not required, it is best that a triangular segment of preaponeurotic tissue be not removed as well.
D. Tissue should be excised layer by layer.
E. The technique relies on maximal fat resection in the upper eyelid.

NONINCISIONAL TECHNIQUES

8. *Which of the following is true regarding nonincisional upper blepharoplasty?*

A. Generally, the desired location of the palpebral crease is slightly superior to the superior margin of the tarsal plate.
B. Incision/suture lines should be slightly wider for younger patients.
C. The palpebral crease is formed by suture apposition and scarring.
D. The closed technique is best suited for eyelids with fat and skin excess.
E. Lower incidence of relapse.

BURIED SUTURE METHODS

9. *Which of the following is a short-term complication of buried sutures in nonincisional blepharoplasty?*

A. Lifted upper lid margin with exaggerated stare.
B. Ptosis.
C. Weakening contractility of the levator aponeurosis.
D. Discrepancy in skin excision.
E. Suture abscess.

ASYMMETRY

10. *A blepharoplasty patient notices asymmetry 4 weeks after surgery. It is noted that the asymmetry is largely due to swelling of the eyelids. When can the patient expect resolution of the swelling?*

A. 1 month.
B. 2 months.
C. 3–6 months.
D. 6–9 months.
E. 9–12 months.

PTOSIS

11. *When is the most appropriate time to perform a revision in the case of ptosis or lid retraction after primary blepharoplasty?*

A. Within 1–2 weeks.
B. Within 1–2 months.
C. After 6 months.
D. After 12 months.
E. There is no time sensitivity; it can be done on an elective basis.

RELAPSE

12. *Which of the following is true regarding eyelid relapse after blepharoplasty surgery?*

A. Eyelid relapse is more likely to occur with incisional techniques.
B. Experienced surgeons can expect a relapse rate of less than 1%.
C. Early relapses should be repaired after 6 months have passed.
D. Eyelid relapse is more likely to occur in bulkier eyelids.
E. Eyelid relapse is more likely to occur in patients with positive vectors.

Answers

PALPEBRAL FOLD

1. ***Which of the following explains why Asians lack a palpebral fold?***

   A. The levator aponeurosis in the Asian eyelid does not penetrate the orbital septum.

   According to the levator-dermal expansion theory,[1,2,3,4,5,6] the lack of a palpebral fold in Asians is due to the low insertion of the levator aponeurosis, which does not cross the orbital septum (**Fig. 36.1**). The Asian eyelid is characterized by increased preseptal fat, low insertion of the levator aponeurosis, and a shorter tarsal height than white eyelids.[7] Although a medial epicanthal fold may be present in the Asian eyelid, this does not account for the lack of a palpebral fold.

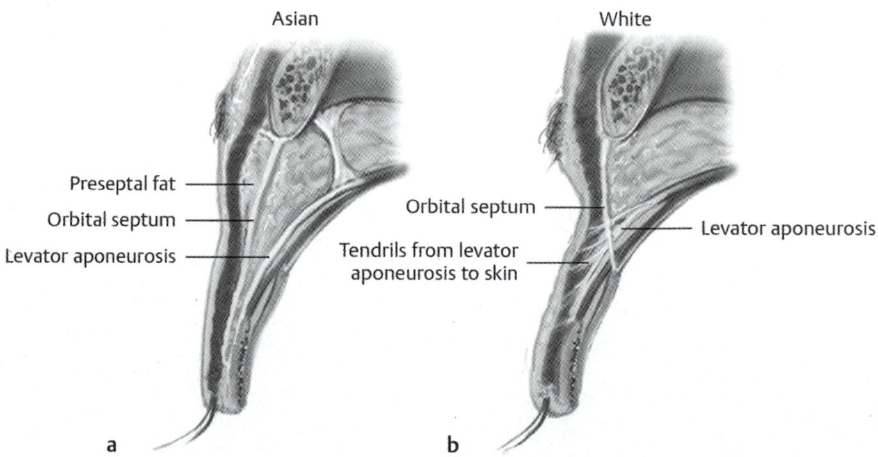

Fig. 36.1 (a) Asian eyelid versus the high fusion in **(b)**, white eyelid. Also note the presence of abundant preseptal fat and the lack of fascial attachments from the levator to the orbicularis and skin. (Source: Epicanthal fold. In: Pu L, ed. Aesthetic Plastic Surgery in Asians: Principles & Techniques. 1st Edition. New York: Thieme; 2015.)

REFERENCES

1. Sayoc BT. Plastic construction of the superior palpebral fold. Am J Ophthalmol 1954;38:556
2. Cheng J, Xu FZ. Anatomic microstructure of the upper eyelid in the Oriental double eyelid. Plast Reconstr Surg 2001;107:1665
3. Sayoc BT. Absence of superior palpebral fold in slit eyes; an anatomic and physiologic explanation. Am J Ophthalmol 1956;42:298
4. Zubiri JS. Correction of the Oriental eyelid. Clin Plast Surg 1981;8:725
5. Morikawa K, Yamamoto H, Uchinuma E, et al. Scanning electron microscopic study on double and single eyelids in Orientals. Aesthetic Plast Surg 2001;25:20
6. Chen WP. The concept of a glide zone as it relates to upper lid crease, lid fold, and application in upper blepharoplasty. Plast Reconstr Surg 2007;119:379
7. Kakisaki H, Goold LA, Casson RJ, et al. Tarsal height. Ophthamology 2009;116:1831

EYELID ANATOMY

2. ***In the upper eyelid, the conjoined fascia is formed by which of the following?***

   C. The orbital septum and the levator aponeurosis.

   In the Asian eyelid, the levator aponeurosis does not penetrate the orbital septum. Instead, the levator joins the orbital septum inferiorly and forms the conjoined fascia (**Fig. 36.2**).[1,2]

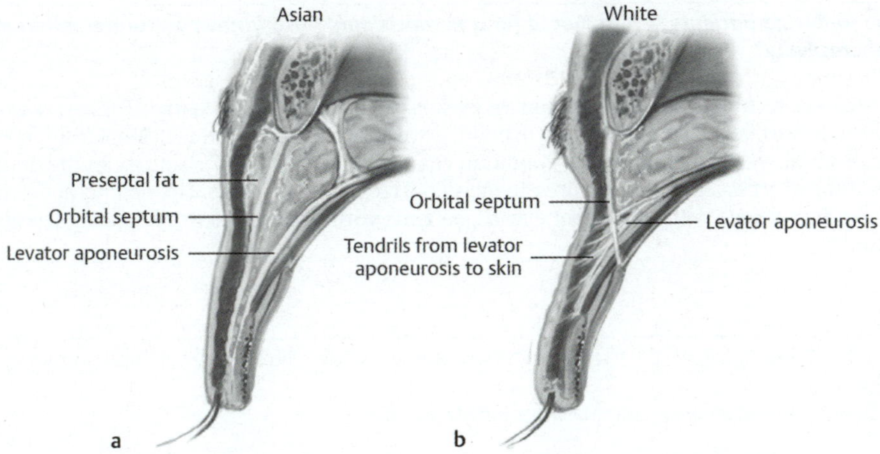

Fig. 36.2 (a) Asian eyelid versus the high fusion in **(b)**, white eyelid. Also note the presence of abundant preseptal fat and the lack of fascial attachments from the levator to the orbicularis and skin. (Source: Epicanthal fold. In: Pu L, ed. Aesthetic Plastic Surgery in Asians: Principles & Techniques. 1st Edition. New York: Thieme; 2015.)

REFERENCES

1. Seiff SR, Seiff BD. Anatomy of the Asian eyelid. Facial Plast Surg Clin North Am 2007;15:309
2. Kakisaki H, Goold LA, Casson RJ, et al. Tarsal height. Ophthamology 2009;116:1831

SOFT TISSUE CHARACTERISTICS

3. ***Which of the following is a characteristic of the Asian eyelid but not the Caucasian eyelid?***

B. More prominent preseptal fibroadipose tissue.

There exist many soft tissue differences between the Asian eyelid and the Caucasian eyelid.[1,2,3] Asian skin has thicker dermis and higher collagen content. The Asian eyelid has more prominent preseptal fibroadipose tissue, thicker pretarsal subcutaneous tissue, and a thicker, bulkier orbicularis oculi muscle. Asian eyelids have a less defined palpebral crease due to the above factors.

REFERENCES

1. Kakisaki H, Goold LA, Casson RJ, et al. Tarsal height. Ophthamology 2009;116:1831
2. Cheng J, Xu FZ. Anatomic microstructure of the upper eyelid in the Oriental double eyelid. Plast Reconstr Surg 2001;107:1665
3. Sayoc BT. Absence of superior palpebral fold in slit eyes; an anatomic and physiologic explanation. Am J Ophthalmol 1956;42:298

PRETARSAL SHOW

4. ***When evaluating the Asian eyelid for aesthetic characteristics, what is the ideal amount of pretarsal show?***

B. 1–4 mm.

Pretarsal show is an important consideration when evaluating the Asian eyelid for aesthetics. It is important to note that the ideal amount of pretarsal show is different for Asian versus white eyelids. Although the amount of pretarsal show is a patient's decision, 1 to 4 mm is recommended.[1,2,3]

REFERENCES

1. Chen WP. The concept of a glide zone as it relates to upper lid crease, lid fold, and application in upper blepharoplasty. Plast Reconstr Surg 2007;119:379
2. Flowers RS. Asian blepharoplasty. Aesthet Surg J 2002;22:558
3. Yoon KC, Park S. Systematic approach and selective tissue removal in blepharoplasty for young Asians. Plast Reconstr Surg 1998;102:502

INCISIONAL VERSUS NONINCISIONAL

5. *Which of the following patients is best suited for a nonincisional (also known as suture, minimal incision, or closed) blepharoplasty?*

E. A young patient with thin upper eyelids who does not want a visible scar.

The nonincisional technique is best reserved for eyelids requiring minimal change. For this reason, eyelids with excess subcutaneous fat or tissue requiring debulking are better suited for an incisional technique, which allows for tissue removal. Dermatochalasis is a condition characterized by loss of elasticity in the dermal connective tissue, resulting in excess skin that requires an incisional technique to excise. The nonincisional approach is best suited for young patients with thin upper eyelids, patients with no excess skin, and patients who do not want a visible scar.[1,2]

REFERENCES

1. Baek SM, Kim SS, Tokunaga S, et al. Oriental blepharoplasty: single-stitch, nonincision technique. Plast Reconstr Surg 1989;83:236
2. Flowers RS. Asian blepharoplasty. Aesthet Surg J 2002;22:558

INCISIONAL TECHNIQUE WITH LEVATOR RELEASE

6. *When reapproximating fascial attachments in the incisional technique with levator release, to which structures is the levator aponeurosis sutured?*

D. Anterior tarsus and dermal margin of lower incision.

When reapproximating fascial attachments, a "fat sling" is formed with the orbital septum and levator aponeurosis. The fat layer between these structures is highly vascularized and should not be sutured to the other structures. Instead, sutures are used to approximate the levator aponeurosis to the anterior tarsus and the dermis at the margin of the lower incision (**Fig. 36.3a,b**).[1,2,3,4]

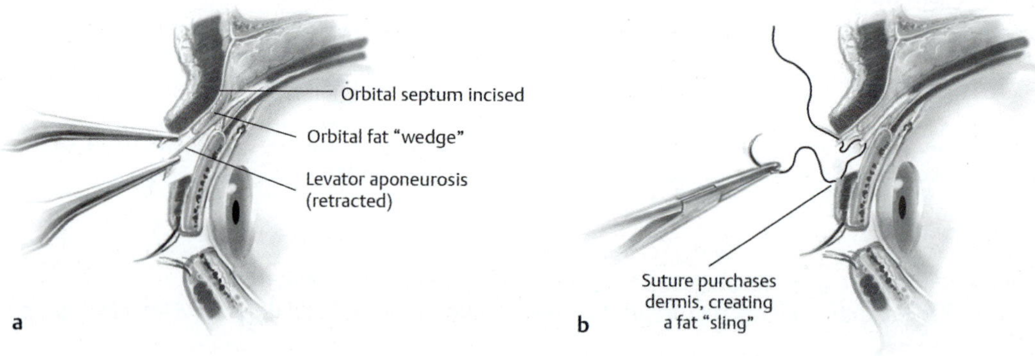

Fig. 36.3 (a) The forceps hold the two components of the fat sling. The upper forceps is on the edge of the orbital septum, while the lower places have the medial free edge of the levator aponeurosis on tension, pulling down and revealing the fibers of the levator muscle. A small, highly vascularized fat wedge separates the two layers. **(b)** After the pretarsal tissues are smoothed and advanced nasally, sutures approximate the free edge of the levator aponeurosis to the pretarsal tissue. In this case, the aponeurosis is sutured to both the anterior tarsus and the dermis at the margin of the lower incision. (Source: Incisional techniques with levator-dermal fixation. In: Janis J, ed. Essentials of Aesthetic Surgery. 1st Edition. New York: Thieme; 2018.)

REFERENCES

1. Yoon KC, Park S. Systematic approach and selective tissue removal in blepharoplasty for young Asians. Plast Reconstr Surg 1998;102:502
2. Fernandez LR. The East Asian eyelid—open technique. Clin Plast Surg 1993;20:247
3. Flowers RS. Upper blepharoplasty by eyelid invagination. Anchor blepharoplasty. Clin Plast Surg 1993;20:193
4. Collin JR, Beard C, Wood I. Experimental and clinical data on the insertion of the levator palpebrae superioris muscle. Am J Ophthalmol 1978;85:792

TRAPEZOIDAL DEBULKING TECHNIQUE

7. *Which of the following regarding trapezoidal debulking of preaponeurotic tissues in Asian blepharoplasty is true?*

A. The technique allows precise, physiologic, on-plane debulking.

Trapezoidal debulking is an upper blepharoplasty technique used to resect preaponeurotic tissue in the Asian eyelid. The technique offers precise, physiologic results and requires few steps compared to other techniques. Generally, some skin excision is required to achieve the desired results—however, when skin excision is not desired, a triangular cross-segment of tissue can be removed instead (**Fig. 36.4**). Clearing of tissue layer by layer is not recommended, as this can result in uneven treatment of layers. Instead, tissue should be cleared in a single, trapezoidal block. A correctly performed trapezoidal debulking technique will result in wound edge approximation without excess tension. In fact, the eyelid crease created by this technique can be observed prior to wound closure. The technique relies on minimal fat excision in order to prevent a sunken sulcus.[1]

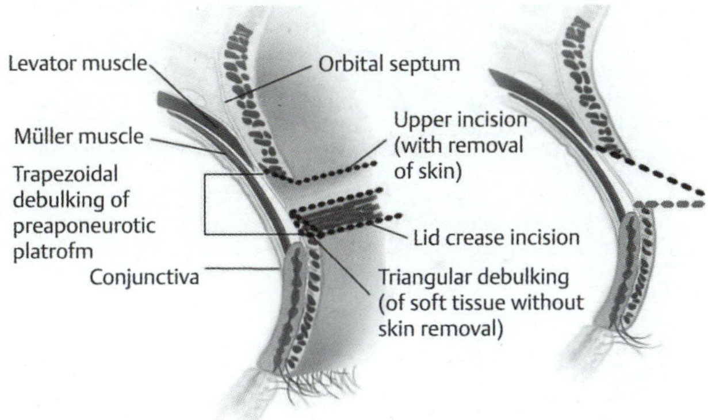

Fig. 36.4 The concept of trapezoidal and triangular debulking of eyelid tissues as applied in Asian upper blepharoplasty. (Source: Trapezoidal debulking of preaponeurotic tissues in Asian blepharoplasty. In: Janis J, ed. Essentials of Aesthetic Surgery. 1st Edition. New York: Thieme; 2018.)

REFERENCE

1. Chen WP. Concept of triangular, trapezoidal, and rectangular debulking of eyelid tissues: application in Asian blepharoplasty. Plast Reconstr Surg 1996;97:212

NONINCISIONAL TECHNIQUES

8. *Which of the following is true regarding nonincisional upper blepharoplasty?*

C. The palpebral crease is formed by suture apposition and scarring.

Nonincisional blepharoplasty fixes eyelid skin to the superficial portion of the tarsal plate via suture apposition and resultant scarring. Because the eyelid is not incised, this approach is best suited for eyelids without fat and skin excess. The desired location for the palpebral fold formed by this technique is at or slightly inferior to the superior margin of the tarsal plate, following the natural curve of the upper eyelid. Wider suture lines are suitable for older patients, and shorter suture lines are suitable for younger patients. Nonincisional techniques have higher rates of relapse.[1]

REFERENCE

1. Baek SM, Kim SS, Tokunaga S, et al. Oriental blepharoplasty: single-stitch, nonincision technique. Plast Reconstr Surg 1989;83:236

BURIED SUTURE METHODS

9. *Which of the following is a short-term complication of buried sutures in nonincisional blepharoplasty?*

A. Lifted upper lid margin with exaggerated stare.

Buried sutures in nonincisional blepharoplasty encircle the orbicularis oculi, levator aponeurosis, and Müller muscle (**Fig. 36.5**). Binding of these structures may lead to lifted upper lid margin and exaggerated stare in the short term—however, fixation of these structures can lead to eventual weakness of the contractility of the levator aponeurosis. For this reason, ptosis is a long-term complication associated with buried sutures in nonincisional blepharoplasty. Skin excision discrepancy is not a complication of nonincisional blepharoplasty because the technique does not involve skin removal.[1,2]

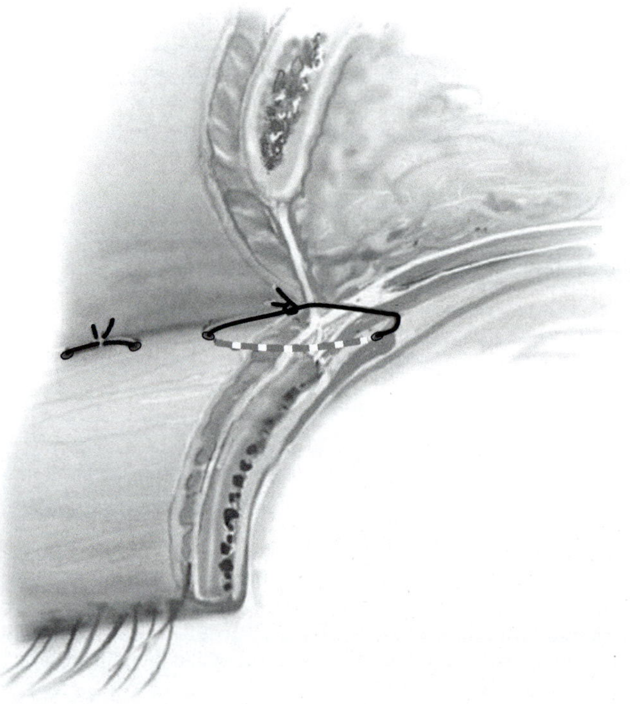

Fig. 36.5 Cross section showing placement of a buried suture that encircles the orbicularis oculi, levator aponeurosis, and underlying Müller muscle. It is a suture loop of 7-0 nylon or polypropylene. Often, a small fragment of preaponeurotic fat pad and orbital septum may be inadvertently included in the ligature. (Source: Technique. In: Janis J, ed. Essentials of Aesthetic Surgery. 1st Edition. New York: Thieme; 2018.)

REFERENCES

1. Wong JK. A method in creation of the superior palpebral fold in Asians using a continuous buried tarsal stitch (CBTS). Facial Plast Surg Clin North Am 2007;15:337
2. Wong JK, Zhou X, Ai T, et al. A simple, minimally invasive method for creation of the superior palpebral fold in Asians with the modified continuous buried tarsal stitch. Arch Facial Plast Surg 2010;12:269

ASYMMETRY

10. *A blepharoplasty patient notices asymmetry 4 weeks after surgery. It is noted that the asymmetry is largely due to swelling of the eyelids. When can the patient expect resolution of the swelling?*

C. 3–6 months.

Asymmetry is one of the most common complications of blepharoplasty; 13 to 35% of patients cite asymmetry as a source of dissatisfaction.[1] One of the most common causes of asymmetry is postoperative swelling. For this reason, it is important to counsel patients during early postoperative visits that swelling will last a minimum of 6 weeks and may take up to 3 to 6 months to resolve. However, it is important to remain vigilant for other sources of eyelid asymmetry. These include resolution of compensatory frontalis activation and discrepancy in skin excision; these may require additional surgery to resolve.

REFERENCE

1. Johnson CC. Epicanthus and epiblepharon. Arch Ophthalmol 1978;96:1030

PTOSIS

11. *When is the most appropriate time to perform a revision in the case of ptosis or lid retraction after primary blepharoplasty?*

A. Within 1–2 weeks.

Ptosis or lid retraction is a possible complication of blepharoplasty. Ptosis can be caused by hemorrhage into the Müller muscle. In the case of ptosis or lid retraction, revision surgery should be performed within 1 to 2 weeks, as the wound can be more readily opened and waiting longer will result in a more difficult revision.[1]

REFERENCE

1. Oestreicher J, Mehta S. Complications of blepharoplasty: prevention and management. Plast Surg Int 2012;2012:252368

RELAPSE

12. *Which of the following is true regarding eyelid relapse after blepharoplasty surgery?*

D. Eyelid relapse is more likely to occur in bulkier eyelids.

Relapse is a known complication of blepharoplasty surgery that occurs in 2.9 to 4.5% of patients of experienced surgeons.[1,2] Risk factors for relapse include bulkier eyelids and use of nonincisional techniques. Early relapses should be repaired within 2 to 3 weeks, while late relapses should be repaired after 3 to 6 months have passed. Relapse and complication rates are higher in patients with negative vectors.

REFERENCES

1. Baek SM, Kim SS, Tokunaga S, et al. Oriental blepharoplasty: single-stitch, nonincision technique. Plast Reconstr Surg 1989;83:236
2. Wong JK. A method in creation of the superior palpebral fold in Asians using a continuous buried tarsal stitch (CBTS). Facial Plast Surg Clin North Am 2007;15:337

37. Correction of the Tear Trough Deformity

Elbert E. Vaca, Anmol Chattha
See *Essentials of Aesthetic Surgery*, pp. 482–489

ANATOMY

1. ***Which of the following is a reason for development of the tear trough deformity?***
   A. Herniation of temple fat.
   B. Zygoma retrusion.
   C. Hypertrophy of the malar fat pad.
   D. Tight attachment of the orbicularis oculi muscle to the arcus marginalis.
   E. Hypertrophy of the procerus.

ANATOMY

2. ***Which of the following techniques decreases the risk of complications with hyaluronic acid fillers to the tear trough?***
   A. Intradermal injection.
   B. Injection until effacement of the tear trough to prevent undercorrection.
   C. Supraperiosteal injection.
   D. Injection using bolus technique.
   E. Injection while the needle is being advanced.

ANATOMY

3. ***A 43-year-old female presents for transconjunctival lower blepharoplasty and orbital fat repositioning to smooth the eyelid–cheek junction. Which of the following structures is released to gain access to the midface?***
   A. Lockwood's ligament.
   B. Orbital septum.
   C. Capsulopalpebral fascia.
   D. Orbicularis retaining ligament.
   E. Zygomatic retaining ligaments.

ANATOMY

4. ***The palpebromalar groove occurs due to skeletonization of which of the following retaining ligaments?***
   A. Orbicularis retaining ligament.
   B. Masseteric retaining ligaments.
   C. Zygomatic retaining ligaments.
   D. Lateral orbital thickening.
   E. Arcus marginalis.

ANATOMY

5. ***Which of the following statements best describes the progression for grading the severity of the tear trough deformity?***
   A. The eyelid–cheek junction first becomes apparent laterally, and then deepens and progresses medially.
   B. The eyelid–cheek junction first becomes apparent in the midpupillary area, and then deepens and progresses medially and laterally.
   C. The eyelid–cheek junction first becomes apparent medially, and then deepens and progresses laterally.
   D. Skeletonization of the eyelid–cheek junction does not usually follow a predictable pattern.
   E. The eyelid–cheek junction is congenital in most patients and is graded based on severity at childbirth.

Answers

ANATOMY

1. *Which of the following is a reason for development of the tear trough deformity?*

D. Tight attachment of the orbicularis oculi muscle to the arcus marginalis.

Development of the nasojugal groove, or tear trough, is due to the triad of: (1) herniation of orbital fat, (2) malar retrusion, and (3) tight attachment of the orbicularis oculi muscle to the arcus marginalis of the inferomedial orbital rim. Volumetric deflation, and not hypertrophy, of the deep malar fat compartment can contribute to midfacial aging changes but is not part of the classic triad of reasons for the development of the tear trough. Hypertrophy of the procerus does not contribute to a tear trough deformity. Herniation of temple fat is not related to the tear trough deformity.[1]

REFERENCE

1. Barton FE, Ha R, Awada M. Fat extrusion and septal reset in patients with the tear trough triad: a critical appraisal. Plast Reconstr Surg 2004;113:2115

ANATOMY

2. *Which of the following techniques decreases the risk of complications with hyaluronic acid fillers to the tear trough?*

C. Supraperiosteal injection.

Supraperiosteal plane injection is recommended. Intradermal injection risks contour irregularities and bumps, as there is little overlying soft tissue in this area. Furthermore, intradermal injection around the tear trough carries a higher risk of intravascular injection and bruising. Similarly, overinjection of hyaluronic acid fillers in the tear trough also risks contour irregularities due to the paucity of overlying soft tissue in this area. Many practitioners prefer to use blunt cannulas in this area to minimize the risk of intravascular injection. Bolus injection technique and injecting while the needle is being advanced should be avoided to minimize the risk of intravascular injection.[1,2]

REFERENCES

1. Lambros VS. Hyaluronic acid injections for correction of the tear trough deformity. Plast Reconstr Surg 2007;120 (6 Suppl):74S
2. Hirmand H. Anatomy and nonsurgical correction of the tear trough deformity. Plast Reconstr Surg 2010;125:699

ANATOMY

3. *A 43-year-old female presents for transconjunctival lower blepharoplasty and orbital fat repositioning to smooth the eyelid–cheek junction. Which of the following structures is released to gain access to the midface?*

D. Orbicularis retaining ligament.

The orbicularis retaining ligament (ORL) separates the lower eyelid from the midface and is responsible for formation of the orbitomalar groove. The ORL is released to gain access to the midface and allow redraping of orbital fat into the midface to smoothen the eyelid–cheek junction.

Lockwood's ligament helps support the globe and functions as a fulcrum to redirect the vector of the capsulopalpebral fascia. The capsulopalpebral fascia functions as a lower eyelid retractor.

The orbital septum helps contain orbital contents and inserts inferiorly on the arcus marginalis.

The zygomatic retaining ligaments span the inferior border of the body of the zygoma. In the periorbita, these ligaments lie at the inferior border of the suborbicularis oculi fat (SOOF) and form the inferior border of malar mounds. These ligaments should be released during a midface lift.[1,2]

REFERENCES

1. Hester TR Jr, Codner MA, McCord CD, et al. Evolution of technique of the direct transblepharoplasty approach for the correction of lower lid and midfacial aging: maximizing results and minimizing complications in a 5-year experience. Plast Reconstr Surg 2000;105:393; discussion 407

2. Haddock NT, Saadeh PB, Boutros S, et al. The tear trough and lid/cheek junction: anatomy and implications for surgical correction. Plast Reconstr Surg 2009;123:1332

ANATOMY

4. *The palpebromalar groove occurs due to skeletonization of which of the following retaining ligaments?*

A. Orbicularis retaining ligament.

Demarcation of the eyelid–cheek junction of the lateral inferior periorbita is due to skeletonization of the orbicularis retaining ligament (ORL). Above the ORL, orbital fat herniation and laxity of the orbital septum contribute to lower eyelid bag formation. Caudal to the ORL, prominence and decent of the suborbicularis oculi fat (SOOF) can contribute to the formation of malar bags. The caudal border of malar bags is the zygomatic retaining ligaments.[1]

REFERENCE

1. Mendelson BC, Muzaffar AR, Adams WP. Surgical anatomy of the midcheek and malar mounds. Plast Reconstr Surg 2002;110:885

ANATOMY

5. *Which of the following statements best describes the progression for grading the severity of the tear trough deformity?*

C. The eyelid–cheek junction first becomes apparent medially, and then deepens and progresses laterally.

With aging, the eyelid–cheek junction first becomes apparent medially. This corresponds to the tear trough or nasojugal groove. The tear trough occurs due to the tight attachment of the inferomedial orbicularis oculi muscle to the arcus marginalis, herniation of orbital fat, and malar retrusion. With further aging changes, the palpebromalar groove develops, which is in continuity with the nasojugal groove. The palpebromalar groove forms due to skeletonization of the orbicularis retaining ligament. With increasing orbital fat herniation and malar retrusion, the eyelid–cheek junction becomes more prominent and can be accompanied by the formation of malar bags. The eyelid–cheek junction is not primarily a congenital problem and is not graded based on severity at childbirth.[1,2,3]

REFERENCES

1. Hester TR Jr, Codner MA, McCord CD, et al. Evolution of technique of the direct transblepharoplasty approach for the correction of lower lid and midfacial aging: maximizing results and minimizing complications in a 5-year experience. Plast Reconstr Surg 2000;105:393; discussion 407
2. Haddock NT, Saadeh PB, Boutros S, et al. The tear trough and lid/cheek junction: anatomy and implications for surgical correction. Plast Reconstr Surg 2009;123:1332
3. Pessa JE. An algorithm of facial aging: verification of Lambros's theory by three-dimensional stereolithography, with reference to the pathogenesis of midfacial aging, scleral show, and the lateral suborbital trough deformity. Plast Reconstr Surg 2000;106:479; discussion 467

38. Lateral Canthopexy

Elbert E. Vaca, Anmol Chattha
See *Essentials of Aesthetic Surgery*, pp. 490–497

SURGICAL JUDGMENT

1. ***Which of the following is an absolute indication to perform a lateral canthopexy?***
   A. Lower lid distraction test of 10 mm.
   B. Orbicularis oculi hypertrophy.
   C. When performing a concomitant skin pinch procedure.
   D. Positive intercanthal tilt.
   E. When performing secondary lower lid procedures.

SURGICAL TECHNIQUE

2. ***Which of the following is considered a canthoplasty procedure?***
   A. Release of the superficial head of the lateral canthal tendon and suture fixation to the lateral orbital rim.
   B. Suturing of the lateral canthus to the lateral orbital rim without release of the lateral canthal tendon.
   C. Suture suspension of the lower lid orbicularis oculi muscle to the superolateral orbital rim periosteum.
   D. Passing of a lateral canthal anchoring suture through a burr hole in the lateral orbital rim without release of the lateral canthal tendon.
   E. Horizontal shortening of a lax lower lid, with suture fixation of the lower lid lateral tarsal strip to the superomedial aspect of the lateral orbital rim periosteum.

PREOPERATIVE EVALUATION

3. ***A 61-year-old male with no prior surgical history presents for blepharoplasty consultation. On examination, lower eyelid malposition is noted with 3 mm of scleral show below the inferior scleral limbus. The patient is able to close both eyes against resistance. The lower eyelid is easily repositioned with cephalic digital manipulation. Which of the following best describes the patient's lower eyelid deformity?***
   A. Eyelid ptosis.
   B. Senile ectropion.
   C. Cicatricial ectropion.
   D. Paralytic ectropion.
   E. Entropion.

SURGICAL TECHNIQUE

4. ***A 37-year-old female with a negative globe vector and 1 mm of scleral show presents for transconjunctival lower blepharoplasty due to orbital fat herniation and bilateral tear trough deformities. Which of the following best describes the most appropriate maneuver to minimize the risk of lower eyelid retraction?***
   A. Orbicularis suspension.
   B. Transcantho-canthopexy, with suture fixation to the inner aspect of the lateral orbital rim periosteum at the level of the lower border of the pupil.
   C. Transcantho-canthopexy, with suture fixation to the inner aspect of the lateral orbital rim periosteum at the level of the mid pupil.
   D. Transcantho-canthopexy, with suture fixation to the inner aspect of the lateral orbital rim periosteum at the level of the upper border of the pupil.
   E. Horizontal lower eyelid shortening.

SURGICAL TECHNIQUE

5. ***The specific technical refinements of a canthopexy for deep-set eyes include placement of fixation point where relative to the lateral orbital rim?***
   A. Superiorly and externally.
   B. Superiorly and internally.
   C. Inferiorly and externally.
   D. Inferiorly and internally.
   E. Laterally and internally.

Answers

SURGICAL JUDGMENT

1. *Which of the following is an absolute indication to perform a lateral canthopexy?*

A. Lower lid distraction test of 10 mm.

A lower lid distraction test of >10 mm, scleral show between the lower lid margin and inferior limbus, an abnormal snap-back test, and canthal dystopia (i.e., negative intercanthal tilt) are absolute indications for lateral canthopexy during blepharoplasty procedures. Orbicularis oculi weakness would be a relative indication for a lateral canthopexy, but hypertrophy has no bearing on the canthus. Performing a concomitant skin pinch procedure would not have any impact on the need to perform canthopexy. Previous procedures are not an absolute indication to perform a lateral canthopexy.[1,2]

REFERENCES

1. Trussler AP, Rohrich RJ. MOC-PSSM CME article: Blepharoplasty. Plast Reconstr Surg 2008;121(1 Suppl):S1
2. Maffi TR, Chang S, Friedland JA. Traditional lower blepharoplasty: is additional support necessary? A 30-year review. Plast Reconstr Surg 2011;128:265

SURGICAL TECHNIQUE

2. *Which of the following is considered a canthoplasty procedure?*

E. Horizontal shortening of a lax lower lid, with suture fixation of the lower lid lateral tarsal strip to the superomedial aspect of the lateral orbital rim periosteum.

Understanding the difference between lateral canthopexy and canthoplasty procedures is important. This can be a source of confusion as there is significant variability in canthopexy procedures. Canthopexy is defined as tightening of the lateral canthus while maintaining attachment of the lateral canthus to the orbital rim, whereas canthoplasty involves complete transection of the lateral canthus and reattachment to the orbital rim. Answer choice E is correct as this describes release of the lower eyelid attachment to the lateral canthus and reattachment of the lower lid to the orbital rim with suture.

Answer choice A describes a superficial retinacular lateral canthopexy, where the superficial lateral canthal tendon is released and fixated to the lateral orbital rim with suture. This is considered a canthopexy as the deep aspect of the lateral canthal tendon is left attached.

Although orbicularis suspension can provide additional lower lid support, this procedure is considered neither a canthopexy nor canthoplasty, as this procedure does not involve manipulation of the lateral canthal tendon.[1,2,3]

REFERENCES

1. Maffi TR, Chang S, Friedland JA. Traditional lower blepharoplasty: is additional support necessary? A 30-year review. Plast Reconstr Surg 2011;128:265
2. Flowers RS, Nassif JM, Rubin PA, et al. A key to canthopexy: the tarsal strap. A fresh cadaveric study. Plast Reconstr Surg 2005;116:1752
3. Tepper OM, Steinbrech D, Howell MH, et al. A retrospective review of patients undergoing lateral canthoplasty techniques to manage existing or potential lower eyelid malposition: identification of seven key preoperative findings. Plast Reconstr Surg 2015;136:40

PREOPERATIVE EVALUATION

3. *A 61-year-old male with no prior surgical history presents for blepharoplasty consultation. On examination, lower eyelid malposition is noted with 3 mm of scleral show below the inferior scleral limbus. The patient is able to close both eyes against resistance. The lower eyelid is easily repositioned with cephalic digital manipulation. Which of the following best describes the patient's lower eyelid deformity?*

B. Senile ectropion.

Senile ectropion results from acquired lower eyelid laxity with aging. These patients benefit from canthopexy procedures, and canthoplasty if eyelid shortening is found to be necessary.

Eyelid ptosis refers to caudal upper eyelid malposition with a marginal reflex distance (MRD-1) of <4 mm. This patient has no history of prior eyelid surgical procedures and the lower eyelid position is easily corrected with digital manipulation; therefore, cicatricial ectropion is incorrect. With cicatricial ectropion, there would be minimal superior excursion of the lower eyelid with upward digital manipulation. Cicatricial ectropion results from scar contracture of the middle (i.e., septum) or external (i.e., skin or orbicularis) eyelid lamella, resulting in lower eyelid retraction and eversion of the eyelid margin.

Orbicularis oculi muscle tone provides support to the lower eyelid. Paralysis can result in power eyelid malposition. However, this patient can close both eyes against resistance; therefore, paralytic ectropion is incorrect.[1,2]

References

1. Barton FE. Eyelids. In: Barton FE, ed. Facial Rejuvenation. New York: Thieme Publishers; 2008
2. Trussler AP, Rohrich RJ. MOC-PSSM CME article: Blepharoplasty. Plast Reconstr Surg 2008;121(1 Suppl):S1

SURGICAL TECHNIQUE

4. *A 37-year-old female with a negative globe vector and 1 mm of scleral show presents for transconjunctival lower blepharoplasty due to orbital fat herniation and bilateral tear trough deformities. Which of the following best describes the most appropriate maneuver to minimize the risk of lower eyelid retraction?*

D. Transcantho-canthopexy, with suture fixation to the inner aspect of the lateral orbital rim periosteum at the level of the upper border of the pupil.

Patients with a negative globe vector (i.e., prominent eyes) typically have scleral show below the inferior limbus and are at an increased risk of lower eyelid retraction after blepharoplasty. Canthopexy is indicated in these patients. There are several options for canthopexy procedures including transcantho-canthopexy. In transconjunctival lower blepharoplasty, transcantho-canthopexy is a convenient option as other forms of canthopexy require a subciliary incision for access to the lateral canthal tendon. An important canthopexy consideration in patients with a negative vector is to choose a higher point of canthopexy fixation to prevent inferior "clotheslining" of the lower eyelid. Therefore, canthopexy fixation at the level of the upper pupillary border is appropriate in this patient.

Although orbicularis suspension helps support the lower eyelid, this is not considered a canthopexy procedure. This patient has lower scleral show and a negative globe vector, which are indications for prophylactic canthopexy to prevent lower eyelid malposition.

Horizontal lower eyelids shortening is considered a form of canthoplasty. There is no indication in the clinical vignette that the patient has horizontal lower eyelid laxity—therefore, horizontal lower eyelid shortening is not indicated.[1]

Reference

1. McCord CD, Boswell CB, Hester TR. Lateral canthal anchoring. Plast Reconstr Surg 2003;112:222

SURGICAL TECHNIQUE

5. *The specific technical refinements of a canthopexy for deep-set eyes include placement of fixation point where relative to the lateral orbital rim?*

D. Inferiorly and internally.

Standard canthal anchoring techniques may result in upward clotheslining of lower eyelid and narrowing of orbital fissure. Deep-set or enophthalmic eyes present a unique challenge since the lateral commissure is usually at or near the orbital rim that requires supraplacement for any lower eyelid support that further narrows the vertical palpebral aperture, and the exaggerated (usually temporary) canthal tilt frequently lasts longer than one would expect.[1]

Reference

1. McCord CD, Boswell CB, Hester TR. Lateral canthal anchoring. Plast Reconstr Surg 2003;112:222

39. Blepharoptosis

Adam Jacoby, Anmol Chattha
See *Essentials of Aesthetic Surgery*, pp. 498–508

PREOPERATIVE EVALUATION

1. ***Prior to a Fasanella-Servat procedure (tarsus muscle–conjunctival resection), what test may help predict the postoperative result?***
   A. Instillation of phenylephrine.
   B. Jones test.
   C. Visual fields testing.
   D. Marginal reflex distance measurement.
   E. Schirmer test.

PREOPERATIVE EVALUATION

2. ***What is the most common cause of eyelid ptosis?***
   A. Involutional (senile).
   B. Traumatic.
   C. Neurogenic.
   D. Mechanical.
   E. Congenital.

TECHNIQUE

3. ***What is the preferred technique of ptosis repair for patients with congenital ptosis with poor levator function?***
   A. Levator advancement.
   B. Frontalis suspension.
   C. Levator resection.
   D. Fasanella-Servat procedure.
   E. Müllerectomy.

PREOPERATIVE EVALUATION

4. ***When planning an eyelid ptosis repair, which of the following is the most important factor in choosing the most appropriate procedure?***
   A. Amount of dermatochalasis.
   B. Levator function.
   C. Visual fields testing.
   D. Epiphora.
   E. Degree of dry eye symptoms.

COMPLICATIONS

5. ***A 50-year-old woman who underwent injection of her glabellar lines with 10 units of botulinum toxin type A 2 weeks ago is now complaining of left eyelid ptosis. Which intervention may help this patient's complaint?***
   A. Scar massage.
   B. Steroid injection.
   C. Alpha-adrenergic eye drops.
   D. Gold weight insertion.
   E. Repeat botulinum toxin injections.

PREOPERATIVE EVALUATION

6. *Which of the following preoperative findings places a patient at risk for corneal ulceration after blepharoplasty?*

A. Asymmetric pupils.
B. Absent Bell's phenomenon.
C. Marcus Gunn pupil.
D. Dermatochalasis.
E. Positive Hering's test.

PREOPERATIVE EVALUATION

7. *The levator palpebrae superioris is innervated by which of the following cranial nerves?*

A. III.
B. IV.
C. V.
D. VI.
E. VII.

PREOPERATIVE EVALUATION

8. *After bilateral upper eyelid blepharoplasty and ptosis repair of the right upper eyelid, a patient comes to the office complaining with new-onset left upper eyelid ptosis. Which of the following explains this new ptosis?*

A. Myogenic ptosis.
B. Involutional ptosis.
C. Ectropion.
D. Hering's law.
E. Bell's phenomenon.

ANATOMY

9. *In the upper eyelid, what structure separates the skin and orbicularis oculi (anterior lamella) from the tarsus and conjunctiva (posterior lamella)?*

A. Whitnall's tubercle.
B. Müller's muscle.
C. Levator aponeurosis.
D. Orbital septum.
E. Frontalis.

ANATOMY

10. *What is the ideal position of the lower border of the upper eyelid?*

A. 5 mm above the lower eyelid.
B. Whitnall's tubercle.
C. Upper limbus.
D. Lower limbus.
E. Mid-pupil line.

Answers

PREOPERATIVE EVALUATION

1. ***Prior to a Fasanella-Servat procedure (tarsus muscle–conjunctival resection), what test may help predict the postoperative result?***

   A. Instillation of phenylephrine.

   The answer is A, instillation of phenylephrine hydrochloride drops into the conjunctival sac, which contracts Müller's muscle, simulating the planned procedure. Jones testing can help evaluate patency of the canalicular drainage system of the eye and is not helpful in patients with isolated ptosis. Visual fields and marginal reflex distance measurements are important parts of the physical examination in patients with ptosis but do not predict or simulate a surgical result. Schirmer test is a good test to evaluate for patients with dry eyes.[1,2]

REFERENCES

1. McCord CD Jr, Codner MA, eds. Eyelid & Periorbital Surgery. New York: Thieme Publishers; 2008
2. Carraway J. Correction of blepharoptosis. In: Achauer BM, Eriksson E, Guyuron B, et al, eds. Plastic Surgery: Indications, Operations, and Outcomes. St Louis: Mosby–Year Book; 2000

PREOPERATIVE EVALUATION

2. ***What is the most common cause of eyelid ptosis?***

   A. Involutional (senile).

   The answer is A, involutional, which is caused by stretching of the levator's attachments to the anterior tarsus, often resulting in a high-appearing eyelid crease; this stretching and loosening of the levator's attachments are associated with aging. Traumatic ptosis is the second most common cause of acquired ptosis. Neurogenic causes of ptosis include Horner syndrome and myasthenia gravis, which are overall less common causes. Eyelid tumors and dermatochalasis can lead to mechanical ptosis, which is less common than involutional or senile ptosis. Congenital ptosis, which refers to eyelid drooping present at birth due to a developmental issue, is one of the primary types of ptosis (eyelid drooping). Although congenital ptosis is not as common as acquired types of ptosis, it remains a significant concern, particularly levator aponeurosis malformation and congenital myogenic ptosis.[1,2]

REFERENCES

1. McCord CD Jr, Codner MA, eds. Eyelid & Periorbital Surgery. New York: Thieme Publishers; 2008
2. Carraway J. Correction of blepharoptosis. In: Achauer BM, Eriksson E, Guyuron B, et al, eds. Plastic Surgery: Indications, Operations, and Outcomes. St Louis: Mosby–Year Book; 2000

TECHNIQUE

3. ***What is the preferred technique of ptosis repair for patients with congenital ptosis with poor levator function?***

   B. Frontalis suspension.

   The answer is B, frontalis suspension, which is the preferred technique for most patients with poor levator excursion (defined as <5 mm of excursion). Levator advancement and resection are reserved for patients with moderate levator excursion (5–10 mm). The Fasanella-Servat procedure (conjunctival approach to excise tarsus, Müller's muscle, and conjunctiva) can only be used in patients with excellent levator function and minimal ptosis. History alone usually can distinguish congenital from acquired ptosis, but if it is questionable, lagophthalmos on downward gaze is characteristic of congenital ptosis because levator fibrosis prevents downward eyelid migration.[1,2,3]

REFERENCES

1. McCord CD Jr, Codner MA, eds. Eyelid & Periorbital Surgery. New York: Thieme Publishers; 2008
2. Carraway J. Correction of blepharoptosis. In: Achauer BM, Eriksson E, Guyuron B, et al, eds. Plastic Surgery: Indications, Operations, and Outcomes. St Louis: Mosby–Year Book; 2000
3. Chang S, Lehrman C, Itani K, et al. A systematic review of comparison of upper eyelid involutional ptosis repair techniques: efficacy and complication rates. Plast Reconstr Surg 2012;129:149

PREOPERATIVE EVALUATION

4. ***When planning an eyelid ptosis repair, which of the following is the most important factor in choosing the most appropriate procedure?***

   B. Levator function.

   The answer is B, levator function, which guides the current treatment algorithm for ptosis repair. Mild dysfunction may only require an aponeurotic repair while poor levator function may only be helped by frontalis suspension. Dermatochalasis or excess skin in the eyelids can be associated with eyelid ptosis but does not help guide ptosis repair techniques. Visual fields testing can help diagnose ptosis but not its severity. Epiphora may indicate a nasolacrimal duct obstruction. Degree of dry eyes may help determine if someone is a surgical candidate or not; however, this would not change the type of ptosis repair indicated as much as levator function would.[1,2]

REFERENCES

1. McCord CD Jr, Codner MA, eds. Eyelid & Periorbital Surgery. New York: Thieme Publishers; 2008
2. Carraway J. Correction of blepharoptosis. In: Achauer BM, Eriksson E, Guyuron B, et al, eds. Plastic Surgery: Indications, Operations, and Outcomes. St Louis: Mosby–Year Book; 2000

COMPLICATIONS

5. ***A 50-year-old woman who underwent injection of her glabellar lines with 10 units of botulinum toxin type A 2 weeks ago is now complaining of left eyelid ptosis. Which intervention may help this patient's complaint?***

   C. Alpha-adrenergic eye drops.

   The answer is C, prescription of alpha-adrenergic eye drops (apraclonidine). Periorbital injections of botulinum toxin A can inadvertently paralyze the levator palpebrae superioris muscle, which is the main muscle responsible for raising the eyelid. Alpha-adrenergic eye drops stimulate Müller's muscle, which is sympathetically innervated and contributes to eyelid elevation. Scar massage is unlikely to affect this new-onset ptosis, as is a steroid injection. Gold weights are inserted as a treatment for lagophthalmos and would worsen ptosis. Repeat botulinum toxin injections may just worsen the underlying ptosis or provide no change.[1,2]

REFERENCES

1. McCord CD Jr, Codner MA, eds. Eyelid & Periorbital Surgery. New York: Thieme Publishers; 2008
2. Carraway J. Correction of blepharoptosis. In: Achauer BM, Eriksson E, Guyuron B, et al, eds. Plastic Surgery: Indications, Operations, and Outcomes. St Louis: Mosby–Year Book; 2000

PREOPERATIVE EVALUATION

6. ***Which of the following preoperative findings places a patient at risk for corneal ulceration after blepharoplasty?***

   B. Absent Bell's phenomenon.

   The answer is B, absent Bell's phenomenon, a reflex which causes the eye to move upwards and outwards when eyelid closure is attempted. When this reflex is absent, dry eyes and corneal ulcerations are potential complications if postoperative lagophthalmos occurs. Pupil abnormalities are unlikely to cause corneal ulcerations after blepharoplasty or ptosis repair. Dermatochalasis refers to excess eyelid skin and should not affect corneal exposure or ulceration after surgery. Hering's test reveals contralateral ptosis to help surgical planning.[1,2]

REFERENCES

1. McCord CD Jr, Codner MA, eds. Eyelid & Periorbital Surgery. New York: Thieme Publishers; 2008
2. Carraway J. Correction of blepharoptosis. In: Achauer BM, Eriksson E, Guyuron B, et al, eds. Plastic Surgery: Indications, Operations, and Outcomes. St Louis: Mosby–Year Book; 2000

PREOPERATIVE EVALUATION

7. ***The levator palpebrae superioris is innervated by which of the following cranial nerves?***

   A. III.

   The answer is A, the third cranial nerve or oculomotor nerve, which innervates the levator muscle, superior rectus, medial rectus, inferior rectus, and inferior oblique muscles. The fourth cranial nerve, or trochlear nerve, innervates the superior oblique muscle. The fifth cranial nerve, or trigeminal nerve, is mostly responsible for sensation of the face but it also innervates the muscles of mastication. The sixth cranial nerve, or abducens nerve, innervates the lateral rectus muscle. The seventh cranial nerve is responsible for innervating the muscles of facial expression.[1,2]

REFERENCES

1. McCord CD Jr, Codner MA, eds. Eyelid & Periorbital Surgery. New York: Thieme Publishers; 2008
2. Carraway J. Correction of blepharoptosis. In: Achauer BM, Eriksson E, Guyuron B, et al, eds. Plastic Surgery: Indications, Operations, and Outcomes. St Louis: Mosby–Year Book; 2000

PREOPERATIVE EVALUATION

8. *After bilateral upper eyelid blepharoplasty and ptosis repair of the right upper eyelid, a patient comes to the office complaining with new-onset left upper eyelid ptosis. Which of the following explains this new ptosis?*

D. Hering's law.

The answer is D, Hering's law, which provides the following explanation: after ptosis repair of the right eyelid, the signal for eyelid elevation decreased, causing new ptosis in the left eyelid. This is caused by equal innervation to both upper eyelid levator muscles. Myogenic and involutional ptosis would not explain new-onset postoperative ptosis. Ectropion is an outward turning of the eyelid usually caused by aging or scarring.[1,2]

REFERENCES

1. McCord CD Jr, Codner MA, eds. Eyelid & Periorbital Surgery. New York: Thieme Publishers; 2008
2. Carraway J. Correction of blepharoptosis. In: Achauer BM, Eriksson E, Guyuron B, et al, eds. Plastic Surgery: Indications, Operations, and Outcomes. St Louis: Mosby–Year Book; 2000

ANATOMY

9. *In the upper eyelid, what structure separates the skin and orbicularis oculi (anterior lamella) from the tarsus and conjunctiva (posterior lamella)?*

D. Orbital septum.

The answer is D, orbital septum, also called the middle lamella. During blepharoplasty and ptosis repair, violation of the septum places patients at higher risk of developing retrobulbar hematomas. Whitnall's tubercle is located on the lateral orbital wall and is not part of the upper eyelid. Müller's muscle is in the posterior lamella. The levator aponeurosis is posterior to the orbital septum. The frontalis is a muscle more cranial than the eyelid.[1,2]

REFERENCES

1. McCord CD Jr, Codner MA, eds. Eyelid & Periorbital Surgery. New York: Thieme Publishers; 2008
2. Carraway J. Correction of blepharoptosis. In: Achauer BM, Eriksson E, Guyuron B, et al, eds. Plastic Surgery: Indications, Operations, and Outcomes. St Louis: Mosby–Year Book; 2000

ANATOMY

10. *What is the ideal position of the lower border of the upper eyelid?*

C. Upper limbus.

The answer is C, upper limbus, also known as the border of the cornea and the sclera. Whitnall's tubercle is on the lateral orbital wall and considered the ideal site of re-attachment of the lateral canthal tendon during a canthoplasty. Positioning 5 mm above the lower eyelid is too low for ideal upper eyelid. The lower limbus of the eye would also be too low for ideal positioning of the upper eyelid. The upper eyelid at the mid-pupil line would denote severe ptosis and is not the ideal eyelid position.[1,2]

REFERENCES

1. McCord CD Jr, Codner MA, eds. Eyelid & Periorbital Surgery. New York: Thieme Publishers; 2008
2. Carraway J. Correction of blepharoptosis. In: Achauer BM, Eriksson E, Guyuron B, et al, eds. Plastic Surgery: Indications, Operations, and Outcomes. St Louis: Mosby–Year Book; 2000

40. Midface Rejuvenation

David A. Sterling, Christopher C. Surek
See *Essentials of Aesthetic Surgery*, pp. 509–527

PERTINENT ANATOMY

1. ***With aging, the midcheek segments become separated by which of the following three cutaneous grooves?***
   A. Palpebromalar, nasolabial, midcheek.
   B. Palpebromalar, nasojugal, midcheek.
   C. Nasojugal, nasolabial, midcheek.
   D. Palpebromalar, nasolabial, nasojugal.
   E. Lateral malar, nasojugal, midcheek.

PERTINENT ANATOMY

2. ***With aging, the relationship between the anterior maxillary wall and the orbital rim leads to what vector type and how does this influence the surgical outcome?***
   A. A positive vector; increased rates of ectropion.
   B. A neutral vector; decreased rates of ectropion.
   C. A negative vector; increased rates of ectropion.
   D. A negative vector; decreased rates of ectropion.
   E. A positive vector; decreased rates of ectropion.

PERTINENT ANATOMY

3. ***The prezygomatic space is bordered by which two retaining ligaments?***
   A. Orbicularis retaining ligament and upper masseteric ligament.
   B. Orbicularis retaining ligament and zygomatic ligament.
   C. Zygomatic ligament and upper masseteric ligament.
   D. Upper masseteric ligament and mandibular ligament.
   E. Upper masseteric ligament and orbicularis retaining ligament.

ASSESSMENT OF THE MIDFACE

4. ***A 62-year-old woman presents with concerns about her aging facial appearance, specifically her sagging cheeks. What physical examination finding would be the biggest indication for operative intervention?***
   A. Soft tissue and fat atrophy.
   B. Skeletal changes and bone loss.
   C. Fat hypertrophy.
   D. Skin pigmentary changes.
   E. Inferior displacement of soft tissue from ligamentous attenuation.

SURGICAL PRINCIPLES

5. ***A 75-year-old male undergoes a skin-only rhytidectomy without fat grafting. The patient is unhappy with his result 2 years after surgery and complains that his nasolabial folds and jowls are still present. Which of the following is a reason for this patient's disappointing result?***
   A. Not performing concomitant fat grafting to nasolabial folds.
   B. Releasing too many ligaments.
   C. Not enough sutures used during the closure.
   D. Not addressing the deeper foundation structures of the face.
   E. Too much early postoperative swelling.

CHARACTERISTICS OF THE IDEAL MIDFACE

6. ***A 45-year-old female presents with concerns about the appearance of midface hollowing and a loss of definition in the lower eyelid–cheek area. On examination, she has mild scleral show, and malar descent with a very pronounced V-shaped interface of the eyelid–cheek junction, including elements of herniated fat and slight negative canthal tilt. Which of the following would best address her concerns?***

A. Transcutaneous skin–muscle blepharoplasty with midface lift.
B. Transcutaneous skin–muscle blepharoplasty with fat repositioning and lateral canthopexy.
C. Fat grafting to the midface.
D. Fat excision of the herniated fat and fat grafting to the midface.
E. Fat excision of the herniated fat, fat grafting to the midface, and lateral canthopexy.

OPERATIVE TECHNIQUES

7. ***Regarding alloplastic implants for midface rejuvenation, the major body of the zygomatic bone is defined by which zone?***

A. I.
B. II.
C. III.
D. IV.
E. V.

OPERATIVE TECHNIQUES

8. ***What are the appropriate anatomic planes or targets for fat grafting?***

A. Subcutaneous, subperiosteal, muscle.
B. Subperiosteal, muscle, sub-SMAS.
C. Subcutaneous, subperiosteal, sub-SMAS.
D. Subcutaneous, muscle, sub-SMAS.
E. Dermal, muscle, supraperiosteal.

OPERATIVE TECHNIQUES

9. ***A 62-year-old male presents to your clinic for facial rejuvenation. He has noticeable descent of the malar fat pads, resulting in a hollowed midface appearance. There is also a loss of skin elasticity and a mild mandibular jowling. The surgeon discusses the possibility of an endoscopic midface lift. What specific aspect of this patient's operation is most important to giving the patient a successful outcome?***

A. Piecewise mobilization of midface structures.
B. Minimal periosteal release in the lower and medial boundaries of the cheek.
C. Strong suspensory element and release of ligaments.
D. Selective subperiosteal and subfascial dissection.
E. Sub-SMAS dissection.

SURGICAL COMPLICATIONS AND TREATMENT

10. ***After 2 days of completing a composite rhytidectomy with malar resuspension on a 58-year-old female, she presents to the clinic with increasing pain and swelling of her left face. You suspect a hematoma. What could have avoided this complication?***

A. Use of cold compress postoperatively.
B. Use of a temporary Frost suture immediately postoperatively.
C. Strict blood pressure control and meticulous hemostasis.
D. Limited tension of skin closure.
E. Use of fibrin glue under advancement flap.

SURGICAL COMPLICATIONS AND TREATMENT

11. ***A 60-year-old male presents with visible swelling of his conjunctiva and a foreign body sensation 5 days following midface rejuvenation. What is the best initial management plan?***

A. Steroid eye drops.
B. Antibiotic eye drops.
C. Placement of a temporary Frost suture.
D. Conjunctivotomy.
E. Observation.

SURGICAL COMPLICATIONS AND TREATMENT

12. *Your patient presents with mild lower eyelid malposition 3 weeks following midface rejuvenation. How would you treat this patient?*

A. No treatment required; this is expected.
B. Surgical canthopexy or canthoplasty.
C. Drill hole canthal anchoring.
D. Postoperative massage and eye lubrication.
E. Filler or fat grafting to support lower eyelid.

Answers

PERTINENT ANATOMY

1. *With aging, the midcheek segments become separated by which of the following three cutaneous grooves?*

B. Palpebromalar, nasojugal, midcheek.

The midface is divided into the anterior and lateral segments. The anterior segment, called the midcheek, extends from the lower eyelid to the nasolabial groove and upper lip. The midcheek represents the aesthetically pleasing fullness of the youthful cheek. As an individual ages, three cutaneous grooves separate the midcheek into the lid–cheek segment, the malar segment, and the nasolabial segment. The nasojugal groove separates the lid–cheek and nasolabial segments. The palpebromalar groove separates the lid–cheek and malar segments. The midcheek groove separates the malar and nasolabial segments. These grooves intersect to form an obliquely oriented Y (**Fig. 40.1**).[1]

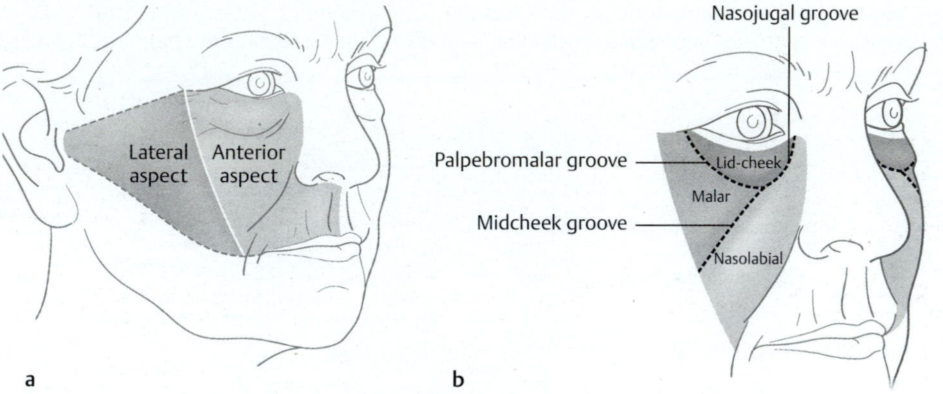

Fig. 40.1 (a,b) Subcutaneous compartments of the midcheek. (Source: Applied Anatomy. In: Janis J, ed. Essentials of Aesthetic Surgery. 1st Edition. New York: Thieme; 2018.)

REFERENCE

1. Mendelson B, Jacobsen S. Surgical anatomy of the midcheek: facial layers, spaces, and the midcheek segments. Clin Plast Surg 2008;35:395

PERTINENT ANATOMY

2. *With aging, the relationship between the anterior maxillary wall and the orbital rim leads to what vector type and how does this influence the surgical outcome?*

C. A negative vector; increased rates of ectropion.

Aging of the midface includes changes in skin quality, loss of fat volume, attenuation of ligamentous structures, and changes in the underlying skeletal support structure. Although historically it was believed that facial skeleton aging consisted of growth and expansion, studies have identified retrusion of key structures that result in the characteristic appearance of the aging face. For instance, there is retrusion of the anterior maxillary wall in relation to the relatively fixed inferior orbital rim. This leads to a "negative vector" appearance of the lid–cheek junction, which is defined as ocular globe located in a more anterior position relative to the lower lid and malar eminence.[1,2,3,4]

REFERENCES

1. Pessa JE, Desvigne LD, Lambros VS, et al. Changes in ocular globe-to-orbital rim position with age: implications for aesthetic blepharoplasty of the lower eyelids. Aesthetic Plast Surg 1999;23:337
2. Mendelson B, Hartley W, Scott M, et al. Age-related changes of the orbit and midcheek and the implications for facial rejuvenation. Aesthetic Plast Surg 2007;31:419

3. Jelks GW, Glat PM. Jelks EB, et al. The inferior retinacular lateral canthoplasty: a new technique. Plast Reconstr Surg 1997;100:1262
4. Shaw RB, Kahn DM. Aging of the midface bony elements: a three-dimensional computed tomographic study. Plast Reconstr Surg 2007;119:675

PERTINENT ANATOMY

3. *The prezygomatic space is bordered by which two retaining ligaments?*

B. Orbicularis retaining ligament and zygomatic ligament.

The topographic anatomy of the midface can be likened to the layers of the scalp—skin, subcutaneous tissue, musculoaponeurotic layer, loose areolar tissue, fixed periosteum, and deep fascia. The loose areolar tissue, which allows gliding movement of the more superficial layers, is maintained in several areas by retaining ligaments. These ligaments serve as fixation points between deep and superficial layers, and between them are specific areas of loose areolar tissue that are important during midface rejuvenation. The roof of these spaces is the underside of the superficial musculoaponeurotic system (SMAS), the floor the deep fascia or periosteum, and the walls of the retaining ligaments. The three important retaining ligaments of the midface are the orbicularis retainingligament, the zygomatic ligament, and the upper masseteric ligament. The four midface spaces between these ligaments are the preseptal, prezygomatic, masticator, and oral cavity spaces. Theprezygomatic space lies between the orbicularis retaining ligament and the zygomatic ligament (**Fig. 40.2**).[1]

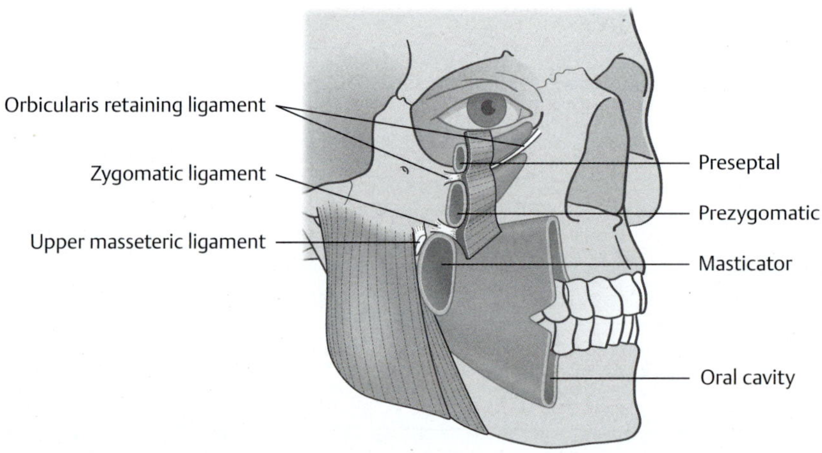

Fig. 40.2 Four major midface spaces. (Source: Nahai F, ed. The Art of Aesthetic Surgery: Principles & Techniques, ed 2. New York: Thieme Publishers, 2011.)

REFERENCE

1. Mendelson B, Jacobsen S. Surgical anatomy of the midcheek: facial layers, spaces, and the midcheek segments. Clin Plast Surg 2008;35:395

ASSESSMENT OF THE MIDFACE

4. *A 62-year-old woman presents with concerns about her aging facial appearance, specifically her sagging cheeks. What physical examination finding would be the biggest indication for operative intervention?*

E. Inferior displacement of soft tissue from ligamentous attenuation.

Facial aging is the result of several factors, including skin laxity, ptosis of soft tissues, volume loss within the soft tissues, and changes within the skeletal structures of the facial bones. According to Hester and Szczerba, four important changes occur during the aging process: (1) There is gradual ptosis of the cheek skin below the inferior orbital rim with descent of the attenuated lower eyelid skin, which creates a skeletonized appearance with infraorbital hollowness; (2) the malar fat pad descends, creating a loss of the malar prominence; (3) the tear trough deepens; and (4) there is exaggeration of the nasolabial fold. In addition to these four changes, there is also laxity and descent of the orbicular oculi muscle, laxity of the orbital septum, descent of the lid–cheek junction, horizontal laxity of the lower eyelid tarsal plate, laxity of the orbitomalar ligament resulting in descent of the cheek fat pad, and laxity of the zygomaticus muscles and otherlipelevators.[1] However, the most important of these is the inferior displacement of soft tissue from ligamentous attenuation.

REFERENCE

1. Hester TR, Szczerba S. Midface rejuvenation. In: Nahai F, ed. The Art of Aesthetic Surgery: Principles and Techniques. New York: Thieme Publishers; 2005

SURGICAL PRINCIPLES

5. ***A 75-year-old male undergoes a skin-only rhytidectomy without fat grafting. The patient is unhappy with his result 2 years after surgery and complains that his nasolabial folds and jowls are still present. Which of the following is a reason for this patient's disappointing result?***

D. Not addressing the deeper foundation structures of the face.

Historically, surgical facial rejuvenation consisted undermining and redraping skin flaps under tension without addressing deeper structures. Inadequate results fueled a major shift toward the modern approach, which focuses on adequately releasing soft tissues with resuspension along appropriate vectors to recreate a youthful appearance while limiting tension on the reconstruction. Adequate mobilization of soft tissues includes release of fixation points (ligamentous attachments). Compartments are then repositioned along vectors that recreate a youthful anatomy, and multiple sutures are used to decrease the load exerted on any one fixation point to improve the longevity of the result (**Fig. 40.3**, **Fig. 40.4**).[1,2]

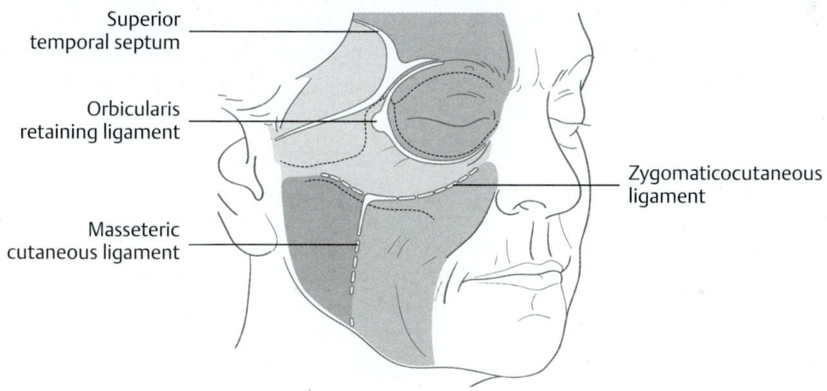

Fig. 40.3 Regions of the face. (Source: Codner MA, McCord CD Jr, eds. Eyelid & Periorbital Surgery, ed 2. New York: Thieme Publishers, 2016.)

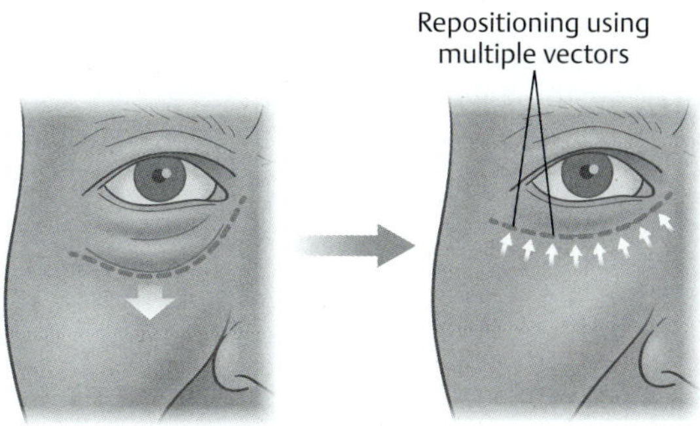

Fig. 40.4 Principle of correction of laxity of the lower lid. (Source: Surgical principles. In: Janis J, ed. Essentials of Aesthetic Surgery. 1st Edition. New York: Thieme; 2018.)

References

1. Marten TJ. High SMAS facelift: combined single flap lifting of the jawline, cheek, and midface. Clin Plast Surg 2008;35:569
2. Mendelson B. Surgery of the superficial musculo-aponeurotic system: principles of release, vectors, and fixation. Plast Reconstr Surg 2001;107:1545

CHARACTERISTICS OF THE IDEAL MIDFACE

6. *A 45-year-old female presents with concerns about the appearance of midface hollowing and a loss of definition in the lower eyelid–cheek area. On examination, she has mild scleral show, and malar descent with a very pronounced V-shaped interface of the eyelid–cheek junction, including elements of herniated fat and slight negative canthal tilt. Which of the following would best address her concerns?*

E. Fat excision of the herniated fat, fat grafting to the midface, and lateral canthopexy.

Ramirez described a list of concepts that are integral to the ideal midface rejuvenation, which supplement the principles of release, vectors, and fixation described by Mendelson.[1] The concepts include providing a volumetric remodeling of the cheek where the skeletal foundation is augmented or released while minimizing incisions and dissection planes, and fat may be injected without the risk of migration or need for fixation or alternative grafts. Fat pad herniation of the lower eyelid and the V deformity of the eyelid–cheek junction should be corrected. The corners of the mouth should be lifted as necessary. The skin should be safely treated in the same operative setting if indicated. Facial edema should be minimized, and nerve injury should be avoided.[2,3]

Given these as ideals, in a patient with an extreme V-shaped cheek–lower eyelid, two main principles apply: smoothing out the eyelid–cheek junction by excising herniated fat and fat grafting to blend that junction. Along with that, doing a lateral canthopexy for the mild scleral show and negative canthal tilt would help her overall aesthetics. Doing a midface lift would not correct her severe midface V-shaped deformity. An isolated blepharoplasty would not correct her midface ptosis and volumization issue. Fat transposition works when fat redistribution is isolated to less than 2 cc; however, in this patient who requires severe volumization, performing midface fat grafting would be the better solution.

References

1. Ramirez OM. Three-dimensional endoscopic midface enhancement: a personal quest for the ideal cheek rejuvenation. Plast Reconstr Surg 2002;109(1):329-340; discussion 341-349
2. Marten TJ. High SMAS facelift: combined single flap lifting of the jawline, cheek, and midface. Clin Plast Surg 2008;35:569
3. Mendelson B. Surgery of the superficial musculoaponeurotic system: principles of release, vectors, and fixation. Plast Reconstr Surg 2001;107:1545

OPERATIVE TECHNIQUES

7. *Regarding alloplastic implants for midface rejuvenation, the major body of the zygomatic bone is defined by which zone?*

A. I.

Alloplastic augmentation of the midface is an option for volumization of this region during rejuvenation. Terino popularized this method and developed the concept of anatomic zones of the face. Five distinct skeletal zones compromise the zygomatic region. The suborbital zygomatic region is defined specifically by Zone I, the major body of the malar bone, and Zone III, the paranasal suborbital zone. Alloplastic augmentation of the midface is usually combined with a subperiosteal lift to allow placement of the implant in this plane (**Fig. 40.5**).[1]

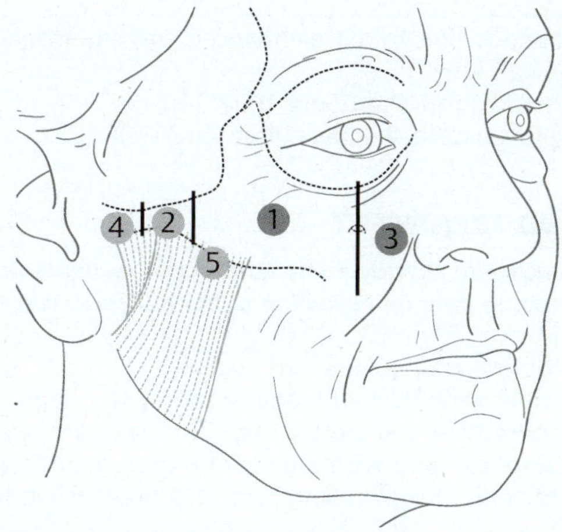

Fig. 40.5 Skeletal zones of the zygomatic region. 1, Major body of the malar bone. 2, Middle third of the zygomatic arch. 3, Paranasal suborbital zone. 4, Zone overlying the posterior third of the zygomatic arch. 5, Submalar zonal triangle. (Source: Alloplastic Implants. In: Janis J, ed. Essentials of Aesthetic Surgery. 1st Edition. New York: Thieme; 2018.)

Reference

1. Terino EO. Alloplastic contouring for suborbital, maxillary, zygomatic deficiencies. In: Fagien S, ed. Putterman's Cosmetic Oculoplastic Surgery. 4th ed. Philadelphia: Saunders Elsevier; 2008

OPERATIVE TECHNIQUES

8. *What are the appropriate anatomic planes or targets for fat grafting?*

C. Subcutaneous, subperiosteal, sub-SMAS.

Fat grafting is a useful technique for addressing volume loss of the midface. Areas that often need augmentation include the tear trough and infraorbital areas, the malar eminence, the submalar region, and the nasolabial crease. Coleman popularized the use of structural fat grafting employing a three-dimensional approach to soft tissue augmentation. Lipoinfiltration is performed in multiple planes, including the subcutaneous, sub-SMAS, and subperiosteal planes. Coleman cautioned against injection into muscle, as it can lead to edema, distortion, undercorrection, muscle fibrosis, and thickening.[1]

Reference

1. Coleman SR. The technique of periorbital lipoinfiltration. Oper Tech Plast Reconstr Surg 1994;1:120

OPERATIVE TECHNIQUES

9. *A 62-year-old male presents to your clinic for facial rejuvenation. He has noticeable descent of the malar fat pads, resulting in a hollowed midface appearance. There is also a loss of skin elasticity and a mild mandibular jowling. The surgeon discusses the possibility of an endoscopic midface lift. What specific aspect of this patient's operation is most important to giving the patient a successful outcome?*

C. Strong suspensory element and release of ligaments.

Endoscopic techniques for midface rejuvenation have been popularized by several surgeons. The main benefit to this approach is avoiding traumatic dissection of the orbicularis oculi. Ramirez outlined several key principles of endoscopic midface surgery. They include wide subperiosteal and subfascial dissection, en bloc mobilization of soft tissue, periosteal release of the lower and medial boundaries of the cheek, and a strong suspensory element to maintain cheek repositioning.[1,2,3]

References

1. Ramirez OM. Three-dimensional endoscopic midface enhancement: a personal quest for the ideal cheek rejuvenation. Plast Reconstr Surg 2002;109:329
2. Isse NG. Endoscopic facial rejuvenation. Clin Plast Surg 1997;24:213
3. Ramirez OM. Endoscopic facial rejuvenation. Perspect Plast Surg 1995;9:22

SURGICAL COMPLICATIONS AND TREATMENT

10. *After 2 days of completing a composite rhytidectomy with malar resuspension on a 58-year-old female, she presents to the clinic with increasing pain and swelling of her left face. You suspect a hematoma. What could have avoided this complication?*

C. Strict blood pressure control and meticulous hemostasis.

Hematoma is a common complication of rhytidectomy, more often seen in men than women. Appropriate blood pressure control perioperatively and meticulous hemostasis are key to avoiding this issue. Use of cold compresses and head elevation can help with edema. A temporary Frost suture postoperatively can help prevent chemosis. Limited tension of skin closure can help prevent wound healing issues.[1]

Reference

1. Cason RW, Avashia YJ, Shammas RL, Savetsky IL, Rohrich RJ. Perioperative approach to reducing hematoma during rhytidectomy: what does the evidence show? Plast Reconstr Surg 2021;147(6):1297–1309

SURGICAL COMPLICATIONS AND TREATMENT

11. *A 60-year-old male presents with visible swelling of his conjunctiva and a foreign body sensation 5 days following midface rejuvenation. What is the best initial management plan?*

A. Steroid eye drops.

This patient's presentation is concerning for chemosis. This is the most common nonsurgical complication from a transpalpebral approach to the midface. It usually presents within 1 week from surgery and can last up to 4 weeks or longer. Prevention is key, starting with lubrication of the eye during surgery and taking care to prevent trauma during exposure. A temporary tarsorrhaphy can help reduce the rate of postoperative chemosis. Treatment is largely conservative with lubricating eye drops. Ophthalmic steroid drops can be helpful. In severe or prolonged cases, conjunctivotomy can be considered.[1,2]

References

1. Weinfeld AB, Burke R, Codner MA. The comprehensive management of chemosis following cosmetic lower blepharoplasty. Plast Reconstr Surg 2008;122(2):579–586
2. Hester TR Jr, Douglas T, Szczerba S. Decreasing complications in lower lid and midface rejuvenation: the importance of orbital morphology, horizontal lower lid laxity, history of previous surgery, and minimizing trauma to the orbital septum: a critical review of 269 consecutive cases. Plast Reconstr Surg 2009;123:1037

SURGICAL COMPLICATIONS AND TREATMENT

12. *Your patient presents with mild lower eyelid malposition 3 weeks following midface rejuvenation. How would you treat this patient?*

D. Postoperative massage and eye lubrication.

Lower eyelid malposition is the most common surgical complication following a transpalpebral approach. It is characterized by eyelid retraction, scleral show, and ectropion. It is caused by a vertical deficiency of the anterior or posterior lamella in patients with laxity of the tarsus. Patients at increased risk include those with lower eyelid laxity, prominent eyes, negative vector, negative canthal tilt, and/or preoperative scleral show. Mild lower eyelid malposition is treated conservatively with postoperative massage, external taping, and eye lubrication. If these treatments fail, the next options include surgical canthopexy or canthoplasty. More severe cases may require drill hole canthal anchoring. Immediate surgical correction may also be required to prevent keratopathy. It would be too early to start thinking about any filler or fat grafting to support the lower eyelid in situations of inferior eyelid retraction. The underlying issue must be a volumelossissue for this to be effective.[1,2]

References

1. Weinfeld AB, Burke R, Codner MA. The comprehensive management of chemosis following cosmetic lower blepharoplasty. Plast Reconstr Surg 2008;122(2):579–586
2. Hester TR Jr, Douglas T, Szczerba S. Decreasing complications in lower lid and midface rejuvenation: the importance of orbital morphology, horizontal lower lid laxity, history of previous surgery, and minimizing trauma to the orbital septum: a critical review of 269 consecutive cases. Plast Reconstr Surg 2009;123:1037

41. Perioral Rejuvenation

Ira L. Savetsky, Anmol Chattha
See *Essentials of Aesthetic Surgery*, pp. 528–539

PREOPERATIVE EVALUATION

1. ***What is the typical size of the upper lip compared to total lip volume?***
   A. 1/5 of the total lip volume.
   B. 1/4 of the total lip volume.
   C. 1/3 of the total lip volume.
   D. 1/2 of the total lip volume.
   E. 2/3 of the total lip volume.

PATIENT EVALUATION

2. ***How many millimeters of upper incisor show in repose is considered aesthetically pleasing?***
   A. 0.5–1 mm.
   B. 1–2 mm.
   C. 2–3 mm.
   D. 3–4 mm.
   E. 4–5 mm.

PATIENT EVALUATION

3. ***A patient has perioral static lines without lip atrophy but with dyschromias. What is the optimal method of perioral enhancement?***
   A. Laser resurfacing with or without dermabrasion.
   B. Fat injection.
   C. Direct lip lift.
   D. Indirect lip lift.
   E. Maxillary lengthening.

PATIENT EVALUATION

4. ***A patient has lip hypoplasia with optimal incisor show. What is the optimal method of perioral enhancement?***
   A. Indirect lip lift.
   B. Fat injection.
   C. Direct lip lift.
   D. Maxillary lengthening.
   E. Neuromodulator "lip flip."

PATIENT EVALUATION

5. ***A patient has lip hypoplasia with excessive incisor show. What is the optimal method of perioral enhancement?***
   A. Indirect lip lift.
   B. Direct lip lift.
   C. Gingival shortening.
   D. Maxillary lengthening.
   E. Laser resurfacing.

PATIENT EVALUATION

6. ***An old patient has lip hypoplasia, inadequate incisor show, a long lip, and an adequate nasolabial angle. What is the optimal method of perioral enhancement?***
   A. Indirect lip lift.
   B. Direct lip lift.
   C. Lip augmentation.
   D. Maxillary lengthening.
   E. Laser resurfacing.

CHEMODENERVATION

7. ***A 67-year-old female is frustrated with the fact that she looks sad all the time and would like to know if there is anything you can do for her downward-slanted oral commisures. What is the best product to use and which of the following muscle is the main target to treat her condition?***
   A. Filler; oribicularis oris.
   B. Filler; levator anguli oris.
   C. Filler; depressor anguli oris.
   D. Neuromodulator; mentalis.
   E. Neuromodulator; depressor anguli oris.

CHEMODENERVATION

8. ***A 23-year-old girl has a "gummy smile" when she smiles and wants to know if there is a way to temporarily treat this. Which of the following muscles are targeted with botulinum toxin to treat her condition?***
   A. Oribicularis oris.
   B. Levator anguli oris.
   C. Levator labii superioris.
   D. Depressor anguli oris.
   E. Mentalis.

SOFT TISSUE FILLERS

9. ***Which of the following soft tissue fillers is best used on patients with HIV lipoatrophy?***
   A. Hyaluronic acid based.
   B. Poly-L-lactic acid.
   C. Bovine collagen.
   D. Human-based collagen.
   E. Calcium hydroxyapatite.

SOFT TISSUE FILLERS

10. ***Which of the following soft tissue fillers requires skin testing prior to use?***
    A. Hyaluronic acid based.
    B. Poly-L-lactic acid.
    C. Bovine collagen.
    D. Human-based collagen.
    E. Calcium hydroxyapatite.

SOFT TISSUE FILLERS

11. ***Which of the following is a permanent soft tissue filler?***
    A. Polymethylmethacrylate.
    B. Poly-L-lactic acid.
    C. Bovine collagen.
    D. Human-based collagen.
    E. Calcium hydroxyapatite.

SOFT TISSUE FILLERS

12. *Which of the following soft tissue fillers should not be used for lip augmentation given the high incidence of nodule formation?*
A. Polymethylmethacrylate.
B. Autologous fat from knee.
C. Bovine collagen.
D. Human-based collagen.
E. Calcium hydroxyapatite.

SOFT TISSUE FILLERS

13. *When correcting nasolabial folds with soft tissue filler, which of the following is the best technique to fill this region?*
A. Inject within the fold directly.
B. Inject slightly medial to the fold.
C. Inject slightly medial and lateral to the fold.
D. Inject slightly lateral to the fold.
E. Inject deep and caudally.

DERMABRASION

14. *What is the most reliable indicator that the operator has reached the optimal depth in dermabrasion?*
A. Erythema.
B. Frost effect.
C. Punctiform, superficial bleeding.
D. Pale yellow color.
E. Visualization of hair follicles.

LASER ABLATIVE RESURFACING

15. *What is the clinical endpoint when performing laser ablative resurfacing with a carbon dioxide laser?*
A. Erythema.
B. Frost effect.
C. Punctiform, superficial bleeding.
D. Pale yellow color.
E. Visualization of hair follicles.

Answers

PREOPERATIVE EVALUATION

1. *What is the typical size of the upper lip compared to total lip volume?*

C. 1/3 of the total lip volume.

The upper lip is smaller than the lower lip and is a third of the total lip volume (**Fig. 41.1**).[1]

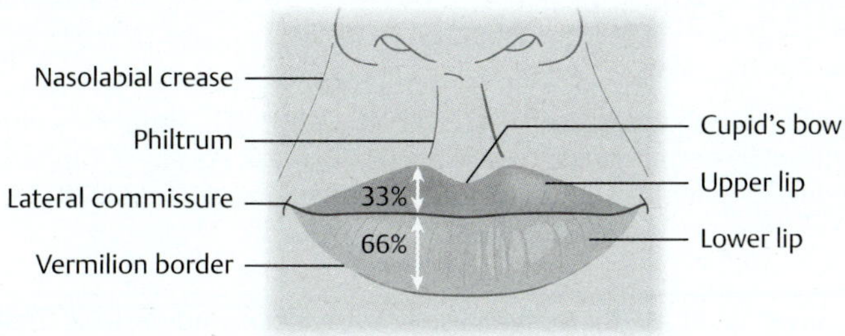

Fig. 41.1 The upper lip is smaller than the lower lip and is a third of the total lip volume. (Source: Anatomy. In: Janis J, ed. Essentials of Aesthetic Surgery. 1st Edition. New York: Thieme; 2018.)

REFERENCE

1. Agarwal A, Dejoseph L, Silver W, et al. Anatomy of the jawline, neck, and perioral area with clinical correlations. Facial Plast Surg 2005;21:3

PATIENT EVALUATION

2. *How many millimeters of upper incisor show in repose is considered aesthetically pleasing?*

C. 2–3 mm.

Aesthetically, 2 to 3 mm of the upper incisors may show in repose, but the full length of the incisors should show while smiling.[1]

REFERENCE

1. Agarwal A, Dejoseph L, Silver W, et al. Anatomy of the jawline, neck, and perioral area with clinical correlations. Facial Plast Surg 2005;21:3

PATIENT EVALUATION

3. *A patient has perioral static lines without lip atrophy but with dyschromias. What is the optimal method of perioral enhancement?*

A. Laser resurfacing with or without dermabrasion.

Perioral lines can be a challenging problem. There are a variety of treatment modalities depending on the type of lines present. In this patient with static lines (with dyschromias), laser resurfacing would be the best option. Use of fat grafting would be the best option if the patient had concomitant atrophy of the lips. Lip lifts or maxillary lengthening is the best for patients with lip hypoplasia or atrophy due to aging (**Fig. 41.2**).[1,2,3]

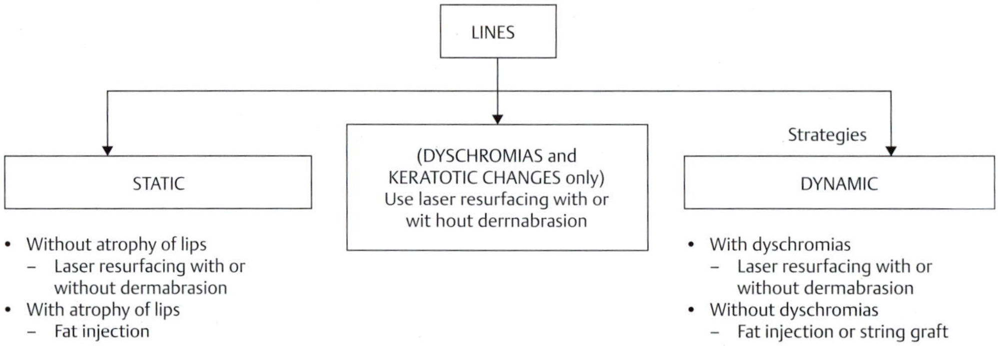

Fig. 41.2 Algorithm for perioral enhancement. (DLL, Direct liplift; ILL, indirect liplift; NLA, nasolabial angle.) (Source: Translated & reproduced by permission of Oxford University Press. Ponsky D, Guyuron B. Comprehensive surgical aesthetic enhancement & rejuvenation of the perioral region. Aesthet Surg J 31:382, 2011.)

REFERENCES

1. Agarwal A, Dejoseph L, Silver W, et al. Anatomy of the jawline, neck, and perioral area with clinical correlations. Facial Plast Surg 2005;21:3
2. Calhoun KH. Lip anatomy and function. In: Calhoun KH, Stiernberg CM, eds. Surgery of the Lip. New York: Thieme Publishers; 1992
3. Leveque JL, Goubanova E. Influence of age on the lips and perioral skin. Dermatology 2004;208:307

PATIENT EVALUATION

4. *A patient has lip hypoplasia with optimal incisor show. What is the optimal method of perioral enhancement?*

B. Fat injection.

In a patient with lip hypoplasia with optimal incisor show, the best method would be fat injection or filler augmentation to improve volume. If the patient had inadequate incisor show and a long lip, then an indirect or direct lip lift would be the ideal surgical decision. If the patient had a short lip, maxillary lengthening would be the procedure of choice (**Fig. 41.3**).[1,2,3]

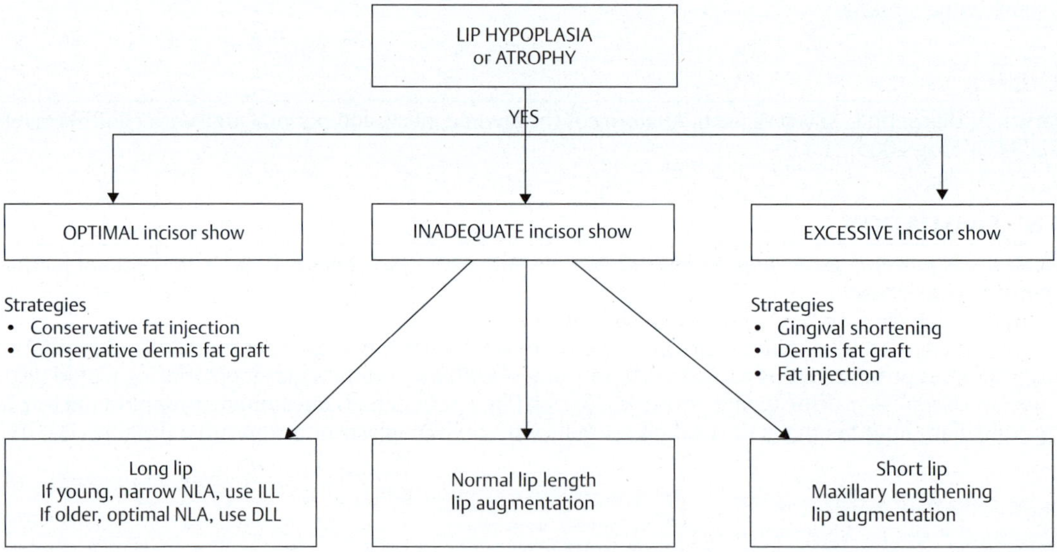

Fig. 41.3 Algorithm for perioral enhancement. (DLL, Direct liplift; ILL, indirect liplift; NLA, nasolabial angle.) (Source: Translated & reproduced by permission of Oxford University Press. Ponsky D, Guyuron B. Comprehensive surgical aesthetic enhancement & rejuvenation of the perioral region. Aesthet Surg J 31:382, 2011.)

REFERENCES

1. Agarwal A, Dejoseph L, Silver W, et al. Anatomy of the jawline, neck, and perioral area with clinical correlations. Facial Plast Surg 2005;21:3
2. Calhoun KH. Lip anatomy and function. In: Calhoun KH, Stiernberg CM, eds. Surgery of the Lip. New York: Thieme Publishers; 1992
3. Leveque JL, Goubanova E. Influence of age on the lips and perioral skin. Dermatology 2004;208:307

PATIENT EVALUATION

5. *A patient has lip hypoplasia with excessive incisor show. What is the optimal method of perioral enhancement?*

C. Gingival shortening.

For a patient with lip hypoplasia with excessive incisor show, the best procedure of choice is gingival shortening, dermal fat grafting, or fat injection. A direct or indirect lip lift or maxillary lengthening would be a good procedure for a patient with inadequate incisor show. Laser resurfacing would be a good option for a patient with static lines and would not correct lip hypoplasia (**Fig. 41.4**).[1,2,3]

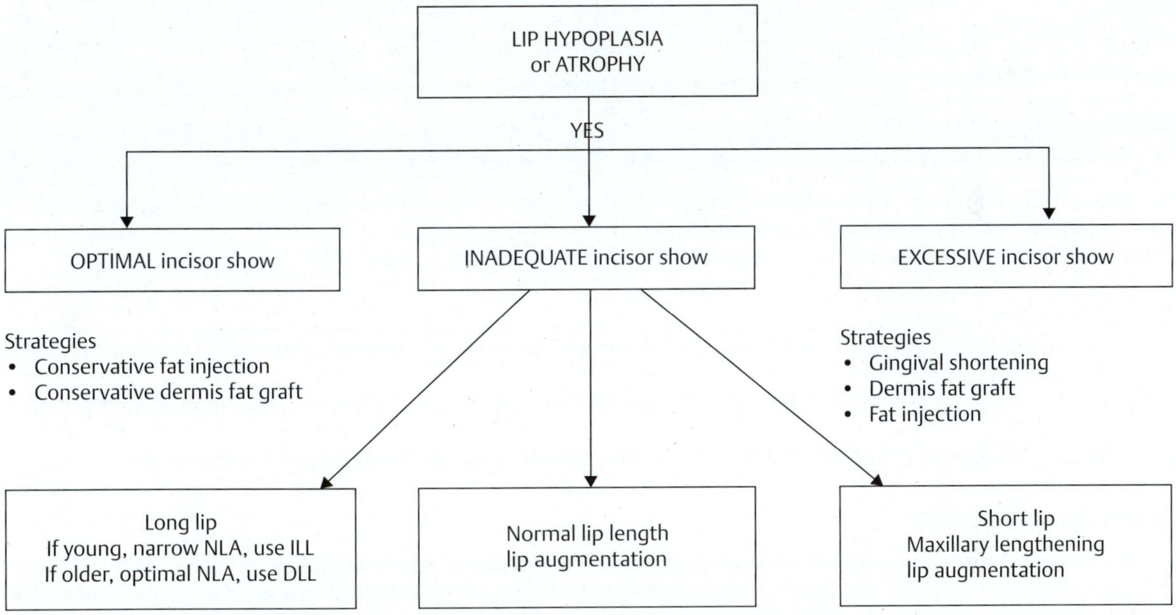

Fig. 41.4 Algorithm for perioral enhancement. (DLL, Direct liplift; ILL, indirect liplift; NLA, nasolabial angle.) (Source: Translated & reproduced by permission of Oxford University Press. Ponsky D, Guyuron B. Comprehensive surgical aesthetic enhancement & rejuvenation of the perioral region. Aesthet Surg J 31:382, 2011.)

REFERENCES

1. Agarwal A, Dejoseph L, Silver W, et al. Anatomy of the jawline, neck, and perioral area with clinical correlations. Facial Plast Surg 2005;21:3
2. Calhoun KH. Lip anatomy and function. In: Calhoun KH, Stiernberg CM, eds. Surgery of the Lip. New York: Thieme Publishers; 1992
3. Leveque JL, Goubanova E. Influence of age on the lips and perioral skin. Dermatology 2004;208:307

PATIENT EVALUATION

6. *An old patient has lip hypoplasia, inadequate incisor show, a long lip, and an adequate nasolabial angle. What is the optimal method of perioral enhancement?*

B. Direct lip lift.

In patients with lip atrophy with inadequate incisor show due to atrophy and ptosis, a direct lip lift is the procedure of choice. The other options would not be the ideal modality of treatment for this patient (**Fig. 41.5**).[1,2,3]

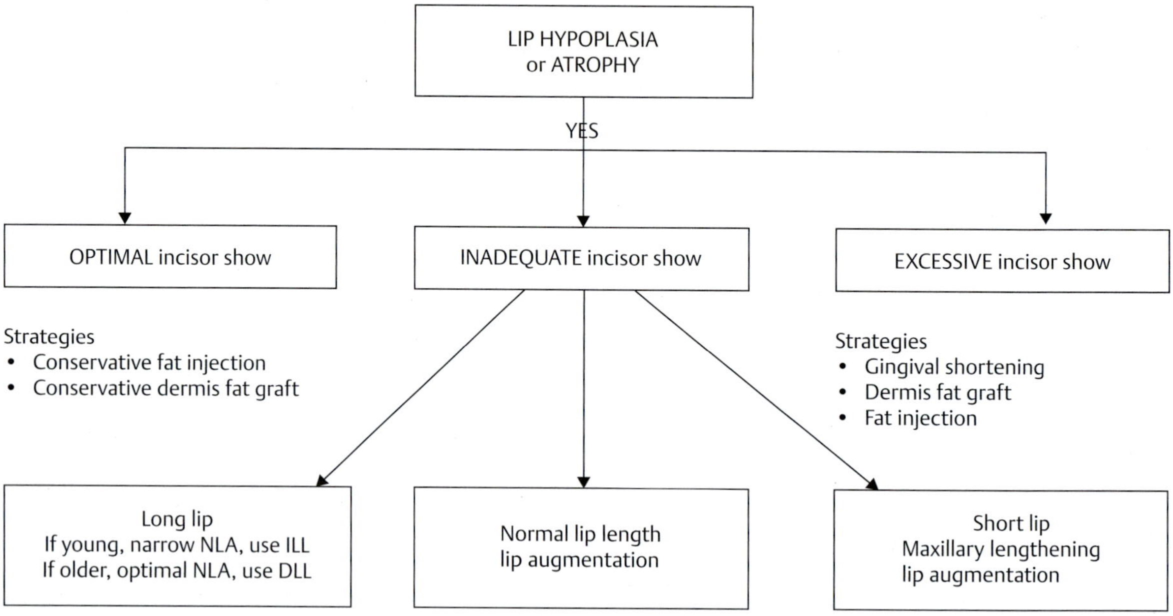

Fig. 41.5 Algorithm for perioral enhancement. (DLL, Direct liplift; ILL, indirect liplift; NLA, nasolabial angle.) (Source: Translated & reproduced by permission of Oxford University Press. Ponsky D, Guyuron B. Comprehensive surgical aesthetic enhancement & rejuvenation of the perioral region. Aesthet Surg J 31:382, 2011.)

References

1. Agarwal A, Dejoseph L, Silver W, et al. Anatomy of the jawline, neck, and perioral area with clinical correlations. Facial Plast Surg 2005;21:3
2. Calhoun KH. Lip anatomy and function. In: Calhoun KH, Stiernberg CM, eds. Surgery of the Lip. New York: Thieme Publishers; 1992
3. Leveque JL, Goubanova E. Influence of age on the lips and perioral skin. Dermatology 2004;208:307

CHEMODENERVATION

7. *A 67-year-old female is frustrated with the fact that she looks sad all the time and would like to know if there is anything you can do for her downward-slanted oral commisures. What is the best product to use and which of the following muscle is the main target to treat her condition?*

E. Neuromodulator; depressor anguli oris.

Neuromodulator to the depressor anguli oris is the target muscle to treat this patient's condition. On each side, 2 to 5 units are used. The needle is inserted into peak of the Cupid's bow, 2 to 3 mm above the vermilion border. Injection of the depressor anguli oris muscle will cause elevation of the oral commissure. This muscle can be found by asking the patient to depress the lower lip or frown. The bulk of the muscle is palpable inferolateral to the oral commissure at the level of the mandible.[1]

Reference

1. Loos BM, Maas CS. Relevant anatomy for botulinum toxin facial rejuvenation. Facial Plast Surg Clin North Am 2003;11:439

CHEMODENERVATION

8. *A 23-year-old girl has a "gummy smile" when she smiles and wants to know if there is a way to temporarily treat this. Which of the following muscles are targeted with botulinum toxin to treat her condition?*

C. Levator labii superioris.

Injecting 1 unit of botulinum toxin into the levator labii superioris muscle at its origin on the maxilla (superolateral to the ala) creates a weakness of the central aspect of the upper lip during smile which helps eliminates gingival show.[1]

Reference

1. Loos BM, Maas CS. Relevant anatomy for botulinum toxin facial rejuvenation. Facial Plast Surg Clin North Am 2003;11:439

SOFT TISSUE FILLERS

9. *Which of the following soft tissue fillers is best used on patients with HIV lipoatrophy?*

B. Poly-L-lactic acid.

Poly-L-lactic acid (PLLA) fillers, often marketed under the brand name Sculptra, are commonly used for patients with HIV lipoatrophy. Lipoatrophy is a condition characterized by the loss of fat tissue, and it can be a side effect of certain HIV medications. PLLA fillers are biocompatible and can help stimulate collagen production, leading to a gradual increase in volume over time. They are particularly well-suited for addressing the facial volume loss associated with HIV lipoatrophy.[1]

Reference

1. Monhian N, Ahn MS, Maas CS. Injectable and implantable materials for facial wrinkles. In: Papel ID, ed. Facial Plastic and Reconstructive Surgery. 2nd ed. New York: Thieme Publishers; 2002

SOFT TISSUE FILLERS

10. *Which of the following soft tissue fillers requires skin testing prior to use?*

C. Bovine collagen.

Collagen fillers (bovine collagen), which are derived from either human or bovine sources, used to require skin testing prior to use. This testing was done to check for potential allergic reactions or sensitivities to the collagen product. However, it is important to note that many modern fillers no longer require skin testing due to advancements in filler formulations.[1]

Reference

1. Monhian N, Ahn MS, Maas CS. Injectable and implantable materials for facial wrinkles. In: Papel ID, ed. Facial Plastic and Reconstructive Surgery. 2nd ed. New York: Thieme Publishers; 2002

SOFT TISSUE FILLERS

11. *Which of the following is a permanent soft tissue filler?*

A. Polymethylmethacrylate.

Polymethylmethacrylate (PMMA) fillers are considered permanent soft tissue fillers. PMMA is a synthetic material that is not absorbed by the body over time, providing long-lasting results. These fillers are often used for deep wrinkles and facial volume loss. However, it is important to note that while PMMA fillers are considered permanent, they may still require touch-up treatments over the years as natural aging processes continue.[1]

Reference

1. Monhian N, Ahn MS, Maas CS. Injectable and implantable materials for facial wrinkles. In: Papel ID, ed. Facial Plastic and Reconstructive Surgery. 2nd ed. New York: Thieme Publishers; 2002

SOFT TISSUE FILLERS

12. *Which of the following soft tissue fillers should not be used for lip augmentation given the high incidence of nodule formation?*

E. Calcium hydroxyapatite.

Calcium hydroxyapatite (Radiesse) and poly-L-lactic acid (Sculptra) should not be used for lip augmentation because of their high incidence of nodule formation.[1]

Reference

1. Monhian N, Ahn MS, Maas CS. Injectable and implantable materials for facial wrinkles. In: Papel ID, ed. Facial Plastic and Reconstructive Surgery. 2nd ed. New York: Thieme Publishers; 2002

SOFT TISSUE FILLERS

13. *When correcting nasolabial folds with soft tissue filler, which of the following is the best technique to fill this region?*

B. Inject slightly medial to the fold.

Filler is injected slightly medial to the actual fold. The filler can then be massaged into the center of the fold. The filler can be placed at angles to the fold, and layering may be done to enhance longevity (cross-medial or cross-hatching technique). Caution should be exercised when attempting to place the filler deep caudally, as the facial artery courses more superficially as it courses toward midline. For very deep folds, more viscous products (Perlane, Cosmoplast, Zyplast) or permanent/semipermanent (Radiesse, Sculptra, Artefill) products may be placed deep under less viscous fillers such as Restylane, Juvéderm, and Cosmoderm. Injection might require two or more syringes for each fold.[1,2]

REFERENCES

1. Monhian N, Ahn MS, Maas CS. Injectable and implantable materials for facial wrinkles. In: Papel ID, ed. Facial Plastic and Reconstructive Surgery. 2nd ed. New York: Thieme Publishers; 2002
2. Guyuron B. The armamentarium to battle the recalcitrant nasolabial crease. Clin Plast Surg 1995;22:253

DERMABRASION

14. *What is the most reliable indicator that the operator has reached the optimal depth in dermabrasion?*

C. Punctiform, superficial bleeding.

Punctiform, superficial bleeding is the most reliable indicator that the grinding procedure has reached the optimal depth.[1]

REFERENCE

1. Shpall R, Beddingfield FC III, Watson D, et al. Microdermabrasion: a review. Facial Plast Surg 2004;20:47

LASER ABLATIVE RESURFACING

15. *What is the clinical endpoint when performing laser ablative resurfacing with a carbon dioxide laser?*

D. Pale yellow color.

The clinical endpoint is a pale yellow color of the skin surface indicative that treatment has reached mid-reticular dermis.[1] The depth of ablation depends on the number of passes and the amount of cooling time allowed between passes. Insufficient cooling time can lead to thermal damage of the skin.[1]

REFERENCE

1. Schwartz RJ, Burns AJ, Rohrich RJ, et al. Long-term assessment of CO_2 facial laser resurfacing: aesthetic results and complications. Plast Reconstr Surg 1999;103:592

42. Facelift

Cameron R. Erickson, Michael R. Lee, Simon Moradian
See *Essentials of Aesthetic Surgery*, pp. 540–550

THE AGING FACE

1. *Which of the following accurately describes the changes found in the aging face?*

A. Over time the dermis will hypertrophy and become more elastic.
B. The superficial musculoaponeurotic system (SMAS) and platysma layer remain unchanged during the aging process.
C. Loss of skeletal support can contribute to facial aging.
D. Over time the facial skeleton increases in volume, particularly in the lower face.
E. Facial fat always increases in volume with age, causing inflation over time.

FACIAL ANALYSIS

2. *Which of the following choices is accurate regarding forehead analysis and potential interventions for aging?*

A. The corrugator supercilii muscles are responsible for the large transverse dynamic rhytids of the forehead.
B. Active wrinkles (dynamic rhytids) of the forehead are always a voluntary response.
C. Passive wrinkles (static rhytids) of the forehead respond well to chemodenervation.
D. The procerus muscle is responsible for the presence of vertical glabellar furrows and responds well to soft tissue fillers.
E. Active wrinkles (dynamic rhytids) occur with animation and may be improved by chemodenervation.

FACIAL ANALYSIS

3. *Lid ptosis is characterized by which of the following?*

A. High resting lid margin, low supratarsal crease.
B. High resting lid margin, high supratarsal crease.
C. Low resting lid margin, low supratarsal crease.
D. Low resting lid margin, unchanged supratarsal crease.
E. Low resting lid margin, high supratarsal crease.

FACIAL ANALYSIS

4. *Which of the following is included in the analysis of the upper eyelid only?*

A. Relationship of the orbital rim to the anterior surface of the globe.
B. Lid snap-back test and lid distraction test.
C. Globe prominence, which may indicate systemic disease.
D. Laxity of orbicularis oculi muscle.
E. Lateral brow ptosis.

FACIAL ANALYSIS

5. *What aging facial feature is accentuated by tethering at the mandibulocutaneous ligament?*

A. Jowling.
B. Marionette lines.
C. Deep perioral rhytids.
D. Platysmal banding.
E. Nasolabial folds.

FACELIFT TECHNIQUES

6. *A 59-year-old woman is interested in a facelift. A rhytidectomy with SMASectomy (superficial musculoaponeurotic system) is planned. Compared with a skin-only facelift, a SMAS tightening procedure is associated with a decrease in which of the following?*

A. Longevity of result.
B. Tension on skin closure.
C. Nerve injury.
D. Hematoma formation.
E. Infection rate.

FACELIFT PLANES

7. *A 52-year-old woman undergoes a rhytidectomy with browlift. Ipsilateral weakness of the forehead muscles is noted in the recovery room. The suspected injury is most likely immediately deep to which of the following?*

A. Subcutaneous tissue.
B. Deep layer of the deep temporal fascia.
C. Superficial layer of the deep temporal fascia.
D. Superficial temporal fat pad.
E. Superficial temporal fascia.

ADJUNCTIVE PROCEDURES

8. *Which is the most appropriate statement(s) regarding autologous fat grafting to the face?*

A. Approximately 10% loss of fat graft over time.
B. Approximately 15% loss of fat graft over time.
C. Approximately 20% loss of fat graft over time.
D. Approximately 30 to 50% loss of fat graft over time.
E. Autologous fat grafts are permanent and usually have 100% take after injection.

OPERATIVE AND FOLLOW-UP CARE

9. *What is the best regimen following a facelift procedure?*

A. Head elevation with neck flexion and bed rest for the first 24 hours.
B. Patients should sleep flat on their back with a pillow to allow for neck flexion.
C. Cold compresses to the eyes with slight neck extension and strict blood pressure control.
D. Directions for high fluid consumption while at home to maintain a systolic BP >120.
E. Alcohol is permissible 48 hours after surgery.

OPERATIVE AND FOLLOW-UP CARE

10. *Which statement regarding postoperative hematoma is true?*

A. Large, expanding hematomas (>5 cc) are best managed at bedside with aspiration.
B. More common in females.
C. Preoperative hypertension is a risk factor.
D. Small, nonexpanding (<5 cc) hematomas should be explored in the operating room emergently.
E. Usually occurs 48 hours post-surgery.

OPERATIVE AND FOLLOW-UP CARE

11. *A 56-year-old female patient presents to your office 8 days after undergoing a primary facelift. She is complaining of subjective fevers at home, increased pain, and redness of her right preauricular incision. On examination her right incision is swollen, warm, erythematous, and tender to palpation. What is the most likely organism responsible for her presentation?*

A. Streptococcus.
B. Klebsiella.
C. Clostridium.
D. Staphylococcus.
E. Escherichia.

OPERATIVE AND FOLLOW-UP CARE

12. ***During a facelift, injury to which of the following nerves occurs most commonly is unrecognized?***

A. Buccal branch of facial nerve.
B. Frontal branch of facial nerve.
C. Great auricular nerve.
D. Accessory nerve.
E. Mental nerve.

TOPICAL SKIN MAINTENANCE

13. ***Which of the following is the mechanism of action of cleansers?***

A. Dermal stimulation.
B. Protects skin from harmful radiation.
C. Slow, gradual exfoliation.
D. Helps to preserve natural lipid barriers between cells.
E. Inhibition of melanin production and deposition.

Answers

THE AGING FACE

1. *Which of the following accurately describes the changes found in the aging face?*

C. Loss of skeletal support can contribute to facial aging.

Over time the dermis will atrophy (not hypertrophy) and become less (not more) elastic. The SMAS layer and platysma will develop laxity over time. The ideal face is described as a youthful heart shape. The facial skeleton loses volume and loss of skeletal support influences the appearance of the aging face.[1,2]

REFERENCES

1. Pessa JE. An algorithm of facial aging: verification of Lambros's theory by three-dimensional stereolithography, with reference to the pathogenesis of midfacial aging, scleral show, and the lateral suborbital trough deformity. Plast Reconstr Surg 2000;106(2):479–488; discussion 489–490
2. Shaw RB Jr, Katzel EB, Kolz PF, et al. Aging of the facial skeleton: aesthetic implications and rejuvenation strategies. Plast Reconstr Surg 2011;127:374

FACIAL ANALYSIS

2. *Which of the following choices is accurate regarding forehead analysis and potential interventions for aging?*

E. Active wrinkles (dynamic rhytids) occur with animation and may be improved by chemodenervation.

The frontalis muscle is responsible for the large transverse rhytids across the forehead, not the corrugator supercilii muscles. Additionally, the procerus is responsible for the presence of horizontal glabellar furrows, not vertical, and is typically addressed with neuromodulators, not fillers. Active rhytids are due to either voluntary or involuntary muscle movements. Passive wrinkles (static rhytids) do not disappear with relaxation. Passive wrinkles are best addressed by skin resurfacing treatments and will only be minimally improved by chemodenervation or surgical lifts. Active wrinkles (dynamic rhytids) occur with animation and can be voluntary or involuntary. Active wrinkles are more likely to be improved with chemodenervation and possibly brow lifting.[1]

REFERENCE

1. Gonyon DL, Barton FE. The aging face: rhytidectomy and adjunctive procedures. Sel Read Plast Surg 2005;10:21

FACIAL ANALYSIS

3. *Lid ptosis is characterized by which of the following?*

E. Low resting lid margin, high supratarsal crease.

Lid ptosis is characterized by a low resting lid margin and a high supratarsal crease. Both brow and eyelid ptosis should be addressed in the surgical plan. Assess the amount of upper eyelid skin. Compensate for excess skin from lateral brow hooding by manual repositioning of the lateral brow. Of note, lateral brow ptosis can give the appearance of excess upper lid skin and should be corrected with a browlift rather than a blepharoplasty.[1]

REFERENCE

1. Shaw RB Jr, Katzel EB, Kolz PF, et al. Aging of the facial skeleton: aesthetic implications and rejuvenation strategies. Plast Reconstr Surg 2011;127:374

FACIAL ANALYSIS

4. *Which of the following is included in the analysis of the upper eyelid only?*

E. Lateral brow ptosis.

Assessment of lateral brow ptosis is only relevant to upper eyelid ptosis. The relationship of the orbital rim to the anterior surface of the globe is important to determine if the patient has a positive vector, where the most anterior projection of the globe is posterior to the lid margin and malar eminence, which aids in a more favorable outcome and better support for lid suspension. On the other hand, a negative vector, defined as when the most anterior projection of the globe is anterior to the lid margin and malar eminence, can result in the orbit lacking the support it needs and therefore should be addressed by planning additional lower eyelid support or midface soft tissue augmentation. Also, prominence of the globe may indicate thyroid disease that should be treated appropriately. Assessment of lid tone and tarsal suspension using a lid snap-back test and lid distraction test is part of lower eyelid analysis, rather than upper eyelid. Additionally, laxityofthe orbicularis muscle is assessed, sometimes evident by the presence of festoons.[1,2]

REFERENCES

1. Shaw RB Jr, Katzel EB, Kolz PF, et al. Aging of the facial skeleton: aesthetic implications and rejuvenation strategies. Plast Reconstr Surg 2011;127:374
2. Gonyon DL, Barton FE. The aging face: rhytidectomy and adjunctive procedures. Sel Read Plast Surg 2005;10:21

FACIAL ANALYSIS

5. *What aging facial feature is accentuated by tethering at the mandibulocutaneous ligament?*

A. Jowling.

Jowling is accentuated by the mandibulocutaneous ligament. With aging, the superior and inferior jowl fat compartments descend secondary to attenuation of the mandibular septum. As the jowl forms, its anterior extension is limited by the mandibulocutaneous ligament. Therefore, the groove that forms just anterior to the jowl corresponds to the mandibulocutaneous ligament. The subcutaneous extension can cause skin indentation with aging. Failure to recognize and correct this deformity by subcutaneous release can lead to patient dissatisfaction after facelift surgery. Platysmal banding is the result of attenuated superficial cervical fascia. Orbicularis oris atrophy, in combination with thinning of the overlying skin, results in formation of deep perioral rhytids.[1,2]

REFERENCES

1. Rohrich RJ, Pessa JE. The fat compartments of the face: anatomy and clinical implications for cosmetic surgery. Plast Reconstr Surg 2007;119:2219
2. Marten TJ. Lamellar high SMAS face and midface lift: a comprehensive technique for natural appearing rejuvenation of the face. In: Nahai F, ed. The Art of Aesthetic Surgery: Principles & Techniques. 2nd ed. New York: Thieme Publishers; 2010

FACELIFT TECHNIQUES

6. *A 59-year-old woman is interested in a facelift. A rhytidectomy with SMASectomy (superficial musculoaponeurotic system) is planned. Compared with a skin-only facelift, a SMAS tightening procedure is associated with a decrease in which of the following?*

B. Tension on skin closure.

When superficial musculoaponeurotic system (SMAS) tightening procedures are performed, the tension of the facelift is secured at the SMAS level rather than the skin. With a skin-only facelift, the lift must depend solely on the skin sutures for support. The more the tension on the skin, the more likely a spread or hypertrophic scar will occur which would be more likely in a skin-only procedure. SMAS procedures do not decrease the longevity of results. Although many surgeons believe that a SMAS facelift will produce better and longer-lasting results given the better dispersion of tension on the final closure/suspension, there are no conclusive evidence-based studies to prove an increase in longevity of results. Hematoma formation is related to hypertension and extent of dissection, not whether a SMASectomy was performed. Although not a significant difference, the incidence of facial nerve injury is more likely to occur with any technique that involves elevationormanipulation of the SMAS layer. Infection rates are low in both procedures.[1,2,3]

REFERENCES

1. Stuzin JM. MOC-PSSM CME article: Face lifting. Plast Reconstr Surg 2008;121(1 Suppl):1–19
2. Marten TJ. Lamellar high SMAS face and midface lift: a comprehensive technique for natural appearing rejuvenation of the face. In: Nahai F, ed. The Art of Aesthetic Surgery: Principles & Techniques. 2nd ed. New York: Thieme Publishers; 2010
3. Mustoe TA, Park E. Evidence-based medicine: face lift. Plast Reconstr Surg 2014;133(5):1206–1213

FACELIFT PLANES

7. *A 52-year-old woman undergoes a rhytidectomy with browlift. Ipsilateral weakness of the forehead muscles is noted in the recovery room. The suspected injury is most likely immediately deep to which of the following?*

E. Superficial temporal fascia.

The temporal branch of the facial nerve is found just deep to the superficial temporal fascia, otherwise known as the temporoparietal fascia. The facial nerve exits the stylomastoid foramen and the main trunk, pes anserinus, can be found 1 cm inferior and posterior, midway between the tragal pointer and the posterior belly of the digastric muscle. It then arborizes into five branches, namely, temporal, zygomatic, buccal, marginal, and cervical. Interconnections between the zygomatic and buccal offer some additional regenerative potential if one of those branches is injured. Injury to the temporal or cervical branches can leave more lasting deformities, so management of injury is important. Avoiding injury is the best way to prevent injury. Therefore, when dissecting in the temporal zone it is critical to avoid entering deep to the superficial temporal fascia. In fact, based on the work of Agarwal et al on cadaveric hemiface dissections, the frontal branchtravelswithin the innominate fascia, which is the layer immediately deep to the superficial temporal fascia as it crosses the zygomatic arch into the temporal region. A fascial transition zone was identified in a region 1.5 to 3.0 cm above the zygomatic arch and 0.9 to 1.4 cm posterior to the lateral orbital rim, where the frontal branches crossed from the innominate fascia to run within the superficial temporal fascia.[1,2,3]

REFERENCES

1. Agarwal CA, Mendenhall SD 3rd, Foreman KB, Owsley JQ. The course of the frontal branch of the facial nerve in relation to fascial planes: an anatomic study. Plast Reconstr Surg 2010;125(2):532–537
2. Rohrich RJ, Pessa JE. The fat compartments of the face: anatomy and clinical implications for cosmetic surgery. Plast Reconstr Surg 2007;119:2219
3. Shaw RB Jr, Katzel EB, Kolz PF, et al. Aging of the facial skeleton: aesthetic implications and rejuvenation strategies. Plast Reconstr Surg 2011;127:374

ADJUNCTIVE PROCEDURES

8. *Which is the most appropriate statement(s) regarding autologous fat grafting to the face?*

D. Approximately 30 to 50% loss of fat graft over time.

You can expect 30 to 50% loss of fat graft over time. However, the results may vary with surgeon and technique.[1]

REFERENCE

1. Gerth DJ, King B, Rabach L, Glasgold RA, Glasgold MJ. Long-term volumetric retention of autologous fat grafting processed with closed-membrane filtration. Aesthet Surg J 2014;34(7):985–994

OPERATIVE AND FOLLOW-UP CARE

9. *What is the best regimen following a facelift procedure?*

C. Cold compresses to the eyes with slight neck extension and strict blood pressure control.

Slight neck extension, low salt diet, strict blood pressure control, preemptive emesis management, and early ambulation are all considered appropriate postoperative steps to reduce complications such as hematomas. Head elevation can help prevent swelling but should not result in neck flexion as this would close the cervicomental angle and potentially obstruct lymphatic flow. Cold compresses can be applied to the eyes for 15 to 20 minutes each hour for the first 3 days. Postoperative hypertension can lead to a hematoma and should be prevented. Clonidine patch (0.2 mg/day) placed preoperatively can offer sustained blood pressure control during and after surgery.[1,2]

REFERENCES

1. Mustoe TA, Park E. Evidence-based medicine: Face lift. Plast Reconstr Surg 2014;133(5):1206–1213
2. Marten TJ. Lamellar high SMAS face and midface lift: a comprehensive technique for natural appearing rejuvenation of the face. In: Nahai F, ed. The Art of Aesthetic Surgery: Principles & Techniques. 2nd ed. New York: Thieme Publishers; 2010

OPERATIVE AND FOLLOW-UP CARE

10. *Which statement regarding postoperative hematoma is true?*

C. Preoperative hypertension is a risk factor.

Large expanding hematomas >5 cc should be managed promptly by returning to the OR for evacuation. Hematomas usually occur in the first 8 hours postoperatively. Small hematomas <5 cc may be managed with needle aspiration. Risk factors for hematoma postoperatively include male sex, preoperative hypertension, qualitative platelet disorders, and postoperative rebound hypertension.[1]

REFERENCE

1. Mustoe TA, Park E. Evidence-based medicine: face lift. Plast Reconstr Surg 2014;133(5):1206–1213

OPERATIVE AND FOLLOW-UP CARE

11. *A 56-year-old female patient presents to your office 8 days after undergoing a primary facelift. She is complaining of subjective fevers at home, increased pain, and redness of her right preauricular incision. On examination her right incision is swollen, warm, erythematous, and tender to palpation. What is the most likely organism responsible for her presentation?*

D. Staphylococcus.

The most common organism that causes surgical site infections after rhytidectomy is *Staphylococcus aureus*. However, these infections are considered uncommon (2%). Most appear at the periauricular incision about 5 to 7 days after surgery. They usually respond well to drainage and oral antibiotic therapy with minimal sequelae.[1]

REFERENCE

1. Sinclair NR, Coombs DM, Kwiecien G, Zins JE. How to prevent and treat complications in facelift surgery, Part 1: short-term complications. Aesthet Surg J Open Forum 2021;3(1):ojab007

OPERATIVE AND FOLLOW-UP CARE

12. *During a facelift, injury to which of the following nerves occurs most commonly is unrecognized?*

A. Buccal branch of facial nerve.

The most common unrecognized nerve injury likely occurs to the buccal branch of the facial nerve. The facial nerve exits the stylomastoid foramen and the main trunk, pes anserinus, can be found 1 cm inferior and posterior, midway between the tragal pointer and the posterior belly of the digastric muscle. It then arborizes into five branches, namely, temporal, zygomatic, buccal, marginal, and cervical. Interconnections between the zygomatic and buccal offer some additional regenerative potential if one of those branches is injured. Injury to the temporal or cervical branches can leave more lasting deformities so management of injury is important. Avoiding injury is the best way to prevent injury. Nerve injury to the great auricular nerve is recognized most commonly (**Fig. 42.1**).[1]

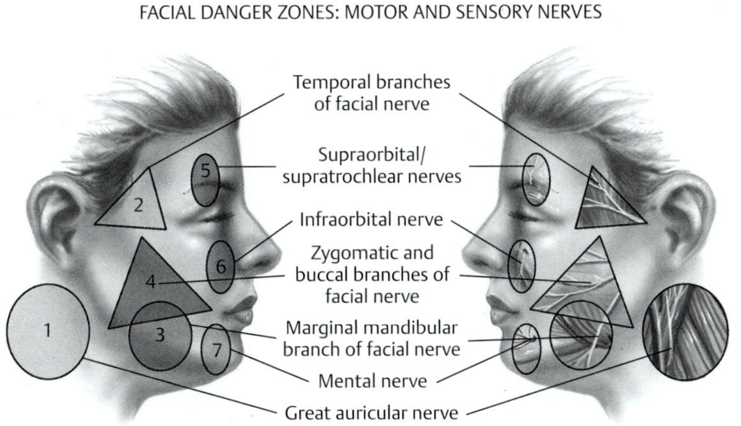

Fig. 42.1 Facial danger zones: Motor and sensory nerves. (Source: Nerve Injury. In: Janis J, ed. Essentials of Aesthetic Surgery. 1st Edition. New York: Thieme; 2018.)

Reference

1. Roostaeian J, Rohrich RJ, Stuzin JM. Anatomical considerations to prevent facial nerve injury. Plast Reconstr Surg 2015;135(5):1318–1327

TOPICAL SKIN MAINTENANCE

13. *Which of the following is the mechanism of action of cleansers?*

D. Helps to preserve natural lipid barriers between cells.

Cleansers help to preserve natural lipid barriers between cells. Exfoliation works by a slow, gradual exfoliation that can be achieved with alpha-hydroxy acids and retinols. Pigment control works by melanin production and deposition which can be inhibited by using hydroquinone, kojic acid, or azelaic acid. Sun protection by the use of a sunscreen and physical blockers with an SPF 30 or greater will absorb up to 97% of harmful radiation. Topical antioxidants such as vitamins C and E can also be applied to protect against photodamage. Other than chemical peels, cell stimulation via only the topical agent tretinoin consistently results in clinically significant dermal stimulation.[1,2,3,4,5]

References

1. Sinno S, Lee DS, Khachemoune A. Vitamins and cutaneous wound healing. J Wound Care 2011;20:287
2. Chatterjee L, Agarwal R, Mukhtar H. Ultraviolet B radiation-induced DNA lesions in mouse epidermis: an assessment using a novel 32P-postlabeling technique. Biochem Biophys Res Commun 1996;229:590
3. Duell EA, Derguini F, Kang S, et al. Extraction of human epidermis treated with retinol yields retro-retinoids in addition to free retinol and retinyl esters. J Invest Dermatol 1996;107:178
4. Torras H. Retinoids in aging. Clin Dermatol 1996;14:207
5. Spencer TS. Dry skin and skin moisturizers. Clin Dermatol 1988;6:24

43. The Nasolabial Fold

Jacob Nathaniel Grow, Christopher C. Surek
See *Essentials of Aesthetic Surgery*, pp. 551–564

OBSERVATIONS ABOUT THE NASOLABIAL FOLD AFTER ANATOMIC DISSECTION

1. ***Anatomically, the nasolabial fold represents the border between which of the following?***
A. Superficial and deep upper lip elevators.
B. Cheek subcutaneous fat and upper lip elevators.
C. Orbicularis oris muscle and the modiolus.
D. Nasal ala and philtral column.
E. Upper lip elevators and upper lip.

THE SMAS AND THE NASOLABIAL FOLD

2. ***During rhytidectomy, what structure serves as the clinical landmark for attenuation of the superficial musculoaponeurotic system?***
A. Orbicularis oris muscle.
B. Modiolus.
C. Zygomaticus major muscle.
D. Nasolabial fold.
E. Buccinator muscle.

DYNAMICS OF THE NASOLABIAL FOLD

3. ***Activation of lip elevators has which of the following effect on the nasolabial fold?***
A. Deepening.
B. Flattening.
C. Effacement.
D. Widening.
E. Accentuates dimpling.

DYNAMICS OF THE NASOLABIAL FOLD

4. ***Which of the following plays a role in both elevation and depression of the mouth during facial expression?***
A. Levator labii superioris.
B. Zygomaticus minor.
C. Platysma.
D. Buccinator.
E. Mentalis.

DYNAMICS OF THE NASOLABIAL FOLD

5. ***Which of the following changes is rarely observed during facial aging with regards to the nasolabial fold?***
A. Deepening of the nasolabial fold.
B. Ptosis of overlying lateral cheek adipose tissue.
C. Development of a midcheek furrow.
D. Progressive shortening of the upper lip.
E. Accentuation of the labiomental groove.

ASSESSING THE NASOLABIAL FOLD

6. *A middle-aged female patient requesting facial rejuvenation presents for evaluation. You note the presence of visible nasolabial folds at rest that deepen significantly on animation. According to the Nahai classification, this patient would be categorized as which of the following with regards to her nasolabial folds?*

A. Grade I.
B. Grade II.
C. Grade III.
D. Grade IV.
E. Grade V.

MANAGEMENT OF THE NASOLABIAL FOLD

7. *A female patient in her late thirties presents for treatment of her nasolabial folds. On examination, her folds are present at rest but do not significantly deepen on animation (Nahai Grade II). She requests a correction that will give the most long-lasting result that is also most appropriate given the severity of her folds. Which of the following is the most appropriate treatment option?*

A. Hyaluronic acid filler in the superficial plane.
B. Silicone in the superficial plane.
C. Autologous fat grafting.
D. Direct nasolabial fold excision.
E. Midface lift.

MANAGEMENT OF THE NASOLABIAL FOLD

8. *During rhytidectomy, improvement of the nasolabial fold requires dissection in which of the following planes anterior to the zygomaticus major muscle?*

A. Subcutaneous tissue.
B. Sub-SMAS.
C. Below zygomaticus major.
D. Subperiosteal.
E. Dual plane.

SURGICAL COMPLICATIONS AND TREATMENT

9. *Following correction of the nasolabial folds with injection of a hyaluronic acid filler, a patient presents 3 weeks later unhappy with the results. On examination, there is an area of prominent and palpable fullness on the right compared with the left. No evidence of erythema, drainage, or open wounds is present. Which of the following is the most appropriate method of treatment?*

A. Conservative massage over the area.
B. Oral antibiotics.
C. Placement of filler into the contralateral fold.
D. Injection of hyaluronidase.
E. Direct excision.

Answers

OBSERVATIONS ABOUT THE NASOLABIAL FOLD AFTER ANATOMIC DISSECTION

1. *Anatomically, the nasolabial fold represents the border between which of the following?*

E. Upper lip elevators and upper lip.

The nasolabial fold (NLF) is a distinct fusion plane that separates the fatty cheek including upper lip elevators from the dense upper lip. These upper lip mimetic muscles insert onto the orbicularis oris at the level of the NLF and are covered by a generous amount of overlying subcutaneous fat. This is in direct contrast to the upper lip where the subcutaneous tissue is minimal, creating a visually distinct transition between these two regions which manifests as a fold. The upper lip mimetic muscles include zygomaticus major and minor, levator labii superioris, and levator labii superioris alaeque nasi in the more superficial plane, in addition to levator anguli oris and buccinator in a deeper plane.[1] Histologically,the NLF is comprised of dense fibrous tissue, muscle fibers branching from these elevating muscles of the upper lip, and striated muscle bundles originating in the fold fascia. The modiolus is a dense, mobile, fibrovascular structureconsisting of terminal muscle fibers that either converge toward (aforementioned labial tractors) or diverge away (orbicularis oris) from its center, located approximately 1.5 cm lateral to the labial commissure.[2]

REFERENCES

1. Yousif NJ, Gosain A, Matloub HS, et al. The nasolabial fold: an anatomic and histologic reappraisal. Plast Reconstr Surg 1994;93:60
2. Zufferey J. Anatomic variations of the nasolabial fold. Plast Reconstr Surg 1992;89:225; discussion 232

THE SMAS AND THE NASOLABIAL FOLD

2. *During rhytidectomy, what structure serves as the clinical landmark for attenuation of the superficial musculoaponeurotic system?*

C. Zygomaticus major muscle.

The relationship between the superficial musculoaponeurotic system (SMAS) and nasolabial fold (NLF) is both complex and incompletely understood. As the SMAS continues anteriorly, it becomes attenuated at the level of the zygomaticus major muscle, representing a common endpoint for dissection during rhytidectomy. At this level, the SMAS invests the anterior and posterior aspects of the zygomaticus major muscle and is indistinguishable from the muscle's investing fascia on the anterior surface. As the attenuated SMAS approaches the NLF, it divides into a superficial and deep leaflet with no separate extensions present.[1]

REFERENCE

1. Barton FE Jr, Gyimesi IM. Anatomy of the nasolabial fold. Plast Reconstr Surg 1997;100:1276

DYNAMICS OF THE NASOLABIAL FOLD

3. *Activation of lip elevators has which of the following effect on the nasolabial fold?*

A. Deepening.

The activation of upper lip elevators results in movement of the nasolabial fold (NLF), an essential component of the human smile and expression of complex emotion. For all humans, activation of the upper lip elevators causes a deepening or accentuation of the NLF. In addition, fold dynamics facilitate a number of other predictable patterns of facial expression including a comma-shaped crease lateral to the oral commissure, a dimple above the modiolus, and a shallow dimple next to the nasal ala in the upper fold. Although dimpling may be accentuated with upper lip elevation, not all people have dimpling; hence, it is viewed as a common anatomic variant.[1]

REFERENCE

1. Barton FE Jr. The SMAS and the nasolabial fold. Plast Reconstr Surg 1992;89:1054

DYNAMICS OF THE NASOLABIAL FOLD

4. *Which of the following plays a role in both elevation and depression of the mouth during facial expression?*

D. Buccinator.

Facial expression involves the complex interplay between many facial muscles responsible for upper lip elevation, lower lip depression, and depression of the angle of the mouth (**Fig. 43.1a–d**). Of note, the upper and lower divisions of the buccinator muscle play a role in perioral elevation and depression, respectively. Levator labii superioris and zygomaticus minor are upper lip elevators, while the mentalis and platysma muscle are lower lip depressors.[1]

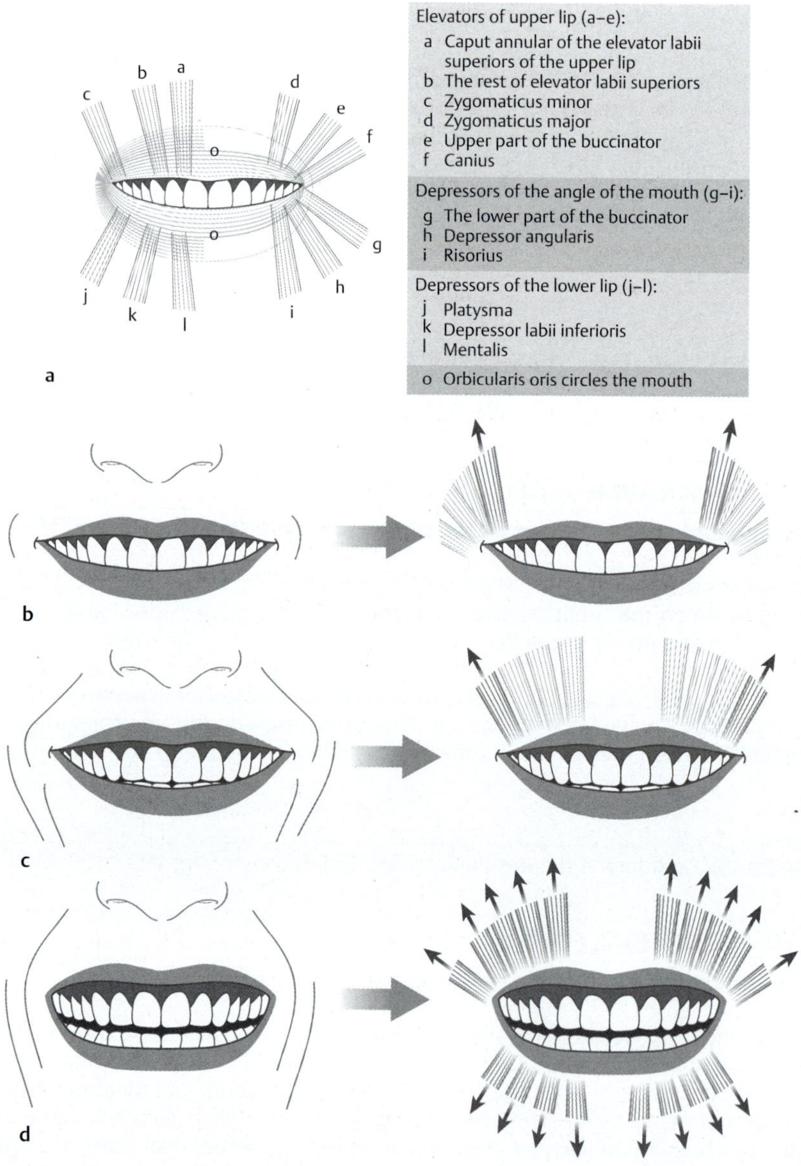

Fig. 43.1 (a–d) Rubin's classic work on smiling. (Source: The Human Smile. In: Janis J, ed. Essentials of Aesthetic Surgery. 1st Edition. New York: Thieme; 2018.)

REFERENCE

1. Rubin LR, Mishriki Y, Lee G. Anatomy of the nasolabial fold: the keystone of the smiling mechanism. Plast Reconstr Surg 1989;83:1

DYNAMICS OF THE NASOLABIAL FOLD

5. *Which of the following changes is rarely observed during facial aging with regards to the nasolabial fold?*

D. Progressive shortening of the upper lip.

Predictable changes involving the midface, specifically as they relate to the nasolabial fold (NLF), are a hallmark of facial aging and have been well-described. With aging, the NLF deepens as the lateral redundant tissue of the cheek becomes lax and ptotic where no skin muscle attachments are present. In contrast, anterior to the fold, extensive muscular attachments aid in providing better support to the upper lip relative to the lateral cheek, causing a more pronounced NLF with age. However, it should be noted that with time, downward descent of the upper lip also causes the NLF to appear both deeper and longer, also contributing to the development of marionette furrows. In addition, loss of midface volume and tissue laxity/descent result in the appearance of an obliquely oriented midcheek furrow. In the lower lip, the mental crease becomes deeper, longer, and downturned forming the labiomental groove.[1]

REFERENCE

1. Mendelson BC. Correction of the nasolabial fold: extended SMAS dissection with periosteal fixation. Plast Reconstr Surg 1992;89:822

ASSESSING THE NASOLABIAL FOLD

6. *A middle-aged female patient requesting facial rejuvenation presents for evaluation. You note the presence of visible nasolabial folds at rest that deepen significantly on animation. According to the Nahai classification, this patient would be categorized as which of the following with regards to her nasolabial folds?*

C. Grade III.

Clinically, the Nahai classification system categorizes the changes that occur with age at the nasolabial fold (NLF) and ultimately helps to dictate the most appropriate operative intervention for improvement. This system involves assessment both in repose and with animation. In Grade I, the NLF is visible only with animation. In Grade II, the fold is also visible at rest. As in the patient in the question prompt, Grade III patients have a visible fold at rest that significantly deepens with animation. Grade IV patients are a more severe form of Grade III, with deep folds at rest that worsen on animation. Finally, Grade V patients have ptotic, overhanging folds. **Fig. 43.2** illustrates clinical examples for each grade.[1]

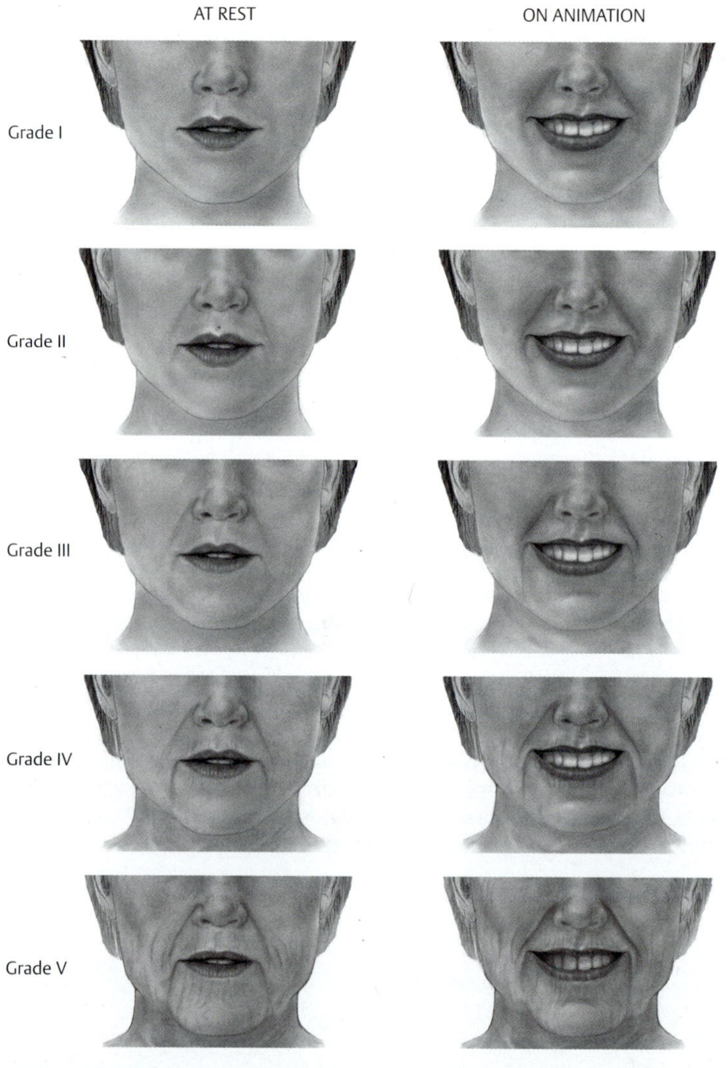

Fig. 43.2 Classification of nasolabial fold aging. (Source: Nahai F, ed. The Art of Aesthetic Surgery: Principles & Techniques, ed 2. New York: Thieme Publishers, 2011.)

REFERENCE

1. Nahai F. Clinical decision-making for nonsurgical cosmetic treatments. In: Nahai F, ed. The Art of Aesthetic Surgery: Principles & Techniques. New York: Thieme Publishers; 2005

MANAGEMENT OF THE NASOLABIAL FOLD

7. ***A female patient in her late thirties presents for treatment of her nasolabial folds. On examination, her folds are present at rest but do not significantly deepen on animation (Nahai Grade II). She requests a correction that will give the most long-lasting result that is also most appropriate given the severity of her folds. Which of the following is the most appropriate treatment option?***

   C. Autologous fat grafting.

   Treatment modality for correction of the nasolabial fold (NLF) must be individualized for each patient and is broadly categorized based on the severity of the folds (**Fig. 43.3**). For patients with mild signs of fold progression (Nahai Grades I–III), surface approaches, which include neurotoxins, injection of filler products, and autologous fat, tend to be the method of choice for fold effacement. In this clinical scenario, the patient is young with only mild deformity, so performing more invasive procedures such as midface lift or direct excision with high scar burden would be inappropriate. Injection of hyaluronic acid fillers is commonly implemented in these cases and would not be unreasonable to offer to this patient. However, compared with autologous fat grafting, the longevity is inferior and therefore not the best choice given this patient's request for a longer-lasting result. Of note, interposition of a dermal fat graft representsa-notherautologous option that may be performed either in isolation or following rhytidectomy procedure once the NLF has been surgically effaced. Acting as a mechanical barrier, the dermal fat graft prevents reattachment of the lip elevators at the prior NLF to the overlying dermis, preventing reformation of the fold. Although effective, complications with this technique include migration and contour irregularities. Injection of silicone is wrought with multiple complications including inflammatory skin reactions, extrusion, and contour irregularities, and therefore should no longer be performed.[1,2]

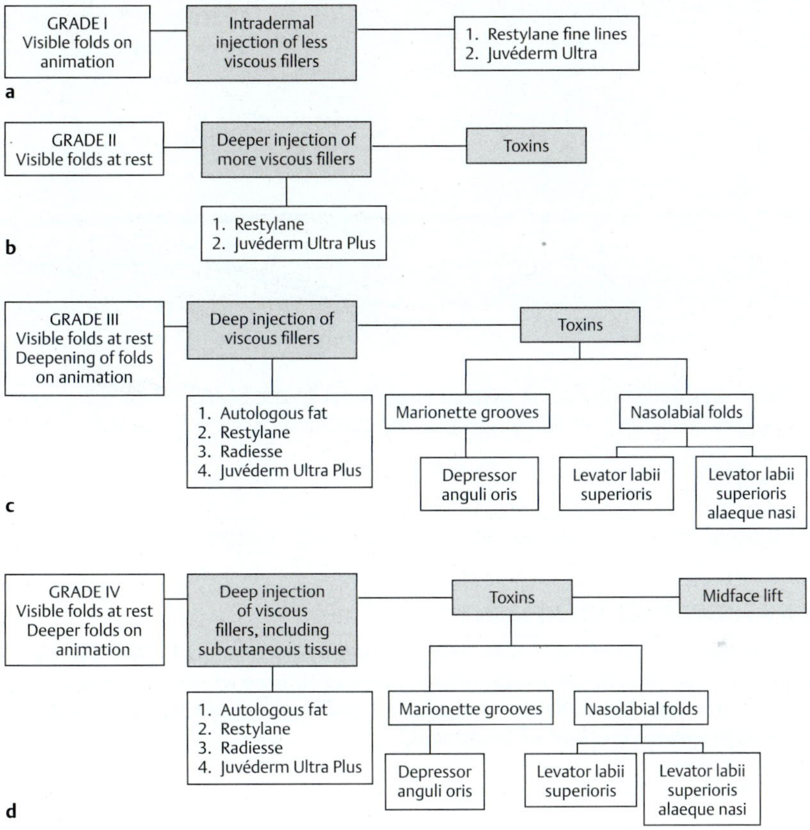

Fig. 43.3 (a–d) Treatment options for nasolabial folds and marionette grooves. A, Grade I. B, Grade II. C, Grade III. D, Grade IV. (Source: Nahai F, ed. The Art of Aesthetic Surgery: Principles & Techniques, ed 2. New York: Thieme Publishers, 2011.)

REFERENCES

1. Marten TJ, Elyassnia D. Fat grafting in facial rejuvenation. Clin Plast Surg 2015;42:219
2. Guyuron B, Michelow B. The nasolabial fold: a challenge, a solution. Plast Reconstr Surg 1994;93:522

MANAGEMENT OF THE NASOLABIAL FOLD

8. *During rhytidectomy, improvement of the nasolabial fold requires dissection in which of the following planes anterior to the zygomaticus major muscle?*

A. Subcutaneous tissue.

Surgical correction of the nasolabial folds (NLFs) through rhytidectomy is effective but requires expertise and familiarity with surgical anatomy. As dissection proceeds anteriorly, the superficial musculoaponeurotic system (SMAS) becomes significantly attenuated and envelopes the zygomaticus major muscle. At this point, the attachment of the SMAS to the underlying muscle should be incised and any further dissection carried out in the subcutaneous plane only, freeing the overlying tissue from the underlying SMAS (**Fig. 43.4**). As a result, the skin over the crease is allowed to move with the rest of the flap, allowing for effacement of the NLF. Of note, the zygomatic branch of the facial nerve is especially vulnerable at the level of the zygomaticus major muscle, so care should be taken to avoid its injury.[1]

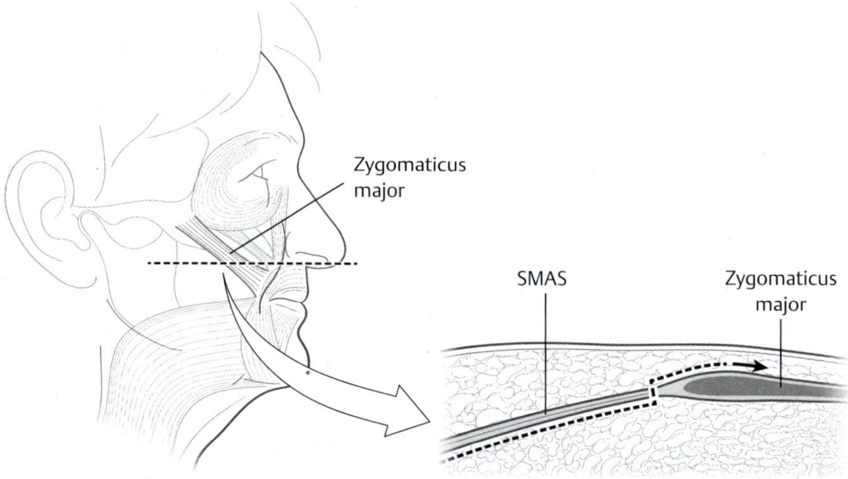

Fig. 43.4 Dissection of the rhytidectomy flap is carried superficial to the SMAS when the zygomatic muscles are encountered. (Source: Facelift. In: Janis J, ed. Essentials of Aesthetic Surgery. 1st Edition. New York: Thieme; 2018.)

Reference

1. Barton FE Jr. The SMAS and the nasolabial fold. Plast Reconstr Surg 1992;89:1054

SURGICAL COMPLICATIONS AND TREATMENT

9. ***Following correction of the nasolabial folds with injection of a hyaluronic acid filler, a patient presents 3 weeks later unhappy with the results. On examination, there is an area of prominent and palpable fullness on the right compared with the left. No evidence of erythema, drainage, or open wounds is present. Which of the following is the most appropriate method of treatment?***

   D. Injection of hylauronidase.

   This patient presenting with contour irregularity following injection of hyaluronic acid–based filler will be most appropriately treated with hyaluronidase injection. This enzyme dissolves hyaluronic acid (HA), which would correct the area of fullness that is causing the patient's complaint. Following initial injection, some "lumps and bumps" are not uncommon in the first 24 to 48 hours and can be gently massaged for manual correction. However, this conservative management is unlikely to correct a deformity present for multiple weeks. There are no signs of infection in the clinical scenario; therefore, oral antibiotics are not indicated. Although injecting the contralateral side would allow for symmetry, this would only accentuate the complication, which is an overfilled area rather than asymmetry. Some non-HA products used for filler that cannot be dissolved may require excision for removal, including silicone and calcium-based products. However, injection of hyaluronidase is less invasive, better tolerated by patients, and avoids surgical scar.[1,2]

References

1. Lupo MP, Smith SR, Thomas JA, et al. Effectiveness of Juvéderm Ultra Plus dermal filler in the treatment of severe nasolabial folds. Plast Reconstr Surg 2008;121:289
2. Cohen SR, Berner CF, Busso M, et al. Five year safety and efficacy of a novel polymethylmethacrylate aesthetic soft tissue filler for the correction of nasolabial folds. Dermatol Surg 2007;33(Suppl 2):S222

44. Necklift

Ira L. Savetsky, Simon Moradian
See *Essentials of Aesthetic Surgery*, pp. 565–580

YOUTHFUL NECK

1. *What is the ideal cervicomental angle?*
A. 90–100 degrees.
B. 100–105 degrees.
C. 105–120 degrees.
D. 120–130 degrees.
E. >130 degrees.

YOUTHFUL NECK

2. *Which of the following can contribute to an obtuse cervicomental angle?*
A. Tight submental skin.
B. Excess subplatysmal fat.
C. Deflated preplatysmal fat.
D. High position of hyoid bone.
E. Prominent submandibular glands.

PREOPERATIVE EVALUATION

3. *Which of the following describes part of the pathogenesis of platysmal banding?*
A. A contracted platysma creates a hammock between the jawline and hyoid bone.
B. The contraction of muscle fibers creates a bow-string effect toward the tubular neck which is countered by superficial cervical fascia.
C. The contraction of muscle fibers creates a bow-string effect toward the tubular neck which is countered by the deep cervical fascia.
D. Age-related changes to the fascia allow contents of platysma (fat and other structures) to "bulge," creating bands.
E. A contracted platysma creates a hammock between the jawline and the inferior aspect of the thyroid cartilage.

NONSURGICAL OPTIONS FOR NECK REJUVENATION

4. *Which of the following is accurate regarding the use of botulinum toxin to treat platysmal bands?*
A. Typically, less than 10 units is required in total.
B. A total of approximately 40 to 100 units is typically required.
C. Best results are in older patients with passive platysmal banding.
D. Best results are in younger patients with passive platysmal banding.
E. Injection should occur adjacent to the band, not directly into the band.

NONSURGICAL OPTIONS FOR NECK REJUVENATION

5. *Which of the following is accurate regarding the use of deoxycholic acid (Kybella, Allergan)?*
A. It is contraindicated in patients with a history of dysphagia.
B. It can be injected around facial nerve branches safely.
C. It can be injected into or around lymph nodes or muscles.
D. It can be used on patients who are on antiplatelet or therapeutic anticoagulation therapy.
E. It can be used safely in areas other than the submental area.

SURGICAL OPTIONS FOR NECK REJUVENATION

6. *Which of the following patients is most likely to benefit from submental liposuction alone?*
A. A young patient with good skin quality, localized submental adiposity, and no platysmal bands at rest.
B. A young patient with good skin quality, significant preplatysmal adiposity, and no platysmal bands at rest.
C. A young patient with poor skin quality, localized submental adiposity, and platysmal bands at rest.
D. An older patient with good skin quality, localized submental adiposity, and no platysmal bands at rest.
E. An older patient with poor skin quality, significant preplatysmal adiposity, and no platysmal bands at rest.

SURGICAL OPTIONS FOR NECK REJUVENATION

7. *Which of the following aspects of a necklift would be difficult to address via an anterior submental approach?*
A. Posterior platysmal bands.
B. Anterior digastric muscle resection.
C. Submental fat.
D. Anterior platysmal neck bands.
E. Submandibular gland resection.

SURGICAL OPTIONS FOR NECK REJUVENATION

8. *In which of the following clinical scenarios is a short-scar facelift and necklift indicated?*
A. A patient with excess skin, jowling, and an aged neck–face interface.
B. A patient with no excess skin, jowling, and an aged neck–face interface.
C. A patient with excess skin, no jowling, and without an aged neck–face interface.
D. A patient with excess skin, jowling, and without an aged neck–face interface.
E. A patient with no excess skin, no jowling, and without an aged neck–face interface.

SURGICAL OPTIONS FOR NECK REJUVENATION

9. *Which of the following is an indication for a full-scar facelift and necklift?*
A. Well-defined neck–face interface.
B. Minimal skin excess of the face.
C. Minimal platysmal bands.
D. Poor and excess skin of the neck.
E. Mild nasolabial folds with localized submental fat.

SURGICAL OPTIONS FOR NECK REJUVENATION

10. *To minimize and prevent notching of the occipital hairline and to remove excess skin in a full-scar facelift and necklift, the retroauricular incision is continued in which direction?*
A. Along the hairline.
B. Below the hairline.
C. Above the hairline.
D. Along for 3 cm and then carried above the hairline.
E. Along for 3 cm and then carried below the hairline.

SURGICAL OPTIONS FOR NECK REJUVENATION

11. *When using a direct approach to treat a "turkey-gobbler" neck deformity, which of the following has been described restore a youthful contour to the cervical angle?*
A. Z-plasty.
B. T-Z incision.
C. Straight incision.
D. Pure-string suture.
E. W-plasty.

COMPLICATIONS AND SUBOPTIMAL RESULTS

12. *Which of the following is considered a major risk factor for developing skin necrosis after a necklift?*
A. Hematoma.
B. Hemostatic net.
C. Minimal tension.
D. Light neck/face compression garment.
E. Postoperative icing of the neck.

COMPLICATIONS AND SUBOPTIMAL RESULTS

13. ***When performing a necklift with submental, preauricular, and retroauricular incisions, in which area is skin slough most likely to occur?***
A. Submental.
B. Preauricular.
C. Retroauricular.
D. Overlying the medial edge of the platysma.
E. Overlying the lateral edge of the platysma.

COMPLICATIONS AND SUBOPTIMAL RESULTS

14. ***Which of the following may contribute to increased risk of contour abnormalities along the anterior neck?***
A. Using small cannulas for liposuction.
B. Limiting passes of suction.
C. Preserving 1 to 2 mm of subcutaneous fat.
D. Performing direct subplatysmal fat lipectomy.
E. Liposuction of subplatysmal fat.

COMPLICATIONS AND SUBOPTIMAL RESULTS

15. ***Which of the following is a major potential contributor to persistent platysmal banding after a necklift with platysmal plication?***
A. Platysmal plication using a running suture.
B. Platsymal plication using interrupted sutures.
C. Use of a nonabsorbable suture.
D. Significant skin excess.
E. Dehiscence.

COMPLICATIONS AND SUBOPTIMAL RESULTS

16. ***Postoperatively after a submental necklift with direct lipectomy and platysmal plication, there is persistent bulging in the submental triangle. This is most likely due to which of the following?***
A. Inadequate fat excision.
B. Digastric muscle.
C. Submandibular gland.
D. Pleating of the platysma.
E. Hematoma.

COMPLICATIONS AND SUBOPTIMAL RESULTS

17. ***After 9 months of a submental necklift with direct lipectomy and bilateral submandibular gland resection, a patient has asymmetry of smile with the right side being higher as well as asymmetric pursing of the lips. Which of the following is likely responsible for this abnormality?***
A. Right-sided marginal mandibular nerve injury.
B. Left-sided marginal mandibular nerve injury.
C. Right-sided cervical nerve injury.
D. Left-sided cervical nerve injury.
E. Right hypoglossal nerve injury.

COMPLICATIONS AND SUBOPTIMAL RESULTS

18. ***Which of the following can be a result of overexcision and skeletonization of subcutaneous tissue?***
A. Nerve injury.
B. Hematoma.
C. Contour deformities.
D. Infection.
E. An obtuse cervicomental angle.

Answers

YOUTHFUL NECK

1. *What is the ideal cervicomental angle?*

C. 105–120 degrees.

The visual criteria for a youthful neck are a distinct inferior mandibular border, a visible subhyoid depression, a visible thyroid cartilage bulge, a visible anterior border of the sternocleidomastoid muscle, and a cervicomental angle of 105 to 120 degrees (**Fig. 44.1**).[1]

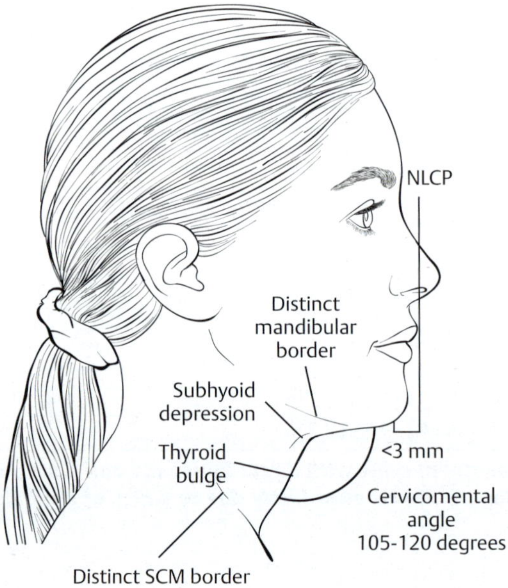

Fig. 44.1 Visual criteria for a youthful neck. (NLCP, Nose-lip-chin plane; SCM, sternocleidomastoid.) (Source: Visual Criteria for A Youthful Neck. In: Janis J, ed. Essentials of Aesthetic Surgery. 1st Edition. New York: Thieme; 2018.)

REFERENCE

1. Ellenbogen R, Karlin JV. Visual criteria for success in restoring the youthful neck. Plast Reconstr Surg 1980;66:826

YOUTHFUL NECK

2. *Which of the following can contribute to an obtuse cervicomental angle?*

B. Excess subplatysmal fat.

Excess or loose skin would contribute to an obtuse cervicomental angle, whereas tight skin would not. Excess subplatysmal and/or preplatysmal fat can contribute to an obtuse cervicomental angle. High position of the hyoid bone would not contribute, whereas a low hyoid bone could. Although prominent submandibular glands may contribute to an overall unfavorable neck contour, they would not be a direct cause of an obtuse cervicomental angle.[1]

REFERENCE

1. Vistnes AM, Souther SG. The anatomical basis for common cosmetic anterior neck deformities. Ann Plast Surg 1979;2(5):381–388

PREOPERATIVE EVALUATION

3. *Which of the following describes part of the pathogenesis of platysmal banding?*

D. Age-related changes to the fascia allow contents of platysma (fat and other structures) to "bulge," creating bands.

Pathogenesis of platysmal banding is controversial; however, a contracted platysma creates a hammock between the jawline and clavicle, not the hyoid bone. In addition, the contraction of muscle fibers creates a bow-string effect away from the tubular neck, not toward. Skin excess often times accompanies platysmal bands. The bow-string effect is countered by superficial cervical fascia. Age-related changes to the fascia allow contents of platysma (fat and other structures) to "bulge," creating bands (**Fig. 44.2a,b**).[1,2,3]

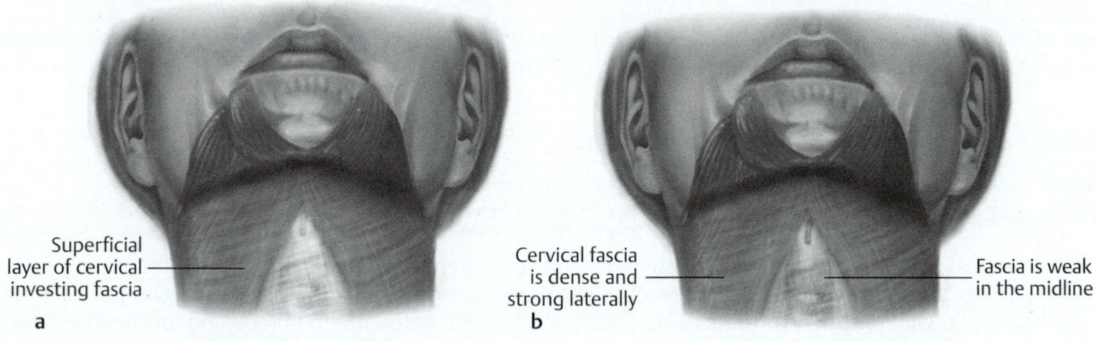

Fig. 44.2 (a,b) Platysmal banding. (Source: Thin Necks with Platysmal Bands. In: Barton F, ed. Facial Rejuvenation. 1st Edition. New York: Thieme; 2008.)

REFERENCES

1. Aston SJ. Platysma muscle in rhytidoplasty. Ann Plast Surg 1979;3:532
2. Guerrerosantos J. The role of platysma muscle in rhytidoplasty. Clin Plast Surg 1979;5:29
3. Guerrerosantos J. Neck lift. Simplified surgical techniques, refinements, and clinical classification. Clin Plast Surg 1983;10:379

NONSURGICAL OPTIONS FOR NECK REJUVENATION

4. *Which of the following is accurate regarding the use of botulinum toxin to treat platysmal bands?*

B. A total of approximately 40 to 100 units is typically required.

Botulinum toxin may delay eventual surgical correction of platysmal bands and may be useful as a supplement to surgery and for postsurgical defects of persistent banding. The technique involves grasping the bands and distracting them away from the neck. The usual starting dose is 10 to 30 units in women and 10 to 40 units in men, with women receiving 2 to 12 injections per band and men receiving 3 to 12 injections. A total of approximately 40 to 100 units is typically used (Botox). The relatively large number of units required makes treatment with toxins very expensive, especially in the long term. The best results are in younger patients with active (rather than passive) bands. It is not to be used where significant excess skin is present, since this would not be corrected by injection. Further, it is not used in older patients with passive platysmal banding. It requires firm, toned skin and youthful subcutaneous tissue. Complications include dysphagia (rare).[1,2,3]

REFERENCES

1. Brandt FS, Bellman B. Cosmetic use of botulinum A exotoxin for the aging neck. Dermatol Surg 1998;24:1232
2. Kane MA. Nonsurgical treatment of platysmal bands with injection of botulinum toxin A. Plast Reconstr Surg 1999;103:656
3. Matarasso A, Matarasso SL, Brandt FS, Bellman B. Botulinum A exotoxin for the management of platysma bands. Plast Reconstr Surg 1999;103(2):645–652; discussion 653–655

NONSURGICAL OPTIONS FOR NECK REJUVENATION

5. *Which of the following is accurate regarding the use of deoxycholic acid (Kybella, Allergan)?*

A. It is contraindicated in patients with a history of dysphagia.

Kybella should not be injected in patients with dysphagia; into or in close proximity to the marginal mandibular branch of the facial nerve; or close to the salivary glands, lymph nodes, or muscles.[1] Injection hematoma/bruising has been reported in up to 72% of patients in clinical trials. A single treatment may consist of up to 50 separate injections and up to 6 single treatments may be performed 1 month apart. Safe and effective use for the treatment of subcutaneous fat outside the submental region has not been established and is not recommended.[1]

Reference

1. Dayan SH, Humphrey S, Jones DH, et al. Overview of ATX-101 (deoxycholic acid injection): a nonsurgical approach for reduction of submental fat. Dermatol Surg 2016;42(Suppl 1):S263–S270

SURGICAL OPTIONS FOR NECK REJUVENATION

6. *Which of the following patients is most likely to benefit from submental liposuction alone?*

A. A young patient with good skin quality, localized submental adiposity, and no platysmal bands at rest.

The cervical–mandibular contours create neck and facial definition which may be obliterated by localized fatty depositions particularly in the submental area. Liposuction of the submental area is best used for younger patients (generally 20–30 years of age) with normal skin and with good tone and localized excess submental subcutaneous fat. The examination should include skin and subcutaneous pinch tests which are the best assessment for selecting appropriate candidates. Isolated submental liposuction can improve a short, fatty neck, and improve the overall contour of the jawline. Additionally, it can be combined with an open neck technique to ease subsequent surgical dissection.[1,2,3,4,5,6] It should be noted that this techniqueis not indicated for patients with subplastysmal fat (too deep for liposuction).

References

1. Jones BM, Grover R. Reducing complications in cervicofacial rhytidectomy by tumescent infiltration: a comparative trial evaluating 678 consecutive face lifts. Plast Reconstr Surg 2004;113:398
2. Courtiss EH. Suction lipectomy of the neck. Plast Reconstr Surg 1985;76:882
3. Tapia A, Ferreira B, Eng R. Liposuction in cervical rejuvenation. Aesthetic Plast Surg 1987;11:95
4. Zins JE, Fardo D. The "anterior only" approach to neck rejuvenation: an alternative to facelift surgery. Plast Reconstr Surg 2005;1155:1761
5. Gryskiewicz JM. Submental suction-assisted lipectomy without platysmaplasty: pushing the (skin) envelope to avoid a facelift for unsuitable patients. Plast Reconstr Surg 2003;112:1393
6. Mladick RA. Neck rejuvenation without facelift. Aesthet Surg J 2005;25:285

SURGICAL OPTIONS FOR NECK REJUVENATION

7. *Which of the following aspects of a necklift would be difficult to address via an anterior submental approach?*

A. Posterior platysmal bands.

Given the usual 2- to 3-cm incision in the submental crease used for accessing the anterior neck, the anterior digastric muscles, submental fat, anterior platysmal neck bands, and submandibular gland resection can all be treated through this incision. Posterior platysmal bands would be difficult to visualize and treat through an anterior submental approach and would best be treated through a posterior exposure, typically in the setting of a necklift incision. Indications for a submental necklift are patients with anterior platysmal bands, if undermining of the skin is necessary for neck contouring, or to access intermediate or deeper tissues. Typically, this is performed as an isolated procedure (rare), or in combination with a facial procedure.[1,2,3,4,5]

References

1. Zins JE, Fardo D. The "anterior only" approach to neck rejuvenation: an alternative to facelift surgery. Plast Reconstr Surg 2005;1155:1761
2. Connell BF. Cervical lifts: the value of platysmal muscle flaps. Ann Plast Surg 1978;1:34
3. Connell BF. Contouring the neck in rhytidectomy by lipectomy and a muscle sling. Plast Reconstr Surg 1978;61:376
4. Hamilton JM. Submental lipectomy with skin excision. Plast Reconstr Surg 1993;92:443
5. Gradinger GP. Anterior lipectomy with skin excision. Plast Reconstr Surg 2000;106:1146

SURGICAL OPTIONS FOR NECK REJUVENATION

8. *In which of the following clinical scenarios is a short-scar facelift and necklift indicated?*

B. A patient with no excess skin, jowling, and without an aged neck–face interface.

Indications for a short-scar facelift and necklift are patients with no excess neck skin, presence of jowling, and an aged neck–face interface.[1] For a subset of patients who only have an isolated neck issue, a short-scar necklift in which no skin is removed can be an ideal method of treating poor neck contour. Typically, these patients include younger women with full, obtuse necks, and young and middle-aged men with poor neck contour. The procedure is performed through a submental incision and relies on modification of deep-layer structures to improve neck contour without any removal of skin. Any excess skin is then allowed to redistribute itself over the increased neck surface area and results in an improved neck contour and deepening of the cervicomental angle. For properly selected patients, a short-scar necklift can produce a marked improvement in facial appearance.

Reference

1. Baker DC. Lateral SMASectomy. Plast Reconstr Surg 1997;100:509

SURGICAL OPTIONS FOR NECK REJUVENATION

9. *Which of the following is an indication for a full-scar facelift and necklift?*

D. Poor and excess skin of the neck.

Indications for a full-scar facelift and necklift are aging changes of face and neck, a poorly defined neck–face interface, inelastic and excess skin of face, poor and excess skin of neck, visible static platysmal bands down to inferior cervical, neck crease below the thyroid, and a visible submandibular gland.[1]

Reference

1. Nahai F, ed. The Art of Aesthetic Surgery: Principles & Techniques. New York: Thieme Publishers; 2010

SURGICAL OPTIONS FOR NECK REJUVENATION

10. *To minimize and prevent notching of the occipital hairline and to remove excess skin in a full-scar facelift and necklift, the retroauricular incision is continued in which direction?*

A. Along the hairline.

In patients with significant excess skin in the lower neck, the retroauricular incision is continued along the hairline to prevent notching the occipital hairline and to remove more excess skin (**Fig. 44.3**).[1]

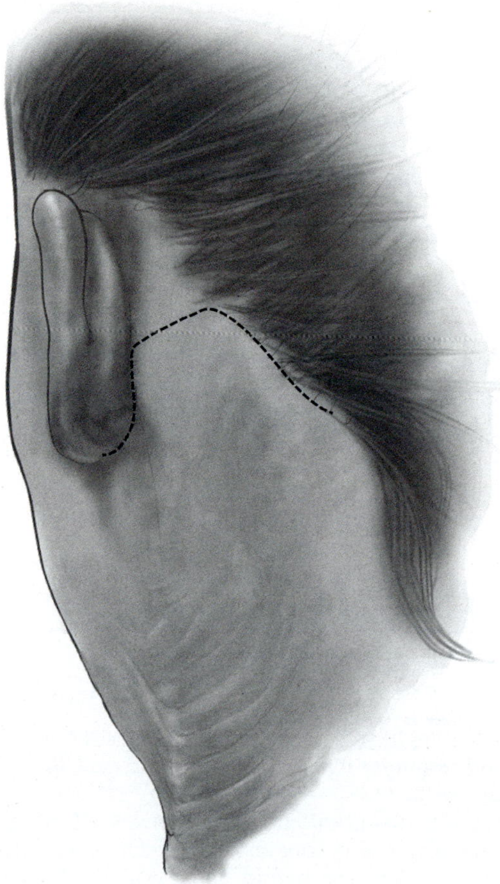

Fig. 44.3 Occipital hairline incision. (Source: Nahai F, ed. The Art of Aesthetic Surgery: Principles & Techniques, ed 2. New York: Thieme Publishers; 2011.)

Reference

1. Nahai F, ed. The Art of Aesthetic Surgery: Principles & Techniques. New York: Thieme Publishers; 2010

SURGICAL OPTIONS FOR NECK REJUVENATION

11. *When using a direct approach to treat a "turkey-gobbler" neck deformity, which of the following has been described restore a youthful contour to the cervical angle?*

B. T-Z incision.

In patients with severe and massive anterior neck redundancy ("turkey-gobbler" neck deformity) skin can be excised using a direct approach. A T-Z incision can restore a youthful contour to the cervical angle. The initial procedure was done through a midcervical skin excision through which preplatysmal and subplatysmal fat was excised and the platysma was closed in the midline.[1,2]

References

1. Adamson JE, Horton CE, Crawford HH. The surgical correction of the "turkey gobbler" deformity. Plast Reconstr Surg 1964;34:598
2. Cronin TD, Biggs TM. The T-Z plasty for the male "turkey gobbler" neck. Plast Reconstr Surg 1971;47:534

COMPLICATIONS AND SUBOPTIMAL RESULTS

12. *Which of the following is considered a major risk factor for developing skin necrosis after a necklift?*

A. Hematoma.

Skin necrosis is more common if significant tension remains laterally at the retroauricular sulcus. Skin slough is usually preceded by hematoma or infection, most commonly in the retroauricular area with hematomas reported in 0 to 14% of facelifts. Some surgeons do not place dressings on the neck to prevent pressure necrosis.[1] Excessive tension, not minimal, could potentially lead to skin necrosis. There is no increased rate of skin necrosis with the use of hemostatic net placements or face and neck compression garments.[1,2]

REFERENCES

1. Meade RA. Neck lift. In Janis JE, ed. Essentials of Plastic Surgery. New York: Thieme Publishers; 2006
2. Janssen TJ, Maheshwari K, Sivadasan A, Waterhouse N. Hemostatic net in facelift surgery: a 5-year single-surgeon experience. Aesthet Surg J 2023;43(10):1106–1111

COMPLICATIONS AND SUBOPTIMAL RESULTS

13. *When performing a necklift with submental, preauricular, and retroauricular incisions, in which area is skin slough most likely to occur?*

C. Retroauricular.

Skin necrosis is more common if significant tension remains laterally at the retroauricular sulcus. Skin slough is usually preceded by hematoma or infection, most commonly in the retroauricular area.[1]

REFERENCE

1. Meade RA. Neck lift. In: Janis JE, ed. Essentials of Plastic Surgery. New York: Thieme Publishers; 2006

COMPLICATIONS AND SUBOPTIMAL RESULTS

14. *Which of the following may contribute to increased risk of contour abnormalities along the anterior neck?*

C. Preserving 1 to 2 mm of subcutaneous fat.

Contour abnormalities, also known as fat interface problems, are usually related to underexcision or overexcision. Overexcision of fat is generally subcutaneous. Liposuction of subplatysmal fat is not indicated as it is in too deep a plane and direct lipectomy is preferred. Fat interface problems can be prevented by using small cannulas, limiting passes of suction, and uniformly preserving 3 to 5 mm (not 1–2 mm) of subcutaneous fat.[1]

REFERENCE

1. Meade RA. Neck lift. In: Janis JE, ed. Essentials of Plastic Surgery. New York: Thieme Publishers; 2006

COMPLICATIONS AND SUBOPTIMAL RESULTS

15. *Which of the following is a major potential contributor to persistent platysmal banding after a necklift with platysmal plication?*

E. Dehiscence.

Persistence of banding from failure of platysmal sutures and postoperative dehiscence is most common. Absorbable sutures should not be generally used for plication. Correction is often needed and requires opening the neck to replicate or resect as indicated.[1]

REFERENCE

1. Meade RA. Neck lift. In: Janis JE, ed. Essentials of Plastic Surgery. New York: Thieme Publishers; 2006

COMPLICATIONS AND SUBOPTIMAL RESULTS

16. *Postoperatively after a submental necklift with direct lipectomy and platysmal plication, there is persistent bulging in the submental triangle. This is most likely due to which of the following?*

C. Submandibular gland.

Postoperative bulging in the submental triangle is often from an enlarged submandibular gland. It is usually present preoperatively that was not surgically addressed. Correction entails opening the neck again and addressing the gland.[1,2,3.] Hematoma would be a rare cause of persistent bulging in the submental area.

References

1. Singer DP, Sullivan PK. Submandibular gland I: an anatomic evaluation and surgical approach to submandibular gland resection for facial rejuvenation. Plast Reconstr Surg 2003;112:1150; discussion 1155
2. Sullivan PK, Freeman MB, Schmidt S, et al. Contouring the aging neck with submandibular gland suspension. Aesthet Surg J 26:465, 2006.
3. Guyuron B, Jackowe D, Lamphongsai S. Basket submandibular gland suspension. Plast Reconstr Surg 122:938, 2008.

COMPLICATIONS AND SUBOPTIMAL RESULTS

17. *After 9 months of a submental necklift with direct lipectomy and bilateral submandibular gland resection, a patient has asymmetry of smile with the right side being higher as well as asymmetric pursing of the lips. Which of the following is likely responsible for this abnormality?*

B. Left-sided marginal mandibular nerve injury.

The submandibular gland may be a reason for bulging in the submental triangle due to an enlarged gland. Correction entails opening the neck and addressing the gland with either a partial or total resection. However, given the close proximity of the marginal mandibular gland with the submandibular gland, a known risk is either a transient neuropraxia or in some rare cases permanent nerve injury. In the above patient scenario, the left-sided marginal mandibular nerve has likely been injured as it innervates the lower lip depressors (depressor anguli oris and depressor labii inferioris), mentalis, and orbicularis. Therefore, injury causes the opposite side to be lower during smile, and asymmetry with pursing of lips due to mentalis and orbicularis. Treatment includes observation, since pseudoparalysis is common; (80% heal within 6 months). If this persists for >6 months, then an anesthetic block of the opposite depressor with botulinum toxin or division of musclecanbe considered. After more than 2 years, it is unlikely the neuromuscular junction will recover function, so nerve repair will not useful.[1,2,3]

References

1. Sinclair NR, Coombs DM, Kwiecien G, Zins JE. How to prevent and treat complications in facelift surgery, Part 1: short-term complications. Aesthet Surg J Open Forum 2021;3(1):ojab007
2. Hazani R, Chowdhry S, Mowlavi A, Wilhelmi BJ. Bony anatomic landmarks to avoid injury to the marginal mandibular nerve. Aesthet Surg J 2011;31(3):286–289
3. Connell BF, Shamoun JM. The significance of digastric muscle contouring for rejuvenation of the submental area of the face. Plast Reconstr Surg 1997;99:1586

COMPLICATIONS AND SUBOPTIMAL RESULTS

18. *Which of the following can be a result of overexcision and skeletonization of subcutaneous tissue?*

C. Contour deformities.

Preserving more fat is better than denuding fat. Do not skeletonize the subcutaneous tissue, which can cause platysmal banding or visible underlying contour irregularities. Endpoint: Use skin-pinch technique and observation of irregularities to ensure soft contour, leaving fat just under skin. Oversuctioning may adhere the skin to underlying platysma, creating unnatural tethering and banding.[1]

Reference

1. Nahai F, ed. The Art of Aesthetic Surgery: Principles & Techniques. New York: Thieme Publishers; 2010

45. Rhinoplasty

Elbert E. Vaca, Simon Moradian
See *Essentials of Aesthetic Surgery*, pp. 581–619

ANATOMY

1. ***After an open rhinoplasty via a transcolumellar incision, which of the following vessels is subsequently principally responsible for perfusion of the nasal tip?***
   A. Columellar artery.
   B. Superior labial artery.
   C. Dorsal nasal artery.
   D. Lateral nasal artery.
   E. Angular artery.

ANATOMY

2. ***Which of the following best describes the most common relationship between the upper lateral and lower lateral cartilage in the scroll area?***
   A. There is end-on-end contact between the upper lateral and lower lateral cartilages.
   B. The upper lateral cartilages overlap the lower lateral cartilages.
   C. The upper lateral cartilages underlap the lower lateral cartilages.
   D. The cephalic border of the upper lateral cartilage lies medial to the caudal border of the lower lateral cartilage.
   E. The upper lateral and lower lateral nasal cartilage do not come in contact.

ANATOMY

3. ***A 24-year-old female presents to your clinic for a rhinoplasty consultation. On examination, the left alar base is noted to be higher than the right. This alar base discrepancy is noted to be more prominent with smiling. Action of which of the following muscles is responsible for this finding?***
   A. Nasalis.
   B. Depressor septi nasi.
   C. Levator labii superioris.
   D. Levator labii alaeque nasi.
   E. Levator angularis oris.

ANATOMY

4. ***A 34-year-old female is displeased with her postoperative result 1 year after an open rhinoplasty. On profile view in repose, she has a smooth dorsum with a nasolabial angle of 95 degrees. However, upon smiling, she complains of a downward pointing nasal tip and her nasolabial angle decreases to 75 degrees. Which of the following maneuvers would have prevented this patient's postoperative complaint?***
   A. Transposition of the depressor septi nasi muscle.
   B. Placement of a columellar strut.
   C. Closed instead of open rhinoplasty approach.
   D. Placement of a caudal septal extension graft.
   E. Transdomal suture placement.

ANATOMY

5. ***The internal nasal valve is formed by which of the following structures?***
   A. Inferior turbinate and septum.
   B. Caudal edge of upper lateral cartilage and septum.
   C. Caudal edge of upper lateral cartilage, inferior turbinate, and septum.
   D. Caudal edge of the lower lateral cartilage and septum.
   E. Caudal edge of the lower lateral cartilage, inferior turbinate, and septum.

ANATOMY

6. *A postoperative rhinoplasty patient is seen in clinic and is diagnosed with "empty nose syndrome." This is most likely a result of aggressive resection of which of the following structures?*

A. Superior turbinate.
B. Middle turbinate.
C. Inferior turbinate.
D. Quadrangular cartilage.
E. Dorsal hump.

ANATOMY

7. *A Caucasian female patient is diagnosed with a wide alar base. On frontal view, which of the following findings best supports the diagnosis of a wide alar base?*

A. Alar base located lateral to the medial canthus.
B. Alar base width >50% the width of the oral aperture.
C. Alar base located lateral to the medial brow margin.
D. Alar base is wider than the bony base of the upper third of the nose.
E. Alar base width is wider than the length of the upper and lower cartilaginous vault combined.

ANATOMY

8. *A patient presents with a deep and inferiorly located nasal radix and a radix graft is planned. What effect will placement of the radix graft have on nasal appearance?*

A. No change in apparent nasal length and decrease in the nasofrontal angle.
B. No change in apparent nasal length and increase in the nasofrontal angle.
C. Shorten the nose and increase the nasofrontal angle.
D. Shorten the nose and decrease the nasofrontal angle.
E. Lengthen the nose and increase the nasofrontal angle.

ANATOMY

9. *Which of the following is an advantage of the open versus closed rhinoplasty approach?*

A. Decreased postoperative nasal edema.
B. Improved visualization of the cartilaginous framework.
C. Cartilage grafts can be placed in precisely sized pockets without fixation.
D. Improved preservation of native tip support structures.
E. Less ability to determine the etiology of asymmetry found on examination.

ANATOMY

10. *Which of the following grafts is used to improve internal nasal valve patency?*

A. Nasal sidewall onlay graft.
B. Spreader graft.
C. Alar spreader graft.
D. Septal extension graft.
E. Alar rim graft.

ANATOMY

11. *When performing nasal osteotomies, what is the reason for preserving the caudal aspect of the frontal process of the maxilla (i.e., Webster's triangle)?*

A. Minimizing the risk of nasal bone instability.
B. Decreasing the risk of injury to the lateral nasal artery.
C. Avoiding disruption of ligamentous attachments of lateral crura to the piriform aperture.
D. Avoiding disruption of the medial canthal tendon.
E. Avoiding infracture of the inferior nasal turbinate.

ANATOMY

12. *An Asian patient presents for rhinoplasty and dorsal nasal augmentation is planned. Which of the following methods of dorsal augmentation is most prone to postoperative warping?*

A. Septum.
B. Diced cartilage fascia graft.
C. Human acellular dermal matrix.
D. Irradiated rib cartilage.
E. Autologous rib cartilage.

ANATOMY

13. *A 30-year-old woman undergoes rhinoplasty to correct a droopy nasal tip. Which of the following suture techniques can help correct this deformity?*

A. Transdomal suture.
B. Interdomal suture.
C. Horizontal mattress suture between the upper lateral cartilage and the septum.
D. Medial crural septal suture.
E. Lateral crural mattress suture.

ANATOMY

14. *A 51-year-old male presents with a droopy and overprojected nasal tip. Which of the following maneuvers can be performed to address both of these deformities?*

A. Lateral crural mattress suture.
B. Spring flap.
C. Lateral crural strut.
D. Subdomal graft.
E. Lateral crural resection/overlay.

ANATOMY

15. *A 19-year-old female presents for rhinoplasty with a deviated nose and an S-shaped septal deformity. Bilateral mucoperichondrial flaps are elevated and septal cartilage is harvested leaving a 12-mm L-strut. Severe convexity of the base of the caudal L-strut is observed. Which of the following maneuvers should be performed next to address this problem?*

A. Spreader grafts.
B. Trimming of the caudal L-strut to 6 mm.
C. Releasing the caudal septum from the anterior nasal spine and caudal septal reduction.
D. Lateral crural strut grafts.
E. Lateral crural mattress sutures.

Answers

ANATOMY

1. *After an open rhinoplasty via a transcolumellar incision, which of the following vessels is subsequently principally responsible for perfusion of the nasal tip?*

D. Lateral nasal artery.

The lateral nasal artery is one of the most important vessels in nasal blood supply, and preserving it mitigate against postoperative complications. The lateral nasal artery originates from the angular artery, coursing 2 to 3 mm cephalad to the alar groove and provides arterial inflow to the nasal tip. The transcolumellar incision during open rhinoplasty results in division of the columellar vessels; therefore, vascularity of the nasal tip is reliant upon inflow from the lateral nasal vessels. The superior labial artery is the source of the columellar artery. The superior labial artery does not supply the nasal tip after open rhinoplasty. The dorsal nasal artery supplies the upper third of the nose and provides axial inflow for the dorsal nasal artery flap. The angular artery is incorrect because the lateral nasal artery branches from the angular artery; therefore, the lateral nasal artery is the better answer choice (**Fig. 45.1**).[1]

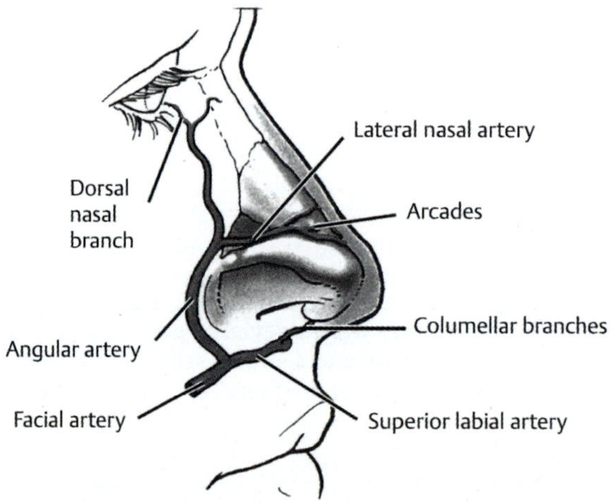

Fig. 45.1 The lateral nasal artery is one of the most important vessels in nasal blood supply, and preserving it promotes healing and helps to prevent deleterious postoperative skin changes. (Source: Blood supply. In: Janis J, ed. Essentials of Aesthetic Surgery. 1st Edition. New York: Thieme; 2018.)

REFERENCE

1. Rohrich RJ, Gunter JP, Friedman RM. Nasal tip blood supply: an anatomic study validating the safety of the transcolumellar incision in rhinoplasty. Plast Reconstr Surg 1995;95:795

ANATOMY

2. *Which of the following best describes the most common relationship between the upper lateral and lower lateral cartilage in the scroll area?*

C. The upper lateral cartilages underlap the lower lateral cartilages.

The anatomy of the lowest portion of the upper lateral cartilage in relation to the lower lateral cartilages can be quite variable. This region is called the *scroll area* and provides significant support to the nasal pyramid, particularly the tip. It is most commonly described as the junction where the upper lateral cartilages underlap the lower lateral cartilages. Although variations may exist, this orientation tends to be the most common form encountered.[1]

REFERENCE

1. Bitik O, Uzun H, Konaş E. Scroll reconstruction: fine tuning of the interface between middle and lower thirds in rhinoplasty. Aesthet Surg J 2019;39(5):481–494

ANATOMY

3. *A 24-year-old female presents to your clinic for a rhinoplasty consultation. On examination, the left alar base is noted to be higher than the right. This alar base discrepancy is noted to be more prominent with smiling. Action of which of the following muscles is responsible for this finding?*

D. Levator labii alaeque nasi.

The levator labii alaeque nasi muscle is innervated by the buccal branch of the facial nerve and is composed of a medial and lateral head, with the lateral head inserting onto the alar base. Contraction of this muscle helps open the external nasal valve and elevates the alar base.[1] Asymmetric hyperactivity or ipsilateral facial nerve palsy can result in alar base height asymmetry. The nasalis muscle has two components which helps both compress and dilate the nostrils. The depressor septi nasi muscle may originate from incisive fossa of the maxilla or orbicularis, inserting into the nasal septum. Contracture of the depressor septi nasi muscle depresses the nasal tip.[2,3] The levator labii superioris does not insert into the nasal base. The levator labii superioris elevates the medial aspect of the upper lip lateral to the piriform aperture. The levator angularis oris inserts into the modiolus and helps elevate the oral commissure (**Fig. 45.2**).

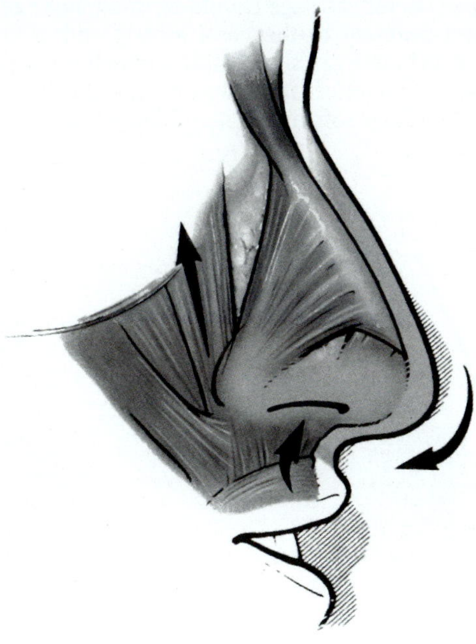

Fig. 45.2 The depressor septi nasi muscle and other musculature can affect nasal shape and the tip position. (Source: Enhancing the Nasal Tip–Upper Lip Relationship: The Importance of the Depressor Septi Nasi Muscle in Rhinoplasty. In: Rohrich R, Adams W, Ahmad J, Gunter J, ed. Dallas Rhinoplasty: Nasal Surgery by the Masters. 3rd Edition. New York: Thieme; 2014.)

REFERENCES

1. Howard BK, Rohrich R J. Understanding the nasal airway principles and practice. Plast Reconstr Surg 2002;109:1128
2. Rohrich RJ, Huynh B, Muzaffar AR, et al. Importance of the depressor septi nasi muscle in rhinoplasty: anatomic study and clinical application. Plast Reconstr Surg 2000;105:376
3. Ghavami A, Janis JE, Guyuron B. Regarding the treatment of dynamic tip ptosis using botulinum toxin A. Plast Reconstr Surg 2006;118:263

ANATOMY

4. *A 34-year-old female is displeased with her postoperative result 1 year after an open rhinoplasty. On profile view in repose, she has a smooth dorsum with a nasolabial angle of 95 degrees. However, upon smiling, she complains of a downward pointing nasal tip and her nasolabial angle decreases to 75 degrees. Which of the following maneuvers would have prevented this patient's postoperative complaint?*

A. Transposition of the depressor septi nasi muscle.

The depressor septi nasi arises from either the incisive foramen of the maxilla or orbicularis oculi muscle and inserts into the caudal septum. Contracture of this muscle depresses the nasal tip, therefore explaining this patient's dynamic nasal tip complaints during smiling. Rohrich et al described a technique to dissect and transpose this muscle to improve dynamic tip descent in the appropriately selected patient.[1]

REFERENCE

1. Rohrich RJ, Huynh B, Muzaffar AR, et al. Importance of the depressor septi nasi muscle in rhinoplasty: anatomic study and clinical application. Plast Reconstr Surg 2000;105:376

ANATOMY

5. *The internal nasal valve is formed by which of the following structures?*

B. Caudal edge of upper lateral cartilage and septum.

The caudal aspect of the upper lateral cartilage should form an angle of >10 to 15 degrees with the nasal septum—this is the narrowest segment of the nasal airway and is known as the internal nasal valve. Although a prominent inferior turbinate can significantly contribute to nasal airflow resistance, the inferior turbinate is not considered part of the internal nasal valve. The external nasal valve is formed by the caudal edge of the lower lateral cartilage, alar soft tissue, membranous septum, and nostril sill (**Fig. 45.3**).[1,2,3,4]

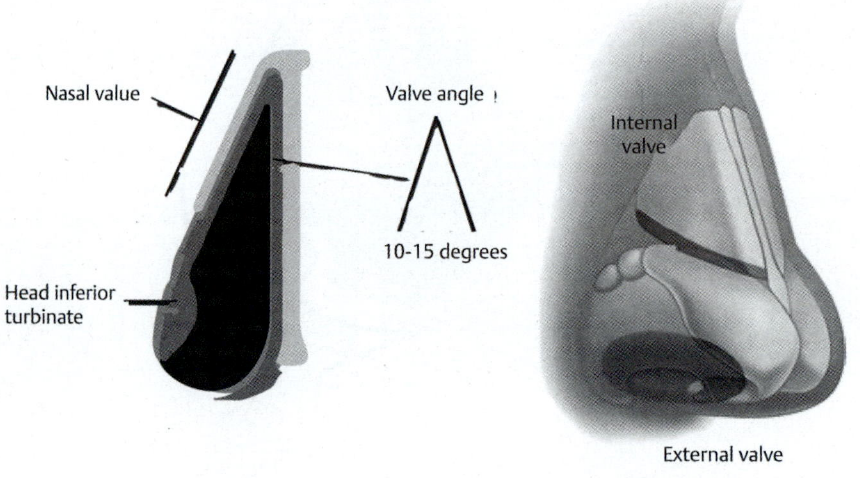

Fig. 45.3 The internal nasal valve is one of the most important aspects in septorhinoplasty and must be maintained open using spreader grafts and/or flaps. (Source: Incrementally Reduce the Dorsum. In: Rohrich R, Adams W, Ahmad J, Gunter J, ed. Dallas Rhinoplasty: Nasal Surgery by the Masters. 3rd Edition. New York: Thieme; 2014.)

REFERENCES

1. Beekhuis GJ. Nasal obstruction after rhinoplasty: etiology, and techniques for correction. Laryngoscope 1976;86:540
2. Howard BK, Rohrich RJ. Understanding the nasal airway: principles and practice. Plast Reconstr Surg 2002;109:1128

3. Gunter JP, Rohrich RJ. Management of the deviated nose. The importance of septal reconstruction. Clin Plast Surg 1988;15:43
4. Rohrich RJ, Gunter JP, Deuber MA, et al. The deviated nose: optimizing results using a simplified classification and algorithmic approach. Plast Reconstr Surg 2002;110:1509

ANATOMY

6. *A postoperative rhinoplasty patient is seen in clinic and is diagnosed with "empty nose syndrome." This is most likely a result of aggressive resection of which of the following structures?*

C. Inferior turbinate.

"Empty nose syndrome" is typically a consequence of aggressive resection of the inferior turbinate, which results in turbulent airflow. The nasal turbinate's help humidify and regulate nasal airflow. If present, preoperative diagnosis of hypertrophied inferior nasal turbinates is critical as they can contribute up to two-thirds of nasal airflow resistance. However, overaggressive resection of the inferior turbinate can result in paradoxical increased airway resistance.[1,2]

REFERENCES

1. Beekhuis GJ. Nasal obstruction after rhinoplasty: etiology, and techniques for correction. Laryngoscope 1976;86:540
2. Howard BK, Rohrich RJ. Understanding the nasal airway: principles and practice. Plast Reconstr Surg 2002;109:1128

ANATOMY

7. *A Caucasian female patient is diagnosed with a wide alar base. On frontal view, which of the following findings best supports the diagnosis of a wide alar base?*

A. Alar base located lateral to the medial canthus.

In Caucasian patients, the alar base should (generally) coincide with the medial intercanthal width, as is shown with facial analysis using vertical fifths (**Fig. 45.4**). The alar base is generally considered wide if it extends lateral to the medial canthus. Generally, the alar base is approximately two-thirds the width of the oral aperture. Although the medial brow margin should approximately coincide with the medial canthi, this is variable and the alar base width is traditionally compared to the medial canthi, not the medial brow margin. The nasal dorsal aesthetic lines should be narrowest at the medial canthi, corresponding to the bony nasal vault. The nasal bony base should be 75 to 80% of the alar base width; therefore, answer D is incorrect. In general, the alar base width will be less than the length of the upper and lower cartilaginous vaults combined; however, comparison of the two is not traditionally used in this assessment of alarbasewidth.[1,2,3]

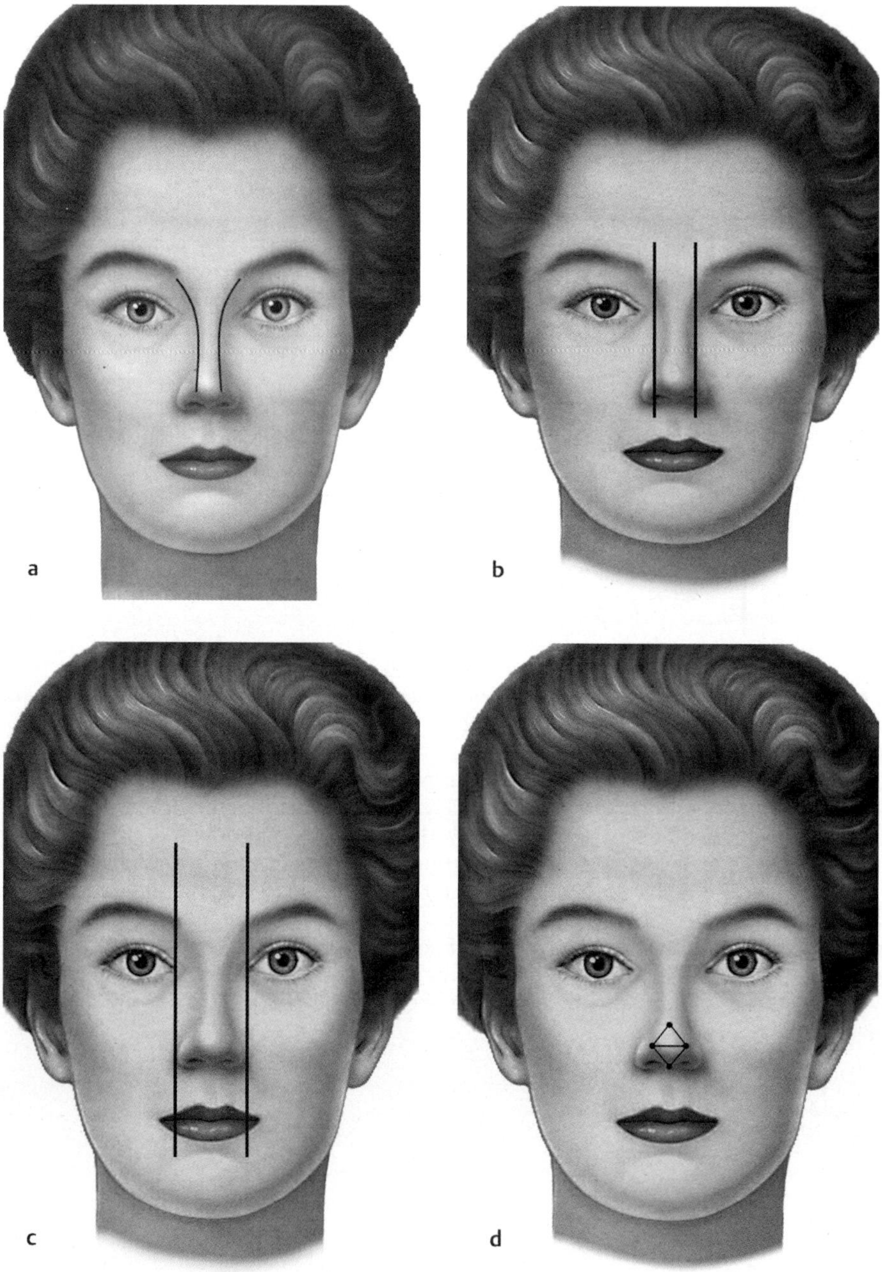

Fig. 45.4 **(a)** Dorsal aesthetic contour lines are curvilinear in females and descend from the medial brow toward the tip-defining points. **(b)** Nasal bones are generally narrower than the alar base width by about 20-25%. **(c)** Alar base width is generally equivalent to the medial canthi; however, many variations exist. **(d)** Generally, aesthetically pleasing nasal tip highlights are diamond shaped. (Source: Incrementally Reduce the Dorsum. In: Rohrich R, Adams W, Ahmad J, Gunter J, ed. Dallas Rhinoplasty: Nasal Surgery by the Masters. 3rd Edition. New York: Thieme; 2014.)

REFERENCES

1. Sheen JH, Sheen A, eds. Aesthetic Rhinoplasty. 2nd ed. St Louis: CV Mosby; 1987
2. Janis JE, Ahmad J, Rohrich RJ. Clinical decision-making in rhinoplasty. In: Nahai F, ed. The Art of Aesthetic Surgery. 2nd ed. New York: Thieme Publishers; 2010
3. Byrd HS, Hobar PC. Rhinoplasty: a practical guide for surgical planning. Plast Reconstr Surg 1993;91:642

ANATOMY

8. *A patient presents with a deep and inferiorly located nasal radix and a radix graft is planned. What effect will placement of the radix graft have on nasal appearance?*

E. Lengthen the nose and increase the nasofrontal angle.

A deep and inferiorly located radix is correlated with a short nose and a more acute nasofrontal angle. Placement of a radix graft will increase the apparent nasal length by raising the location of the radix superiorly. Furthermore, a radix graft will decrease the apparent depth of the radix and therefore make the nasofrontal angle more obtuse. Radix grafts are useful for treatment of the short nose with an acute nasofrontal angle (**Fig. 45.5**).[1,2,3]

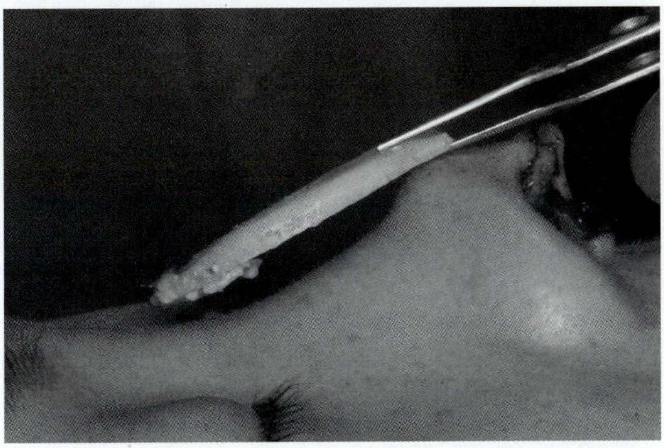

Fig. 45.5 Dorsal graft orientation. Placed with concave side down. If concave side is up, warping can occur resulting in fullness in the radix and supratip. (Source: Dorsal grafting. In: Janis J, ed. Essentials of Aesthetic Surgery. 1st Edition. New York: Thieme; 2018.)

REFERENCES

1. Rohrich RJ, Muzaffar AR. Rhinoplasty in the African-American patient. Plast Reconstr Surg 2003;111:1322
2. Daniel RK. Hispanic rhinoplasty in the United States with emphasis on the Mexican American nose. Plast Reconstr Surg 2003;112:244
3. Rohrich RJ, Ghavami A. Rhinoplasty for Middle Eastern noses. Plast Reconstr Surg 2009;123:1343

ANATOMY

9. *Which of the following is an advantage of the open versus closed rhinoplasty approach?*

B. Improved visualization of the cartilaginous framework.

There are several advantages and disadvantages to open rhinoplasty. Advantages of open rhinoplasty include improved visualization and correlation of internal deformities with external appearance. Disadvantages include an external nasal scar, prolonged nasal edema, and the need for suture stabilization of most grafts. Advantages of closed rhinoplasty included decreased tip edema, faster recover, the ability to limit dissection and place grafts in precisely dissected pockets without fixation, and possible preservation of more nasal support structures due to more limited dissection. Disadvantages of closed rhinoplasty included decreased visualization and greater reliance on experience and preoperative diagnosis.[1]

REFERENCE

1. Gunter JP. The merits of open approach in rhinoplasty. Plast Reconstr Surg 1997;99:863

ANATOMY

10. *Which of the following grafts is used to improve internal nasal valve patency?*

B. Spreader graft.

Spreader grafts are placed between the upper lateral cartilage and cartilaginous septum and can serve several roles including maintaining patency of the internal nasal valve, straightening of a deviated dorsal septum, and improvement of dorsal aesthetic lines (**Fig. 45.6**). Furthermore, extended spreader grafts can be used to lengthen the nose and provide an additional method to fixate a columellar strut or caudal septal extension graft to control tip rotation and projection.

Nasal sidewall onlay grafts can be used to improve the contour of a narrow middle vault. Alar spreader grafts are placed between the lateral crura of the lower lateral cartilage and vestibular skin to improve patency of the external nasal valve. The septal extension graft is used to control tip rotation and projection. The alar rim graft is placed in a subcutaneous pocket along the alar rim to treat alar retraction.[1,2,3]

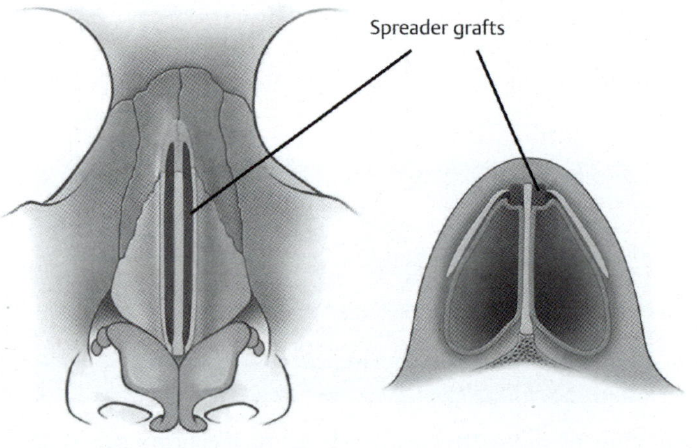

Fig. 45.6 Spreader grafts allow internal nasal valve patency. (Source: Spreader graft. In: Rohrich R, Adams W, Ahmad J, Gunter J, ed. Dallas Rhinoplasty: Nasal Surgery by the Masters. 3rd Edition. New York: Thieme; 2014.)

References

1. Sheen JH. Spreader graft: a method of reconstructing the roof of the middle nasal vault following rhinoplasty. Plast Reconstr Surg 1984;73:230
2. Gunter JP, Rohrich RJ. Management of the deviated nose. The importance of septal reconstruction. Clin Plast Surg 1988;15:43
3. Rohrich RJ, Gunter JP, Deuber MA, et al. The deviated nose: optimizing results using a simplified classification and algorithmic approach. Plast Reconstr Surg 2002;110:1509

ANATOMY

11. *When performing nasal osteotomies, what is the reason for preserving the caudal aspect of the frontal process of the maxilla (i.e., Webster's triangle)?*

E. Avoid infracture of the inferior nasal turbinate.

The caudal aspect of the frontal process of the maxilla, i.e., Webster's triangle, should be preserved if nasal osteotomies are planned as this corresponds to the location of the anterior aspect of the inferior turbinate. Infracture of Webster's triangle results in nasal airway collapse due to inferior turbinate infracture (**Fig. 45.7**).[1,2]

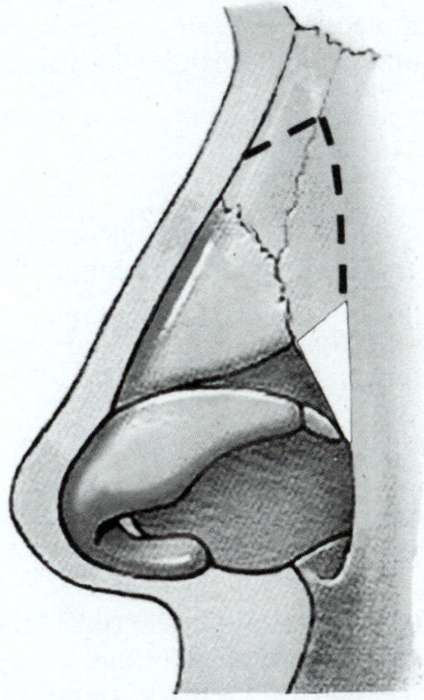

Fig. 45.7 Various starting points and endpoints of osteotomy patterns exist. (Source: Rohrich RJ, Adams WP Jr, Ahmad J, Gunter JP, eds. Dallas Rhinoplasty: Nasal Surgery by the Masters, ed 3. New York: Thieme Publishers, 2014.)

REFERENCES

1. Guyuron B. Nasal osteotomy and airway changes. Plast Reconstr Surg 1998;102:856
2. Gruber R, Chang TN, Kahn D, et al. Broad nasal bone reduction: an algorithm for osteotomies. Plast Reconstr Surg 2007;119:1044

ANATOMY

12. ***An Asian patient presents for rhinoplasty and dorsal nasal augmentation is planned. Which of the following methods of dorsal augmentation is most prone to postoperative warping?***

E. Autologous rib cartilage.

Autologous rib is the strongest cartilage source and useful when >3 mm of dorsal augmentation is required; however, warping is common and likely underreported. Suture stabilization and threading with a K-wire is recommended to help prevent movement and warping. Furthermore, it is recommended that rib cartilage sculpting be performed a minimum of 30 minutes prior to graft placement to predict warping characteristics. Septal cartilage is less prone to warping than rib cartilage. Acellular dermal matrix may be used for minimal dorsal enhancement or to camouflage underlying surface irregularities. Irradiated rib cartilage has the convenience of avoiding non-nasal donor site and is less prone to warping; however, resorption may be unpredictable.[1,2,3]

REFERENCES

1. Gruber RP, Nahai F, Bogdan MA, et al. Changing the convexity and concavity of nasal cartilages and cartilage grafts with horizontal mattress sutures: part II. Clinical results. Plast Reconstr Surg 2005;115:595
2. Byrd S, Andochick S, Copit S, et al. Septal extension grafts: a method of controlling tip projection, rotation, and shape. Plast Reconstr Surg 1997;100:999
3. Lee MJ, Song HM. Asian rhinoplasty with rib cartilage. Semin Plast Surg 2015;29(4):262–268

ANATOMY

13. ***A 30-year-old woman undergoes rhinoplasty to correct a droopy nasal tip. Which of the following suture techniques can help correct this deformity?***

D. Medial crural septal suture.

Medial crural septal sutures attach the medial crura to the septum and assist with tip positioning, columellar show, and changing the columellar and nasolabial angles. Medial crural septal sutures help to reposition the drooping nasal tip. Transdomal sutures are horizontal mattress sutures placed at the lateral and medial genu of the middle crura to help sharpen and refine the dome and can moderately increase tip projection. Interdomal sutures are placed between the domes of each lower lateral cartilage to decrease interdomal width or improve symmetry in domal height. Lateral crural mattress sutures can be used to correct lateral crural convexity.[1,2,3,4]

REFERENCES

1. Gruber RP, Friedman GD. Suture algorithm for the broad or bulbous nasal tip. Plast Reconstr Surg 2002;110:1752
2. Ghavami A, Janis JE, Acikel C, et al. Tip shaping in primary rhinoplasty: an algorithmic approach. Plast Reconstr Surg 2008;122:1229
3. Behmand RA, Ghavami A, Guyuron B. Nasal tip sutures part I: the evolution. Plast Reconstr Surg 2003;112:1125
4. Guyuron B, Behmand RA. Nasal tip sutures part II: the interplays. Plast Reconstr Surg 2003;112:1130

ANATOMY

14. *A 51-year-old male presents with a droopy and overprojected nasal tip. Which of the following maneuvers can be performed to address both of these deformities?*

E. Lateral crural resection/overlay.

The nasal tripod is defined by the medial crura and lateral crura of the paired lower lateral cartilage. Variation in the length and structural support of each of these structures influences tip position and shape. In the droopy and overprojected nasal tip, transection and overlay of the lateral crura will help cephalically rotate the nasal tip and decrease projection.[1] Lateral crural mattress sutures can be used to correct lateral crural convexity. A spring flap is an autospreader flap technique in which the cephalic margin of the upper lateral cartilage is turned in without scoring and sutured to the dorsal septum to open the internal nasal valve. Lateral crural strut grafts are secured to the undersurface of the lateral crura and are a powerful technique to inferiorly position cephalically oriented lateral crura and can extend to the piriform aperture to increase tip projection. A subdomal graft is a bar-shaped graft placed beneath the domes tocorrect domeasymmetry and a pinched nasal tip. Interdomal sutures are placement between the domes of each lower lateral cartilage to decrease interdomal width or improve symmetry in domal height (**Fig. 45.8**).

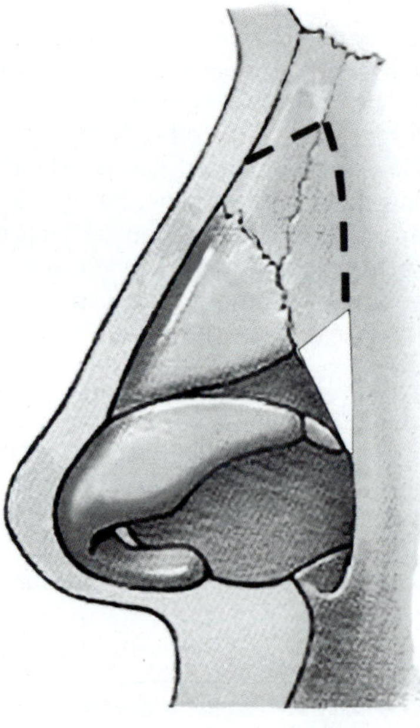

Fig. 45.8 The nasal tip "tripod concept" helps when trying to understand dynamic changes in nasal tip shape and position defined by the central medial crura and bilateral lower lateral cartilages. (Source: Background. In: Rohrich R, Adams W, Ahmad J, Gunter J, ed. Dallas Rhinoplasty: Nasal Surgery by the Masters. 3rd Edition. New York: Thieme; 2014.)

REFERENCE

1. Toriumi DM. New concepts in nasal tip contouring. Arch Facial Plast Surg 2006;8:156

ANATOMY

15. *A 19-year-old female presents for rhinoplasty with a deviated nose and an S-shaped septal deformity. Bilateral mucoperichondrial flaps are elevated and septal cartilage is harvested leaving a 12-mm L-strut. Severe convexity of the base of the caudal L-strut is observed. Which of the following maneuvers should be performed next to address this problem?*

C. Releasing the caudal septum from the anterior nasal spine and caudal septal reduction.

Caudal septal deviations should be addressed by release of the caudal septum from the anterior nasal spine. This deformity is usually associated with buckling due to excessive length of the caudal septum, which requires detachment and reduction of this excess in order to centralize and fixate the caudal septum to the anterior nasal spine.

Spreader grafts can be used to help straighten deviations of the dorsal septum. Spreader grafts do not address caudal septal deviations. Leaving a 6-mm caudal L-strut could result in nasal collapse due to insufficient support and is not recommended. Lateral crural strut grafts can be used to correct cephalically oriented lower lateral crura, alar notching, and to support the nasal tip. Neither a lateral crural strut graft nor lateral crural mattress sutures will correct a caudal septal deviation.[1,2]

REFERENCES

1. Beekhuis GJ. Nasal obstruction after rhinoplasty: etiology, and techniques for correction. Laryngoscope 1976;86:540
2. Guyuron B, Behmand RA. Caudal nasal deviation. Plast Reconstr Surg 2003;111:2449

46. Secondary Rhinoplasty

Sammy Sinno, Michael E. Nissan, Simon Moradian
See *Essentials of Aesthetic Surgery*, pp. 620–633

ENDONASAL/CLOSED APPROACH

1. ***Which of the following applies to the endonasal/closed approach in secondary rhinoplasty?***
   A. It results in increased postoperative edema and scarring.
   B. It is effective when changes to the overall framework of the nose are required.
   C. It can be used in patients with multiple prior nasal incisions.
   D. It is the preferred approach for secondary rhinoplasty, in general.
   E. It is the preferred approach for situations that require addressing multiple underlying framework issues.

EXTERNAL/OPEN APPROACH

2. ***Which of the following applies to the external/open approach to secondary rhinoplasty?***
   A. The transcolumellar incision should always be placed over the original scar.
   B. If the original transcolumellar scar is inconspicuous but incorrectly located, it should be ignored, and a new incision should be placed at the correct location.
   C. It is more difficult to achieve hemostatic control when compared with endonasal/closed rhinoplasty.
   D. External/open rhinoplasty provides limited tissue exposure.
   E. Results in decreased postoperative edema.

BODY DYSMORPHIC DISORDER

3. ***Which of the following is a consideration when treating rhinoplasty patients who have body dysmorphic disorder (BDD)?***
   A. BDD is more prevalent in secondary rhinoplasty patients than primary rhinoplasty patients.
   B. A patient who is experiencing significant stress due to a visually apparent nasal deformity after primary rhinoplasty is likely to have the diagnosis of BDD.
   C. Psychiatry consultation is rarely helpful for BDD patients.
   D. The nose is rarely the primary complaint of BDD patients.
   E. The nose is the primary complaint in 25% of BDD patients desiring secondary rhinoplasty.

ROCKER DEFORMITY

4. ***Which of the following maneuvers is most likely to result in a rocker deformity?***
   A. Inadequate placement of medial osteotomy.
   B. Overresection of dorsal midvault and upper lateral cartilages.
   C. Overresection of the noncartilaginous caudal dorsum or underresection.
   D. Underresection of the cartilaginous nasal dorsum.
   E. Disruption of lateral crural support.

INVERTED-V DEFORMITY

5. ***Which of the following maneuvers is most likely to result in an inverted-V deformity?***
   A. Inadequate alignment of bones after osteotomy.
   B. Overresection of dorsal midvault and upper lateral cartilages.
   C. Unplanned osteotomy fracture sites.
   D. Incorrect placement of transcolumellar incision.
   E. Disruption of lateral crural support.

POSTOPERATIVE DEFORMITY

6. *Overresection of the noncartilaginous caudal dorsum and underresection of the cartilaginous nasal dorsum are most likely to result in which of the following deformities?*
A. Boxy tip deformity.
B. Pinched nasal tip deformity.
C. Alar retraction.
D. Alar notching.
E. Polly beak deformity.

ALAR DEFORMITY

7. *Which of the following is crucial in understanding and assessing alar deformities?*
A. Alar rim collapse is usually caused by loss of upper lateral cartilage integrity.
B. Alar rim collapse can be assessed clinically by palpating resistance of alae to gentle compressive force.
C. Alar flaring is characterized by a narrowed base.
D. Alar notching is more likely when supporting alar grafts are used.
E. Alar rim collapse can result in impaired internal nasal valve competency.

PATIENT CONCERNS

8. *Which of the following is the most common complaint in patients presenting for revision?*
A. Nasal deviation.
B. Supratip deformity.
C. Tip deformity.
D. Alar deformity.
E. Breathing difficulty.

SURGICAL PLANNING

9. *A patient presents to the clinic 60 days after primary rhinoplasty with asymmetry concerns. When is the earliest possible time to reevaluate for revision rhinoplasty?*
A. 3 months.
B. 6 months.
C. 9 months.
D. 12 months.
E. 18 months.

EARLY INTERVENTION

10. *In the case of the presence of a gross anomaly or a surgical error, when the surgeon must intervene within?*
A. 2 days.
B. 10 days.
C. 12 days.
D. 20 days.
E. 40 days.

SUPRATIP

11. *What differential height between the tip and the septum must be present in order to have an appreciable supratip break for desirable results?*
A. 0–2 mm.
B. 2–6 mm.
C. 6–10 mm.
D. 10–12 mm.
E. 12–14 mm.

GRAFTS

12. ***A patient has a short columella but sufficient infratip volume. Which graft is most appropriate to address this deformity?***
    A. Columellar strut.
    B. Tip graft.
    C. Spreader graft.
    D. Alar spreader graft.
    E. Dorsal onlay graft.

OVERRESECTION OF DORSUM

13. ***Which of the following is most appropriate for correction of an overresected dorsum that requires little (less than 3 mm) augmentation?***
    A. Dorsal rib graft.
    B. Extended spreader grafts.
    C. Septal extension graft.
    D. Columellar strut graft.
    E. Cantilever bone graft.

ALAR RETRACTION

14. ***Alar retraction is identified in a secondary rhinoplasty patient. There is minimal vestibular lining loss and 5 mm of residual lower lateral cartilage rim. Which of the following is the most appropriate corrective maneuver?***
    A. Alar contour graft.
    B. Alar spreader graft.
    C. Lateral crural strut graft.
    D. Intercartilaginous graft.
    E. Z-plasty scar revision of the internal nasal mucosal lining.

PROSTHETIC COMPLICATIONS

15. ***A dorsal prosthetic implant becomes palpable and visible beneath the skin. What is the most appropriate corrective action?***
    A. No action is needed unless the prosthetic is extruded.
    B. External repositioning of the implant.
    C. Starting a short course of antibiotics.
    D. Removal of the implant and replacement with a new prosthetic.
    E. Removal of the implant and replacement with autologous tissue.

RIB GRAFT

16. ***Injury to the parietal pleura is identified during rib graft extraction. What is the correct course of action by the surgeon?***
    A. Consult general surgery for assistance immediately.
    B. Close the pleura and overlying tissues in layers and obtain chest radiograph postoperatively.
    C. Insert a chest tube and close the overlying layers.
    D. Place red rubber catheter into the cavity, close the incision in layers, and remove catheter with suction while providing positive pressure ventilation.
    E. Do not attempt repair but have anesthesia increase FiO_2 to 100% and obtain an upright CXR in the PACU.

Answers

ENDONASAL/CLOSED APPROACH

1. ***Which of the following applies to the endonasal/closed approach in secondary rhinoplasty?***
   C. It can be used in patients with multiple prior nasal incisions.
   There are two surgical approaches for secondary rhinoplasty: the endonasal/closed approach and the external/open approach. For secondary rhinoplasty, the external/open approach is preferred for its complete exposure of the underlying nasal framework.[1] However, the endonasal/closed approach does have some advantages, as it results in less edema and scarring due to its decreased disruption of the nasal anatomy. For this reason, it can be used to address isolated deformities that do not require changes to the overall nasal framework. Additionally, it is preferred in the case of a severely scarred nose in which additional incisions and scarring from open rhinoplasty may further compromise vasculature.[1]

REFERENCE

1. Gunter JP, Rohrich RJ. External approach for secondary rhinoplasty. Plast Reconstr Surg 1987;80:161

EXTERNAL/OPEN APPROACH

2. ***Which of the following applies to the external/open approach to secondary rhinoplasty?***
   B. If the original transcolumellar scar is inconspicuous but incorrectly located, it should be ignored, and a new incision should be placed at the correct location.
   The advantage of the external/open approach is the surgeon's ability to reflect the skin superiorly, providing increased tissue exposure, greater ability to manipulate the underlying nasal framework, and increased ease of achieving hemostasis under direct visualization. For the external/open approach, the transcolumellar incision should be strategically placed to provide adequate tissue visualization and to leave an inconspicuous scar postoperatively. In the case of a previously incorrectly placed transcolumellar scar that is well-hidden, a new incision should be placed in the correct location.[1]

REFERENCE

1. Gunter JP, Rohrich RJ. External approach for secondary rhinoplasty. Plast Reconstr Surg 1987;80:161

BODY DYSMORPHIC DISORDER

3. ***Which of the following is a consideration when treating rhinoplasty patients who have body dysmorphic disorder (BDD)?***
   A. BDD is more prevalent in secondary rhinoplasty patients than primary rhinoplasty patients.
   Surgeons should screen for BDD in all patients prior to operation, particularly for secondary rhinoplasty; incidence of BDD is 12% (not 25%) for secondary rhinoplasty and 2 to 7% for primary cosmetic consultations. In half of patients with BDD, the nose is the primary concern.[1,2] Reoperation should be avoided in cases of BDD, and psychiatry consult can help to improve the condition. The condition is characterized by an extreme preoccupation with an imagined or minor physical deformity. In the case of a patient experiencing significant stress due to a visually apparent nasal deformity, BDD is not a likely diagnosis because the deformity is significant enough to be visible.

REFERENCES

1. Constantian MB. Identify BDD patients prior to rhinoplasty. Cosmetic Surgery Times, June 2001
2. Constantian MB. Emotional matters. Presented at the Rhinoplasty Symposium at the Annual Meeting of the American Society for Aesthetic Plastic Surgery, New York, April 2007

ROCKER DEFORMITY

4. *Which of the following maneuvers is most likely to result in a rocker deformity?*

A. Inadequate placement of medial osteotomy.

Rocker deformity is a defect in the nasal bony pyramid, resulting from inadequate placement of medial osteotomy. The result is a wide upper dorsum due to the incorrectly placed nasal bone fracture (**Fig. 46.1**). Overresection of the dorsal midvault and upper lateral cartilages may result in an inverted-V deformity. Overresection of the noncartilagenous caudal dorsum or undersection may result in a polly beak deformity. Underresection of the cartilaginous nasal dorsum may result in a persistent dorsal hump or contour irregularity. Disruption of the lateral crural support may result in a pinched nasal deformity.[1,2,3]

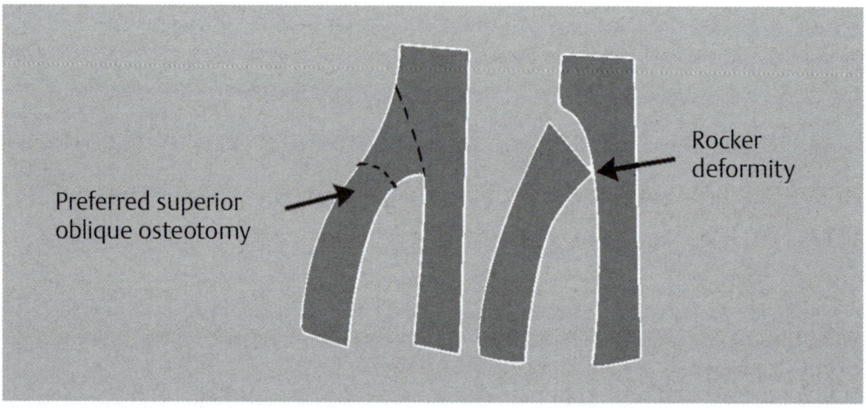

Fig. 46.1 Rocker deformity. (Source: Medial Osteotomies. In: Rohrich R, Adams W, Ahmad J, Gunter J, ed. Dallas Rhinoplasty: Nasal Surgery by the Masters. 3rd Edition. New York: Thieme; 2014.)

REFERENCES

1. Byrd HS, Constantian MB, Guyuron B, et al. Revision rhinoplasty. Aesthet Surg J 2007;27:175
2. Gunter JP, Rohrich RJ. External approach for secondary rhinoplasty. Plast Reconstr Surg 1987;80:161
3. Constantian MB. The two essential elements for planning tip surgery in primary and secondary rhinoplasty: observations based on review of 100 consecutive patients. Plast Reconstr Surg 2004;114:1571; discussion 1582

INVERTED-V DEFORMITY

5. *Which of the following maneuvers is most likely to result in an inverted-V deformity?*

B. Overresection of dorsal midvault and upper lateral cartilages.

Inverted-V deformity is a defect in the nasal midvault, in which collapse of the midvault causes visibility of the caudal edge of the nasal bones, forming an upside-down V (**Fig. 46.2**). This is a result of overresection of the dorsal midvault and upper lateral cartilages or inadequate infracture of the nasal bones. Inadequate alignment of bones or unplanned osteotomy fracture sites after osteotomy may result in an unfavorable narrowing or convexity, irregularity, step off, or rocker deformity. Disruption of the lateral crural support system may result in a pinched nasal deformity due to collapsed alar rims.[1,2,3]

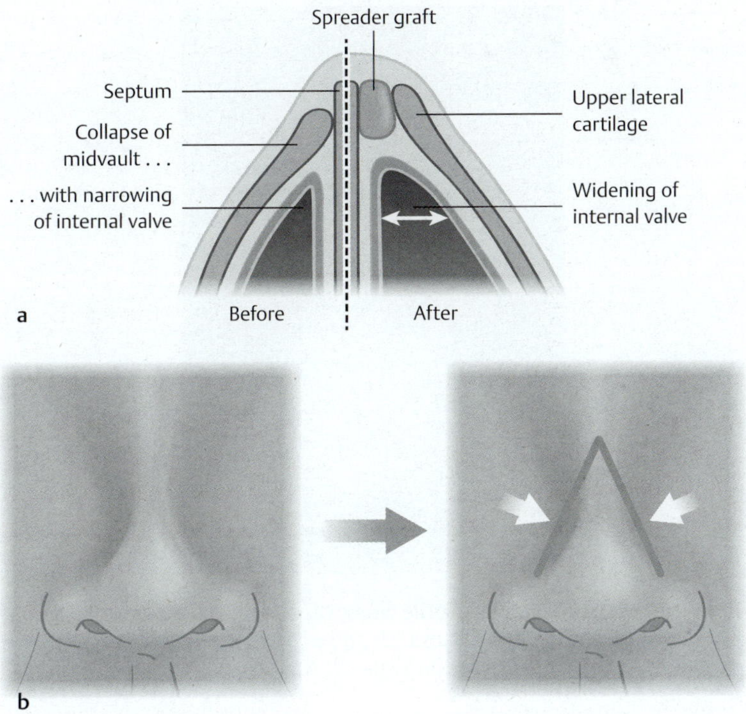

Fig. 46.2 (a,b) Inverted-V deformity. (Source: Comprehensive Nasal and Facial Analysis. In: Janis J, ed. Essentials of Aesthetic Surgery. 1st Edition. New York: Thieme; 2018.)

REFERENCES

1. Byrd HS, Constantian MB, Guyuron B, et al. Revision rhinoplasty. Aesthet Surg J 2007;27:175
2. Gunter JP, Rohrich RJ. External approach for secondary rhinoplasty. Plast Reconstr Surg 1987;80:161
3. Constantian MB. The two essential elements for planning tip surgery in primary and secondary rhinoplasty: observations based on review of 100 consecutive patients. Plast Reconstr Surg 2004;114:1571; discussion 1582

POSTOPERATIVE DEFORMITY

6. ***Overresection of the noncartilaginous caudal dorsum and underresection of the cartilaginous nasal dorsum are most likely to result in which of the following deformities?***

   E. Polly beak deformity.

   Polly beak deformity, a supratip deformity, is a convexity located just superior to the nasal tip (**Fig. 46.3**). It is a result of overresection of the caudal nasal dorsum.[1] Prevention of polly beak deformity postoperatively involves vigorous taping of the supratip area and triamcinolone injections deep into the supratip if taping alone does not prevent the deformity. Boxy tip deformity may be a result of an inadequate cephalic trim of the lower lateral cartilages (LLCs). Pinched nasal deformity results from disruption of the lateral crural support after collapse of the alar rims. Alar notching is a resultof inadequate placement or closure of previous incisions, scarring, and failure of supporting grafts. Alar retraction may result from a widened alar base.

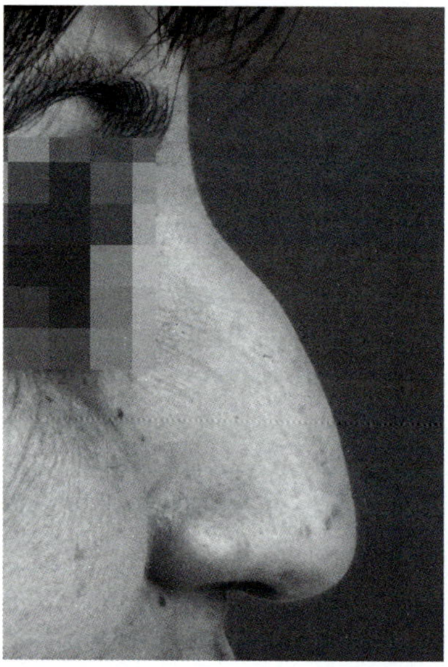

Fig. 46.3 Polly beak deformity. Postoperative profile view of a secondary rhinoplasty patient with a supratip deformity caused by both an underprojected tip and an underresected caudal dorsum. (Source: Case Analysis. In: Rohrich R, Adams W, Ahmad J, Gunter J, ed. Dallas Rhinoplasty: Nasal Surgery by the Masters. 3rd Edition. New York: Thieme; 2014.)

Reference

1. Guyuron B, DeLuca L, Lash R. Supratip deformity: a closer look. Plast Reconstr Surg 2000;105:1140

ALAR DEFORMITY

7. *Which of the following is crucial in understanding and assessing alar deformities?*

B. Alar rim collapse can be assessed clinically by palpating resistance of alae to gentle compressive force.

Alar rim collapse is a deformity in the caudal nose caused by loss of integrity of the lower lateral cartilages (**Fig. 46.4**). The degree of alar rim collapse may not be evident by visual inspection alone—for this reason, it is important to clinically assess the degree of alar collapse by applying gentle compressive force to the alae when palpating. This will reveal the degree of alar collapse or potential alar collapse. Other alar deformities include alar flaring, which is characterized by a widened base, and alar notching, which is caused by inadequate placement or closure of incisions or failure to place supporting grafts. Treatment for alar notching often involves placement of an alar rim graft. Additionally, alar rim collapse can result in impaired external nasal valve competency.[1,2]

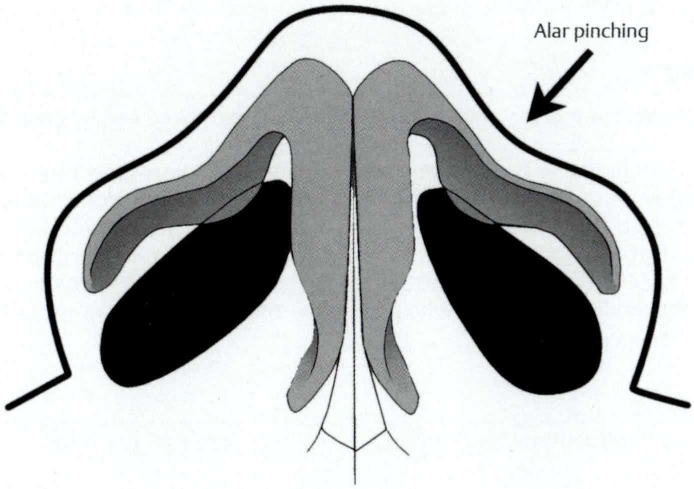

Fig. 46.4 Alar rim collapse. Alar rim collapse caused by lack of lower lateral cartilage support. (Source: Anatomy. In: Rohrich R, Adams W, Ahmad J, Gunter J, ed. Dallas Rhinoplasty: Nasal Surgery by the Masters. 3rd Edition. New York: Thieme; 2014.)

REFERENCES

1. Constantian MB. The boxy nasal tip, the ball tip, and alar cartilage malposition: variations on a theme—a study in 200 consecutive primary and secondary rhinoplasty patients. Plast Reconstr Surg 2005;116:268
2. Constantian MB.The two essential elements for planning tip surgery in primary and secondary rhinoplasty: observations based on review of 100 consecutive patients. Plast Reconstr Surg 2004;114:1571; discussion 1582

PATIENT CONCERNS

8. *Which of the following is the most common complaint in patients presenting for revision?*

E. Breathing difficulty.

Breathing difficulty and asymmetry are the most common complaints of patients presenting for secondary rhinoplasty. A retrospective analysis of 100 secondary rhinoplasty patients showed that 65% of patients complained of breathing difficulties and 33% complained of nasal asymmetry.[1] However, airway occlusion is the most common underdiagnosed and untreated deformity in secondary rhinoplasty. For this reason, it is important for the surgeon to remain vigilant to preserve or improve the function of the nose while enhancing its aesthetics.

REFERENCE

1. Lee M, Zwiebel S, Guyuron B. Frequency of the preoperative flaws and commonly required maneuvers to correct them: a guide to reducing the revision rhinoplasty rate. Plast Reconstr Surg 2013;132:769

SURGICAL PLANNING

9. *A patient presents to the clinic 60 days after primary rhinoplasty with asymmetry concerns. When is the earliest possible time to reevaluate for revision rhinoplasty?*

D. 12 months.

Any secondary surgery must be delayed for at least 12 months. This ensures maximal resolution of edema, scar maturation, and improved vascularity. It is important to explain to the patient that even 60 days after surgery the nose has not yet reached its final appearance and asymmetry concerns at this time may be due to residual edema that cannot be fully assessed until 1 year has passed.[1,2]

REFERENCES

1. Guyuron B, Bokhari F. Patient satisfaction following rhinoplasty. Aesthetic Plast Surg 1996;20:153

2. Lee M, Zwiebel S, Guyuron B. Frequency of the preoperative flaws and commonly required maneuvers to correct them: a guide to reducing the revision rhinoplasty rate. Plast Reconstr Surg 2013;132:769

EARLY INTERVENTION

10. *In the case of the presence of a gross anomaly or a surgical error, when the surgeon must intervene within?*

C. 12 days.

Generally, revision rhinoplasty is not performed until at least 1 year after primary rhinoplasty. However, there are a few exceptions to this rule: (1) grossly suboptimal nasal appearance that was not apparent at the time of surgery, (2) significant malposition of parts of the nose, such as a graft shift, and (3) recognition that an important surgical maneuver was not performed.[1] Early intervention within 12 days is important in these cases in order to remediate the error before the nasal tissues become adherent and difficult to reposition. This also benefits patients, who are spared the anxiety of waiting 12 months with a suboptimal primary rhinoplasty result.

REFERENCE

1. Gruber RP. Early surgical intervention after rhinoplasty. Aesthet Surg J 2001;21:549

SUPRATIP

11. *What differential height between the tip and the septum must be present in order to have an appreciable supratip break for desirable results?*

C. 6–10 mm.

Patients with weak nasal cartilages are prone to supratip deformities, including weak midvault and plunging tip with polly beak deformity. A study of 20 patients showed that control of the position of the nasal tip relative to the nasal dorsum can be achieved by septal extension grafts, which helped to maintain tip projection in all but one of the patients.[1]

REFERENCE

1. Byrd HS, Andochick S, Copit S, et al. Septal extension grafts: a method of controlling tip projection shape. Plast Reconstr Surg 1997;100:999

GRAFTS

12. *A patient has a short columella but sufficient infratip volume. Which graft is most appropriate to address this deformity?*

A. Columellar strut.

A columellar strut is used when the columella is short. Tip grafts are used when infratip volume is deficient. Spreader grafts maintain septal alignment, support the upper lateral cartilages, and support the internal nasal valve. Alar spreader grafts can be used to repair a pinched-appearing tip. Dorsal onlay grafts may be used for improved dorsal contour.[1,2]

REFERENCES

1. Constantian MB. The boxy nasal tip, the ball tip, and alar cartilage malposition: variations on a theme—a study in 200 consecutive primary and secondary rhinoplasty patients. Plast Reconstr Surg 2005;116:268
2. Byrd HS, Constantian MB, Guyuron B, et al. Revision rhinoplasty. Aesthet Surg J 2007;27:175

OVERRESECTION OF DORSUM

13. *Which of the following is most appropriate for correction of an overresected dorsum that requires little (less than 3 mm) augmentation?*

B. Extended spreader grafts.

Extensive overresection of the nasal dorsum can result in saddle nose or inverted-V deformity. However, when there is only minor overresection requiring less than 3 mm of augmentation, correction can be achieved with extended spreader grafts. Dorsal rib grafts and cantilever bone grafts are reserved for the nasal dorsum that requires more extensive augmentation. The columellar strut graft corrects a short columella—it has no role in augmentation of the nasal dorsum.[1,2]

References

1. Gunter JP, Rohrich RJ. External approach for secondary rhinoplasty. Plast Reconstr Surg 1987;80:161
2. Constantian MB. Four common anatomic variants that predispose to unfavorable rhinoplasty results: a study based on 150 consecutive secondary rhinoplasties. Plast Reconstr Surg 2005;105:316; discussion 332

ALAR RETRACTION

14. *Alar retraction is identified in a secondary rhinoplasty patient. There is minimal vestibular lining loss and 5 mm of residual lower lateral cartilage rim. Which of the following is the most appropriate corrective maneuver?*

A. Alar contour graft.

The deformity described is mild alar retraction, which is characterized by minimal vestibular lining loss and at least 3 mm of residual lower lateral cartilage rim. Mild alar retraction is an indication for an alar contour graft, which reestablishes a functional external nasal valve and an aesthetically desirable alar contour (**Fig. 46.5**).[1] Although a Z-plasty of the internal nasal mucosal lining may help in a more appropriate redistribution of forces, this alone would be unlikely to correct this deformity. Alar spreader grafts and lateral crural strut grafts are used for moderate alar retraction for patients with increased lining loss or scarring.[2] Intercartilaginous grafts are used to span the space between the upper and lower lateral cartilages when there is even more significant skin or lining deficiency (**Fig. 46.6**).[3]

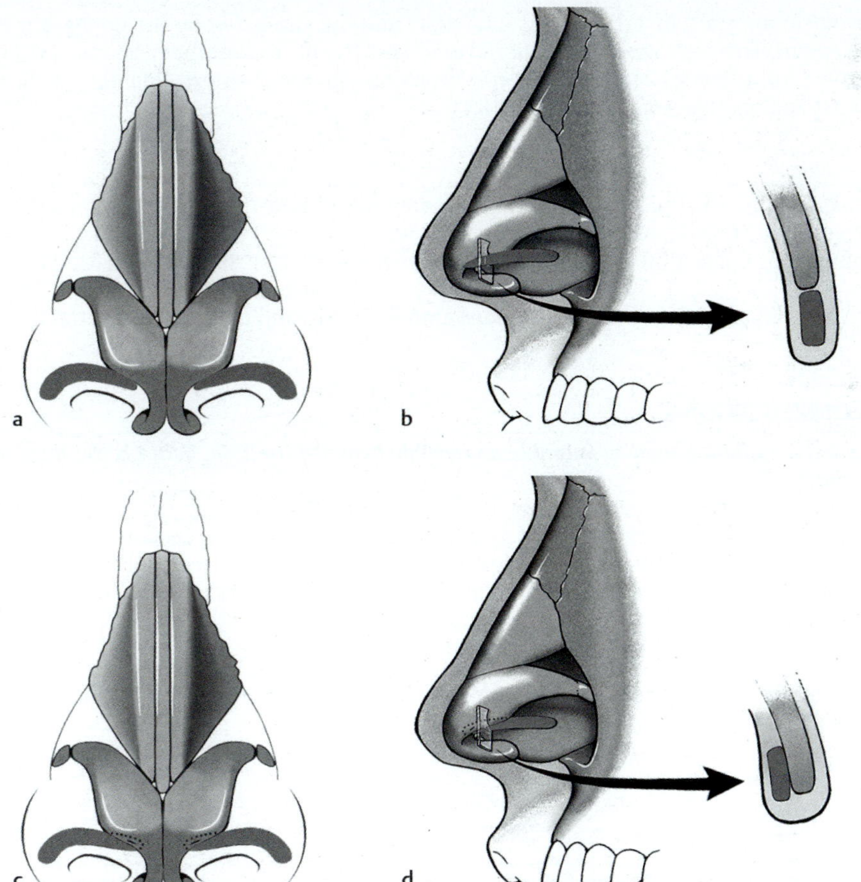

Fig. 46.5 (a–d) Alar contour graft. A key element is proper placement and shape of the alar contour graft immediately above the alar rim and spanning the alar notched area. (Source: Alar Contour Graft. In: Rohrich R, Adams W, Ahmad J, Gunter J, ed. Dallas Rhinoplasty: Nasal Surgery by the Masters. 3rd Edition. New York: Thieme; 2014.)

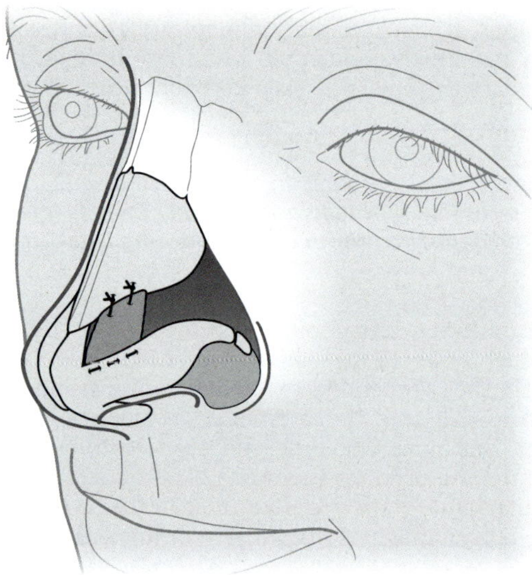

Fig. 46.6 Intercartilaginous graft. Insertion of a septal graft into the gap between the upper lateral cartilage and the lateral crus element. The cephalic end of it is sutured end-to-end to the upper lateral cartilage. The caudal end slips under (deep to) the edge of the lateral crus element. (Source: Overresection. In: Janis J, ed. Essentials of Aesthetic Surgery. 1st Edition. New York: Thieme; 2018.)

References

1. Rohrich RJ, Raniere J Jr, Ha RY. The alar contour graft: correction and prevention of alar rim deformities in rhinoplasty. Plast Reconstr Surg 2002;109:2495; discussion 2506
2. Gunter JP, Rohrich RJ. Correction of the pinched nasal tip with alar spreader grafts. Plast Reconstr Surg 1992;90:821
3. Gruber RP, Kryger G, Chang D. The intercartilaginous graft for actual and potential alar retraction. Plast Reconstr Surg 2008;121:288e

PROSTHETIC COMPLICATIONS

15. *A dorsal prosthetic implant becomes palpable and visible beneath the skin. What is the most appropriate corrective action?*

D. Removal of the implant and replacement with a new prosthetic.

When prosthetic implants become extruded, palpable, or visible, there is increased risk of infection even if the skin remains intact. For this reason, they must be removed and replaced with autologous tissue, which carries a lower risk of infection. There is no indication in the case described above to start antibiotics.[1,2]

References

1. Gryskiewicz JM, Rohrich RJ, Reagan BJ. The use of AlloDerm for the correction of nasal contour deformities. Plast Reconstr Surg 2001;107:561; discussion 571
2. Cochran CS, Gunter JP. Secondary rhinoplasty and the use of autogenous rib cartilage grafts. Clin Plast Surg 2010;37:371

RIB GRAFT

16. *Injury to the parietal pleura is identified during rib graft extraction. What is the correct course of action by the surgeon?*

D. Place red rubber catheter into the cavity, close the incision in layers, and remove catheter with suction while providing positive pressure ventilation.

Collection of rib graft carries the risk of pneumothorax, as the parietal pleura lies just beneath the ribs and is prone to injury when the overlying rib is extracted. In the case of injury to the parietal pleura, a red rubber catheter should be placed into the pleural cavity, the incision should be closed in layers, and the catheter should be removed with suction while positive pressure ventilation is provided. This should be followed by a chest radiograph postoperatively to monitor for pneumothorax.[1]

Reference

1. Marin VP, Landecker A, Gunter JP. Harvesting rib cartilage grafts for secondary rhinoplasty. Plast Reconstr Surg 2008;121:1442

47. Ethnic Rhinoplasty

Anup Patel, Simon Moradian
See *Essentials of Aesthetic Surgery*, pp. 634–644

PREOPERATIVE PLANNING

1. ***To ensure patient satisfaction following ethnic cosmetic rhinoplasty, which of the following must be routinely addressed during the preoperative evaluation?***
   A. Payment plans.
   B. Skip over sensitive history such as previous facial trauma or prior nasal/sinus surgery.
   C. CT of the head looking for any abnormalities.
   D. Rhinometry results.
   E. Determine whether the goal is for Westernization of features versus maintenance of natural characteristics.

PREOPERATIVE PLANNING

2. ***What tool should surgeons use to demonstrate potential changes preoperatively that can help patients comment on desired modifications, and allow the surgeon to better understand the patient's goals and desires?***
   A. CT head.
   B. Digital image-morphing software.
   C. Pencil/paper sketches.
   D. Clay carvings.
   E. Rhinometry.

ETHNIC ANATOMIC PRINCIPLES

3. ***What are anatomic variations in ethnic patients when compared to Western patients?***
   A. Skin is usually thicker, more sebaceous, and relatively inelastic in ethnic patients.
   B. The fibrofatty layer is thinner and less prominent over the lower lateral cartilages and between the medial crura.
   C. Alar base usually has a decreased base width with insertion lateral to the medial canthal lines. There is minimal flaring where the alae extend less than 1 mm lateral to the alar facial grove.
   D. The soft tissue facet between the medial crura and lower lateral cartilages is often acute and has minimal fat.
   E. The fibrofatty layer does not contribute to the tip definition.

ETHNIC ANATOMIC PRINCIPLES

4. ***Which of the following is characteristic of a Black nose?***
   A. Short nasal bones, wide nose, low dorsum, wide bimalar distance, horizontally oriented nostrils, deficient premaxilla, limited septal cartilage.
   B. Thick sebaceous skin, low dorsum, weak lower lateral cartilage, less septal cartilage, deficient premaxilla, wide nasal base, and retracted columella.
   C. Long nasal bones, low radix, large hump, hanging columella, septal deviation.
   D. Long nasal bones, low dorsum, narrow nose.
   E. Low radix height, near-normal bridge, dependent tip.

ETHNIC ANATOMIC PRINCIPLES

5. *Which of the following is characteristic of an Asian nose?*

A. Short nasal bones, wide nose, low dorsum, wide bimalar distance, horizontally oriented nostrils, deficient premaxilla, limited septal cartilage.
B. Thick sebaceous skin, low dorsum, weak lower lateral cartilage, less septal cartilage, deficient premaxilla, wide nasal base, and retracted columella.
C. Long nasal bones, low radix, large hump, hanging columella, septal deviation.
D. Low radix height, near-normal bridge, dependent tip.
E. High radix, near-normal bridge, dependent tip.

ETHNIC ANATOMIC PRINCIPLES

6. *Which of the following is characteristic of a Middle Eastern nose?*

A. Short nasal bones, wide nose, low dorsum, wide bimalar distance, horizontally oriented nostrils, deficient premaxilla, limited septal cartilage.
B. Thick sebaceous skin, low dorsum, weak lower lateral cartilage, less septal cartilage, deficient premaxilla, wide nasal base, and retracted columella.
C. Long nasal bones, low radix, large hump, hanging columella, septal deviation.
D. Low radix height, near-normal bridge, dependent tip.
E. Thick sebaceous skin, low dorsum, weak lower lateral cartilage, wide nasal base.

ETHNIC ANATOMIC PRINCIPLES

7. *Which of the following is characteristic of a type II (Mexican American) nose?*

A. Short nasal bones, wide nose, low dorsum, wide bimalar distance, horizontally oriented nostrils, deficient premaxilla, limited septal cartilage.
B. Thick sebaceous skin, low dorsum, weak lower lateral cartilage, less septal cartilage, deficient premaxilla, wide nasal base, retracted columella.
C. Long nasal bones, low radix, large hump, hanging columella, septal deviation.
D. Low radix height, near-normal bridge, dependent tip.
E. Long nasal bones, low dorsum, deficient premaxilla, septal deviation, horizontally oriented nostrils, wide nasal base.

ANATOMIC PRINCIPLES/PREOPERATIVE PLANNING

8. *Which of the following is an advantage to using costal cartilage as grafting material?*

A. Overall infection risk of 5%.
B. Grafts tend to be straighter compared to septal grafts.
C. Higher vascular demand making it less likely to resorb.
D. Low donor site morbidity.
E. Lower vascular demand making it less likely to resorb.

PREOPERATIVE PLANNING

9. *Which of the following is an advantage of using allografts such as silicone, ePTFE, and porous polyethylene?*

A. Decreased lifetime risk of infection.
B. No additional surgical site, and minimal change in operative time.
C. Decreased lifetime risk of extrusion.
D. Less prolonged edema after implantation.
E. Less nasal stiffness after structural grafting.

PERIOPERATIVE CONSIDERATIONS

10. *Which of the following is correct regarding injecting local anesthetic before prepping and draping?*

A. It allows ample time for vasodilation.
B. Injection can create hydrostatic dissection for ease of elevation of mucoperichondrial flaps.
C. 2% lidocaine without epinephrine is preferred.
D. 2% Marcaine with epinephrine is preferred.
E. An infraorbital block (V2) is preferred.

ANATOMIC PRINCIPLES/PREOPERATIVE PLANNING

11. *Which of the following is true when harvesting auricular cartilage?*
A. Infection prophylaxis is not required if auricular cartilage is to be harvested.
B. It takes longer to harvest than costal cartilage.
C. Infection prophylaxis is required if auricular cartilage is to be harvested.
D. If auricular cartilage is to be harvested, the surgeon does not have to change gloves to prevent contamination.
E. Auricular cartilage has a lower vascular demand when compared to costal cartilage.

PREOPERATIVE PLANNING/PERIOPERATIVE CONSIDERATIONS

12. *What is the benefit of sharp dissection while opening the nose?*
A. A large, loose subperiosteal pocket is created in anticipation of a secure dorsal augmentation graft.
B. Helps preserve the subdermal plexus and prevent excessive swelling.
C. Helps preserve the columellar artery.
D. Minimizes destabilization of septal cartilage.
E. Minimizes intraoperative blood loss.

ANATOMIC PRINCIPLES/PERIOPERATIVE CONSIDERATIONS

13. *Why is it important to avoid injury to soft tissue triangles during tip exposure?*
A. They are likely to cause excessive intraoperative bleeding.
B. They contain the neurovascular bundle.
C. Injury can lead to destabilization of the junction between the upper and lower cartilages.
D. They are extremely difficult to repair.
E. They protect and support the lower lateral cartilages.

ANATOMIC PRINCIPLES/PERIOPERATIVE CONSIDERATIONS

14. *When harvesting septal cartilage after the upper third of the nose is addressed to prevent destabilization, how much cartilaginous L-strut should be preserved to ensure adequate support?*
A. 2.5 mm.
B. 5 mm.
C. 10 mm.
D. 15 mm.
E. 20 mm.

ANATOMIC PRINCIPLES/PERIOPERATIVE CONSIDERATIONS

15. *What is true when performing an osteotomy?*
A. They are performed from lateral to medial.
B. They should be performed if using a large dorsal graft greater than 3.5 mm in height.
C. They are used to narrow the dorsum or correct deviations or dorsal hump.
D. They should only be performed in revision rhinoplasty.
E. They should only be used in primary rhinoplasty.

ANATOMIC PRINCIPLES/PERIOPERATIVE CONSIDERATIONS

16. *Which of the following is a benefit of using spreader grafts?*
A. They allow for retraction of the columella.
B. Unilateral placement of a spread graft is used to add curvature to the nose.
C. They increase the area of the internal nasal valve and provide foundation to prevent saddling.
D. They are used to decrease the internal nasal valve angle.
E. They are primarily used to help correct septal deviation.

OPERATIVE TECHNIQUE

17. *What technique is used to reset the caudal septum to midline?*
A. With a swinging-door maneuver or by shifting the nasal spine.
B. By placing 4–0 Silk sutures in the columella, and using as a lever to shift the spine.
C. By placing a curved caudal septal extension graft.
D. Costal cartilage is preferred to septal cartilage for caudal septal extension grafts as it is straighter.
E. Placement of spreader grafts.

OPERATIVE TECHNIQUE

18. ***Which of the following is an appropriate technique for tip contouring?***
A. Tip onlay grafts are used when no change to the infratip is needed.
B. A shield graft is used to decrease tip projection in thin-skinned patients.
C. Lateral crural strut grafts are used to enhance convexity.
D. Tip bulbosity can be corrected through the use of alar batten grafts.
E. Malpositioned lateral crura and alar retraction are corrected through repositioning of asymmetrical or caudally oriented lateral crura.

PREOPERATIVE PLANNING/ETHNIC ANATOMIC PRINCIPLES

19. ***Which of the following is a good example of why an individualized approach is crucial to tip management in ethnic patients?***
A. Repositioning of the lateral crus may be effective for flared nostrils caused by the large convex lower lateral cartilages common to Middle Eastern patients.
B. Repositioning of the lateral crus may be effective for flared nostrils caused by the large convex lower lateral cartilages common to Asian patients.
C. Repositioning of the lateral crus may worsen the appearance of flared nostrils caused by large convex lower lateral cartilages seen in Middle Eastern patients that commonly have weak lower lateral cartilages and hanging alar lobules.
D. Repositioning of the lateral crus may be effective for narrowed nostrils caused by the large convex lower lateral cartilages common to African American patients.
E. Repositioning of the lateral crus may worsen the appearance of flared nostrils caused by large convex lower lateral cartilages commonly seen in Mexican American patients.

PERIOPERATIVE CONSIDERATIONS/ETHNIC ANATOMIC PRINCIPLES

20. ***Which of the following is an important principle to keep in mind when closing darker-skinned patients?***
A. Absorbable sutures are most appropriate as they will minimize swelling, erythema, and scarring.
B. Nonabsorbable sutures are not appropriate as they will result in prolonged swelling, erythema, and possible suture tracking when compared to absorbable sutures.
C. The use of absorbable sutures will result in prolonged erythema and possible suture tracking.
D. Chromic gut sutures are the most appropriate sutures for closing dark-skinned patients as it minimizes inflammation, erythema, and possible suture tracking.
E. Plain gut sutures will result in minimal inflammation, erythema, and possible suture tracking.

PERIOPERATIVE CONSIDERATIONS

21. ***Radiopaque 0.25-mm septal splints are placed if turbinate work is performed to prevent what potential postoperative complication?***
A. Hematoma.
B. Infection.
C. Empty nose syndrome.
D. Synechiae formation.
E. Suture breakdown.

PERIOPERATIVE CONSIDERATIONS

22. ***When are lateral wall splints appropriate?***
A. If turbinate work is performed.
B. If lateral crural strut grafts were used.
C. If auricular grafts were exclusively used.
D. If a radix graft is placed.
E. If the patient has any previous history of facial trauma.

OPERATIVE TECHNIQUE

23. ***Which is a key to successful base reduction?***
A. The use of cautery.
B. Injecting local anesthetic prior to base reduction.
C. Taping of nose postoperatively to guide remolding.
D. Perpendicular incision to discourage eversion of skin edges.
E. Plan incision slightly adjacent to alar/facial or alar/vestibular junction.

POSTOPERATIVE CARE

24. *Which of the following is an effective strategy to avoid complications following rhinoplasty?*

A. Infection is managed aggressively with the patients returning to OR for a washout and drain placement along with broad spectrum antibiotic coverage.
B. Dermal sutures are not recommended for the columellar incision as they increase scar width.
C. Visible grafts and warping should not be managed during the initial procedure—they should be returned to the OR in 3 to 4 months.
D. Local anesthetic reduces the incidence of keloid formation following rhinoplasty.
E. Any base reduction should be performed prior to complete closure.

Answers

PREOPERATIVE PLANNING

1. ***To ensure patient satisfaction following ethnic cosmetic rhinoplasty, which of the following must be routinely addressed during the preoperative evaluation?***

   E. Determine whether the goal is for Westernization of features versus maintenance of natural characteristics.

   Patient consultation should include discussion of aesthetic preferences and cultural concerns. Patient expectations and preferences should be assessed, and the surgeon should determine whether the goal is for Westernization of features versus maintenance of natural characteristics. Problem-specific surgical history must be obtained as history may greatly alter surgical plan. Palpation of the cartilaginous and bony structures should also be performed.[1,2,3,4,5]

REFERENCES

1. Toriumi DM, Pero CD. Asian rhinoplasty. Clin Plast Surg 2010;37:335
2. Rohrich RJ, Muzaffar AR. Rhinoplasty in the African-American patient. Plast Reconstr Surg 2013;111:1322; discussion 1340
3. Kontis TC, Papel ID. Rhinoplasty on the African-American nose. Aesthetic Plast Surg 2002;26(Suppl1):S12
4. Rohrich RJ, Ghavami A. Rhinoplasty for Middle Eastern noses. Plast Reconstr Surg 2009;123:1343
5. Bizrah MB. Rhinoplasty for Middle Eastern patients. Facial Plast Surg Clin North Am 2002;10:381

PREOPERATIVE PLANNING

2. ***What tool should surgeons use to demonstrate potential changes preoperatively that can help patients comment on desired modifications, and allow the surgeon to better understand the patient's goals and desires?***

   B. Digital image-morphing software.

   Three-dimensional stereophotogrammetry facilitates objective comparison of preoperative and postoperative results. Digital image-morphing software allows direct communication of proposed changes to all parameters (dorsal height, nasal length, tip rotation/projection, and base width). Patients may comment on desired modifications based on the morphed image. The use of a computer-imaging program can demonstrate potential changes preoperatively and aid in communication between patients and surgeons regarding expectations and possible outcomes.[1,2,3]

REFERENCES

1. Afrooz PN, Amirlak B. Digital imaging and standardized photography. In: Rohrich RJ, Adams WP Jr, Gunter JP, eds. Dallas Rhinoplasty: Nasal Surgery by the Masters. 3rd ed. New York: Thieme Publishers; 2014
2. Dixon TK, Caughlin BP, Manaretto N, Toriumi DM. Three-dimensional evaluation of unilateral cleft rhinoplasty results. Facial Plast Surg 2013;29:106
3. Toriumi DM, Dixon TK. Assessment of rhinoplasty techniques by overlay of before-and-after 3D images. Facial Plast Surg Clin North Am 2011;19:711

ETHNIC ANATOMIC PRINCIPLES

3. ***What are anatomic variations in ethnic patients when compared to Western patients?***

   A. Skin is usually thicker, more sebaceous, and relatively inelastic in ethnic patients.

   Ethnic patients generally have thicker skin that is more sebaceous and relatively inelastic when compared to their Western counterparts. The fibrofatty layer is also thicker (2–4 mm) and more prominent over the lower lateral cartilages and between the medial crura. It plays a significant role in lack of tip definition. Alar base usually has an increased base width with insertion lateral to the medial canthal lines. There is excess flaring where the alae extend more than 2 mm lateral to the alar facial groove. Additionally, the soft tissue facet between the medial crura and the lower lateral cartilages is obtuse and filled with fat.[1,2,3,4,5]

REFERENCES

1. Rohrich RJ, Muzaffar AR. Rhinoplasty in the African-American patient. Plast Reconstr Surg 2013;111:1322; discussion 1340

2. Kontis TC, Papel ID. Rhinoplasty on the African-American nose. Aesthetic Plast Surg 2002;26(Suppl1):S12
3. Rohrich RJ, Ghavami A. Rhinoplasty for Middle Eastern noses. Plast Reconstr Surg 2009;123:1343
4. Bizrah MB. Rhinoplasty for Middle Eastern patients. Facial Plast Surg Clin North Am 2002;10:381
5. Beheri GE. Rhinoplasty in Egyptians. Aesthetic Plast Surg 1984;8:145

ETHNIC ANATOMIC PRINCIPLES

4. *Which of the following is characteristic of a Black nose?*

A. Short nasal bones, wide nose, low dorsum, wide bimalar distance, horizontally oriented nostrils, deficient premaxilla, limited septal cartilage.

The Black nose is characterized by short nasal bones, wide nose, low dorsum, wide bimalar distance, horizontally oriented nostrils, deficient premaxilla, limited septal cartilage (**Table 47.1**).[1]

Table 47.1 *Specific Ethnic Characteristics*

Ethnicity	Characteristics
Black nose	Short nasal bones
	Wide nose
	Low dorsum
	Wide bimalar distance
	Horizontally oriented nostrils, wide base
	Deficient premaxilla
	Limited septal cartilage
Asian nose	Thick sebaceous skin
	Low dorsum
	Weak lower lateral cartilage
	Less septal cartilage
	Deficient premaxilla
	Wide nasal base
	Retracted columella
Middle Eastern nose	Long nasal bones
	Low radix
	Large hump
	Hanging columella
	Septal deviation
Hispanic nose (types described by Daniel[1])	**Type I (Castilian):** Normal radix height, high bridge, normal tip projection
	Type II (Mexican American)—most common: Low radix height, near-normal bridge, dependent tip
	Type III (Mestizo): Broad base, thick skin, wide tip
	Type IV (Creole)—predominantly black features: Broad, flat lower third, short columella, transversely oriented nostrils, flaring alae

REFERENCE

1. Daniel RK. Hispanic rhinoplasty in the United States, with emphasis on the Mexican American nose. Plast Reconstr Surg 2003;112:244; discussion 257

ETHNIC ANATOMIC PRINCIPLES

5. *Which of the following is characteristic of an Asian nose?*

B. Thick sebaceous skin, low dorsum, weak lower lateral cartilage, less septal cartilage, deficient premaxilla, wide nasal base, and retracted columella.

The Asian nose is characterized by thick sebaceous skin, low dorsum, weak lower lateral cartilage, less septal cartilage, deficient premaxilla, wide nasal base, and retracted columella (**Table 47.2**).[1,2,3]

Table 47.2 *Specific Ethnic Characteristics*

Ethnicity	Characteristics
Black nose	Short nasal bones
	Wide nose
	Low dorsum
	Wide bimalar distance
	Horizontally oriented nostrils, wide base
	Deficient premaxilla
	Limited septal cartilage
Asian nose	Thick sebaceous skin
	Low dorsum
	Weak lower lateral cartilage
	Less septal cartilage
	Deficient premaxilla
	Wide nasal base
	Retracted columella
Middle Eastern nose	Long nasal bones
	Low radix
	Large hump
	Hanging columella
	Septal deviation
Hispanic nose (types described by Daniel[1])	**Type I (Castilian):** Normal radix height, high bridge, normal tip projection
	Type II (Mexican American)—most common: Low radix height, near-normal bridge, dependent tip
	Type III (Mestizo): Broad base, thick skin, wide tip
	Type IV (Creole)—predominantly black features: Broad, flat lower third, short columella, transversely oriented nostrils, flaring alae

REFERENCES

1. Daniel RK. Hispanic rhinoplasty in the United States, with emphasis on the Mexican American nose. Plast Reconstr Surg 2003;112:244; discussion 257
2. Rohrich RJ, Muzaffar AR. Rhinoplasty in the African-American patient. Plast Reconstr Surg 2013;111:1322; discussion 1340
3. Kontis TC, Papel ID. Rhinoplasty on the African-American nose. Aesthetic Plast Surg 2002;26(Suppl 1):S12

ETHNIC ANATOMIC PRINCIPLES

6. *Which of the following is characteristic of a Middle Eastern nose?*

C. Long nasal bones, low radix, large hump, hanging columella, septal deviation.

The Middle Eastern nose is characterized by long nasal bones, low radix, large hump, hanging columella, septal deviation (**Table 47.3**).[1]

Table 47.3 *Specific Ethnic Characteristics*

Ethnicity	Characteristics
Black nose	Short nasal bones
	Wide nose
	Low dorsum
	Wide bimalar distance
	Horizontally oriented nostrils, wide base
	Deficient premaxilla
	Limited septal cartilage
Asian nose	Thick sebaceous skin
	Low dorsum
	Weak lower lateral cartilage
	Less septal cartilage
	Deficient premaxilla
	Wide nasal base
	Retracted columella
Middle Eastern nose	Long nasal bones
	Low radix
	Large hump
	Hanging columella
	Septal deviation
Hispanic nose (types described by Daniel[1])	**Type I (Castilian):** Normal radix height, high bridge, normal tip projection
	Type II (Mexican American)—most common: Low radix height, near-normal bridge, dependent tip
	Type III (Mestizo): Broad base, thick skin, wide tip
	Type IV (Creole)—predominantly black features: Broad, flat lower third, short columella, transversely oriented nostrils, flaring alae

REFERENCE

1. Daniel RK. Hispanic rhinoplasty in the United States, with emphasis on the Mexican American nose. Plast Reconstr Surg 2003;112:244; discussion 257

ETHNIC ANATOMIC PRINCIPLES

7. *Which of the following is characteristic of a type II (Mexican American) nose?*

D. Low radix height, near-normal bridge, dependent tip.

Hispanic nose, type II Mexican American nose is characterized by low radix height, near-normal bridge, dependent tip (**Table 47.4**).[1]

Table 47.4 *Specific Ethnic Characteristics*

Ethnicity	Characteristics
Black nose	Short nasal bones Wide nose Low dorsum Wide bimalar distance Horizontally oriented nostrils, wide base Deficient premaxilla Limited septal cartilage
Asian nose	Thick sebaceous skin Low dorsum Weak lower lateral cartilage Less septal cartilage Deficient premaxilla Wide nasal base Retracted columella
Middle Eastern nose	Long nasal bones Low radix Large hump Hanging columella Septal deviation
Hispanic nose (types described by Daniel[1])	**Type I (Castilian):** Normal radix height, high bridge, normal tip projection **Type II (Mexican American)—most common:** Low radix height, near-normal bridge, dependent tip **Type III (Mestizo):** Broad base, thick skin, wide tip **Type IV (Creole)—predominantly black features:** Broad, flat lower third, short columella, transversely oriented nostrils, flaring alae

Reference

1. Daniel RK. Hispanic rhinoplasty in the United States, with emphasis on the Mexican American nose. Plast Reconstr Surg 2003;112:244; discussion 257

ANATOMIC PRINCIPLES/PREOPERATIVE PLANNING

8. *Which of the following is an advantage to using costal cartilage as grafting material?*

E. Lower vascular demand making it less likely to resorb.

The overall infection rate is less than 1% (not 5%). Also, costal cartilage is stronger therefore can be cut thinner with less bulk in the nose, has lower vascular demand making it less likely to resorb (not higher), and surgeons are able to harvest a larger amount of cartilage. Septal grafts tend to be straighter when compared to costal cartilage grafts. The disadvantages to costal cartilage harvest include increased operative time, warping, and donor site morbidity.[1,2,3,4,5,6]

References

1. Ozaki W, Buchman SR. Volume maintenance of onlay grafts in the craniofacial skeleton: microarchitecture versus embryologic origin. Plast Reconstr Surg 1998;102:291
2. Lin KY, Bartlett SP, Yaremchuck MJ, et al. The effect of rigid fixation on the survival of onlay bone grafts: an experimental study. Plast Reconstr Surg 1990;86:449
3. Vuyk HD, Adamson PA. Biomaterials in rhinoplasty. Clin Otolaryngol 1998;23:209

4. Peer LA. Diced cartilage grafts. Arch Otolaryngol 1943;38:156
5. Peer LA. Cartilage grafting. Br J Plast Surg 1954;7:250
6. Toriumi DM, Asher SA. Primary rhinoplasty techniques: use of costal cartilage. In: Cobo R, ed. Ethnic Considerations in Facial Plastic Surgery. New York: Thieme Publishers; 2015

PREOPERATIVE PLANNING

9. *Which of the following is an advantage of using allografts such as silicone, ePTFE, and porous polyethylene?*

B. No additional surgical site, and minimal change in operative time.

Advantages of using allografts include ease of use, no additional surgical site, and minimal change in operative time. Disadvantages include increased lifetime risk of infection, displacement/extrusion, thinning of skin over implant site, and implant translucency and pain. Often times, allografts, particularly porous polyethylene, are associated with significant postoperative edema. Additionally, structural grafting can lead to nasal stiffness which should be addressed with the patient during the initial consultation.[1]

REFERENCE

1. Toriumi DM, Asher SA. Primary rhinoplasty techniques: use of costal cartilage. In: Cobo R, ed. Ethnic Considerations in Facial Plastic Surgery. New York: Thieme Publishers; 2015

PERIOPERATIVE CONSIDERATIONS

10. *Which of the following is correct regarding injecting local anesthetic before prepping and draping?*

B. Injection can create hydrostatic dissection for ease of elevation of mucoperichondrial flaps.

Local anesthetic (1% lidocaine with 1:100,000 epinephrine) is injected before prepping and draping, which allows ample time for vasoconstriction. Injection also creates hydrostatic dissection for ease of elevation of mucoperichondrial flaps.[1]

REFERENCE

1. Decker JR, Dutton JM. Local anesthesia for nasal and sinus surgery. Ear Nose Throat J 2013;92(3):107–108

ANATOMIC PRINCIPLES/PREOPERATIVE PLANNING

11. *Which of the following is true when harvesting auricular cartilage?*

C. Infection prophylaxis is required if auricular cartilage is to be harvested.

Infection prophylaxis with first-generation cephalosporin and fluoroquinolone is required if costal or auricular cartilage is to be harvested. The entire face and intranasal area are prepared with dilute povidone-iodine, and the patient is draped to maintain sterility throughout the procedure. If cartilage is to be harvested, then surgeons must change gloves to prevent contamination. Auricular cartilage actually has a higher vascular demand when compared to costal cartilage making it more likely to resorb.[1]

REFERENCE

1. Toriumi DM, Asher SA. Primary rhinoplasty techniques: use of costal cartilage. In: Cobo R, ed. Ethnic Considerations in Facial Plastic Surgery. New York: Thieme Publishers; 2015

PREOPERATIVE PLANNING/PERIOPERATIVE CONSIDERATIONS

12. *What is the benefit of sharp dissection while opening the nose?*

B. Helps preserve the subdermal plexus and prevent excessive swelling.

Sharp dissection while opening the nose helps to preserve the subdermal plexus and prevent excessive swelling that occurs with tearing of the tissue during blunt dissection. By limiting blunt dissection over the nasal dorsum, a tight subperiosteal pocket is preserved in anticipation of a secure dorsal augmentation graft.[1]

REFERENCE

1. Toriumi DM. New concepts in nasal tip contouring. Arch Facial Plast Surg 2006;8:42

ANATOMIC PRINCIPLES/PERIOPERATIVE CONSIDERATIONS

13. *Why is it important to avoid injury to soft tissue triangles during tip exposure?*

D. They are extremely difficult to repair.

The soft-tissue triangle is located between the dome of alar cartilage superiorly and the nostril margin inferiorly. There is a lack of cartilage support in this area as it is formed only of skin and soft tissue. The triangle is made of two juxtaposed layers of skin, the external nasal skin and the internal vestibular skin, separated by loose areolar tissue and some terminal fibers of nasalis and depressor septi nasi muscles. It does not contain any neurovascular structures. Any postoperative retraction, notching, or asymmetries of soft triangles can seriously affect the rhinoplasty outcome. Tip exposure should be achieved with Converse scissors, making every attempt to avoid injury to soft tissue triangles, as these are extremely difficult to repair.[1,2,3]

REFERENCES

1. Toriumi DM. New concepts in nasal tip contouring. Arch Facial Plast Surg 2006;8:42
2. Gunter JP, Friedman RM. Lateral crural strut graft: technique and clinical applications in rhinoplasty. Plast Reconstr Surg 1997;99:943; discussion 953
3. Losquardro WD, Bared A, Toriumi DM. Correction of the retracted alar base. Facial Plast Surg 2012;28:218

ANATOMIC PRINCIPLES/PERIOPERATIVE CONSIDERATIONS

14. *When harvesting septal cartilage after the upper third of the nose is addressed to prevent destabilization, how much cartilaginous L-strut should be preserved to ensure adequate support?*

C. 10 mm.

In order to decrease the potential for loss of the tip and dorsal nasal support, it is imperative to preserve at least a 1-cm (10 mm) width portion of the dorsal and caudal septal segment which is deemed the L-strut. Deformities of the septal L-strut create functional and aesthetic problems such as a twisted nose, malpositioned tip, saddle deformity, and internal valve insufficiency.[1,2]

REFERENCES

1. Jeong JY. Obtaining maximal stability with a septal extension technique in East Asian rhinoplasty. Arch Plast Surg 2014;41(1):19–28
2. Lee J-S, Lee D, Ha D-H, Kim S. Redefining the septal L-strut in septal surgery. PloS one 2015;10:e0119996

ANATOMIC PRINCIPLES/PERIOPERATIVE CONSIDERATIONS

15. *What is true when performing an osteotomy?*

C. They are used to narrow the dorsum or correct deviations or dorsal hump.

Osteotomies are used to narrow the dorsum or to correct deviations or dorsal hump. They are performed medial to lateral and should be avoided if major dorsal augmentation (large dorsal graft >3 mm in height) is planned to prevent a tubular, narrowed appearance of the dorsum.[1]

REFERENCE

1. Toriumi DM, Pero CD. Asian rhinoplasty. Clin Plast Surg 2010;37:335

ANATOMIC PRINCIPLES/PERIOPERATIVE CONSIDERATIONS

16. *Which of the following is a benefit of using spreader grafts?*

C. They increase the area of the internal nasal valve and provide foundation to prevent saddling.

Spreader grafts increase the area of the internal nasal valve and provide foundation to prevent saddling and postoperative rotation/shortening. They also work to lengthen a short nose or retracted columella. Unilateral placement of a spreader graft is used to straighten the nose.[1,2]

REFERENCES

1. Sheen JH. Spreader graft: a method of reconstructing the roof of the middle nasal vault following rhinoplasty. Plast Reconstr Surg 1984;73:230
2. Guyuron B. Nasal osteotomy and airway changes. Plast Reconstr Surg 1998;102:856

OPERATIVE TECHNIQUE

17. *What technique is used to reset the caudal septum to midline?*

A. With a swinging-door maneuver or by shifting the nasal spine.

The caudal septum is reset to midline with swinging-door maneuver or by shifting the nasal spine. This can be achieved with a 5-mm straight osteotome placed at a slight angle toward the desired position. Once engaged, the osteotome acts as a lever to shift the spine. Caudal septal extension/replacement grafts are the only cartilage grafts in structure rhinoplasty that must be straight. Septal cartilage may be preferred over costal cartilage in this case. Caudal septal extension grafts are preferred because they minimize postoperative loss of tip projection and help to control rotation and length.[1,2,3]

REFERENCES

1. Byrd HS, Andochick S, Copit S, et al. Septal extension grafts: a method of controlling tip projection shape. Plast Reconstr Surg 1997;100:999
2. Ha RY, Byrd HS. Septal extension grafts revisited: 6-year experience in controlling nasal tip projection and shape. Plast Reconstr Surg 2003;112:1929
3. Toriumi DM, Asher SA. Primary rhinoplasty techniques: use of costal cartilage. In: Cobo R, ed. Ethnic Considerations in Facial Plastic Surgery. New York: Thieme Publishers; 2015

OPERATIVE TECHNIQUE

18. *Which of the following is an appropriate technique for tip contouring?*

A. Tip onlay grafts are used when no change to the infratip is needed.

Tip onlay grafts are used when no change to the infratip is needed. A shield graft is used to increase projection in thick-skinned patients for appropriate tip definition. Lateral crural grafts prevent alar collapse and control overrotation. They also prevent visibility of the shield graft. Lateral crural strut grafts flatten the convexity. Tip bulbosity can be corrected through alteration of the dome and use of lateral crural strut grafts. Malpositioned lateral crura and alar retraction are corrected through repositioning of asymmetrical or cephalically oriented (not caudally oriented) lateral crura.[1,2]

REFERENCES

1. Toriumi DM. New concepts in nasal tip contouring. Arch Facial Plast Surg 2006;8:42
2. Gunter JP, Friedman RM. Lateral crural strut graft: technique and clinical applications in rhinoplasty. Plast Reconstr Surg 1997;99:943; discussion 953

PREOPERATIVE PLANNING/ETHNIC ANATOMIC PRINCIPLES

19. *Which of the following is a good example of why an individualized approach is crucial to tip management in ethnic patients?*

A. Repositioning of the lateral crus may be effective for flared nostrils caused by the large convex lower lateral cartilages common to Middle Eastern patients.

An individualized approach is crucial to tip management in ethnic patients. Repositioning of the lateral crus may be effective for flared nostrils caused by large convex lower lateral cartilages in Middle Eastern patients but may worsen the appearance in Asian patients with weak lower lateral cartilages and hanging alar lobules.[1,2]

REFERENCES

1. Toriumi DM. New concepts in nasal tip contouring. Arch Facial Plast Surg 2006;8:42
2. Gunter JP, Friedman RM. Lateral crural strut graft: technique and clinical applications in rhinoplasty. Plast Reconstr Surg 1997;99:943; discussion 953

PERIOPERATIVE CONSIDERATIONS/ETHNIC ANATOMIC PRINCIPLES

20. *Which of the following is an important principle to keep in mind when closing darker-skinned patients?*

C. The use of absorbable sutures will result in prolonged erythema and possible suture tracking.

In darker-skinned patients, the use of absorbable sutures will result in prolonged erythema and possible suture tracking. In the early healing period, the inflammatory response in conjunction with the inflammation related to the gradual breakdown of the absorbable suture material can lead to abnormal hypertrophic scarring, hypo- or hyperpigmentation, stitch abscess, and granulomas particularly in dark-skinned patients. In regard to dyspigmentation, these differences in healing between white and darker skin types is likely related to melanocyte regulation. Although black skin and white skin contain almost equal numbers of melanocytes and melanosomes, the cells do differ in terms of structure and function. As melanosomes mature, stage I and II lightly pigmented melanosomes are found in higher ratios in people with paler skin types and more densely laden, pigmented stage III and IV melanosomes in higher ratios in people with darker skin types. Melanocytes withinblackskin are also larger and more dendritic than those of white skin which may contribute to these differences in scarring and dyspigmentation.[1,2,3,4]

REFERENCES

1. Daniel RK. Hispanic rhinoplasty in the United States, with emphasis on the Mexican American nose. Plast Reconstr Surg 2003;112:244; discussion 257
2. Rohrich RJ, Muzaffar AR. Rhinoplasty in the African-American patient. Plast Reconstr Surg 2013;111:1322; discussion 1340
3. Kontis TC, Papel ID. Rhinoplasty on the African-American nose. Aesthetic Plast Surg 2002;26(Suppl 1):S12
4. Chadwick S, Heath R, Shah M. Abnormal pigmentation within cutaneous scars: A complication of wound healing. Indian J Plast Surg 2012;45(2):403-411

PERIOPERATIVE CONSIDERATIONS

21. *Radiopaque 0.25-mm septal splints are placed if turbinate work is performed to prevent what potential postoperative complication?*

D. Synechiae formation.

Synechiae is an adherence with subsequent scarring between the two mucosal surfaces in the nasal cavity which may cause nasal obstruction which may lead to rhinitis and rhinosinusitis that can occur after any turbinate manipulation or trauma. In the setting of functional rhinoplasty with turbinate work, radiopaque 0.25-mm septal splints are placed to prevent synechiae formation.[1]

REFERENCE

1. Losquardro WD, Bared A, Toriumi DM. Correction of the retracted alar base. Facial Plast Surg 2012;28:218

PERIOPERATIVE CONSIDERATIONS

22. *When are lateral wall splints appropriate?*

B. If lateral crural strut grafts were used.

Lateral wall splints are placed if lateral crural strut grafts were used to ensure redraping of vestibular mucosa. They are fashioned from 0.25 bivalve splints.[1]

REFERENCE

1. Losquardro WD, Bared A, Toriumi DM. Correction of the retracted alar base. Facial Plast Surg 2012;28:218

OPERATIVE TECHNIQUE

23. *Which is a key to successful base reduction?*

D. Perpendicular incision to discourage eversion of skin edges.

The key steps to successful base reduction are as follows: Plan incision slightly adjacent to alar/facial or alar/vestibular junction. Forego injecting local anesthetic because it may deform anatomy. Avoid all cautery. Slightly beveled incisions to promote eversion of skin edges. Close incisions meticulously.[1]

REFERENCE

1. Losquardro WD, Bared A, Toriumi DM. Correction of the retracted alar base. Facial Plast Surg 2012;28:218

POSTOPERATIVE CARE

24. *Which of the following is an effective strategy to avoid complications following rhinoplasty?*

A. Infection is managed aggressively with the patients returning to the OR for a washout and drain placement along with broad spectrum antibiotic coverage.

Infection is managed aggressively to prevent graft resorption. These patients usually return to the operating room for washout and placement of drains. Broad spectrum antibiotic coverage is crucial. Dermal sutures at the columellar incision reduce the probability of widened scars if significant augmentation and stretch were required. History of keloid should be determined. They are less likely to form on the face and are managed with massage and steroids—local anesthetic does not reduce the incidence of keloid. Base reductions should be performed after closure is complete (not before). This provides the greatest potential to leave irreversible deformity if not done correctly. If performing a base reduction is questionable, the surgeon should defer this irreversible technique. The decision to forgo base reduction and possibly return at a later date should not be faulted.[1,2]

References

1. Toriumi DM, Asher SA. Primary rhinoplasty techniques: use of costal cartilage. In: Cobo R, ed. Ethnic Considerations in Facial Plastic Surgery. New York: Thieme Publishers; 2015
2. Amici JM. Hypertrophie cicatricielle précoce post-chirurgicale de la région nasale: intérêt des injections de corticoïde retard [Early hypertrophic scar after surgery on the nasal region: value of long-acting corticosteroid injections]. Ann Dermatol Venereol 2014;141(1):7–13

48. Lip Augmentation

David A. Sterling, Christopher C. Surek
See *Essentials of Aesthetic Surgery*, pp. 645–675

PREOPERATIVE EVALUATION

1. *When evaluating a patient for lip augmentation, what is true regarding the ideal lip dimensions?*
A. The length of the lips should equal the distance between the midpupillary lines.
B. The length of the lips should be equal to the double the size of the alar-to-alar base width.
C. The ratio of the upper/lower vermillion show should be 1:1.6.
D. With the lips slightly parted, the ideal incisor show should be 4 mm.
E. The subnasale to stomion and stomion to menton distances should be approximately equal.

AUGMENTATION USING INJECTABLE FILLERS

2. *A patient comes to your office looking for lip augmentation with injectable filler. Which product requires skin testing for hypersensitivity reactions?*
A. Zyderm (Allergan).
B. Restylane (Galderma).
C. Juvéderm (Allergan).
D. Radiesse (Merz).
E. Poly-L-lactic acid (Sculptra).

AUGMENTATION USING INJECTABLE FILLERS

3. *You injected a patient's lips with a hyaluronic acid–based filler on the first appointment of the day. She calls your office in the early afternoon complaining of worsening pain and bruising. She has been injected with fillers on several occasions and has never experienced this. What is the most appropriate response?*
A. Inform her that this is expected after injecting fillers and to keep her normal appointment in 2 weeks.
B. Instruct her to apply ice intermittently to the area.
C. Instruct her to apply intermittent warm compresses and to call the following day.
D. Ask her to come to your office immediately for evaluation.
E. Instruct her to immediately proceed to the nearest emergency department.

AUGMENTATION WITH GRAFTS

4. *You are injecting a patient with autologous fat for augmentation of her lips. What technique is used in an attempt to improve graft survival and overall result?*
A. Injection of large aliquots followed by massage.
B. Injecting with a small cannula under high pressure.
C. Processing of the fat via gravity separation or high-speed centrifugation to produce small aliquot grafts.
D. Undercorrection of the deformity in anticipation of swelling of the graft.
E. Long-term splint and subsequent taping of the fat-grafted area.

AUGMENTATION WITH GRAFTS

5. *What are some important considerations when using dermal fats grafts for augmentation of the lips?*
A. Deepithilializing prior to harvesting the graft.
B. Harvesting precisely as much tissue as needed.
C. Remove 50% of the hair follicles.
D. Preserve as much fat as possible on the underside of the dermis.
E. Has more absorption than just using fat alone.

AUGMENTATION WITH V-Y ADVANCEMENT

6. *A 72-year-old female presents for lip rejuvenation. On examination she has a long, thin upper lip with an inverted vermillion. She is interested in shortening her upper cutaneous lip and would prefer a permanent option with no visible scars. What augmentation option is best for this patient?*

A. V-Y advancement.
B. Direct lift lip.
C. Indirect lift lip.
D. Subnasal lip lift.
E. Anguloplasty.

INDIRECT LIP LIFT (ILL), SUBNASAL LIFT, "BULLHORN LIP LIFT"

7. *When performing an indirect lip lift, how much skin should be left from the nasal base to Cupid's bow?*

A. 7 mm.
B. 10 mm.
C. 12 mm.
D. 15 mm.
E. 17 mm.

DIRECT LIP LIFT, GULL-WING LIP LIFT, VERMILLION LIP LIFT

8. *You are performing a direct lip lift on a 68-year-old female. What modification can be performed to reduce the risk of perioral stricture?*

A. Excising only skin and minimal subcutaneous tissue.
B. Limit the medial extent of the corner mouth lift to Cupid's bow.
C. Using interrupted rather than a running suture for closure.
D. Dermabrasion of the scar postoperatively.
E. Avoiding the use of nonabsorbable sutures for anchoring.

CORNER MOUTHLIFT, ANGULOPLASTY

9. *A 70-year-old female presents to discuss lip augmentation. She has significantly downturned corners of her mouths, which distresses her. She seeks the most permanent option for correction. What technique is best for this patient?*

A. Injectable hyaluronic acid filler to the corners of the mouth.
B. Indirect lip lift.
C. V-Y advancement.
D. Placement of a dermal fat graft at the commissures.
E. Anguloplasty.

Answers

PREOPERATIVE EVALUATION

1. *When evaluating a patient for lip augmentation, what is true regarding the ideal lip dimensions?*

C. The ratio of the upper/lower vermillion show should be 1:1.6.

Like in other areas of aesthetic surgery, it is imperative to know the ideal lip dimensions. There are several important structures in the lower third of the face, as well as important relationships between the middle and lower thirds that contribute to the ideal lip. The length of the lip should equal the distance between the medial corneal limbi. The ratio of the upper/lower vermillion show should be 1:1.6 (golden ratio). The upper cutaneous lip/upper vermillion ratio should be 1.1 to 2.3. The interpupillary line and commissural line should be parallel and horizontal. The subnasale–stomion distance should be half the stomion–menton distance. With the lips slightly parted the incisor show should be about 2 mm. Cupids bow should form a "gentle M," the stomion should form a "lazy M," and the lower lip vermillion should form a "gentle W." There are three thickenings of the upper lip: a central tubercle and lateral thickenings. There are two paramedian thickenings ofthelower lip. The nasolabial angle should be 85 to 105 degrees and there should be a gentle "ski jump" transition at the vermillion border. The upper lip should overly the lower lip by about 2 mm (**Fig. 48.1**, **Fig. 48.2**).[1,2]

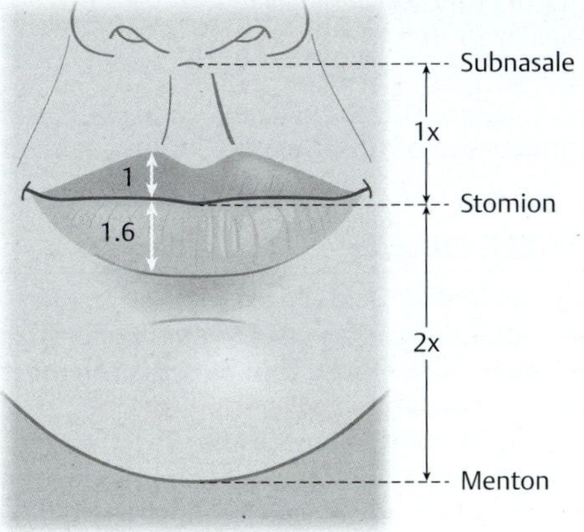

Fig. 48.1 Frontal lip view. (Source: Ideal Lip Dimensions. In: Janis J, ed. Essentials of Aesthetic Surgery. 1st Edition. New York: Thieme; 2018.)

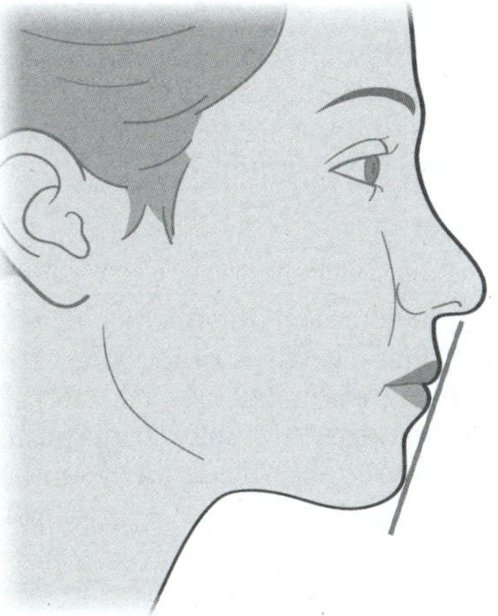

Fig. 48.2 Profile view of the lips. The *line* depicts the Riedel line, connecting upper lip, lower lip, and chin. (Source: Ideal Lip Dimensions. In: Janis J, ed. Essentials of Aesthetic Surgery. 1st Edition. New York: Thieme; 2018.)

References

1. Raphael P, Harris R, Harris SW. Analysis and classification of the upper lip aesthetic unit. Plast Reconstr Surg 2013;132:543
2. Guyuron B, Eriksson E, Persing J, eds. Plastic Surgery: Indications and Practice. Philadelphia: Elsevier; 2009

AUGMENTATION USING INJECTABLE FILLERS

2. *A patient comes to your office looking for lip augmentation with injectable filler. Which product requires skin testing for hypersensitivity reactions?*

A. Zyderm (Allergan).

Injectable fillers are excellent options for mild to moderate lip augmentation. There are many different fillers, with various compositions, properties, and duration of effect. The most commonly used fillers are hyaluronic acid–based, such as Restylane (Galderma) and Juvéderm (Allergan). Hyaluronic acid is a natural, hydrophilic component of the extracellular matrix that draws in fluid to cause volumization. They typically last 6 to 12 months. Radiesse (Merz) is a calcium hydroxyapatite–based filler that has a long duration of action (>12 months). Neither of the above fillers requires hypersensitivity testing prior to use. Zyderm (Allergan), however, is a bovine collagen–based filler that can cause allergic reactions in 3 to 5% of patients. Therefore, hypersensitivity skin testing must be performed several weeks prior to use. Collagen injectable typically have a shorter duration of action, around 3 to 6 months. Other options for injectable fillersincludepoly-L-lactic acid (Sculptra, Galderma), Silicone (Silikon 1000, Alcon), polymethylmethacrylate (Bellafill, Suneva Medical).[1]

Reference

1. Sarnoff DS, Saini R, Gotkin RH. Comparison of filling agents for lip augmentation. Aesthet Surg J 2008;28:556

AUGMENTATION USING INJECTABLE FILLERS

3. *You injected a patient's lips with a hyaluronic acid–based filler on the first appointment of the day. She calls your office in the early afternoon complaining of worsening pain and bruising. She has been injected with fillers on several occasions and has never experienced this. What is the most appropriate response?*

D. Ask her to come to your office immediately for evaluation.

Injectable fillers are associated with several complications that range from mild to severe. Patient's often experience pain, swelling, and bruising after filler injection. These symptoms are usually self-limited and resolve within a week. On the other end of the spectrum, vascular occlusion is a severe complication that can result in tissue necrosis and deformity, and even blindness or stroke. Although estimated to be very rare, occurring in <0.001% of cases, vascular occlusion should be considered in any patient with significant pain, erythema that transitions to duskiness, and/or excessive bruising. Vascular occlusion should be treated immediately with hyaluronidase injection, massage, and warm compresses. Patients with more severe presentations including vision loss or stroke should be sent to the emergency department where targeted hyaluronidase injection via interventional radiology can be considered. Although it is unclear how severe thispatient'scomplaints are over the phone, it is always appropriate to evaluate in the office. At this point, sending her to the emergency department is probably unnecessary in the absence of vision changes or stroke-like symptoms.[1,2,3,4]

References

1. de Vries CG, Geertsma RE. Clinical data on injectable tissue fillers: a review. Expert Rev Med Devices 2013;10:835
2. DeLorenzi C. Complications of Injectable Fillers, part I. Aesthet Surg J 2013;33:561
3. Glogau R, Bank D, Brandt F, et al. A randomized, evaluator-blinded, controlled study of the effectiveness and safety of a small gel particle hyaluronic acid for lip augmentation. Dermatol Surg 2012;38:1180
4. Ozturk CN, Li Y, Tung R, et al. Complications following injection of soft-tissue fillers. Aesthet Surg J 2013;33:862

AUGMENTATION WITH GRAFTS

4. *You are injecting a patient with autologous fat for augmentation of her lips. What technique is used in an attempt to improve graft survival and overall result?*

C. Processing of the fat via gravity separation or high-speed centrifugation to produce small aliquot grafts.

Autologous fat grafting is an excellent tool for longer term augmentation of the lips. Injectable fat grafting can also be employed in the office, which limits the overall cost to the patient. Resorption rates vary, however, and multiple treatments are often necessary to achieve the desired results. There are several important technical factors that should be employed to decrease trauma to the adipocytes and improve take. This includes utilization of a large harvesting cannula (17 gauge) under low negative pressure and with multiple gentle passes. The aspirate can be processed via gentle centrifugation or gravity separation. The fat is injected in small aliquots (0.1–0.2 mL) using a large blunt cannula. Furthermore, the augmentation is usually overcorrected by 30% in anticipation of resorption.[1,2]

REFERENCES

1. Churukian M. Red lip augmentation using fat injections. Clin Facial Plast Surg 1997;5:61
2. Metzinger S, Parrish J, Guerra A, et al. Autologous fat grafting to the lower one-third of the face. Facial Plast Surg 2012;28:21

AUGMENTATION WITH GRAFTS

5. *What are some important considerations when using dermal fats grafts for augmentation of the lips?*

A. Deepithilializing prior to harvesting the graft.

Dermal fat grafting is a useful tool for lip augmentation. Grafts are easily harvested and can be taken from tissue discarded during the operation or from preexisting scars. Dermal fat grafts also undergo less resorption than fat alone. Although a relatively simple graft to harvest, employing several techniques can help with efficiency and improve results. The graft should be deepithelialized prior to harvesting as it is much more difficult to do afterwards, and more tissue should be taken than anticipated. Hair follicles should be avoided in the graft and care should be taken to remove as much fat from the dermis to improve take and limit contour irregularities.[1]

REFERENCE

1. Tabrizi R, Shafiei E, Danesteh H. Dimensional changes of the upper lip using dermis fat graft for lip augmentation. J Oral Maxillofac Surg 2015;73(10):2030–2037

AUGMENTATION WITH V-Y ADVANCEMENT

6. *A 72-year-old female presents for lip rejuvenation. On examination she has a long, thin upper lip with an inverted vermillion. She is interested in shortening her upper cutaneous lip and would prefer a permanent option with no visible scars. What augmentation option is best for this patient?*

A. V-Y advancement.

Some patients require a more significant lip augmentation than can be achieved with fillers or autologous grafting. There are two general options for these patients: V-Y advancement and lip lift. There are several technical variations within each category. Broadly speaking, V-Y advancements utilize intraoral, labial mucosal incisions to advance tissue away from the sulcus. Lip lifts, on the other hand, involve excision of cutaneous lip skin above the upper vermillion to elevate the lip. The benefit of the V-Y advancement is that the scars are not visible. However, both techniques are not without their disadvantages. Complications include debilitating edema, asymmetry, over- and undercorrection, paresthesias, infection, dehiscence, hypertrophic scarring (lip lift). They are also technically challenging with a steep learning curve (**Fig. 48.3**).[1,2,3]

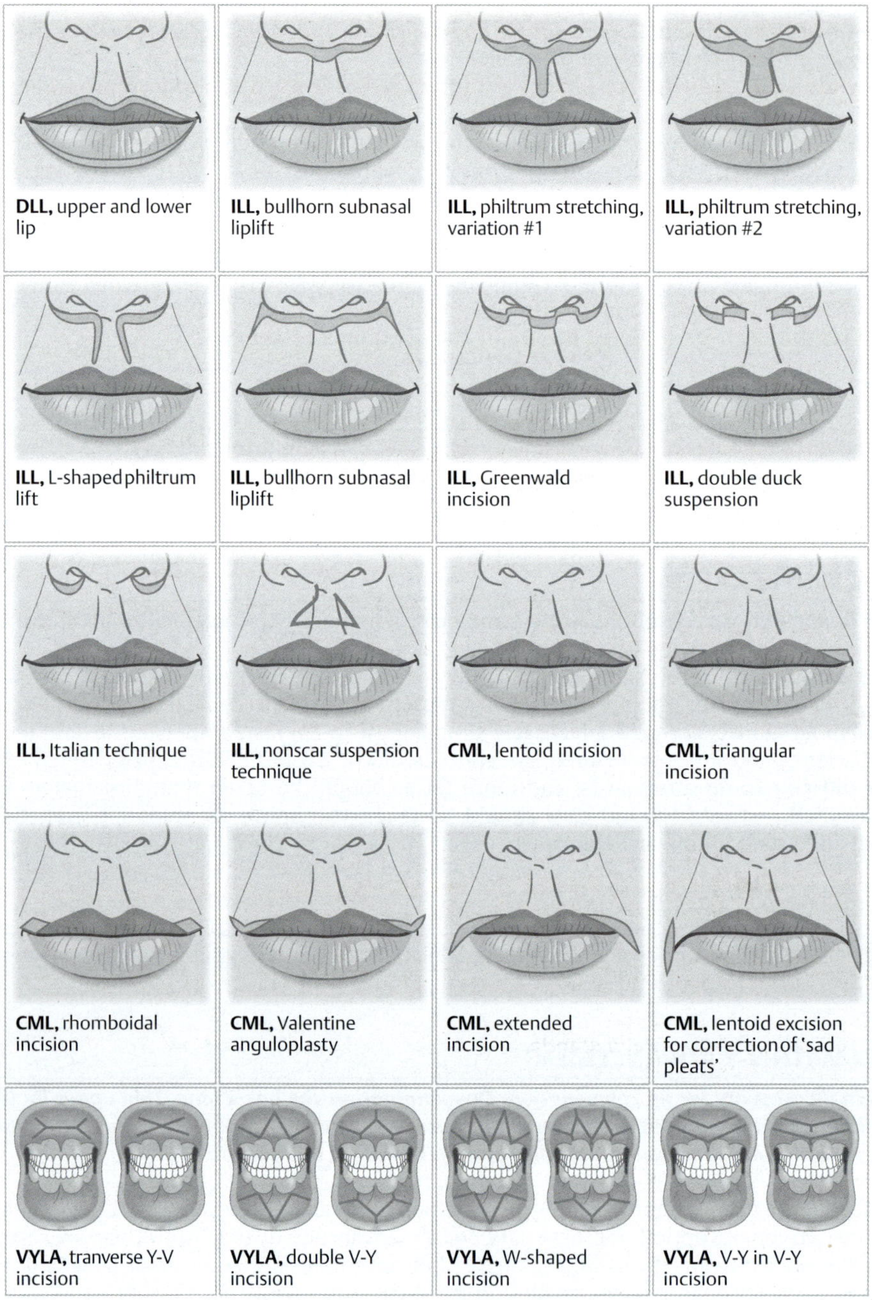

Fig. 48.3 V-Y advancement patterns. The areas shaded indicate incisions or areas to be resected. (CML, Corner of the mouthlift; DLL, direct liplift; ILL, indirect liplift; VYLA, V-Y lip augmentation.) (Source: Technique. In: Janis J, ed. Essentials of Aesthetic Surgery. 1st Edition. New York: Thieme; 2018.)

References

1. Meyer R, Kesserling UK. Aesthetic surgery in the perioral region. Aesthet Plast Surg 1976;1:61
2. Cardoso AD, Sperli AE. Rhytidoplasty of the upper lip. In: Hueston JT, ed. Transactions of the Fifth International Congress of Plastic and Reconstructive Surgery, 1971 Feb 22–26. Melbourne, Australia: Butterworths; 1971
3. Weston GW, Poindexter BD, Sigal RK, et al. Lifting lips: 28 years of experience using the direct excision approach to rejuvenating the aging mouth. Aesthet Surg J 2009;29:83

INDIRECT LIP LIFT (ILL), SUBNASAL LIFT, "BULLHORN LIP LIFT"

7. *When performing an indirect lip lift, how much skin should be left from the nasal base to Cupid's bow?*

C. 12 mm.

It is important to leave at least 12 mm of cutaneous lip between the nasal base and Cupid's bow to prevent the lip from looking too short. This typically translates to 3 to 5 mm of skin excised, regardless of incisor show. Although the indirect lip lift is a powerful technique for augmentation of the lip, it is not without complications. Prolonged edema of >3 months is seen in 8.3%, undercorrection occurs in 2.4%, approximately 1.6 to 2.1% of patients experience an infection, and 5.3% have hypertrophic scarring and 20% undergo scar revision with dermabrasion.[1,2,3]

REFERENCES

1. Moragas JSM, Vercruysse HJ, Mommaerts MY. "Non-filling" procedures for lip augmentation: a systematic review of contemporary techniques and their outcomes. J Craniomaxillofac Surg 2014;42:943
2. Holden PK, Sufyan AS, Perkins SW. Long-term analysis of surgical correction of the senile upper lip. Arch Facial Plast Surg 2011;13:332
3. Knize DM. Lifting of the upper lip: Personal technique [discussion]. Plast Reconstr Surg 2004;113:1836

DIRECT LIP LIFT, GULL-WING LIP LIFT, VERMILLION LIP LIFT

8. *You are performing a direct lip lift on a 68-year-old female. What modification can be performed to reduce the risk of perioral stricture?*

B. Limit the medial extent of the corner mouth lift to Cupid's bow.

Direct lip lifts offer the best control of the desired vermillion placement compared with indirect liplifting and V-Y advancement. Traditionally, a direct lip lift involves excising skin along the vermillion from commissure to commissure. An unfortunate consequence of such a long scar is stricture that can be very difficult to fix. To avoid this, the excision can be limited medially by Cupid's bow, leaving the central lip intact. This area can be augmented instead with an indirect lift.[1,2,3]

REFERENCES

1. Moragas JSM, Vercruysse HJ, Mommaerts MY. "Non-filling" procedures for lip augmentation: a systematic review of contemporary techniques and their outcomes. J Craniomaxillofac Surg 2014;42:943
2. Yoskovitch A, Fanous N. Correction of thin lips: a 17-year follow-up of the original technique. Plast Reconstr Surg 2003;112:670
3. Weston GW, Poindexter BD, Sigal RK, et al. Lifting lips: 28 years of experience using the direct excision approach to rejuvenating the aging mouth. Aesthet Surg J 2009;29:83

CORNER MOUTHLIFT, ANGULOPLASTY

9. *A 70-year-old female presents to discuss lip augmentation. She has significantly downturned corners of her mouths, which distresses her. She seeks the most permanent option for correction. What technique is best for this patient?*

E. Anguloplasty.

This patient is seeking a permanent option for correction of significantly downturned corners of her mouth. The best option for her would be a corner mouthlift, or anguloplasty. This technique involves excision of tissue above the vermillion at the corners of the mouth. There are various patterns that have been described, which differ in shape of skin excised as well as the length of the excision along the vermillion. A simple ellipse along the lateral lip is the most basic pattern. Complications of the anguloplasty include scar hypertrophy, misplaced scar above the vermillion, infection, undercorrection, and depressed scar. Injection of filler and placement of a dermal fat graft at the commissures would likely not create the same correction as an anguloplasty. An indirect lip lift focuses on the central lip below the nose and has little effect on the corner of the mouth.[1,2]

REFERENCES

1. Echo A, Momoh AO, Yuksel E. The no-scar lip-lift: upper lip suspension technique. Aesthet Plast Surg 2011;35:617
2. Moragas JSM, Vercruysse HJ, Mommaerts MY. "Non-filling" procedures for lip augmentation: a systematic review of contemporary techniques and their outcomes. J Craniomaxillofac Surg 2014;42:943

49. Genioplasty

Sammy Sinno, Michael E. Nissan
See *Essentials of Aesthetic Surgery*, pp. 676–690

ANATOMY

1. ***A chin dimple represents a midline void between fibers of which muscle?***
   A. Mentalis.
   B. Orbicularis oris.
   C. Depressor anguli oris.
   D. Quadratus (depressor) labii inferioris.
   E. Anterior belly of digastric.

NERVE SUPPLY

2. ***To prevent injury to nerve branches or tooth apices, where should osteotomies be placed with respect to the mental foramen?***
   A. 1–3 mm superiorly.
   B. 3–4 mm superiorly.
   C. 5–6 mm superiorly.
   D. 1–3 mm inferiorly.
   E. 5–6 mm inferiorly.

BLOOD SUPPLY

3. ***Which of the following branches of the facial artery represents the dominant blood supply to the chin?***
   A. Inferior labial artery.
   B. Superior labial artery.
   C. Lateral nasal branch.
   D. Submandibular artery.
   E. Angular artery.

OSSEOUS GENIOPLASTY

4. ***Which of the following patients is the best candidate for osseous genioplasty?***
   A. A young patient wanting to correct horizontal asymmetry of the chin.
   B. An elderly patient with osteoporosis.
   C. A middle-aged patient with abnormal dentition.
   D. A middle-aged patient with a vertical asymmetry of any magnitude.
   E. A young patient with a mild isolated sagittal deficiency.

ALLOPLASTIC GENIOPLASTY

5. ***Which of the following patients is the best candidate for alloplastic augmentation?***
   A. A young, male patient with excess horizontal deficiency.
   B. A young, male patient with a long face for which only the labiomental fold depth must be increased.
   C. An old, female patient with vertical deficiency undergoing planned necklift/facelift.
   D. A young, female patient with a vertical deficiency.
   E. An old, male patient with mandibular asymmetry.

OCCLUSION TYPE

6. *Preoperative evaluation is performed, and it is observed that the mesiobuccal cusp of a patient's maxillary first molar occludes medial to the buccal groove. Which type of occlusion describes this patient's bite?*
A. Angle class I.
B. Angle class II.
C. Angle class III.
D. Angle class IV.
E. Angle class V.

RIEDEL LINE

7. *The Riedel line is defined by connecting which two anatomical landmarks?*
A. The nasal tip and the anterior lower lip.
B. The nasal tip and the anterior upper lip.
C. The pogonion and the anterior upper lip.
D. The pogonion and the nasal tip.
E. The anterior upper and lower lips.

CERVICOMENTAL ANGLE

8. *The angle between the chin and neck on sagittal view is ideally how large?*
A. Less than 90 degrees.
B. 90–105 degrees.
C. 105–120 degrees.
D. 120–135 degrees.
E. Greater than 135 degrees.

WITCH'S-CHIN DEFORMITY

9. *A witch's-chin deformity is best repaired via which surgical maneuvers?*
A. Osteotomy and resection.
B. Osteotomy with advancement.
C. Alloplastic augmentation.
D. Soft tissue correction.
E. Osteotomy and setback.

POROUS POLYETHYLENE IMPLANT

10. *Which of the following is an advantage of the porous polyethylene implant?*
A. Lower infection rates than other implant types possibly due to increased vascular ingrowth.
B. Easier removal when compared with silicone implants.
C. Easier placement when compared with silicone implants.
D. Is associated with a small/minimal inflammatory response post placement.
E. Requires smaller soft tissue pocket than silicone implants.

SURGICAL TECHNIQUES: OSSEOUS GENIOPLASTY

11. *A patient presents for correction of significant excess vertical chin height. Which of the following osseous genioplasty techniques is most appropriate in this case?*
A. Reduction genioplasty.
B. Sliding genioplasty.
C. Jumping genioplasty.
D. Centralizing genioplasty.
E. Interpositional bone graft placement.

SURGICAL APPROACH: IMPLANT GENIOPLASTY

12. *For implant genioplasty, which of the following is true regarding the extraoral approach when compared with the intraoral approach?*
A. Lower infection rate.
B. More precise implant placement.
C. No visible scars.
D. No direct visualization of pocket.
E. Less tendency for implant to migrate.

IMPLANT POSITION

13. *Which of the following is accurate with regards to chin implant position?*
A. A superiorly misplaced implant will result in an aesthetic defect but will not interfere with dentition.
B. The implant should be placed directly over the menton.
C. The implant should be placed directly over the pogonion.
D. The implant should be placed deep to the mentalis muscle, but superficial to the periosteum.
E. The implant should be placed superficial to the mentalis muscle.

POSTOPERATIVE CARE

14. *Which of the following should be considered for postoperative care after genioplasty?*
A. Patients should wear elastic chin support garment for 24 hours a day for the first 2 days and then at night for 1 to 2 weeks.
B. Patients should be instructed to limit activity that increases heart rate for 5 to 7 days.
C. For the first 3 to 4 days, patients should sleep supine without head elevation.
D. Corticosteroids are not recommended postoperatively.
E. Antibiotics are not recommended postoperatively.

REOPERATION

15. *For a patient who underwent implant genioplasty 1 day prior, which circumstance is an indication for surgical revision?*
A. Transient loss of motor function up to 6 weeks.
B. Transient loss of sensory function up to 6 weeks.
C. Significant paresthesias and/or neuropraxia.
D. Mild lower lip paresthesias for 2 weeks.
E. Postoperative edema lasting greater than 5 to 7 days after alloplastic implant placement.

Answers

ANATOMY

1. ***A chin dimple represents a midline void between fibers of which muscle?***

   A. Mentalis.

   There are many muscles attaching to the mental protuberance that contribute to the appearance of the chin. A chin dimple is seen when there is a void in the midline of the cone-like mentalis muscle, whose vertical fibers span from the incisive fossa to the overlying skin. Other muscles that contribute to the function and aesthetics of the chin include orbicularis oris, depressor anguli oris, quadratus (depressor) labii inferioris, geniohyoid, genioglossus, mylohyoid, and the anterior belly of the digastric. Although these muscles do not contribute to the chin dimple, they are responsible for various chin and face movements. Orbicularis oris closes and puckers the oral commissure. Depressor anguli oris is associated with frowning. Quadratus (depressor) labii inferioris lowers the bottom lip. Geniohyoid, genioglossus, mylohyoid, and the anterior belly of the digastric attach to the posterior aspect of the chin.[1,2]

REFERENCES

1. Cohen SR. Genioplasty. In: Achauer BM, Eriksson E, GuyuronB, et al, eds. Plastic Surgery: Indications, Operations, and Outcomes. Vol. 5. St Louis, Mosby–Year Book; 2000
2. Guyuron B, ed. Genioplasty. Boston: Little Brown, 1993.

NERVE SUPPLY

2. ***To prevent injury to nerve branches or tooth apices, where should osteotomies be placed with respect to the mental foramen?***

   E. 5–6 mm inferiorly.

   The mental nerve is a terminal branch of the inferior alveolar nerve, a branch of V3 that supplies sensation to the mandible. The mental nerve emerges from the mental foramen and divides into three branches deep to depressor anguli oris. These branches supply sensation to the chin and lower lip. During genioplasty, osteotomy puts the mental nerve at risk. Reducing this risk is achieved by placing osteotomies 5 to 6 mm below the mental foramen. This reduces the risk of injury not only to the mental nerve, but also to tooth apices.[1,2,3]

REFERENCES

1. Cohen SR. Genioplasty. In: Achauer BM, Eriksson E, Guyuron B, et al, eds. Plastic Surgery: Indications, Operations, and Outcomes. Vol. 5. St Louis, Mosby–Year Book; 2000
2. Guyuron B, ed. Genioplasty. Boston: Little Brown; 1993
3. Rosen HM. Osseous genioplasty. In: Aston SJ, Beasley RW, Thorne CN, eds. Grabb and Smith's Plastic Surgery. 5th ed. Philadelphia: Lippincott-Raven; 1997

BLOOD SUPPLY

3. ***Which of the following branches of the facial artery represents the dominant blood supply to the chin?***

   A. Inferior labial artery.

   Blood supply to the chin is predominantly provided by two sources: the inferior labial artery and the inferior alveolar artery. The inferior labial artery is a branch of the facial artery which arises from the external carotid artery. The inferior alveolar artery is a branch of the maxillary artery, which also arises from the external carotid.[1,2]

REFERENCES

1. Cohen SR. Genioplasty. In: Achauer BM, Eriksson E, Guyuron B, et al, eds. Plastic Surgery: Indications, Operations, and Outcomes. Vol. 5. St Louis, Mosby–Year Book; 2000
2. Guyuron B, ed. Genioplasty. Boston: Little Brown; 1993

OSSEOUS GENIOPLASTY

4. *Which of the following patients is the best candidate for osseous genioplasty?*

A. A young patient wanting to correct horizontal asymmetry of the chin.

Osseous genioplasty is appropriate to correct horizontal asymmetries of any magnitude. It is also appropriate when there is severe deficiency or excess in the vertical or sagittal planes. In contrast, mild isolated sagittal deficiencies are better corrected by alloplastic augmentation. Contraindications to osseous genioplasty include inadequate bone stock, often found in elderly patients with bone disease, and abnormal dentition.[1]

REFERENCE

1. Rosen HM. Osseous genioplasty. In: Aston SJ, Beasley RW, Thorne CN, eds. Grabb and Smith's Plastic Surgery. 5th ed. Philadelphia: Lippincott-Raven; 1997

ALLOPLASTIC GENIOPLASTY

5. *Which of the following patients is the best candidate for alloplastic augmentation?*

B. A young, male patient with a long face for which only the labiomental fold depth must be increased.

Indications for alloplastic augmentation include mild isolated sagittal deficiencies and need to increase only the labiomental fold length. For the young, male patient with a long face, a deeper fold is a desired characteristic,[1] and can be achieved with alloplastic augmentation alone. Although concomitant necklift/facelift is a relative indication for alloplastic augmentation, vertical deficiency is a contraindication for alloplastic augmentation and thus may be addressed via osseous genioplasty. Excess horizontal deficiency and mandibular asymmetry are likewise contraindications for alloplastic augmentation.[1]

REFERENCE

1. Rosen HM. Osseous genioplasty. In: Aston SJ, Beasley RW, Thorne CN, eds. Grabb and Smith's Plastic Surgery. 5th ed. Philadelphia: Lippincott-Raven; 1997

OCCLUSION TYPE

6. *Preoperative evaluation is performed, and it is observed that the mesiobuccal cusp of a patient's maxillary first molar occludes medial to the buccal groove. Which type of occlusion describes this patient's bite?*

B. Angle class II.

Occlusion describes the relationship of the maxillary teeth with respect to the mandibular teeth (**Fig. 49.1**). For these patients, whose maxillary first molar occludes medial to the buccal groove, further evaluation and orthognathic surgery with maxillary and mandibular osteotomies are possibly warranted. In this case, the diagnosis is angle class II malocclusion, known colloquially as "overbite" (option B). Genioplasty alone often cannot correct the functional and aesthetic defects present in patients with this type of malocclusion. In contrast, angle class III malocclusion, "underbite," is diagnosed when the mesiobuccal cusp of the maxillary first molar occludes distal to the buccal groove of the mandibular first molar (option C). Normal occlusion (angle class I) is characterized by a maxillary first molar whose mesiobuccal cusp occludes into the buccal groove of the mandibular first molar (option A). There is no such thing as angle class IVorV.[1,2,3,4]

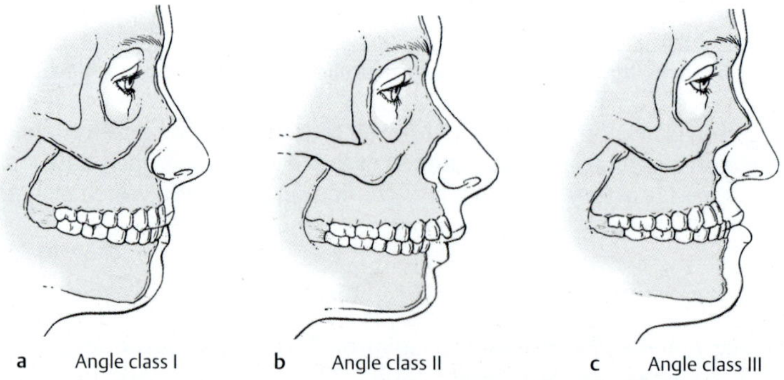

Fig. 49.1 Occlusion types. **(a)** Angle class I. **(b)** Angle class II. **(c)** Angle class III. (Source: Preoperative Evaluation. In: Janis J, ed. Essentials of Aesthetic Surgery. 1st Edition. New York: Thieme; 2018.)

References

1. Zide BM, Pfeifer TM, Longaker MT. Chin surgery: I. Augmentation—the allures and the alerts. Plast Reconstr Surg 1999;104:1843
2. Michelow BJ, Guyuron B. The chin: skeletal and soft tissue components. Plast Reconstr Surg 1995;95:473
3. Guyuron B, Michelow BJ, Willis L. Practical classification of chin deformities. Aesthetic Plast Surg 1995;19:257
4. Yaremchuk MJ. Facial skeletal augmentation. In: Mathes SJ, Hentz VR, eds. Plastic Surgery: The Head and Neck. 2nd ed. Philadelphia: Saunders Elsevier; 2006

RIEDEL LINE

7. *The Riedel line is defined by connecting which two anatomical landmarks?*

E. The anterior upper and lower lips.

The Riedel line is a vertical line defined by connecting the anterior upper and lower lips on sagittal view of the face (**Fig. 49.2**). In a balanced face, the pogonion should not project beyond the Riedel line.[1]

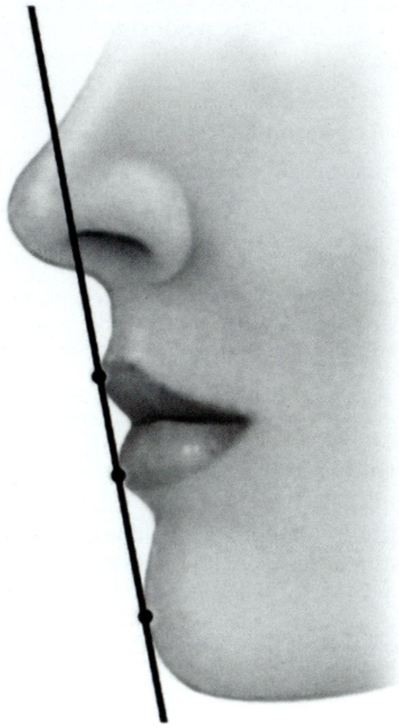

Fig. 49.2 Riedel plane is a simple *line* that connects the most prominent portion of the upper and lower lip, which on a balanced face should touch the pogonion. (Source: Preoperative Evaluation. In: Janis J, ed. Essentials of Aesthetic Surgery. 1st Edition. New York: Thieme; 2018.)

Reference

1. Lee EI. Aesthetic alteration of the chin. Semin Plast Surg 2013;27(3):155–160

CERVICOMENTAL ANGLE

8. *The angle between the chin and neck on sagittal view is ideally how large?*

C. 105–120 degrees.

The cervicomental angle ideally should not be very obtuse or acute. Soft tissue techniques such as submental lipectomy, platysmaplasty, anterior digastric resection, or submandibular gland resection can be used to address aesthetic issues pertaining to the neck and submental region.[1,2,3]

REFERENCES

1. Cohen SR. Genioplasty. In: Achauer BM, Eriksson E, Guyuron B, et al, eds. Plastic Surgery: Indications, Operations, and Outcomes. Vol. 5. St Louis, Mosby–Year Book; 2000
2. Guyuron B, ed. Genioplasty. Boston: Little Brown; 1993
3. Yaremchuk MJ. Facial skeletal augmentation. In: Mathes SJ, Hentz VR, eds. Plastic Surgery: The Head and Neck. 2nd ed. Philadelphia: Saunders Elsevier; 2006

WITCH'S-CHIN DEFORMITY

9. *A witch's-chin deformity is best repaired via which surgical maneuvers?*

D. Soft tissue correction.

Witch's-chin deformity is caused by ptosis of soft tissue caudal to the menton. As such, correction involves soft-tissue techniques only, such as soft tissue or muscle resection (**Table 49.1**). In fact, augmentation may exaggerate the deformity.[1]

Table 49.1 *Classification System for Chin Deformity and Correction*

Type	Deformity	Vector and Surgical Treatment
Class I	Macrogenia	Horizontal: Osteotomy with setback or osteotomy Vertical: Osteotomy and resection Both horizontal and vertical: Osteotomy, resection, and setback
Class II	Microgenia	Horizontal: Osteotomy with advancement, autogenous or alloplastic augmentation Vertical: Osteotomy and lengthening, with or without graft Both horizontal and vertical: Osteotomy, lengthening, and advancement, with or without graft
Class III	Combined	Horizontal macrogenia with vertical microgenia: Osteotomy with lengthening and setback Horizontal microgenia with vertical macrogenia: Osteotomy with resection of horizontal segment and advancement
Class IV	Asymmetrical	Short anterior lower face: Addition of wedge of bone to short side Normal lower facial height: Removal of wedge of bone from long side; add to short side Long anterior facial height: Removal of wedge of bone based on long side
Class V	Witch's-chin	Soft tissue correction
Class VI	Pseudomacrogenia	Soft tissue adjustment (not predictable)
Class VII	Pseudomicrogenia	Maxillary osteotomy

(Source: Reprinted with permission from Guyuron B, Michelow BJ, Willis L. Practical classification of chin deformities. Aesthetic Plast Surg 19:257, 1995.)

REFERENCE

1. Guyuron B, Michelow BJ, Willis L. Practical classification of chin deformities. Aesthetic Plast Surg 1995;19:257

POROUS POLYETHYLENE IMPLANT

10. *Which of the following is an advantage of the porous polyethylene implant?*

A. Lower infection rates than other implant types possibly due to increased vascular ingrowth.

The distinguishing characteristic of porous polyethylene implants is that they contain microscopic pores that allow vascular ingrowth. The advantages conferred are a lower tendency to migrate and erode underlying bone, and lower infection rates when compared with other types of implants, which are incorporated into the tissue via encapsulation. However, there are disadvantages inherent to this implant material and the resulting tissue architecture: placement is more difficult, requiring a larger soft tissue pocket, and removal is likewise more difficult, as vascular ingrowth results in an implant that is more tightly adherent to the surrounding tissues. Porous polyethylene implants can cause prolonged edema/inflammatory reaction.[1,2]

REFERENCES

1. Warren SM, Spector JA, Zide BM. Chin surgery VII: the textured secure implant—a recipe for success. Plast Reconstr Surg 2007;120:1378
2. Guyuron B, Raszewski RL. A critical comparison of osteoplastic and alloplastic augmentation genioplasty. Aesthetic Plast Surg 1990;14:199

SURGICAL TECHNIQUES: OSSEOUS GENIOPLASTY

11. *A patient presents for correction of significant excess vertical chin height. Which of the following osseous genioplasty techniques is most appropriate in this case?*

A. Reduction genioplasty.

Osseous genioplasty can be categorized into three common types: reduction, sliding, and jumping (**Fig. 49.3**). To correct increased vertical height or sagittal excess, reduction genioplasty (option A) is indicated. For this patient with excess vertical height, angling the osteotomy inferiorly will produce the desired result of vertical reduction. Sliding genioplasty (option B) is the standard operation for horizontal (sagittal) deficiency. Jumping genioplasty (option C) is indicated for correction of minor chin height excess. It is less appropriate for the patient in question, whose chin height excess is more significant. Interpositonal bone grafting is used for adding more vertical length which would be inappropriate for this patient. A centralizing genioplasty is best indicated to correct asymmetry using wedges of autologous bone graft.[1,2]

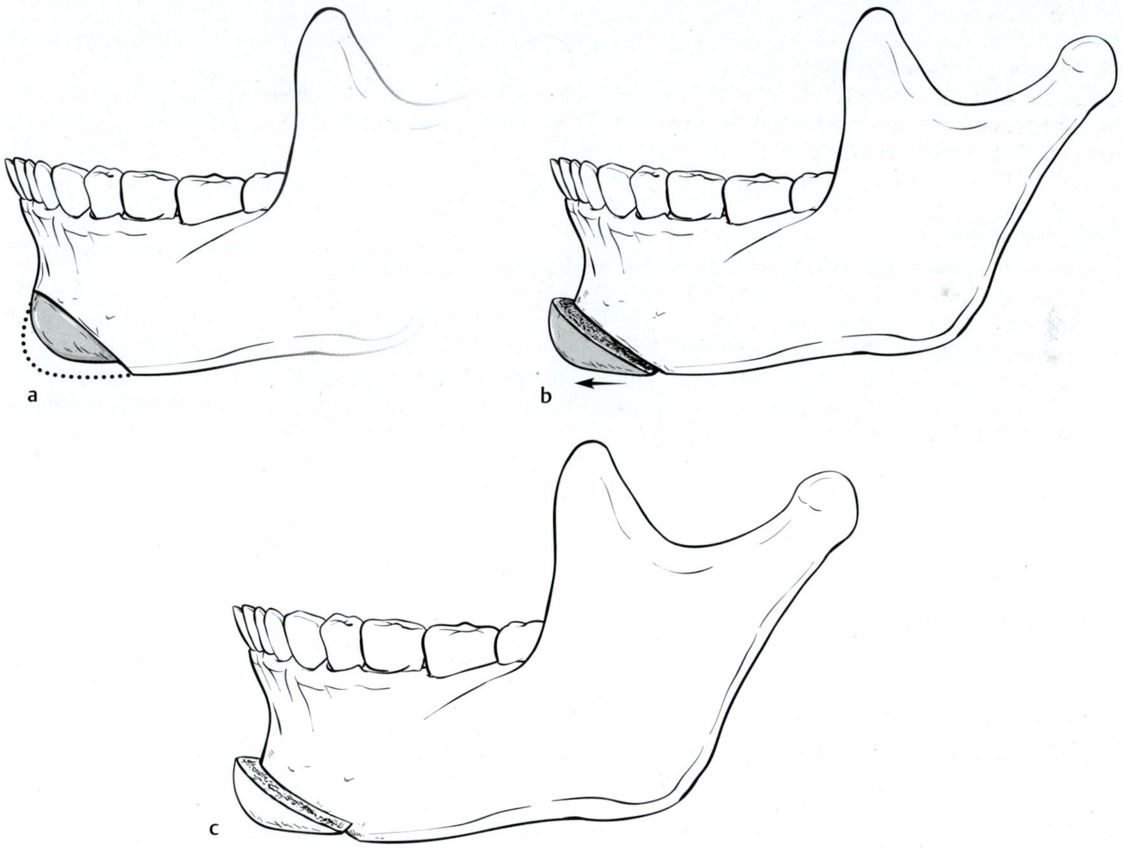

Fig. 49.3 Common types of osseous genioplasty. **(a)** Reduction genioplasty. **(b)** Sliding genioplasty. **(c)** Jumping genioplasty. (Source: Reprinted with permission from Cohen SR. Genioplasty. In Achauer BH, Eriksson E, Guyuron B, et al, eds. Plastic Surgery: Indications, Operations, and Outcomes, vol 5. St Louis: Mosby-Elsevier, 2000.)

REFERENCES

1. Zide BM, Warren SM, Spector JA. Chin surgery IV: the large chin—key parameters for successful chin reduction. Plast Reconstr Surg 2007;120:530
2. Warren SM, Spector JA, Zide BM. Chin surgery V: treatment of the long, nonprojecting chin. Plast Reconstr Surg 2007;120:760

SURGICAL APPROACH: IMPLANT GENIOPLASTY

12. *For implant genioplasty, which of the following is true regarding the extraoral approach when compared with the intraoral approach?*

B. More precise implant placement.

For implant genioplasty, there are two main surgical approaches: intraoral (where the incision is placed in the anterior gingivobuccal sulcus) and extraoral (where the incision is placed on the submental skin). The intraoral approach has the advantage of no visible scars while maintaining a similar infection rate to the extraoral approach. However, the disadvantages of this approach include a higher risk of improper implant position and higher chance of plate/screw extrusion. These are due to a lack of direct visualization of the pocket when compared with the extraoral approach, and implants that are improperly placed via the intraoral approach often are located superior to the proper position. The extraoral approach allows more precise implant placement and possibly lower risk of malposition or mental nerve injury. Closure of soft tissue and muscle during this approach should be strong in order to prevent ptosis. The extraoral approach is relatively indicatedwhenundergoing concomitant procedures that use the submental incision such as submental liposuction or platysma plication.[1,2,3]

REFERENCES

1. Yaremchuk MJ. Facial skeletal augmentation. In: Mathes SJ, Hentz VR, eds. Plastic Surgery: The Head and Neck. 2nd ed. Philadelphia: Saunders Elsevier; 2006
2. Terino EO. Alloplastic facial contouring by zonal principles of skeletal anatomy. Clin Plast Surg 1992;19:487
3. Zide BM, Warren SM, Spector JA. Chin surgery IV: the large chin key parameters for successful chin reduction. Plast Reconstr Surg 2007;120:530

IMPLANT POSITION

13. *Which of the following is accurate with regards to chin implant position?*

C. The implant should be placed directly over the pogonion.

For augmentation genioplasty with implant, the proper position of the implant is subperiosteal, directly over the pogonion. The pogonion is the most projecting portion of the mandible and defines chin excess or deficiency in relation to the surrounding anatomy. Placing the implant directly over this point achieves the aesthetic outcome by increasing chin projection to the desired amount. Placing the implant superior to this position carries the risk of poor aesthetic outcome and damage to dentition, including bone resorption, tooth erosion, and tooth asymmetry. This risk increases with the use of the intraoral approach. Inferior misplacement over the menton, for example, does not sufficiently contribute to chin projection and thus may not result in a good aesthetic outcome. It is likewise important to ensure that implant position is sufficiently deep, with the target tissue pocket between the bone and the periosteum. Placement superficial to this layer risksimplantpalpability and visibility.[1]

REFERENCE

1. Yaremchuk MJ. Improving aesthetic outcomes after alloplastic chin augmentation. Plast Reconstr Surg 2003;112:1422

POSTOPERATIVE CARE

14. *Which of the following should be considered for postoperative care after genioplasty?*

B. Patients should be instructed to limit activity that increases heart rate for 5 to 7 days.

Postoperative care after genioplasty is essential to ensure patient safety and maximize aesthetic outcome. Patients should wear an elastic chin support 24 hours a day for the first 5 to 7 days and then at night for the next 1 to 2 weeks. They should also limit activity that increases heart rate for 5 to 7 days and sleep supine with the head of the bed elevated to 45 degrees for 3 to 5 days. Hard foods should be avoided for 3 days after osseous genioplasty. Limiting salt intake and rinsing mouth after meals with water and/or Peridex is also useful. Preoperatively, one dose of a first-generation cephalosporin such as cefazolin is administered. This regimen is continued postoperatively for 3 to 5 days every 8 hours with oral dosing. Glucocorticoids are also recommended—one intravenous dose should be given perioperatively, and a steroid taper regimen is recommended postoperatively.[1,2]

REFERENCES

1. Cohen SR. Genioplasty. In: Achauer BM, Eriksson E, Guyuron B, et al, eds. Plastic Surgery: Indications, Operations, and Outcomes. Vol. 5. St Louis, Mosby–Year Book; 2000
2. Guyuron B, ed. Genioplasty. Boston: Little Brown; 1993

REOPERATION

15. *For a patient who underwent implant genioplasty 1 day prior, which circumstance is an indication for surgical revision?*

C. Significant paresthesias and/or neuropraxia.

Nerve symptoms such as motor or sensory deficit are not uncommon after genioplasty. Neurapraxia is often a result of retraction injury due to stretching and pulling of tissues intraoperatively and on its own does not necessitate immediate reoperation since spontaneous resolution often occurs within 2 to 6 weeks. Permanent nerve deficits are extremely rare. Certain implants may cause a significant inflammatory response such as porous polyethylene which can cause edema for several weeks after placement which then subsides. Causes include inadvertent nerve transection or avulsion during surgery, or compression injury from an implant impinging on the nerve. For this reason, immediate reoperation is indicated for any significant neurapraxia in which implant nerve compression is suspected in order to prevent permanent deficits.[1,2,3]

REFERENCES

1. Warren SM, Spector JA, Zide BM. Chin surgery VII: the textured secure implant—a recipe for success. Plast Reconstr Surg 2007;120:1378
2. Guyuron B, Raszewski RL. A critical comparison of osteoplastic and alloplastic augmentation genioplasty. Aesthetic Plast Surg 1990;14:199
3. Yaremchuk MJ. Improving aesthetic outcomes after alloplastic chin augmentation. Plast Reconstr Surg 2003;112:1422

50. Otoplasty

Stelios C. Wilson
See *Essentials of Aesthetic Surgery*, pp. 691–708

EAR ANATOMY AND DEVELOPMENT

1. *The ear is 85% of its adult size by what age?*
A. 1 year old.
B. 3 years old.
C. 6 years old.
D. 13 years old.
E. 18 years old.

EAR ANATOMY AND DEVELOPMENT

2. *The vascular supply to the ear is mainly supplied by which two arteries?*
A. Superficial temporal and posterior auricular arteries.
B. Superficial temporal and occipital arteries.
C. Facial and occipital arteries.
D. Transverse facial and posterior auricular arteries.
E. Descending facial artery and superficial temporal artery.

EAR ANATOMY AND DEVELOPMENT

3. *The tragus is innervated by which of the following nerves?*
A. Auriculotemporal nerve (CN V).
B. Great auricular nerve (C2–3).
C. Arnold's nerve (CN X).
D. Lesser occipital nerve (CN2–3).
E. Greater occipital nerve (CN2).

EAR ANATOMY AND DEVELOPMENT

4. *The external acoustic meatus is innervated by which of the following nerves?*
A. Auriculotemporal nerve (CN V).
B. Great auricular nerve (C2–3).
C. Arnold's nerve (CN X).
D. Lesser occipital nerve (CN2–3).
E. Greater occipital nerve (CN2).

EAR ANATOMY AND DEVELOPMENT

5. *The great auricular nerve (C2–3) innervates which portion of the ear?*
A. Tragus.
B. Helix.
C. Antihelix.
D. Scapha.
E. Lobule.

EAR ANATOMY AND DEVELOPMENT

6. *In the ideal proportions of an adult ear, long axis of the ear inclines how many degrees from vertical?*
A. 0 degrees.
B. 5–10 degrees.
C. 15–20 degrees.
D. 25–30 degrees.
E. >30 degrees.

EAR ANATOMY AND DEVELOPMENT

7. *In the ideal proportions of an adult, the helix-to-mastoid distance in the upper third of the ear should be which of the following?*
A. 5–8 mm.
B. 10–12 mm.
C. 16–18 mm.
D. 20–22 mm.
E. 25–30 mm.

EPIDEMIOLOGY|PATHOLOGY

8. *What is the incidence of abnormal ear morphology?*
A. 1%.
B. 5%.
C. 10%.
D. 15%.
E. 25%.

EPIDEMIOLOGY|PATHOLOGY

9. *Which of the follow is considered to be normal ear morphology?*
A. A lobule that is parallel to the antihelical fold.
B. Obtuse conchomastoid angle.
C. The helix should project 2 to 5 mm more medially than the antihelix in frontal view.
D. Conchal wall depth of 1.8 cm.
E. Conchoscaphal angle <90 degrees.

INDICATIONS|CONTRAINDICATIONS

10. *At what minimum age would surgical correction be advised?*
A. 1–2 years of age.
B. 6–7 years of age.
C. 12–13 years of age.
D. 15 years of age.
E. 18 years of age.

SURGICAL TECHNIQUE

11. *Mustardé technique refers to which of the following?*
A. Mattress suturing to better define the antihelix.
B. Suture fixation of the conchal cartilage to the mastoid fascia.
C. Cartilage-breaking technique for severe prominent ear deformities.
D. Posterior lower 1/3 skin resection.
E. Technique for proper harvesting of auricular cartilage.

SURGICAL TECHNIQUE

12. *The Furnas technique refers to which of the following?*
A. Mattress suturing to better define the antihelix.
B. Suture fixation of the conchal cartilage to the mastoid fascia.
C. Cartilage-breaking technique for severe prominent ear deformities.
D. Posterior lower 1/3 skin resection.
E. Technique for proper harvesting of auricular cartilage.

SURGICAL TECHNIQUE

13. *The Converse-Wood-Smith technique refers to which of the following?*

A. Mattress suturing to better define the antihelix.
B. Suture fixation of the conchal cartilage to the mastoid fascia.
C. Cartilage-breaking technique for severe prominent ear deformities.
D. Posterior lower 1/3 skin resection.
E. Technique for proper harvesting of auricular cartilage.

SURGICAL TECHNIQUE

14. *The Modified fishtail excision refers to which of the following?*

A. Mattress suturing to better define the antihelix.
B. Suture fixation of the conchal cartilage to the mastoid fascia.
C. Cartilage-breaking technique for severe prominent ear deformities.
D. Posterior lower 1/3 skin resection.
E. Technique for proper harvesting of auricular cartilage.

COMPLICATIONS

15. *An 18-year-old male patient who had an otoplasty performed yesterday calls the office complaining of sudden onset of persistent, unilateral pain. What is the appropriate next step?*

A. Reassure the patient that the pain will likely be worse on postoperative day 2 and then will start to get better.
B. Have the patient apply ice to the area.
C. Add NSAIDs to the pain regimen.
D. Have the patient come to the ED or office to be evaluated.
E. Prescribe methylprednisolone to help with postoperative edema.

COMPLICATIONS

16. *A 20-year-old female patient who had an otoplasty performed 4 days ago calls the office complaining of sudden onset of persistent, unilateral pain. What complication do you suspect based on timing?*

A. Hematoma.
B. Infection.
C. Suture rupture.
D. Late deformity.
E. Nerve pain.

Answers

EAR ANATOMY AND DEVELOPMENT

1. *The ear is 85% of its adult size by what age?*

C. 6 years old.

The ear begins to protrude at 3 to 4 months of gestation and continues to grow during childhood. Neonatal cartilage is malleable and soft and becomes stiffer and more brittle with age. By the age of 6, the ear is 85% of its adult size. The average length of a 10-year-old male ear is 60 mm.[1,2,3,4,5]

REFERENCES

1. Allison GR. Anatomy of the external ear. Clin Plast Surg 1978;5:419
2. Tan ST, Abramson DL, MacDonald DM, et al. Molding therapy for infants with deformational auricular anomalies. Ann Plast Surg 1997;38:263
3. Tan ST, Shibu M, Gault DT. A splint for correction of congenital ear deformities. Br J Plast Surg 1994;47:575
4. Farkas LG, Posnick JC, Hreczko TM. Anthropometric growth study of the ear. Cleft Palate Craniofac J 1992;29:324
5. Adamson JE, Horton CE, Crawford HH. The growth pattern of the external ear. Plast Reconstr Surg 1965;36:466

EAR ANATOMY AND DEVELOPMENT

2. *The vascular supply to the ear is mainly supplied by which two arteries?*

A. Superficial temporal and posterior auricular arteries.

The vascular supply of the ear is predominantly from two branches of the external carotid system: the superficial temporal artery and the posterior auricular artery (**Fig. 50.1**).[1]

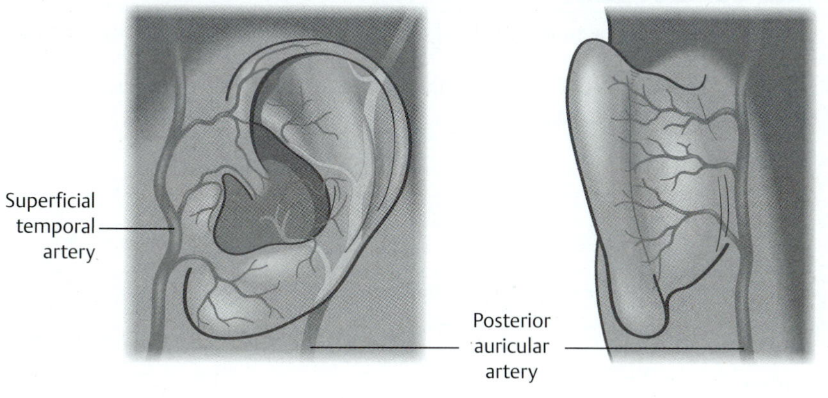

Fig. 50.1 Vascularity of the external ear. (Source: Vascularity. In: Janis J, ed. Essentials of Aesthetic Surgery. 1st Edition. New York: Thieme; 2018.)

REFERENCE

1. Allison GR. Anatomy of the external ear. Clin Plast Surg 1978;5:419

EAR ANATOMY AND DEVELOPMENT

3. *The tragus is innervated by which of the following nerves?*

A. Auriculotemporal nerve (CN V).

The tragus and the crus helicis are innervated by the auriculotemporal nerve (CN V, V3 to be exact). The great auricular nerve (C2–3) divides into anterior and posterior branches and innervates the remaining scapha and lobule. Arnold's nerve (CN X) innervates the external acoustic meatus and medial conchal bowl. The lesser occipital nerve innervates the middle one-third helix and antihelix.[1]

REFERENCE

1. Allison GR. Anatomy of the external ear. Clin Plast Surg 1978;5:419

EAR ANATOMY AND DEVELOPMENT

4. *The external acoustic meatus is innervated by which of the following nerves?*

C. Arnold's nerve (CN X).

The tragus and the crus helicis are innervated by the auriculotemporal nerve (CN V, and specifically V3). The great auricular nerve (C2–3) divides into anterior and posterior branches and innervates the remaining scapha and lobule. Arnold's nerve (CN X) innervates the external acoustic meatus and medial conchal bowl. The lesser occipital nerve innervates the middle one-third helix and antihelix.[1]

REFERENCE

1. Allison GR. Anatomy of the external ear. Clin Plast Surg 1978;5:419

EAR ANATOMY AND DEVELOPMENT

5. *The great auricular nerve (C2–3) innervates which portion of the ear?*

E. Lobule.

The tragus and the crus helicis are innervated by the auriculotemporal nerve (CN V, specifically V3). The great auricular nerve (C2–3) divides into anterior and posterior branches and innervates the remaining scapha and lobule. Arnold's nerve (CN X) innervates the external acoustic meatus and medial conchal bowl. The lesser occipital nerve innervates the middle one-third helix and antihelix.[1]

REFERENCE

1. Allison GR. Anatomy of the external ear. Clin Plast Surg 1978;5:419

EAR ANATOMY AND DEVELOPMENT

6. *In the ideal proportions of an adult ear, long axis of the ear inclines how many degrees from vertical?*

C. 15–20 degrees.

In the ideal adult ear, the long axis of the ear inclines 15 to 20 degrees from vertical. Reference for ideal proportions of the ear is shown (**Fig. 50.2**).[1,2]

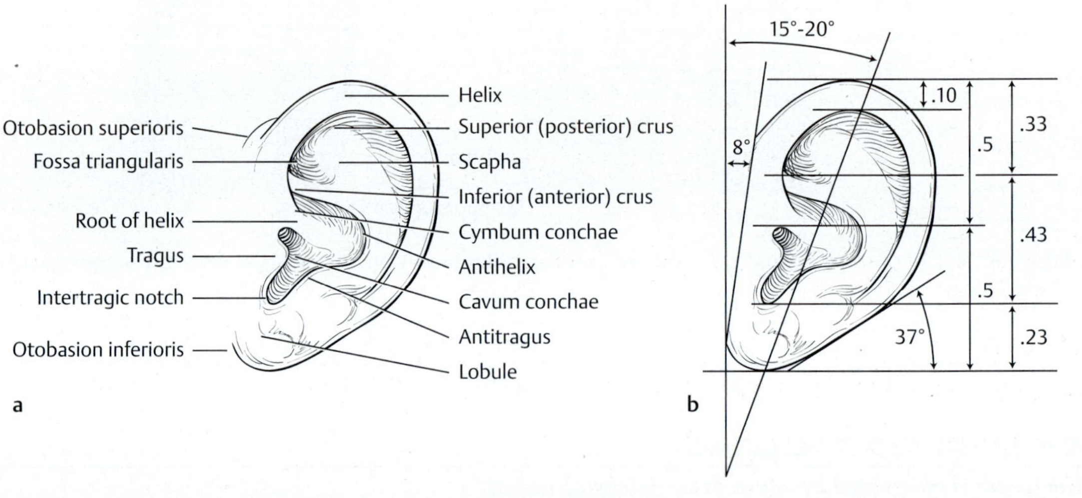

Fig. 50.2 Proportions of the ear. **(a)** The normal ear and its parts. **(b)** The ear's critical proportions. (Source: Ear anatomy. In: Bentz M, Bauer B, Zuker R, ed. Principles & Practice of Pediatric Plastic Surgery. 2nd Edition. New York: Thieme; 2016.)

REFERENCES

1. Farkas LG, Posnick JC, Hreczko TM. Anthropometric growth study of the ear. Cleft Palate Craniofac J 1992;29:324
2. Macgregor FC. Ear deformities: social and psychological implications. Clin Plast Surg 1978;5:347

EAR ANATOMY AND DEVELOPMENT

7. *In the ideal proportions of an adult, the helix-to-mastoid distance in the upper third of the ear should be which of the following?*

B. 10–12 mm.

In the ideal adult ear, the helix-to-mastoid distance should be in the range of 10 to 12 mm in the upper third, 16 to 18 mm in the middle third, and 20 to 22 mm in the lower third.[1]

REFERENCE

1. McDowell AJ. Goals in otoplasty for protruding ears. Plast Reconstr Surg 1968;41:17

EPIDEMIOLOGY/PATHOLOGY

8. *What is the incidence of abnormal ear morphology?*

B. 5%.

The incidence of abnormal ear morphology in the Caucasian populations is approximately 5%. This tends to be an autosomal dominant pattern of transmission in families. The three major contributing factors to the abnormal ear morphology are underdeveloped antihelical fold, prominent concha, and protruding earlobe.[1,2,3,4]

REFERENCES

1. Macgregor FC. Ear deformities: social and psychological implications. Clin Plast Surg 1978;5:347
2. Hao W, Chorney JM, Bezuhly M, et al. Analysis of health-related quality-of-life outcomes and their predictive factors in pediatric patients who undergo otoplasty. Plast Reconstr Surg 2013;132:811e
3. Braun T, Hainzinger T, Stelter K, et al. Health-related quality of life, patient benefit, and clinical outcome after otoplasty using suture techniques in 62 children and adults. Plast Reconstr Surg 2010;126:2115
4. McDowell AJ. Goals in otoplasty for protruding ears. Plast Reconstr Surg 1968;41:17

EPIDEMIOLOGY/PATHOLOGY

9. *Which of the follow is considered to be normal ear morphology?*

E. Conchoscaphal angle <90 degrees.

Absent tragus is not a major contributing factor to abnormal ear morphology. The three major contributing factors to the abnormal ear morphology are underdeveloped antihelical fold, prominent concha, and protruding earlobe. An underdeveloped antihelical fold generally has an an obtuse conchoscaphal angle (>90 degrees) and the scapha and helical rim protrude causing a prominent upper and middle third of the ear. The helix should project 2 to 5 mm more laterally, not medially than the antihelix in the frontal view. A prominent concha can be either from excessively deep conchal wall (>1.5 cm) or obtuse conchamastoid angle causing a prominent middle third of the ear. Additionally, the lobule and antihelical fold should lie in a parallel plane at an acute angle to the mastoid process. A protruding earlobe causes prominent lower third of the ear.[1,2,3,4,5]

REFERENCES

1. Macgregor FC. Ear deformities: social and psychological implications. Clin Plast Surg 1978;5:347
2. Hao W, Chorney JM, Bezuhly M, et al. Analysis of health-related quality-of-life outcomes and their predictive factors in pediatric patients who undergo otoplasty. Plast Reconstr Surg 2013;132:811e
3. Braun T, Hainzinger T, Stelter K, et al. Health-related quality of life, patient benefit, and clinical outcome after otoplasty using suture techniques in 62 children and adults. Plast Reconstr Surg 2010;126:2115
4. McDowell AJ. Goals in otoplasty for protruding ears. Plast Reconstr Surg 1968;41:17
5. Campobasso P, Belloli G. [Protruding ears: the indications for surgical treatment] Pediatr Med Chir 1993;15:151

INDICATIONS/CONTRAINDICATIONS

10. *At what minimum age would surgical correction be advised?*

B. 6–7 years of age.

In general, surgical intervention should not be performed before patients are 4 years of age. The ear is nearly fully developed by 6 to 7 years of age, at which time surgery should be considered in appropriate candidates. However, it is important to address timing on a patient-to-patient basis as some patients may experience significant bullying at a young age and earlier intervention may be necessary.[1,2,3,4,5,6]

REFERENCES

1. Adamson JE, Horton CE, Crawford HH. The growth pattern of the external ear. Plast Reconstr Surg 1965;36:466
2. Macgregor FC. Ear deformities: social and psychological implications. Clin Plast Surg 19785:347
3. Hao W, Chorney JM, Bezuhly M, et al. Analysis of health-related quality-of-life outcomes and their predictive factors in pediatric patients who undergo otoplasty. Plast Reconstr Surg 2013;132:811e
4. McDowell AJ. Goals in otoplasty for protruding ears. Plast Reconstr Surg 1968;41:17
5. Bradbury ET, Hewison J, Timmons MJ. Psychological and social outcome of prominent ear correction in children. Br J Plast Surg 1992;45:97
6. Balogh B, Millesi H. Are growth alterations a consequence of surgery for prominent ears? Plast Reconstr Surg 1992;89:623

SURGICAL TECHNIQUE

11. *Mustardé technique refers to which of the following?*

A. Mattress suturing to better define the antihelix.

Mustardé technique refers to a cartilage-shaping technique using mattress suturing to correct a poorly defined antihelical fold. This helps better shape the upper third of the ear. Of note, this technique is almost never performed in isolation (**Fig. 50.3**).[1]

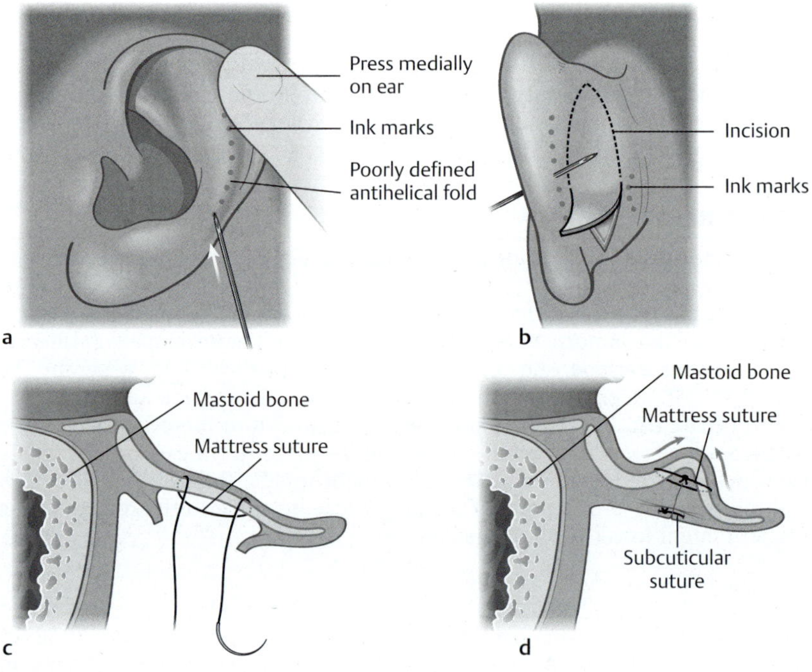

Fig. 50.3 The Mustardé technique. **(a)** Several pairs of ink marks are made on the concha and outer aspect of the antihelix. **(b)** Several 25-gauge needles dipped in ink are used to transfer the ink marks to the postauricular skin. **(c)** The skin excision is carried down to cartilage. After hemostasis is obtained, several sutures are placed through the full thickness of cartilage. Usually only two or three well-placed sutures are required. **(d)** The sutures are tied simultaneously. A subcuticular 4-0 nylon suture is used for closure. (Source: Mustardé technique. In: Janis J, ed. Essentials of Aesthetic Surgery. 1st Edition. New York: Thieme; 2018.)

REFERENCE

1. Mustardé JC. The correction of prominent ears using mattress sutures. Br J Plast Surg 1963;16:170

SURGICAL TECHNIQUE

12. *The Furnas technique refers to which of the following?*

B. Suture fixation of the conchal cartilage to mastoid fascia.

The Furnas technique is used to correct deformities of the superior two-thirds of the ear by addressing conchal excess. In general, an ellipse of skin is excised in the postauricular sulcus in the upper two-thirds of the ear, not the lower one-third. This will then expose the posterior auricular muscles and ligaments which are then divided and resected. Several mattress sutures are then used to attach conchal cartilage to the mastoid fascia (**Fig. 50.4**). Another conchal shaping maneuver is the Mustardé technique which is used to correct the prominent ear deformity with a poorly defined antihelical fold by creating and securing an antihelical fold with two to four horizontal mattress fixation sutures. A posterior skin excision is made once again, exposing the cartilage at which point full-thickness sutures are placed in order to better define the antihelical fold. This maneuver is almost never performed in isolation (**Fig. 50.5**).[1]

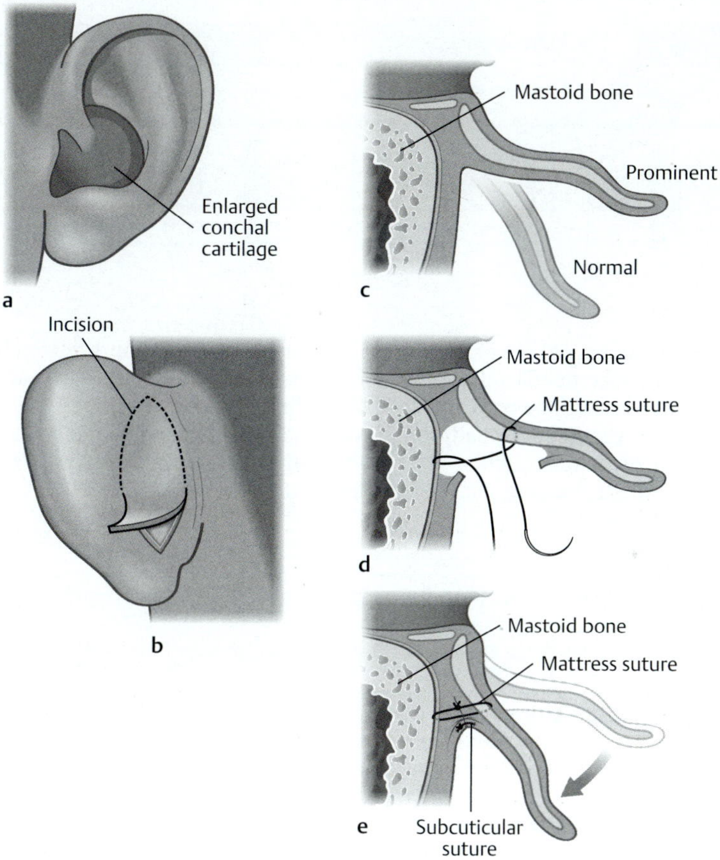

Fig. 50.4 The Furnas technique. **(a)** The Furnas technique is best used for patients with prominence of the superior two thirds of the ear. **(b)** The deeply cupped and enlarged conchal cartilage of the prominent ear is contrasted with normal conchal cartilage in cross section. **(c)** An ellipse of skin is excised in the postauricular sulcus, exposing the posterior auricular muscles and ligaments. These are divided and resected. **(d, e)** Several mattress sutures are used to attach conchal cartilage to the mastoid fascia. The mattress sutures should be placed through the full thickness of the conchal cartilage. The sutures are tied simultaneously. Enlarged conchal. (Source: Furnas technique. In: Janis J, ed. Essentials of Aesthetic Surgery. 1st Edition. New York: Thieme; 2018.)

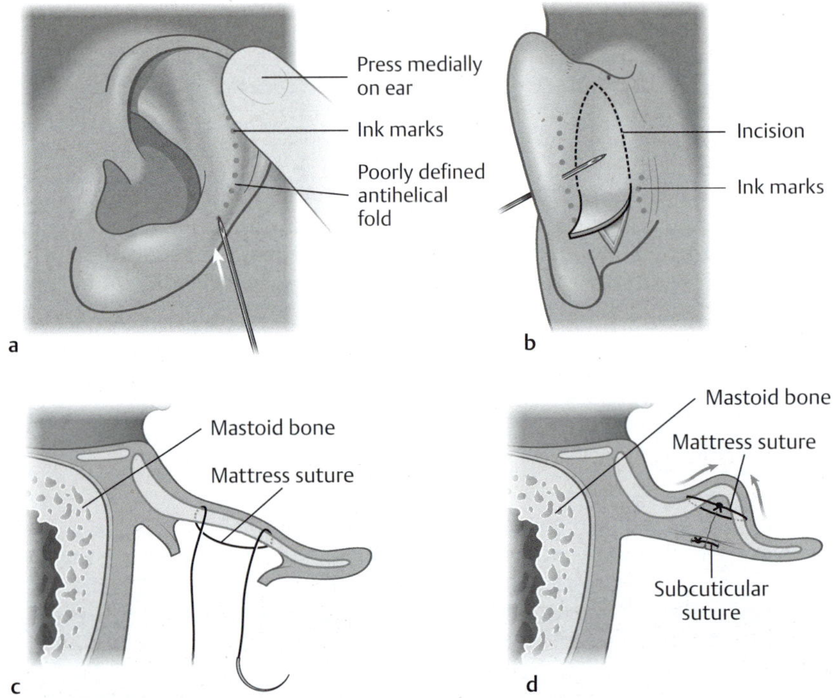

Fig. 50.5 The Mustardé technique. **(a)** Several pairs of ink marks are made on the concha and outer aspect of the antihelix. **(b)** Several 25-gauge needles dipped in ink are used to transfer the ink marks to the postauricular skin. **(c)** The skin excision is carried down to cartilage. After hemostasis is obtained, several sutures are placed through the full thickness of cartilage. Usually only two or three well-placed sutures are required. **(d)** The sutures are tied simultaneously. A subcuticular 4-0 nylon suture is used for closure. (Source: Mustardé technique. In: Janis J, ed. Essentials of Aesthetic Surgery. 1st Edition. New York: Thieme; 2018.)

REFERENCE

1. Furnas DW. Correction of prominent ears by conchamastoid sutures. Plast Reconstr Surg 1968;42:189

SURGICAL TECHNIQUE

13. *The Converse-Wood-Smith technique refers to which of the following?*

C. Cartilage-breaking technique for severe prominent ear deformities.

The Converse-Wood-Smith technique refers a cartilage-breaking technique for severe prominent ear deformities and involves an incision along the entire posterior ear with cartilage removal and resuspension to correct the prominent ear. The pinna is folded back to define the superior

crus of the antihelix, as well as the crural junction. Although this is a powerful technique, one of the drawbacks is that it may cause cartilaginous ridging and sharp edges leading to a "postoperative" appearance (**Fig. 50.6**).[1] This is in contrast to the cartilage-molding techniques like the Mustardé or Furnas techniques which are used for contour shaping of the upper two-thirds of the ear. Both techniques involve a posterior skin excision with mattress sutures being taken from the cartilage to the mastoid fascia in the setting of Furnas sutures which corresponds to answer B. The Mustardé technique involves horizontal mattress sutures being performed along the posterior ear cartilage to better define the antihelical fold. A posterior lower third skin resection is used for lobule prominence correction. Proper auricular cartilage harvesting is by placing an incision along the posterior or anterior mid conchal edge; cartilage resuspensionisnot always required nor is skin excision.

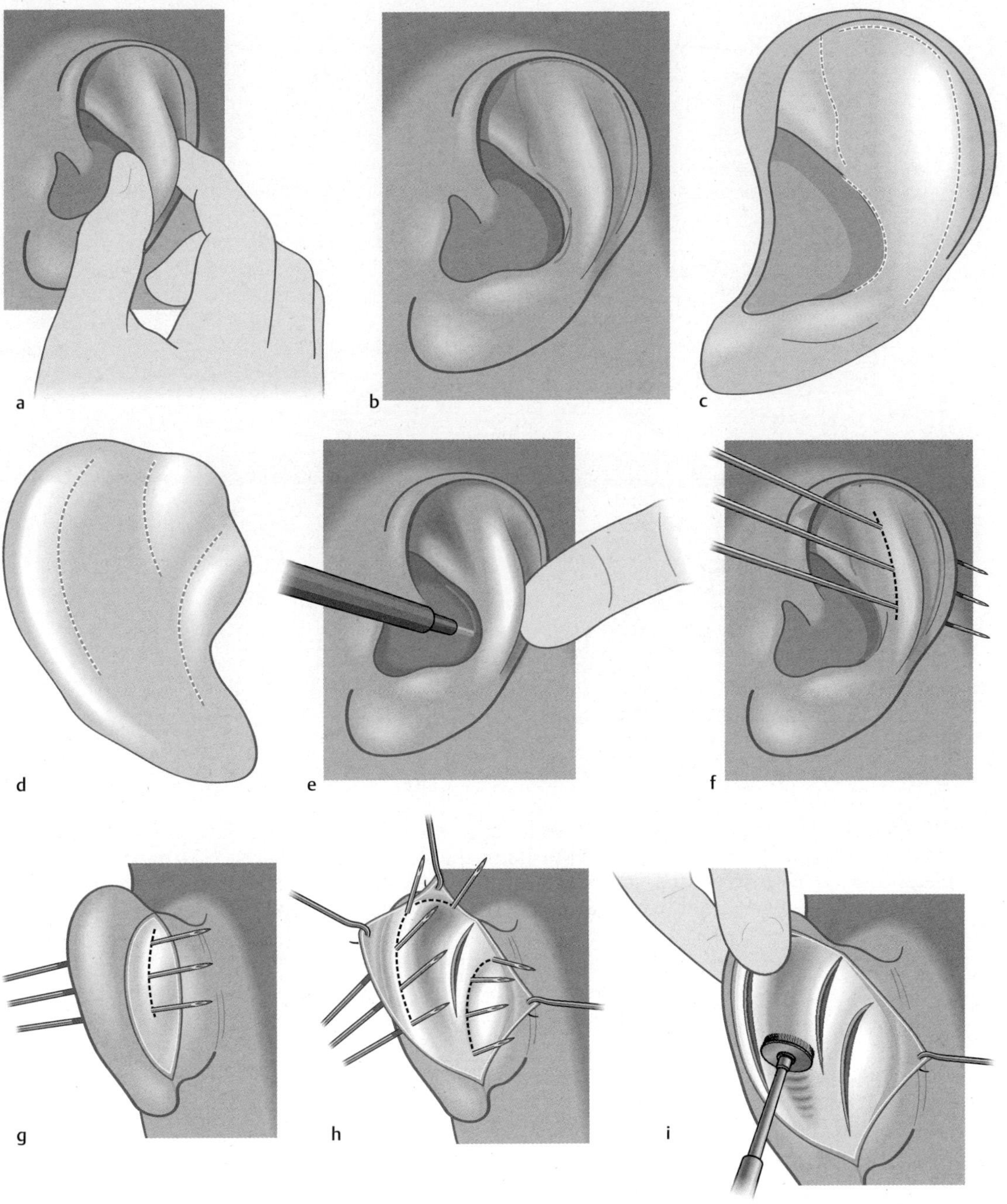

Fig. 50.6 The Converse–Wood-Smith technique. **(a)** The pinna is folded back to define the superior crus of the antihelix, as well as the crural junction. **(b)** The anterior and posterior borders of the antihelix, the superior border of the superior crus, and the conchal rim are outlined with ink. **(c,d)** The planned cartilaginous incisions. **(e)** Conchal rim definition may be facilitated with pressure applied to the scapha. **(f,g)** The center line of the superior crus and antihelix is marked by 25-gauge needles. An ellipse of skin is fashioned to incorporate these and excised. **(h)** The skin is undermined in a subperichondrial plane and the cartilaginous segments marked with needles. The cartilage is incised full thickness, without merging the incisions. **(i)** If necessary, a wire brush may be used to thin thick and rigid cartilage. (*Continued*)

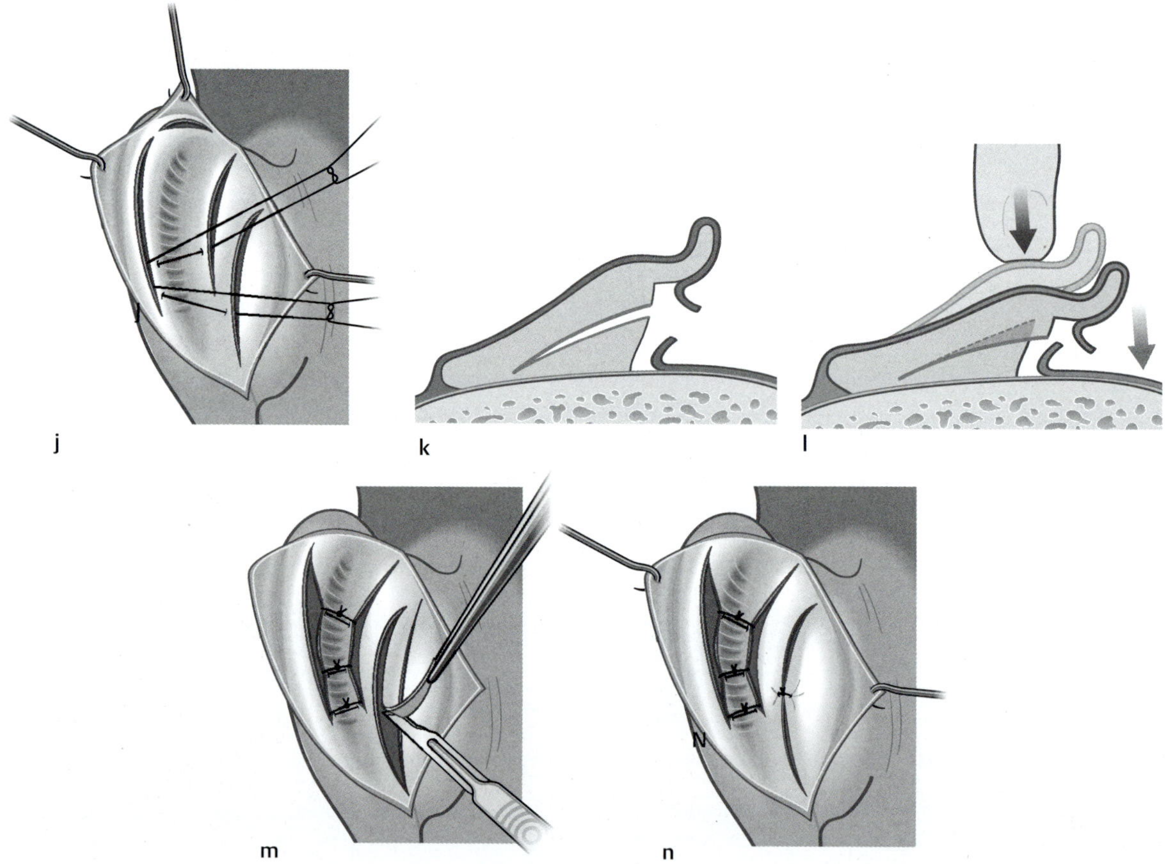

Fig. 50.6 (*Continued*) **(j)** Mattress sutures are placed to form the superior crus and body of the antihelix. **(k)** The conchal rim is incised. **(l)** Digital pressure is used to assess the amount of conchal excess. **(m,n)** The appropriate amount of conchal cartilage is excised, and the antihelix and conchal rim are approximated with a single suture. (Source: Converse–Wood-Smith technique. In: Janis J, ed. Essentials of Aesthetic Surgery. 1st Edition. New York: Thieme; 2018.)

Reference

1. Converse JM, Wood-Smith D. Technical details in the surgical correction of the lop ear deformity. Plast Reconstr Surg 1963;31:118

SURGICAL TECHNIQUE

14. *The Modified fishtail excision refers to which of the following?*

D. Posterior lower 1/3 skin resection.

The modified fishtail excision is a posterior excision for the correction of a prominent lobule. A "V extension" is added inferior to the posterior skin excision and this is pressed against the mastoid fascia to give a mirror image. This segment is then removed bringing the lower third and the lobule closer to the mastoid (**Fig. 50.7**).[1] Mattress suturing to better define the antihelical fold refers to the Mustardé technique. Suture fixation of the conchal cartilage to the mastoid fascia refers to the Furnas technique. Cartilage-breaking technique for severe prominent ears refers to the Converse-Wood-Smith technique. Finally, the technique for proper harvesting of auricular cartilage would not be best performed through modified fishtail excision but rather a posterior or anterior conchal skin incision to expose the cartilage.

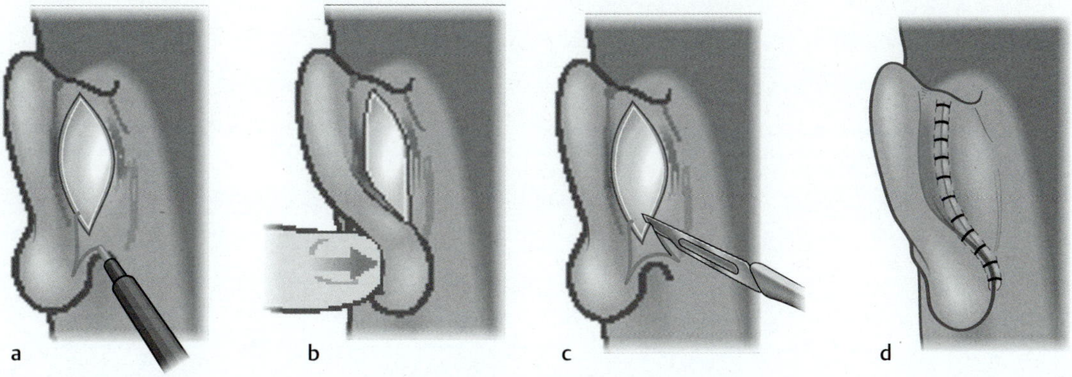

Fig. 50.7 Correction of a prominent lobule using a modified fishtail excision. **(a)** A V extension of the posterior auricular incision is drawn on the posterior surface of the lobule. **(b)** While the ink is still wet, the lobule is pressed against the mastoid skin. **(c)** The mirror impression of the V is transposed to the mastoid skin. All skin within the borders of the modified fishtail design is excised. **(d)** Closure is performed with a running 4-0 nylon suture. (Source: Correction of lobule prominence (lower third). In: Janis J, ed. Essentials of Aesthetic Surgery. 1st Edition. New York: Thieme; 2018.)

REFERENCE

1. Wood-Smith D. Otoplasty. In Rees T, ed. Aesthetic Plastic Surgery. Philadelphia: Saunders; 1980

COMPLICATIONS

15. ***An 18-year-old male patient who had an otoplasty performed yesterday calls the office complaining of sudden onset of persistent, unilateral pain. What is the appropriate next step?***

D. Have the patient come to the ED or office to be evaluated.

The most immediate and pressing postoperative complication is hematoma. This presents as a sudden-onset, persistent, unilateral pain. The patient should be seen as soon as possible, the dressing should be removed, sutures should be removed, the clot should be evacuated, and reapplication of a dressing should be done with mild compression. Hematoma that is not managed quickly and appropriately will jeopardize the patient's result.[1]

REFERENCE

1. Spira M. Otoplasty: what I do now—a 30-year perspective. Plast Reconstr Surg 1999;104:834

COMPLICATIONS

16. ***A 20-year-old female patient who had an otoplasty performed 4 days ago calls the office complaining of sudden onset of persistent, unilateral pain. What complication do you suspect based on timing?***

B. Infection.

If a patient has sudden increased unilateral pain on postoperative day 3 or 4, infection should be suspected. This is usually from *Staphylococcus* or *Streptococcus*, and occasionally *Pseudomonas*. Some advocate liberal use of hospital admission and IV antibiotics for purulent infections to prevent progression to chondritis. Sulfamylon can be useful in preventing spread of infection and chondritis.[1]

REFERENCE

1. Spira M. Otoplasty: what I do now—a 30-year perspective. Plast Reconstr Surg 1999;104:834

Part VIII

Breast Surgery

51. Breast Anatomy

Ara A. Salibian, Anmol Chattha
See *Essentials of Aesthetic Surgery*, pp. 711–722

EMBRYOLOGY, DEVELOPMENT, AND PHYSIOLOGY

1. ***The mammary gland is derived from which of the following cell lines?***
A. Endoderm.
B. Mesoderm.
C. Ectoderm.
D. Neuroectoderm.
E. Neural crest origin.

EMBRYOLOGY, DEVELOPMENT, AND PHYSIOLOGY

2. ***A 19-year-old female presents with complete absence of the right breast and nipple. She has no abnormalities of her extremities or pectoralis muscle. Her chest wall is in good position and size. Which of the following terms best describes the anatomic variation?***
A. Amastia.
B. Amazia.
C. Athelia.
D. Poland syndrome.
E. Anterior thoracic hypoplasia.

EMBRYOLOGY, DEVELOPMENT, AND PHYSIOLOGY

3. ***A 20-year-old female presents with complaints of polymastia. Which is the most likely area of accessory breast tissue found on examination?***
A. Shoulder.
B. Overlying the sternum.
C. Lower lateral chest wall.
D. On the back overlying the latissimus dorsi muscle.
E. Thigh.

EMBRYOLOGY, DEVELOPMENT, AND PHYSIOLOGY

4. ***A young female patient is brought in by her parents regarding concerns of breast asymmetry. She has absence of any breast tissue but presence of the nipple of one side of her chest. On the contralateral chest, she has presence of glandular tissue and areolar pigmentation with a secondary mound formed by the nipple above the level of the breast. What stage of breast development is this patient by the Tanner classification?***
A. 1.
B. 2.
C. 3.
D. 4.
E. 5.

EMBRYOLOGY, DEVELOPMENT, AND PHYSIOLOGY

5. ***A 5-year-old girl's parents are concerned as their daughter has started to develop breasts. Upon examination, the patient has bilateral stage 4 Tanner breast development but no other signs of puberty or skeletal maturation. This patient's condition is best represented by which of the following?***
A. Premature thelarche.
B. Poland syndrome.
C. Jeune syndrome.
D. Supernumerary breast.
E. Delayed maturation.

VASCULAR SUPPLY

6. *During a mastectomy, which of the following vessels is the most critical to preserve perfusion to the skin and nipple-areola complex?*
A. 2nd internal mammary artery perforator.
B. Lateral thoracic artery.
C. Thoracoacromial artery.
D. Intercostal perforators.
E. Thoracodorsal artery.

INNERVATION

7. *Which of the following nerves primarily supplies sensation to the nipple-areolar complex?*
A. Intercostobrachial nerve.
B. T3 branch of intercostal nerve.
C. T4 branch of intercostal nerve.
D. T5 branch of intercostal nerve.
E. T6 branch of intercostal nerve.

SKIN AND PARENCHYMA

8. *A 63-year-old female presents for consultation for mastopexy. On examination, she has deflated breasts, with grade III ptosis of the nipple bilaterally. Attenuation of which of the following structures is responsible for this presentation?*
A. Ductal tissue.
B. Glandular tissue.
C. Fatty tissue.
D. Cooper's ligaments.
E. Dermis.

UNDERLYING MUSCULATURE

9. *Which of the following muscles is used as a landmark to identify different nodal zones during an axillary dissection?*
A. Pectoralis major.
B. Pectoralis minor.
C. Serratus anterior.
D. Intercostal.
E. Latissimus dorsi.

BREAST EXAMINATION

10. *A 43-year-old female presents for consultation for reduction mammoplasty. At which time is it most comfortable for the patient to perform a full breast examination?*
A. Premenstrual.
B. Follicular phase.
C. Luteal phase.
D. Menstruation.
E. Postmenstrual phase.

Answers

EMBRYOLOGY, DEVELOPMENT, AND PHYSIOLOGY

1. *The mammary gland is derived from which of the following cell lines?*

C. Ectoderm.

The mammary glands form from ingrowths of ectoderm that become lactiferous glands and ducts. Around weeks 6 to 7 of gestation, the milk ridge develops beginning with 15 to 20 buds that then undergo apoptosis to leave a single pair of buds at the fourth or fifth intercostal space. The nipple develops with surrounding circular smooth muscle fibers derived from mesoderm.[1]

REFERENCE

1. Lemaine V, Simmons PS. The adolescent female: breast and reproductive embryology and anatomy. Clin Anat 2013;26(1):22–28

EMBRYOLOGY, DEVELOPMENT, AND PHYSIOLOGY

2. *A 19-year-old female presents with complete absence of the right breast and nipple. She has no abnormalities of her extremities or pectoralis muscle. Her chest wall is in good position and size. Which of the following terms best describes the anatomic variation?*

A. Amastia.

There are several congenital breast anomalies that the plastic surgeon should be familiar with. Amastia is the congenital absence of both the breast and the nipple. Patients with amazia have absence of the breast but presence of a nipple, and those with athelia have presence of a breast, but absence of the nipple. Patients with Poland syndrome will have an absent or hypoplastic breast, as well as other anomalies of other chest wall components including the latissimus dorsi, ribs, and serratus muscle, among others. The most common limb abnormality is brachysyndactyly on the affected side. Treatment is typically with a tissue expander initially, followed by a submuscular implant and latissimus dorsi flap after the contralateral breast stops growing.[1] Anterior thoracic hypoplasia presents with unilateral sunken anterior chest wall, hypoplasia of the breast, superiorly placed nipple-areola complex, normal pectoralis muscle, and normalsternalposition.[1]

REFERENCE

1. Hatono A, Nagasao T, Sotome K, et al. A case of congenital unilateral amastia. J Plast Reconstr Aesthet Surg 2012;65(5):671–674

EMBRYOLOGY, DEVELOPMENT, AND PHYSIOLOGY

3. *A 20-year-old female presents with complaints of polymastia. Which is the most likely area of accessory breast tissue found on examination?*

C. Lower lateral chest wall.

Accessory breast tissue (supernumerary breast, polymastia) is common. Polymastia most commonly presents along the mammary line, with the most common location along the lateral inframammary fold. Another common location is the groin. Patients will present with cyclical pain as this breast tissue is responsive to hormonal influence. Treatment is surgical excision.[1,2]

REFERENCES

1. Bourguignon JP, Juul A. Normal female puberty in a developmental perspective. Endocr Dev 2012;22:11–23
2. Gusterson BA, Stein T. Human breast development. Semin Cell Dev Biol 2012;23(5):567–573

EMBRYOLOGY, DEVELOPMENT, AND PHYSIOLOGY

4. *A young female patient is brought in by her parents regarding concerns of breast asymmetry. She has absence of any breast tissue but presence of the nipple of one side of her chest. On the contralateral chest, she has presence of glandular tissue and areolar pigmentation with a secondary mound formed by the nipple above the level of the breast. What stage of breast development is this patient by the Tanner classification?*

D. 4.

The Tanner scale (Tanner stages) is a scale of physical development in children based on external primary and secondary sex characteristics. The patient in this question has development of subareolar breast tissue with a second mound formed by the nipple and areola above the level of the breast which occurs in Tanner stage 4 breasts. In Tanner stage 5 breasts, the areola returns to the contour of the surrounding breast with a central projecting papilla. Tanner stage 3 breasts have elevation of the breast mound; however, the areola remains in contour with the surrounding breast.[1]

REFERENCE

1. Tanner JM, ed. Growth at Adolescence. 2nd ed. Oxford: Blackwell Scientific; 1978

EMBRYOLOGY, DEVELOPMENT, AND PHYSIOLOGY

5. *A 5-year-old girl's parents are concerned as their daughter has started to develop breasts. Upon examination, the patient has bilateral stage 4 Tanner breast development but no other signs of puberty or skeletal maturation. This patient's condition is best represented by which of the following?*

A. Premature thelarche.

Premature thelarche occurs when breast development starts before the age of 8 years without evidence of other signs of puberty including pubic hair or vaginal mucosal thickening. Symptoms are typically bilateral and end after 3 to 5 years. In Poland syndrome there will be an absent or hypoplastic breast, as well as other anomalies of other chest wall components including the latissimus dorsi, ribs, and serratus muscle, among others. Jeune syndrome presents with a narrow, immobile breast and renal disease. Supernumerary breast is accessory mammary tissue forming along the embryonic milk line (axilla to groin).[1]

REFERENCE

1. Bostwick J III. Anatomy and physiology. In: Bostwick J III, ed. Plastic and Reconstructive Breast Surgery. 2nd ed. New York: Thieme Publishers; 2000

VASCULAR SUPPLY

6. *During a mastectomy, which of the following vessels is the most critical to preserve perfusion to the skin and nipple-areola complex?*

A. 2nd internal mammary artery perforator.

The soft tissue of the breast has a rich vascular supply through a diffuse subdermal plexus that communicates with underlying deeper vessels supplying the breast parenchyma. These vessels include perforators from the lateral thoracic artery, thoracoacromial, intercostal, internal mammary, and thoracodorsal vessels. The 2nd and 3rd interspace perforators of the internal mammary are typically the dominant blood supply to the breast skin and nipple-areola complex and should be preserved during mastectomy and reconstruction to minimize the risk of ischemic complications of the skin envelope.[1,2]

REFERENCES

1. Bostwick J III. Anatomy and physiology. In: Bostwick J III, ed. Plastic and Reconstructive Breast Surgery. 2nd ed. New York: Thieme Publishers; 2000
2. Shermak MA. Female breast anatomy. In: Shermak MA, ed. Body Contouring. New York: McGraw-Hill Professional; 2011:60–61

INNERVATION

7. *Which of the following nerves primarily supplies sensation to the nipple-areolar complex?*

C. T4 branch of intercostal nerve.

The breast has a dermatomal innervation supplied by the anterior and lateral cutaneous branches of the T2–T6 (primarily T3–T5) intercostal nerves. The supraclavicular nerves of the cervical plexus also provide innervation to the upper and lateral portions of the breast. The nipple-areolar complex is primarily supplied by the T4 branch. The lateral branch usually runs deep along the pectoral fascia while the anterior cutaneous branch runs superficially, and therefore is the only preserved branch after a mastectomy is performed.[1]

Reference

1. Schlenz I, Kuzbari R, Gruber H, et al. The sensitivity of the nipple-areola complex: an anatomic study. Plast Reconstr Surg 2000;105:905

SKIN AND PARENCHYMA

8. ***A 63-year-old female presents for consultation for mastopexy. On examination, she has deflated breasts, with grade III ptosis of the nipple bilaterally. Attenuation of which of the following structures is responsible for this presentation?***

D. Cooper's ligaments.

The breast parenchyma extends from the second to seventh ribs and from the sternocostal junction to midaxillary line with an additional extension into the axilla. The breast parenchyma is enveloped by a superficial layer of superficial fascia as well as a deep layer of the superficial fascia. The inframammary fold at the lower border of the breast is the fusion of the deep and superficial fascia with the dermis and is a zone of adherence. Cooper's ligaments are fibrocollagenous septa that penetrate the deep layer of the superficial fascia through breast parenchyma to the dermis. It is the attenuation of these ligaments that results in breast ptosis.[1,2]

References

1. Jones G, ed. Bostwick's Plastic and Reconstructive Breast Surgery. 3rd ed. New York: Thieme Publishers; 2010
2. Hall-Findlay EJ, ed. Aesthetic Breast Surgery: Concepts & Techniques. New York: Thieme Publishers; 2011

UNDERLYING MUSCULATURE

9. ***Which of the following muscles is used as a landmark to identify different nodal zones during an axillary dissection?***

B. Pectoralis minor.

The pectoralis minor muscle originates on the surfaces of the third through sixth ribs and inserts onto the coracoid process of the scapula to draw the scapula inferiorly and anteriorly. This muscle serves as a landmark during axillary dissection as its lateral margin divides the superficial from the deep axillary nodes. The majority of lymph nodes from the breast drain into the axillary lymph node basin and are classified as Level I, lateral to the lateral border of the pectoralis minor; level II, behind the pectoralis minor and below the axillary vein; and level III, medial to the medial border of the pectoralis minor.[1,2]

References

1. Jones G, ed. Bostwick's Plastic and Reconstructive Breast Surgery. 3rd ed. New York: Thieme Publishers; 2010
2. Hall-Findlay EJ, ed. Aesthetic Breast Surgery: Concepts & Techniques. New York: Thieme Publishers; 2011

BREAST EXAMINATION

10. ***A 43-year-old female presents for consultation for reduction mammoplasty. At which time is it most comfortable for the patient to perform a full breast examination?***

E. Postmenstrual phase.

The breast examination and patient's breast symptoms change with the menstrual cycle. The follicular phase (days 4–14) involves mitosis and proliferation of breast epithelial cells. In the luteal phase (days 5–28), the mammary ducts dilate and estrogen increases blood flow to the breast. The breast involutes with decrease in circulating hormones during menstruation. Breast engorgement and sensitivity peaks during the premenstrual phase and hits a nadir around 5 to 7 days after menstruation at which point palpation is most sensitive for detecting masses and the breast examination is most comfortable for the patient.[1,2]

References

1. Bostwick J III. Anatomy and physiology. In: Bostwick J III, ed. Plastic and Reconstructive Breast Surgery. 2nd ed. New York: Thieme Publishers; 2000
2. August DA, Sondak VK. Breast. In: Greenfield LJ, Mulholland M, Oldham KT, et al, eds. Surgery: Scientific Principles and Practice. 2nd ed. Philadelphia: Lippincott-Raven; 1997

52. Breast Augmentation

Nima Khosravani, Anup Patel, Anmol Chattha

See *Essentials of Aesthetic Surgery*, pp. 723–750

SILICONE IMPLANTS

1. ***Which of the following is true of silicone implants?***
   A. Saline implants lost popularity during the 1990s as a result of the silicone scare.
   B. In 1999, the NIH Institute of Medicine and the National Academy of Sciences reviewed 17 epidemiologic studies and were unable to link silicone implants with autoimmune, systemic, and prenatal disease.
   C. Fifth-generation silicone implants consist of a thick (0.25 mm) shell, with thick viscous gel, and a Dacron patch.
   D. First-generation silicone implants consist of a cohesive silicone gel–filled device with inner laminar layer to prevent gel bleeds.
   E. Saline implants were introduced first before silicone implants.

PREOPERATIVE PLANNING

2. ***A 19-year-old female comes in desiring breast augmentation. She would like silicone implants. She has a past medical history of anxiety, Poland syndrome, and depression. She notes she does not have any social pressure to get a breast augmentation; however, all of her friends in college have saline implants. Which of the following is a contraindication for silicone breast augmentation?***
   A. Her past medical history of anxiety and depression.
   B. Patient's age.
   C. Her relationship status.
   D. Poland syndrome.
   E. The fact that all her friends have saline implants.

PREOPERATIVE PLANNING

3. ***Which of the following is not important during the preoperative evaluation of the patient?***
   A. Motivation for surgery.
   B. Psychological state of mind and stability.
   C. Expectations.
   D. Household income.
   E. Self-esteem.

PREOPERATIVE PLANNING

4. ***What is an advantage to using silicone implants versus saline implants?***
   A. Adjusts quickly to body core temperature.
   B. Leaks are easily detected and safely absorbed by the body.
   C. Sizes are more customizable, and easier to adjust for size and correct breast asymmetries.
   D. More natural feel and appearance.
   E. Ability to fill implants in clinic postoperatively.

PREOPERATIVE PLANNING

5. ***Which of the following is an advantage to using saline versus silicone implants?***
   A. More natural feel and appearance.
   B. Historically lower contracture rates.
   C. Complete deflation with leak.
   D. Wrinkling.
   E. Increased viscosity.

PREOPERATIVE PLANNING

6. *What volume increases volume by one cup size in an average body frame?*
A. 50–75 cc.
B. 125–150 cc.
C. 200–225 cc.
D. 250–275 cc.
E. 300–325 cc.

PREOPERATIVE PLANNING

7. *What is an advantage to using textured implants over smooth implants?*
A. Thinner capsule is formed.
B. Less palpable.
C. Lower contracture rate.
D. Easy postoperative manipulation to achieve desired positioning.
E. Lower risk of BIA-ALCL.

PREOPERATIVE PLANNING

8. *Which type of implant has the lowest rate of contracture?*
A. Smooth.
B. Textured.
C. Polyurethane-covered.
D. Silicone.
E. Round.

PREOPERATIVE PLANNING

9. *A 34-year-old female wants to undergo a large breast augmentation with 450 cc bilateral implants. Which of the following is true of implants >400 cc?*
A. They are considered medium–volume implants and are less prone to complications.
B. They are considered medium–volume implants and are more prone to complications.
C. They are considered high–volume implants and are less prone to complications.
D. They are considered high–volume implants and are more prone to complications.
E. They are considered ultra-high-volume implants; however, do not have any increased complication rates.

PREOPERATIVE PLANNING

10. *Which of the following is an advantage of a subglandular/subfascial implant?*
A. Has the lowest capsular contracture rate.
B. Avoids implant distortion with pectoralis activity (in a muscular patient).
C. Prevents double-bubble formation.
D. Does not interfere with mammography.
E. Has a lower infection rate.

PREOPERATIVE PLANNING/ANATOMIC PRINCIPLES

11. *What is a disadvantage to performing dual plane II and dual plane III?*
A. Usually restricted to IMF incisions.
B. Usually restricted to periareolar incision.
C. Usually restricted to axillary incision.
D. Does not allow for complete visualization of subglandular or submuscular pocket.
E. Decreased lower pole arc stretch.

ANATOMIC PRINCIPLES/OPERATIVE TECHNIQUE

12. *Which of the following differentiates dual plane type I, II, and III?*
A. Thickness of the pectoralis muscle.
B. Proximity of the dissection to the areolar tissue.
C. The extent and level of separation of pectoralis from parenchyma.
D. Position of the incision.
E. Subcutaneous undermining level.

ANATOMIC PRINCIPLES/OPERATIVE TECHNIQUE

13. *Which type of dissection involves separation of pectoralis from breast parenchyma in the retromammary plane to the level of the inferior NAC?*
A. Dual plane I.
B. Dual plane II.
C. Dual plane III.
D. Subglandular.
E. Total submuscular.

OPERATIVE TECHNIQUE

14. *A surgeon is looking to minimize contamination of a breast implant he or she is inserting. Which maneuver is the best one to prevent implant contamination?*
A. Postoperative antibiotics.
B. No touch technique.
C. Rinsing the implant in saline before insertion.
D. Using drains.
E. Using sizers.

PREOPERATIVE PLANNING/POSTOPERATIVE CARE

15. *What percentage of patients will experience permanent sensory changes following breast augmentation?*
A. 3%.
B. 7%.
C. 15%.
D. 22%.
E. 30%.

POSTOPERATIVE CONSIDERATIONS

16. *Which of the following is true of postoperative rippling?*
A. It is most commonly due to overfilling.
B. It is most commonly found in the upper pole of underfilled implants.
C. It is most commonly seen in silicone implants.
D. Traction rippling is seen in smooth implants.
E. It is primarily due to preoperative patient risk factors.

POSTOPERATIVE CARE

17. *What is the leak/rupture rate associated with saline implants at 10 years?*
A. 2–5%.
B. 5–10%.
C. 10–15%.
D. 15–20%.
E. 20–25%.

CAPSULAR CONTRACTURE/POSTOPERATIVE CARE

18. *Which of the following Baker classifications is characterized by severe contracture and pain?*
A. Grade I.
B. Grade II.
C. Grade III.
D. Grade IV.
E. Grade V.

CAPSULAR CONTRACTURE/POSTOPERATIVE CARE

19. *Which of the following is historically true of capsular contractures?*
A. The majority will occur within 3 to 4 months.
B. Subglandular implants have a significantly lower contracture rate at 10 years when compared to subpectoral implants.
C. Textured implants have a significantly lower contracture rate at 10 years when compared to smooth implants.

D. Silicone implants have a significantly lower contracture rate at 10 years when compared to saline implants.
E. Closed capsulotomy is the treatment of choice.

BIA-ALCL: POSTOPERATIVE CARE

20. *Which of the following is true of breast implant associated anaplastic large cell lymphoma (BIA-ALCL)?*
A. It is a cancer of the breast tissue.
B. It is associated with only silicone implants.
C. It is associated with only saline implants.
D. It is associated with CD30 positive and ALK-negative T-cell lymphocytes.
E. It is associated only with smooth implants.

Answers

SILICONE IMPLANTS

1. *Which of the following is true of silicone implants?*

B. In 1999, the NIH Institute of Medicine and the National Academy of Sciences reviewed 17 epidemiologic studies and were unable to link silicone implants with autoimmune, systemic, and prenatal disease.

In 1999, the NIH Institute of Medicine and the National Academy of Sciences reviewed 17 epidemiologic studies and were unable to detect any link between silicone implants and autoimmune, systemic, and prenatal disease. Saline implants increased in popularity during the 1990s because of the silicone scare. First-generation silicone implants consist of a thick (0.25 mm) shell, thick viscous gel, and Dacron patch whereas fifth-generation silicone implants consist of a cohesive silicone gel–filled device with inner laminar layer to prevent gel bleed.[1,2]

REFERENCES

1. American Society of Plastic Surgeons. Procedural statistics trends 1992–2004. Available at www.plasticsurgery.org/public_education/Statistical-Trends.cfm
2. Silicone gel-filled breast implants approved. FDA Consum 2007;41:8

PREOPERATIVE PLANNING

2. *A 19-year-old female comes in desiring breast augmentation. She would like silicone implants. She has a past medical history of anxiety, Poland syndrome, and depression. She notes she does not have any social pressure to get a breast augmentation; however, all of her friends in college have saline implants. Which of the following is a contraindication for silicone breast augmentation?*

B. Patient's age.

Silicone implants are not FDA approved for women <22 years of age. Poland syndrome would be a good indication for breast augmentation. The desire to improve body image, symmetry and balance, rejuvenation after postpartum deflation, and the desire to correct breast asymmetry are all indications for breast augmentation. Social instability (e.g., divorce or separation, searching for a relationship) is a contraindication.[1,2]

REFERENCES

1. Rohrich R. Streamlining cosmetic surgery patient selection—just say No! Plast Reconstr Surg 1999;104:220
2. Gorney M. Patient selection criteria. Medicolegal issues in plastic surgery. Clin Plast Surg 1999;26:37

PREOPERATIVE PLANNING

3. *Which of the following is not important during the preoperative evaluation of the patient?*

D. Household income.

During the preoperative evaluation, the following should be assessed: motivation for surgery, psychological state of mind and stability, level of understanding, expectations, and self-esteem. Household income is not typically assessed directly by the surgeon preoperatively, although financial details of surgery would be discussed with the patient through the surgeon's office staff.[1,2]

REFERENCES

1. Rohrich R. Streamlining cosmetic surgery patient selection—just say No! Plast Reconstr Surg 1999;104:220
2. Gorney M. Patient selection criteria. Medicolegal issues in plastic surgery. Clin Plast Surg 1999;26:37

PREOPERATIVE PLANNING

4. *What is an advantage to using silicone implants versus saline implants?*

D. More natural feel and appearance.

Silicone implants have a more natural feel and appearance than saline implants; however, saline implants adjust quickly to body core temperature, leaks are easily detected and safely absorbed, and are more customizable. Filling saline implants and tissue expanders is possible in clinic; it is not an advantage of using silicone implants.

PREOPERATIVE PLANNING

5. *Which of the following is an advantage to using saline versus silicone implants?*

B. Historically lower contracture rates.

The benefits of saline compared to silicone are a historically lower contracture rate, adjusting quickly to body core temperature, leaks are easily detected and safely absorbed by the body, and the sizes are more customizable. Silicone implants have a more natural feel and appearance. Complete deflation with leak and wrinkling are disadvantages of saline implants.[1]

REFERENCE

1. Gutowski KA, Mesna GT, Cunningham BL. Saline-filled breast implants: a Plastic Surgery Educational Foundation multicenter outcomes study. Plast Reconstr Surg 1997;100:1019

PREOPERATIVE PLANNING

6. *What volume increases volume by one cup size in an average body frame?*

B. 125–150 cc.

To increase by one cup size, 125 to 150 cc is required. However, larger body frames may require larger implant volumes to increase cup size.[1,2]

REFERENCES

1. Tebbetts JB, Adams WP. Five critical decisions in breast augmentation using five measurements in 5 minutes. The high five decision support process. Plast Reconstr Surg 2005;116:2005
2. Tebbetts JB. Dual plane breast augmentation: optimizing implant-soft-tissue relationships in a wide range of breast types. Plast Reconstr Surg 2001;107:1255

PREOPERATIVE PLANNING

7. *What is an advantage to using textured implants over smooth implants?*

C. Lower contracture rate.

Textured implants have lower contracture rates due to surface disorienting collagen deposition. It also has less migration and implant rotation, which make intraoperative positioning of implant critical as textured surface resists migration or movement in pocket. Smooth implants form thinner capsules and are less palpable. Textured implants require precise pocket dissection, are more palpable, develop traction rippling more commonly, and have a greater association with breast implant associated anaplastic large cell lymphoma (BIA-ALCL) based on current data.[1,2,3]

REFERENCES

1. Rohrich RJ, Kenkel JM, Adams WP. Preventing capsular contracture in breast augmentation: in search of the Holy Grail. Plast Reconstr Surg 1999;103:1759
2. Doren EL, Miranda RN, Selber JC, et al. Breast implant-associated anaplastic large cell lymphoma: a systematic review. JAMA Surg 2019;154(12):1161–1168
3. Leberfinger AN, Behar BJ, Williams NC, Rakszawski KL, Potochny JD, Mackay DR. Breast implant-associated anaplastic large cell lymphoma: a comprehensive review. Plast Reconstr Surg 2017;139(3):682e–691e

PREOPERATIVE PLANNING

8. *Which type of implant has the lowest rate of contracture?*

C. Polyurethane-covered.

Polyurethane-covered implants have the lowest rate of contractures (<1% over 10 years) but these were pulled from US market because polyurethane breaks down as carcinogenic compound, although levels are likely insignificant.[1,2]

REFERENCES

1. Collis N, Coleman D, Foo IT, et al. Ten-year review of a prospective randomized controlled trial of textured versus smooth subglandular silicone gel breast implants. Plast Reconstr Surg 2000;106:786

2. Marotta JS, Widenhouse CW, Habal MB, et al. Silicone gel breast implant failure and frequency of additional surgeries: analysis of 35 studies reporting examination of more than 800 explants. J Biomed Mater Res 1999;48:354

PREOPERATIVE PLANNING

9. *A 34-year-old female wants to undergo a large breast augmentation with 450 cc bilateral implants. Which of the following is true of implants >400 cc?*

D. They are considered high–volume implants and are more prone to complications.

High–volume implants >400 cc are more prone to complications and many surgeons have special consent forms for such implants. Some of these complications in particular include double bubble deformity, bottoming out of the implant, lateral displacement especially if placed in the submuscular plane, implant rupture, and postoperative asymmetries.[1,2]

REFERENCES

1. Collis N, Coleman D, Foo IT, et al. Ten-year review of a prospective randomized controlled trial of textured versus smooth subglandular silicone gel breast implants. Plast Reconstr Surg 2000;106:786
2. Marotta JS, Widenhouse CW, Habal MB, et al. Silicone gel breast implant failure and frequency of additional surgeries: analysis of 35 studies reporting examination of more than 800 explants. J Biomed Mater Res 1999;48:354

PREOPERATIVE PLANNING

10. *Which of the following is an advantage of a subglandular/subfascial implant?*

B. Avoids implant distortion with pectoralis activity (in a muscular patient).

The advantages of subglandular/subfascial implants include: Avoids implant distortion with pectoralis activity and, in muscular patients, is more anatomic and has better implant projection. However, it has a higher contracture rate when compared to subpectoral and dual plane dissections. Dual plane increases implant–parenchymal interface, which expands lower pole and prevents double-bubble deformity. Finally, subglandular/subfascial implants can interfere with mammography.[1]

REFERENCE

1. Li S, Mu D, Liu C, et al. Complications following subpectoral versus prepectoral breast augmentation: a meta-analysis. Aesthetic Plast Surg 2019;43(4):890–898

PREOPERATIVE PLANNING/ANATOMIC PRINCIPLES

11. *What is a disadvantage to performing dual plane II and dual plane III?*

A. Usually restricted to IMF incisions.

Dual plane II and dual plane III are usually restricted to inframammary fold (IMF) incisions. This allows for complete visualization of subglandular and submuscular pocket. Dual plane II and dual plane III dissections release the muscle more cephalically resulting in less inferior pole muscle coverage, thus increasing, not decreasing, lower pole arc stretch.[1]

REFERENCE

1. Tebbetts JB. Dual plane breast augmentation: optimizing implant-soft-tissue relationships in a wide range of breast types. Plast Reconstr Surg 2001;107:1255

ANATOMIC PRINCIPLES/OPERATIVE TECHNIQUE

12. *Which of the following differentiates dual plane type I, II, and III?*

C. The extent and level of separation of pectoralis from parenchyma.

In a dual plane dissection, the pectoralis major is completely divided from its origin at the level of the inframammary fold (IMF), stopping at the medial aspect of the IMF. The upper pole of the implant is placed under the pectoralis, and the lower pole is placed subglandularly. The attachments of the pectoralis to the breast parenchyma are selectively divided and the amount of dissection differentiates dual plane type I, II, and III.[1]

REFERENCE

1. Tebbetts JB. Dual plane breast augmentation: optimizing implant-soft-tissue relationships in a wide range of breast types. Plast Reconstr Surg 2001;107:1255

ANATOMIC PRINCIPLES/OPERATIVE TECHNIQUE

13. *Which type of dissection involves separation of pectoralis from breast parenchyma in the retromammary plane to the level of the inferior NAC?*

B. Dual plane II.

In a dual plane dissection, the pectoralis major is completely divided from its origin at the level of the inframammary fold (IMF), stopping at the medial aspect of the IMF. The upper pole of the implant is placed under the pectoralis, and the lower pole is placed subglandularly. In Type I, there is no dissection in the retromammary plane to free the breast parenchyma muscle interface. In Type II, there is separation of pectoralis from breast parenchyma in the retromammary plane to the level of the inferior nipple areolar complex (NAC). In Type III, separation of pectoralis from breastparenchyma in the retromammary plane is continued to the level of the superior NAC.[1]

REFERENCE

1. Tebbetts JB. Dual plane breast augmentation: optimizing implant-soft-tissue relationships in a wide range of breast types. Plast Reconstr Surg 2001;107:1255

OPERATIVE TECHNIQUE

14. *A surgeon is looking to minimize contamination of a breast implant he or she is inserting. Which maneuver is the best one to prevent implant contamination?*

B. No touch technique.

To prevent implant contamination from the skin during surgical procedures, it is important to follow strict aseptic techniques. Aseptic techniques are practices used to minimize the risk of introducing harmful microorganisms (such as bacteria) into a surgical environment. The purpose of the no touch technique is to eliminate contact with the surgeon's glove and patient's skin, as skin contamination is thought to be a significant cause of capsular contracture. Use of a Keller funnel may help as well by allowing minimal contact time with surgeon's gloves. Use of sizers has no proven impact on final implant contamination. Rinsing the pocket out with betadine or triple antibiotic solution rather than saline alone will minimize contamination. Use of drains may actually increase implant contamination, as the implants are now exposed to the outside environment. Postoperative antibiotics do not confer any improvement in implant contamination risk.[1]

REFERENCE

1. Mladick RA. "No-touch" submuscular saline breast augmentation technique. Aesthetic Plast Surg 1993;17:183

PREOPERATIVE PLANNING/POSTOPERATIVE CARE

15. *What percentage of patients will experience permanent sensory changes following breast augmentation?*

C. 15%.

About 15% of patients have permanent sensory changes. This is secondary to traction or transection of lateral intercostal cutaneous nerve. Incidence and severity are the same with all techniques.[1,2]

REFERENCES

1. Courtiss EH, Goldwyn RM. Breast sensation before and after plastic surgery. Plast Reconstr Surg 1976;58:1
2. Mofid MM, Klatsky SA, Singh NK, et al. Nipple-areola complex sensitivity after primary breast augmentation: a comparison of periareolar and inframammary incision approaches. Plast Reconstr Surg 2006;117:1694

POSTOPERATIVE CONSIDERATIONS

16. *Which of the following is true of postoperative rippling?*

B. It is most commonly found in the upper pole of underfilled implants.

Rippling occurs secondary to underfilling or traction. It is seen in the upper pole of underfilled implants and can be prevented by filling saline implants to recommended fill or overfilling. Traction rippling is seen in textured implants and can be prevented by ensuring adequate soft tissue over implant and matching pocket size with implant.[1]

Reference

1. Allergan Corporation. Saline implant premarket approval information, 2001. Available at www.fda.gov//downloads/medicaldevices/productsandmedicalprocedures/implantsandprosthetics/breast-implants/ucm064457.pdf

POSTOPERATIVE CARE

17. *What is the leak/rupture rate associated with saline implants at 10 years?*

B. 5–10%.

The risk of rupture for saline implants is at the rate of 2 to 5% at 5 years and 5 to 10% at 10 years. The rate of leak/rupture per year is 1%. The risk factors are underfilling (<25 cc), using intraluminal antibiotics, or employing steroids. Management is complex often requiring implant exchange.[1]

Reference

1. Allergan Corporation. Saline implant premarket approval information, 2001. Available at www.fda.gov//downloads/medicaldevices/productsandmedicalprocedures/implantsandprosthetics/breast-implants/ucm064457.pdf

CAPSULAR CONTRACTURE/POSTOPERATIVE CARE

18. *Which of the following Baker classifications is characterized by severe contracture and pain?*

D. Grade IV.

The Baker classification is a system used to categorize the severity of capsular contracture, a complication that can occur after breast augmentation surgery involving the use of implants. Capsular contracture is the formation of scar tissue around the breast implant, and its severity can range from mild to severe. The Baker classification helps to standardize the assessment of these complications. There are four grades in the Baker classification:

Grade I (Normal): The breast is soft and looks natural. The implant is not palpable, and there is no visible distortion of the breast.

Grade II (Mild): The breast is still relatively soft, but there might be slight firmness when palpated. The appearance of the breast is generally normal, but there might be some minor distortion.

Grade III (Moderate): The breast feels firm to the touch, and there is noticeable distortion of the breast's appearance. This might involve visible changes in shape, position, or texture of the breast. Grade III is often associated with discomfort or pain.

Grade IV (Severe): The breast is hard to the touch, and there is significant distortion in the breast's appearance. The breast might feel very firm and unnatural. This grade is usually accompanied by pain or discomfort.

There is no Grade V in the Baker classification. Capsulectomy is indicated for grade III and grade IV capsular contracture.[1]

Reference

1. Gylbert L, Asplund O, Jurell G. Capsular contracture after breast reconstruction with silicone gel and saline-filled implants: a 6-year follow-up. Plast Reconstr Surg 1990;85:373

CAPSULAR CONTRACTURE/POSTOPERATIVE CARE

19. *Which of the following is historically true of capsular contractures?*

C. Textured implants have a significantly lower contracture rate at 10 years when compared to smooth implants.

Capsular contracture is the tightening of the capsule, with compression and distortion of the implant leading to asymmetry, pain, and implant rupture. The majority of capsular contractures will occur within 1 year, although late occurrences may occur secondary to systemic bacterial seeding or capsular maturation. Subglandular implants have a 32% contracture rate at 10 years compared to subpectoral implants, which have a 12% contracture rate. Smooth implants have a 58% contracture rate at 10 years compared to the 11% contracture rate seen with textured implants. Silicone implants have a 50% contracture rate at 10 years compared to saline implants, which have a 16% rate of contracture. However, these rates are from earlier generation implants and currently newer implants have lower rates of capsular contracture.[1]

Reference

1. Gylbert L, Asplund O, Jurell G. Capsular contracture after breast reconstruction with silicone gel and saline-filled implants: a 6-year follow-up. Plast Reconstr Surg 1990;85:373

BIA-ALCL: Postoperative Care

20. *Which of the following is true of breast implant associated anaplastic large cell lymphoma (BIA-ALCL)?*

D. It is associated with CD30 positive and ALK-negative T-cell lymphocytes.

BIA-ALCL is a rare and treatable type of T cell lymphoma that can develop around breast implants. It is not a cancer of the breast tissue itself. It should be discussed with any patient considering breast implants as part of the informed consent process. It has been associated with both silicone and saline implants in aesthetic as well as reconstructive patients. Diagnosis is based on ultrasound-guided fine needle aspiration (FNA) of the peri-implant fluid, which is assessed with immunohistochemistry for CD30-positive and ALK-negative T-cell lymphocytes.[1,2]

References

1. Clemens MW, Miranda FN, Butler CE. Breast implant informed consent should include the risk of anaplastic large cell lymphoma. Plast Reconstr Surg 2016;137:1117
2. Clemens MW, Medeiros LJ, Butler CE, et al. Complete surgical excision is essential for the management of patients with breast implant-associated anaplastic large-cell lymphoma. J Clin Oncol 2016;34:160

53. Mastopexy

Shervin Etemad, Salam Kassis, Jacob G. Unger
See *Essentials of Aesthetic Surgery*, pp. 751–761

BREAST PTOSIS

1. ***A 47-year-old woman, gravida 4 para 4, is considering mastopexy. On examination, bilateral nipple-areola complexes (NAC) are well below the inframammary fold (IMF) and sit at the inferior contour of the breast. A significant glandular portion of her breasts is also located below the IMF. Based on this description, how would you classify her ptosis?***
   A. Grade I ptosis (mild).
   B. Grade II ptosis (moderate).
   C. Grade III ptosis (severe).
   D. Pseudoptosis.
   E. Does not fit into any classification scheme.

INDICATIONS AND CONTRAINDICATIONS

2. ***A 70-year-old woman with a history of reduction mammaplasty 20 years ago is interested in mastopexy to address grade III ptosis. She has a history of transient ischemic attacks, for which she takes 325 mg of aspirin daily. She currently smokes one half-pack of cigarettes per day, and despite multiple attempts, has been unable to stop. She also has a history of hypothyroidism. Which of the following is a contraindication to mastopexy in this patient?***
   A. Age.
   B. History of prior mastopexy.
   C. Aspirin use.
   D. Active smoking status.
   E. Hypothyroidism.

INDICATIONS AND CONTRAINDICATIONS

3. ***In which of the following scenarios will a patient have the least benefit from mastopexy alone?***
   A. Grade I ptosis with low breast position on chest wall.
   B. Grade II ptosis with skin striae.
   C. Grade II ptosis with significant asymmetry of the areola.
   D. Grade III ptosis with fatty parenchyma.
   E. Grade III ptosis with history of massive weight loss.

PATIENT COUNSELING

4. ***A patient with grade II ptosis is undergoing bilateral vertical mastopexy. In your initial discussion with her, she expresses concern for "losing too much volume" as a result of the operation and asks what postoperative cup size she should expect. An appropriate response to this concern would include which of the following?***
   A. She will maintain her current cup size.
   B. On average, a decrease of 2 cup sizes should be expected.
   C. On average, a decrease of 1 cup size should be expected.
   D. She will most likely have an increase of 1 cup size.
   E. She will most likely have an increase of 2 cup sizes.

MASTOPEXY TECHNIQUES

5. ***A patient presents with a significant concern for ptosis and a desire for a more "perky" breast appearance. On examination, she has adequate upper pole fullness, fibrous parenchyma, and a nipple-areola complex (NAC) that is at the level of the inframammary fold (IMF). Which of the following approaches is most appropriate?***
   A. Inframammary fold wedge excision.
   B. Vertical mastopexy.

C. Wise-pattern mastopexy.
D. Augmentation-mastopexy.
E. Periareolar mastopexy.

MASTOPEXY TECHNIQUES

6. *A 47-year-old woman is interested in mastopexy to address grade II ptosis. She expresses concern because her 54-year-old sister underwent mastopexy 10 years ago and recently required a second operation for recurrence of ptosis. You share that effects of mastopexy are often temporary, and recurrence is common in the long term. Which of the following techniques would limit the risk of recurrent ptosis most in this patient?*
A. Periareolar deepithelialization and closure.
B. Vertical mastopexy without undermining (Lassus).
C. Inframammary fold wedge resection.
D. Superior repositioning of inferior parenchyma.
E. Inferior closure of medial and lateral breast pillars.

MASTOPEXY TECHNIQUES

7. *A 59-year-old woman with a history of silicone gel implants 15 years ago expresses fear of implant rupture and would "like them removed as soon as possible." She is not interested in simultaneous implant exchange but would like to you to address her breast ptosis. On examination, she has grade II ptosis and adequate soft tissue coverage over the implant. In addition to explantation, you plan to perform mastopexy. Which of the following is the best approach to addressing this patient's ptosis?*
A. Simultaneous mastopexy and explantation.
B. Mastopexy 3 months after explantation.
C. Mastopexy 6 months after explantation.
D. Mastopexy 1 year after explantation.
E. This patient does not have an indication for mastopexy.

MASTOPEXY TECHNIQUES

8. *A 27-year-old woman is in your clinic for a second opinion regarding mastopexy. On examination, you note disproportionately large areola and suspect parenchymal herniation into the areola bilaterally. Additional findings include a narrow breast base and high inframammary folds bilaterally. She shares her original surgeon's plan for bilateral inverted-T mastopexy and asks you to comment on the appropriateness of this operation. Which of the following is the best recommendation?*
A. Inverted-T mastopexy.
B. Periareolar mastopexy.
C. Vertical mastopexy with undermining and liposuction (Lejour).
D. Augmentation alone.
E. Further evaluation and planning for correction of tuberous breast deformity.

PATIENT COUNSELING

9. *Patient dissatisfaction following mastopexy is most often regarding which of the following?*
A. Infection.
B. Hematoma.
C. Wound-healing problems.
D. Visible scars.
E. Skin laxity.

Answers

BREAST PTOSIS

1. ***A 47-year-old woman, gravida 4 para 4, is considering mastopexy. On examination, bilateral nipple-areola complexes (NAC) are well below the inframammary fold (IMF) and sit at the inferior contour of the breast. A significant glandular portion of her breasts is also located below the IMF. Based on this description, how would you classify her ptosis?***

   C. Grade III ptosis (severe).

   This patient's ptosis would most appropriately be classified as grade III ptosis (severe ptosis). The Regnault classification of ptosis is based on the relative position of the nipple-areola complex (NAC) to the inframammary fold.[1] In grade I ptosis (A), the NAC is **at** the level of the inframammary fold (A). Grade II ptosis (B) is characterized by an NAC that lies **below** the inframammary fold, but above the most dependent breast parenchyma. In grade III ptosis (C), the NAC lies **well below** the inframammary fold and at the most inferior part of the breast parenchyma. Pseudoptosis is characterized by an increased nipple-to-inframammary fold distance, an NAC that is **above or at** the level of the inframammary fold, and the presence of the bulk of dependent breast parenchyma below the level of the fold (**Fig. 53.1**).[2]

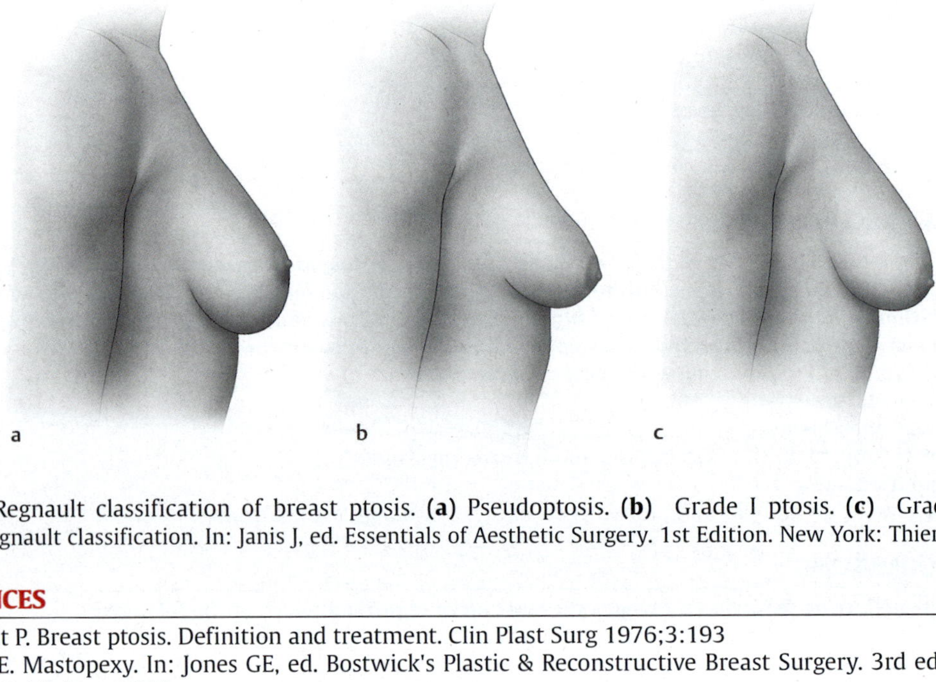

Fig. 53.1 Regnault classification of breast ptosis. **(a)** Pseudoptosis. **(b)** Grade I ptosis. **(c)** Grade II ptosis. (Source: Regnault classification. In: Janis J, ed. Essentials of Aesthetic Surgery. 1st Edition. New York: Thieme; 2018.)

REFERENCES

1. Regnault P. Breast ptosis. Definition and treatment. Clin Plast Surg 1976;3:193
2. Jones GE. Mastopexy. In: Jones GE, ed. Bostwick's Plastic & Reconstructive Breast Surgery. 3rd ed. New York: Thieme Publishers; 2010

INDICATIONS AND CONTRAINDICATIONS

2. ***A 70-year-old woman with a history of reduction mammaplasty 20 years ago is interested in mastopexy to address grade III ptosis. She has a history of transient ischemic attacks, for which she takes 325 mg of aspirin daily. She currently smokes one half-pack of cigarettes per day, and despite multiple attempts, has been unable to stop. She also has a history of hypothyroidism. Which of the following is a contraindication to mastopexy in this patient?***

   D. Active smoking status.

   This patient's **active smoking status** (D) is a contraindication to mastopexy. Wound-healing complications are highly prevalent in smokers and an elective operation such as mastopexy should not be performed in active smokers. Age (A) is not a contraindication to mastopexy, nor is history of prior mastopexy (B). In fact, mastopexy provides a temporary solution for ptosis, and long-term recurrence of ptosis should be an expectation as aging and gravity continue to affect the breast after mastopexy.[1] Hematoma formation is a relatively infrequent complication of mastopexy and the rate of hematoma formation is increased in patients on aspirin.[2] When feasible, patients should hold aspirin (C) and antiplatelet medications for 10 days prior to their operation.

References

1. Bostwick J III. Mastopexy. In: Bostwick J III, ed. Plastic and Reconstructive Breast Surgery. 2nd ed. New York: Thieme Publishers; 1999
2. Grotting JC, Chen SM. Control and precision in mastopexy. In: Nahai F, ed. The Art of Aesthetic Surgery: Principles and Techniques. New York: Thieme Publishers; 2005

INDICATIONS AND CONTRAINDICATIONS

3. *In which of the following scenarios will a patient have the least benefit from mastopexy alone?*

A. Grade I ptosis with low breast position on chest wall.

Patients with low breast position on chest wall without significant ptosis (A) will not benefit from mastopexy alone.[1,2] Striae are a sign of skin laxity (B), and are common skin findings in patients with ptosis, especially as they age. Patients with ptosis often have variations in areola size and shape (C), for which symmetry can be obtained with planned skin incisions during mastopexy. Parenchymal quality is important to consider, as inverted-T techniques may be more appropriate in patients with severe ptosis and fatty parenchyma (D). Recurrence of some degree of ptosis after mastopexy (E) is not uncommon, as gravity and aging continue to influence breast shape.

References

1. Hidalgo DA, Spector JA. Mastopexy. Plast Reconstr Surg 2013;132:642e
2. Ibrahim AM, Sinno HH, Izadpanah A, et al. Mastopexy for breast ptosis: utility outcomes of population preferences. Plast Surg (Oakv) 2015;23:103

PATIENT COUNSELING

4. *A patient with grade II ptosis is undergoing bilateral vertical mastopexy. In your initial discussion with her, she expresses concern for "losing too much volume" as a result of the operation and asks what postoperative cup size she should expect. An appropriate response to this concern would include which of the following?*

C. On average, a decrease of 1 cup size should be expected.

On average, patients experience a decrease of one brassiere cup size (C) following mastopexy alone due to small-volume parenchymal resection combined with skin envelope reduction.[1] A retrospective study of 20 patients with at least a C cup undergoing mastopexy alone for grade II or III ptosis found an average decrease of 1 cup size following their operation.[2] Maintenance of current cup size (A) or decrease of more than one cup size (B) are less likely. It is unlikely that patients undergoing mastopexy alone will have an increase in cup size (D, E). This is an important point to review in the patient counseling process and should be conveyed to patients at their initial visit.

References

1. Swanson E. Prospective outcome study of 106 cases of vertical mastopexy, augmentation/mastopexy and breast reduction. J Plast Reconstr Aesthet Surg 2013;66:937–994
2. Weichman K, Doft M, Matarasso A. The impact of mastopexy on brassiere cup size. Plast Reconstr Surg 2014;134:34e

MASTOPEXY TECHNIQUES

5. *A patient presents with a significant concern for ptosis and a desire for a more "perky" breast appearance. On examination, she has adequate upper pole fullness, fibrous parenchyma, and a nipple-areola complex (NAC) that is at the level of the inframammary fold (IMF). Which of the following approaches is most appropriate?*

B. Vertical mastopexy.

Based on the Regnault classification of breast ptosis,[1] this patient has grade I ptosis (mild ptosis) in which the NAC is at the level of the IMF. Grade I ptosis is best addressed with either periareolar or vertical (B) mastopexy techniques. A survey of board-certified plastic surgeons found periareolar techniques to have the highest rates of surgeon dissatisfaction and revision.[2] Inframammary fold wedge excision (A) may be appropriate for patients with pseudoptosis in which the NAC is above or at the level of the inframammary fold and excess parenchyma has descended below the level of the fold. Wise-pattern mastopexy (C) may be employed in cases of more severe ptosis with the presence of excess skin, and it shares a skin incision pattern with the prevalent reduction mammoplasty technique. Augmentation-mastopexy (D) would be appropriate in cases where restoration of upper pole fullness is desired. Periareolar mastopexy (E) would flattenthebreast to some degree and can only achieve approximately 1 cm of lift.

REFERENCES

1. Regnault P. Breast ptosis. Definition and treatment. Clin Plast Surg 1976;3:193
2. Rohrich RJ, Gosman AA, Brown SA, et al. Mastopexy preferences: a survey of board-certified plastic surgeons. Plast Reconstr Surg 2006;118:1631

MASTOPEXY TECHNIQUES

6. *A 47-year-old woman is interested in mastopexy to address grade II ptosis. She expresses concern because her 54-year-old sister underwent mastopexy 10 years ago and recently required a second operation for recurrence of ptosis. You share that effects of mastopexy are often temporary, and recurrence is common in the long term. Which of the following techniques would limit the risk of recurrent ptosis most in this patient?*

E. Inferior closure of medial and lateral breast pillars.

Although recurrent ptosis is an unavoidable risk in mastopexy, the risk can be mitigated with inferior parenchymal support, which may be obtained through inferior closure of medial and lateral breast pillars (E).[1] Simple periareolar deepithelialization and closure (A) would not be appropriate in a patient with grade II ptosis. Vertical mastopexy without undermining (B) involves en bloc resection of ptotic skin, fat, and gland with superior transposition of the nipple, and will not contribute to inferior parenchymal support.[2] Inframammary fold wedge resection (C) is a technique that addresses pseudoptosis. Superior repositioning of inferior parenchyma (D) would contribute to restoration of superior pole fullness most.

REFERENCES

1. Rohrich RJ, Thornton JF, Jakubietz RG, et al. The limited scar mastopexy: current concepts and approaches to correct breast ptosis. Plat Reconstr Surg 2004;114(6):1622–1630
2. Lassus C. A 30-year experience with vertical mammaplasty. Plast Reconstr Surg 1996;97:373

MASTOPEXY TECHNIQUES

7. *A 59-year-old woman with a history of silicone gel implants 15 years ago expresses fear of implant rupture and would "like them removed as soon as possible." She is not interested in simultaneous implant exchange but would like to you to address her breast ptosis. On examination, she has grade II ptosis and adequate soft tissue coverage over the implant. In addition to explantation, you plan to perform mastopexy. Which of the following is the best approach to addressing this patient's ptosis?*

A. Simultaneous mastopexy and explantation.

In a patient with adequate (>4 cm) soft tissue coverage and moderate ptosis who desires explantation and mastopexy, simultaneous procedures (A) are an appropriate consideration.[1,2] Staging mastopexy 3 months after explantation (B) may be appropriate in cases of severe ptosis and sparse soft tissue coverage. In cases of staged mastopexy following explantation, it is not necessary to prolong staging beyond 3 months (C, D), and the choice of mastopexy technique should be based on preoperative ptosis classification.

REFERENCES

1. Rohrich RJ, Beran SJ, Restifo RJ, et al. Aesthetic management of the breast following explantation: evaluation and mastopexy options. Plast Reconstr Surg 1998;101:827
2. Rohrich RJ, Kenkel JM, Adams WP, et al. A prospective analysis of patients undergoing silicone breast implant explantation. Plast Reconstr Surg 2000;105(7):2529–2537

MASTOPEXY TECHNIQUES

8. *A 27-year-old woman is in your clinic for a second opinion regarding mastopexy. On examination, you note disproportionately large areola and suspect parenchymal herniation into the areola bilaterally. Additional findings include a narrow breast base and high inframammary folds bilaterally. She shares her original surgeon's plan for bilateral inverted-T mastopexy and asks you to comment on the appropriateness of this operation. Which of the following is the best recommendation?*

E. Further evaluation and planning for correction of tuberous breast deformity.

This patient's physical examination reveals key characteristics of a tuberous breast deformity (E): constricted breast base, high inframammary fold, and parenchymal herniation into the areola. The tuberous breast deformity encompasses a spectrum of presentations with variability in the aforementioned characteristics, stemming from inadequate breast development in the horizontal and vertical dimensions.[1,2,3] It is important to identify patients with tuberous breasts, as typical mastopexy techniques are inadequate and more complex surgical planning is required. These patients may benefit from periareolar mastopexy (B), with parenchymal modification through inferior pole radial scoring, and augmentation (D) to restore parenchymal volume. Inverted-T mastopexy (A) would be appropriate for cases of severe ptosis. Likewise, vertical mastopexy with undermining and liposuction (C) may be appropriate in cases of ptosis with larger breast size to reduceparenchymalvolume.

REFERENCES

1. von Heimburg HD, Exner K, Kruft S, et al. The tuberous breast deformity: classification and treatment. Br J Plast Surg 1996;49:339
2. Nahabedian MY. Breast deformities and mastopexy. Plast Reconstr Surg 2011;127:91e–102e
3. Kolker AR, Collins MS. Tuberous breast deformity: classification and treatment strategy for improving consistency in aesthetic correction. Plast Reconstr Surg 2015;135(1):73–86

PATIENT COUNSELING

9. *Patient dissatisfaction following mastopexy is most often regarding which of the following?*

D. Visible scars.

Postoperative scars are a frequent source of patient dissatisfaction as well as litigation following mastopexy. In fact, mastopexy procedures have the greatest incidence of litigation among aesthetic breast procedures.[1] The informed consent process should discuss, in detail, the risk of visible scarring, scar placement, and scar quality. Both periareolar scar widening and medial horizontal inframammary fold scars are common sources of patient dissatisfaction. In the postoperative period, scar treatment should begin at 3 weeks with the surgeon's preferred approach, and scar revisions may be performed 1 year after the initial operation. Infection (A) is an uncommon complication for which prophylactic antibiotics are given in the perioperative period. Hematoma (B) is also uncommon in patients who are off aspirin and antiplatelet medications in the 10-day preoperative period. A tight hematoma is an indication for urgent reoperation for evacuationandhemostasis. Wound-healing problems (C) are more common with inverted-T mastopexy techniques and in smokers. For this reason, mastopexy should not be performed in active smokers.[2] Skin laxity (E) often accompanies ptosis and is not a complication of mastopexy.

REFERENCES

1. Hidalgo DA, Spector JA. Mastopexy. Plast Reconstr Surg 2013;132:642e
2. Stevens WG, Soker DA, Freeman ME, et al. Mastopexy revisited: a review of 150 consecutive cases for complication and revision rates. Aesthet Surg J 2007;27(3):150–154

54. Augmentation-Mastopexy

Shervin Etemad, Salam Kassis, Jacob G. Unger
See *Essentials of Aesthetic Surgery*, pp. 763–768

STAGING

1. ***You are discussing the possibility of one-stage augmentation-mastopexy for a patient with grade II ptosis who desires increased breast fullness. What is the reoperation rate you share for simultaneous augmentation and mastopexy can be?***
   A. Approximately 2%.
   B. Approximately 3–8%.
   C. Approximately 10–20%.
   D. Approximately 20–30%.
   E. Greater than 30%.

INDICATIONS AND CONTRAINDICATIONS

2. ***You are evaluating a 55-year-old woman as a potential candidate for augmentation-mastopexy. She has a history of periareolar mastopexy 10 years ago for grade I ptosis complicated by periareolar scar widening which was surgically revised. She is also a former smoker, who quit 6 months ago after 35 pack-years. Past medical history includes history of asthma and mild hypertension controlled on medication. She last had a mammogram 3 years ago. There is no family history of high-risk breast cancer, and no personal history of breast cancer. Which of the following aspects of her history is a contraindication to augmentation-mastopexy?***
   A. Periareolar mastopexy.
   B. Complications following mastopexy.
   C. Smoking within the past year.
   D. Last mammography 3 years ago.
   E. Hypertension.

STAGING

3. ***Which of following measurements is the most important component to determine staging the procedure in augmentation-mastopexy?***
   A. Pinch thickness.
   B. Skin stretch.
   C. Nipple-to-inframammary fold distance.
   D. Vertical excess.
   E. Base diameter.

SKIN INCISIONS

4. ***You have planned single-stage augmentation-mastopexy for a 47-year-old woman. Her nipples sit 3 cm below the inframammary fold, vertical excess is 4 cm, and additional measurements indicate significant skin excess in both the horizonal and vertical dimensions. Which of the following mastopexy incisions is most appropriate?***
   A. Periareolar.
   B. Vertical.
   C. Wise pattern.
   D. No mastopexy required.
   E. Stage the procedure as the patient is high risk.

PERIAREOLAR MASTOPEXY

5. ***A 40-year-old patient asks about the possibility for a periareolar mastopexy with augmentation to minimize visible scarring. In which of the following scenarios would periareolar augmentation-mastopexy be most appropriate?***
   A. Nipple-areola complex (NAC) at the lower contour of the breast, pointing inferiorly.
   B. Nipple 1 cm below the level of inframammary fold (IMF).
   C. Nipple 3 cm below the level of the IMF.
   D. Nipple at the level of the IMF with the majority of parenchyma below the IMF.
   E. Nipple 5 cm below the level of the IMF.

SURGICAL APPROACHES

6. ***A 35-year-old woman presents for evaluation of hypomastia and post-pregnancy breast changes. Light traction on the nipples produces approximately 2 cm of nipple excursion, with nipple-to-inframammary fold (N-IMF) distances of approximately 5 cm. Which of the following surgical approaches is most appropriate for this patient?***
   A. Staged augmentation followed by mastopexy.
   B. Staged mastopexy followed by augmentation.
   C. One-stage augmentation-mastopexy.
   D. Augmentation alone.
   E. Mastopexy alone.

SURGICAL APPROACHES

7. ***You plan a single-stage augmentation-mastopexy for a 35-year-old woman. On evaluation, you note skin stretch of 5 cm with a nipple-to-inframammary fold distance of 12 cm. She has approximately 3 cm of vertical excess. Which of the following surgical approaches is most appropriate for this patient?***
   A. Breast augmentation only.
   B. One-stage augmentation-mastopexy.
   C. Augmentation followed by staged mastopexy.
   D. Mastopexy followed by staged augmentation.
   E. Mastopexy alone.

SURGICAL APPROACHES

8. ***Which of the following is true regarding one-stage augmentation-mastopexy?***
   A. It is recommended to place the implant prior to mastopexy.
   B. It is recommended to perform mastopexy prior to implant placement.
   C. There is a very low likelihood for needing revision surgery.
   D. There is a high likelihood for implant malposition.
   E. There is a high likelihood for capsular contracture compared to two-stage augmentation-mastopexy.

Answers

STAGING

1. *You are discussing the possibility of one-stage augmentation-mastopexy for a patient with grade II ptosis who desires increased breast fullness. What is the reoperation rate you share for simultaneous augmentation and mastopexy can be?*

C. Approximately 10–20%.

The reoperation rate for single-stage augmentation-mastopexy can range from about 8% to as high as 20% (C), contributing to it being one of the most common causes for malpractice claims in plastic surgery.[1,2] Augmentation and mastopexy subject the breast to opposing forces of skin and parenchymal expansion and reduction resulting in outcomes that are less predictable than those following each procedure alone. A review of 23 studies on single-stage augmentation-mastopexy found an overall complication rate of 13.1% with a revision rate of 10.7%.[3] In this review, the most common complications were recurrent ptosis followed by poor scar formation, capsular contracture, and tissue-related asymmetry. It is therefore important to set an expectation that there is a high revision rate for combined augmentation-mastopexy and critically evaluate the possible need for a two-stage procedure.

REFERENCES

1. Calobrace MB, Herdt DR, Cothron KJ. Simultaneous augmentation/mastopexy: a retrospective 5-year review of 332 consecutive cases. Plast Reconstr Surg 2013;131:145
2. Gorney M. Ten years' experience in aesthetic surgery malpractice claims. Aesthet Surg J 2001;21:569
3. Khavanin N, Jordan SW, Rambachan A, Kim JY. A systematic review of single-stage augmentation-mastopexy. Plast Reconstr Surg 2014;134:922–931

INDICATIONS AND CONTRAINDICATIONS

2. *You are evaluating a 55-year-old woman as a potential candidate for augmentation-mastopexy. She has a history of periareolar mastopexy 10 years ago for grade I ptosis complicated by periareolar scar widening which was surgically revised. She is also a former smoker, who quit 6 months ago after 35 pack-years. Past medical history includes history of asthma and mild hypertension controlled on medication. She last had a mammogram 3 years ago. There is no family history of high-risk breast cancer, and no personal history of breast cancer. Which of the following aspects of her history is a contraindication to augmentation-mastopexy?*

D. Last mammography 3 years ago.

The fact that this patient's last mammogram was 3 years ago is a contraindication to augmentation-mastopexy (D). According to AMA and ACOG guidelines, a mammogram within the last year is required for the following patients: age over 40 years, or age over 35 years with high risk for breast cancer, or a personal history of breast cancer.[1] She should have a mammogram prior to moving forward with the operation. A history of periareolar mastopexy with complications (A, B) is not a contraindication. This patient should, however, be counseled regarding the possibility that she may need revision—especially in the case of a single-stage procedure.[2] This patient is not a current smoker, and therefore option C is not a contraindication to surgery since she quit 6 months ago.Hypertension that is controlled is not a contraindication to surgery.

REFERENCES

1. American College of Obstetricians-Gynecologists. Practice bulletin no. 122: breast cancer screening. Obstet Gynecol 2011;118(2 Pt 1):372
2. Doshier LJ, Eagan SL, Shock LA et al. The subtleties of success in simultaneous augmentation-mastopexy. Plast Reconstr Surg 2016;138(3):585–592

STAGING

3. *Which of following measurements is the most important component to determine staging the procedure in augmentation-mastopexy?*

D. Vertical excess.

All of the above are important considerations of tissue-based planning in augmentation-mastopexy; however, vertical excess of >6 cm is indication for staging procedure. Upper pole pinch thickness (A) may inform pocket plane and implant selection as it provides insight into soft tissue coverage. Skin stretch (B) provides valuable information regarding anteroposterior laxity, while nipple-to-inframammary fold distance (C) provides information regarding laxity in the vertical dimension. Vertical excess (D) is an important measurement as it provides information on the amount of skin/parenchyma to be resected and may inform a consideration of one-stage versus two-stage augmentation-mastopexy.[1,2]

REFERENCES

1. Lee MR, Unger JG, Adams WP Jr. The tissue-based triad: a process approach to augmentation mastopexy. Plast Reconstr Surg 2014;245:215
2. Sanniec K, Adams WP. The tissue-based triad in augmentation mastopexy: single-stage technical refinements [published online ahead of print January 9, 2019]. Aesthet Surg J doi: 10.1093/asj/sjz006

SKIN INCISIONS

4. *You have planned single-stage augmentation-mastopexy for a 47-year-old woman. Her nipples sit 3 cm below the inframammary fold, vertical excess is 4 cm, and additional measurements indicate significant skin excess in both the horizonal and vertical dimensions. Which of the following mastopexy incisions is most appropriate?*

C. Wise pattern.

In cases where the nipple is >2 cm below the level of the inframammary fold (IMF) and there is skin excess in both vertical and horizontal dimensions, a Wise pattern mastopexy (C) incision is most appropriate. Periareolar incision (A) would be appropriate in cases of minimal ptosis and a nipple-areola complex at or above the breast border.[1,2] Vertical pattern (B) would provide acceptable results in cases where the nipple is >2 cm below the IMF with horizontal skin excess but minimal vertical skin excess. Staging the procedure (E) is something to consider once the vertical excess is >6 cm.

REFERENCES

1. Davison SP, Spear SL. Simultaneous breast augmentation with periareolar mastopexy. Semin Plast Surg 2004;18:189
2. Kirwan L. A classification and algorithm for treatment of breast ptosis. Aesthet Surg J 2002;22:355

PERIAREOLAR MASTOPEXY

5. *A 40-year-old patient asks about the possibility for a periareolar mastopexy with augmentation to minimize visible scarring. In which of the following scenarios would periareolar augmentation-mastopexy be most appropriate?*

B. Nipple 1 cm below the level of inframammary fold (IMF).

Periareolar augmentation-mastopexy would be most appropriate in the following cases: less than 3 to 4 cm of breast ptosis, NAC at or above the breast border and not pointing inferiorly, and nipple no more than 2 cm below the IMF (B).[1,2] The presence of an NAC pointing inferiorly at the inferior contour of the breast (A) and low nipple position relative to the IMF (C) are not appropriate cases for periareolar mastopexy as they indicate increased degrees of ptosis which may warrant vertical or Wise-pattern approaches. Choice D describes a case of pseudoptosis, and inferior wedge resection would be indicated in this situation.

REFERENCES

1. Kirwan L. Augmentation of the ptotic breast: simultaneous periareolar mastopexy/breast augmentation. Aesthet Surg J 1999;19:34
2. Stoff-Khalili MA, Schoze R, Morgan WR, et al. Subfascial periareolar augmentation mammaplasty. Plast Reconstr Surg 2003;114:1280–1288

SURGICAL APPROACHES

6. *A 35-year-old woman presents for evaluation of hypomastia and post-pregnancy breast changes. Light traction on the nipples produces approximately 2 cm of nipple excursion, with nipple-to-inframammary fold (N-IMF) distances of approximately 5 cm. Which of the following surgical approaches is most appropriate for this patient?*

D. Augmentation alone.

Breast augmentation alone (D) is most appropriate for this patient. Tissue-based planning should take into consideration superior pole pinch thickness, skin stretch (SS), nipple-to-inframammary fold (N-IMF) distance, vertical excess (VE), and base diameter (BD).[1] In a patient with combined hypomastia and ptosis, tissue-based planning approaches can help the surgeon identify the most appropriate operative approach to maximize patient satisfaction and minimize probability for reoperation.[2] This patient's SS of 2 cm and N-IMF distance of 5 cm suggest minimal anteroposterior and vertical laxity, respectively. Her lack of significant ptosis and minimal skin laxity indicate that she is unlikely to benefit from mastopexy (A, B, C, E).

REFERENCES

1. Lee MR, Unger JG, Adams WP Jr. The tissue-based triad: a process approach to augmentation mastopexy. Plast Reconstr Surg 2014;245:215
2. Sarosiek K, Maxwell PG, Unger JG. Getting the most out of augmentation-mastopexy. Plast Reconstr Surg 2018;142 (5):742e–759e

SURGICAL APPROACHES

7. *You plan a single-stage augmentation-mastopexy for a 35-year-old woman. On evaluation, you note skin stretch of 5 cm with a nipple-to-inframammary fold distance of 12 cm. She has approximately 3 cm of vertical excess. Which of the following surgical approaches is most appropriate for this patient?*

B. One-stage augmentation-mastopexy.

This patient is an appropriate candidate for single-stage augmentation-mastopexy (B). In patients with combined hypomastia and ptosis, skin stretch (SS), nipple-to-inframammary fold (N-IMF) distance, and vertical excess (VE) provide the basis for a tissue-based triad approach to staging, as developed by Lee et al.[1] Her SS and N-IMF distance indicate excess skin laxity and that she would benefit from mastopexy in addition to augmentation (A) for hypomastia. The amount of VE should inform whether or not one should stage the procedures. Vertical excess of <6 cm suggests one-stage augmentation-mastopexy would be effective, thereby avoiding a staged operation (C, D). Contraindications to a single-stage combined approach include: constricted breast or skin deficiency, lack of necessity of either procedure, significant asymmetry requiring asymmetrical mastopexy, and significant vertical skin excess requiring large skin resection.[2]

REFERENCES

1. Lee MR, Unger JG, Adams WP Jr. The tissue-based triad: a process approach to augmentation mastopexy. Plast Reconstr Surg 2014;245:215
2. Stevens WG, Macias LH, Spring M, et al. One-stage augmentation mastopexy: a review of 1192 simultaneous breast augmentation and mastopexy procedures in 615 consecutive patients. Aesthet Surg J 2014;34:723–732

SURGICAL APPROACHES

8. *Which of the following is true regarding one-stage augmentation-mastopexy?*

A. It is recommended to place the implant prior to mastopexy.

In single-stage procedures, the implant should be placed prior to mastopexy (A). This allows an evaluation for whether augmentation alone may provide effective ptosis correction and helps avoid the consequence of being skin-short as a result of the mastopexy. The reoperation rate (C) for one-stage procedures can be as high as 20%, and a discussion of this possibility is an important component of the informed consent process.[1] In a review of 321 cases of one-stage augmentation-mastopexy, complications included reoperation (14.6%), implant rupture (3.7%), unattractive scarring (2.5%), recurrent ptosis or bottoming out (2.2%), nipple malposition or asymmetry (2.2%), and <2% rates of capsular contraction, breast asymmetry, infection, loss of nipple sensation, nipple loss or depigmentation, implant malposition, and hematoma.[2]

REFERENCES

1. Calobrace MB, Herdt DR, Cothron KJ. Simultaneous augmentation/mastopexy: a retrospective 5-year review of 332 consecutive cases. Plast Reconstr Surg 2013;131:145
2. Stevens WG, Freeman ME, Stoker DA, et al. One-stage mastopexy with breast augmentation: a review of 321 patients. Plast Reconstr Surg 2007;120:1674

55. Breast Reduction

Juan L. Rendon, Anmol Chattha
See *Essentials of Aesthetic Surgery*, pp. 769–785

BREAST PHYSIOLOGY

1. ***Breast hypertrophy is associated with which of the following?***
   A. Increased estrogen receptors.
   B. Increased circulating estrogens.
   C. Increase estrogen sensitivity.
   D. Increase estrogen sensitivity and excess adiposity.
   E. Excess adiposity.

BREAST PHYSIOLOGY

2. ***Disadvantages to suction lipectomy of the breast include which of the following?***
   A. Disruption of the vascular supply to the nipple-areolar complex.
   B. Inability for precise pathologic examination of evacuated breast tissue.
   C. Disruption to nipple-areolar complex sensation.
   D. Contraindication in elderly patients.
   E. Must be performed under general anesthesia.

SURGICAL TECHNIQUE

3. ***The inferior pedicle resection is associated with which of the following?***
   A. Variable neurovascular supply and high complication rate.
   B. Impaired lactation and high rate of bottoming out.
   C. Ideal only for small reductions.
   D. Boxy breast appearance and high rate of bottoming out.
   E. Large learning curve compared to other breast reduction techniques.

SURGICAL TECHNIQUE

4. ***The superior and superomedial pedicle resections are associated with which of the following?***
   A. Variable neurovascular supply and high complication rate.
   B. Impaired lactation and high rate of bottoming out.
   C. Upper pole fullness and limited bottoming out.
   D. Boxy breast appearance and high rate of bottoming out.
   E. Easier inset comparted to inferior pedicle.

SURGICAL TECHNIQUE

5. ***Lactation is best preserved with which of the following reduction techniques?***
   A. Superior pedicle.
   B. Central pedicle.
   C. Superomedial pedicle.
   D. Inferior pedicle.
   E. Lateral pedicle.

SURGICAL TECHNIQUE

6. *In an inferior pedicle breast reduction, what should be the typical measure of the vertical limbs?*
A. 5–6 cm.
B. 7–8 cm.
C. 9–10 cm.
D. 11–12 cm.
E. 12–15 cm.

SURGICAL TECHNIQUE

7. *In a superomedial pedicle breast reduction, what should be the width of the pedicle?*
A. 2–4 cm.
B. 4–6 cm.
C. 6–10 cm.
D. 10–12 cm.
E. 12–15 cm.

SURGICAL JUDGMENT

8. *Which of the following statements regarding the breast meridian and Pitanguy's point is correct?*
A. The breast meridian determines the new vertical nipple position while Pitanguy's point determines the new horizontal nipple position.
B. The breast meridian determines the new horizontal nipple position while Pitanguy's point determines the new vertical nipple position.
C. The breast meridian and Pitanguy's point both determine the new horizontal nipple position.
D. The breast meridian and Pitanguy's point both determine the new vertical nipple position.
E. Pitanguy's point overestimates nipple vertical height.

SURGICAL JUDGMENT

9. *Which is the following is the recommended surgical approach for the treatment of recurrent hypermastia in patients requiring large resections (>500 g) with unknown primary pedicle?*
A. Liposuction alone.
B. Inferior wedge resection.
C. Inferior pedicle reduction.
D. Superomedial pedicle reduction.
E. Free-nipple graft technique.

SURGICAL JUDGMENT

10. *A key principle to maintaining vascularity to the nipple-areolar complex during re-reduction includes which of the following?*
A. Developing a new pedicle.
B. Deepithelializing only around the nipple-areolar complex.
C. Excising excess breast tissue under the nipple-areolar complex.
D. Excising excess skin below the inframammary fold.
E. Dissect down through the subdermal plexus around the nipple-areolar complex.

SURGICAL TECHNIQUE

11. *Wetting solution in breast reduction surgery should be infiltrated into which of the following areas?*
A. Retroglandular space and peri-incisional.
B. Retroglandular space only.
C. Peri-incisional only.
D. Circumferentially around the breast footprint taking care not to infiltrate the retroglandular space.
E. Around the pedicle of choice.

SURGICAL JUDGMENT

12. *Strategies for reducing the tension in the T region of an inverted-T skin excision breast reduction include which of the following?*

A. Marking a 90-degree superior keyhole angle.
B. Marking 6 cm vertical limbs.
C. Leaving a small wedge of skin at the T region closure site.
D. Placement of closed suction drains.
E. Leaving some permanent sutures in place.

SURGICAL TECHNIQUE

13. *The use of closed suction drains in breast reductions is associated with which of the following?*

A. Decreased rates of hematomas.
B. Decreased rates of nipple loss.
C. Decreased rates of wound complications.
D. No difference in complications or hematomas.
E. Increased infection rates.

SURGICAL JUDGMENT

14. *When is pathological examination of excised breast tissue warranted?*

A. All specimens should undergo pathological examination.
B. In patients >50 years old.
C. In patients with family history of breast malignancy.
D. In patients with BMI >30 kg/m^2.
E. In patients <50 years old.

Answers

BREAST PHYSIOLOGY

1. *Breast hypertrophy is associated with which of the following?*

D. Increase estrogen sensitivity and excess adiposity.

Normal number of estrogen receptors and normal levels of circulating estrogens have been found in women with hypermastia. Thus, an increased sensitivity to the hormone is thought to be responsible for breast hypertrophy. Additionally, with the increasing obesity epidemic, breast hypertrophy is often from excess adipose tissue rather than just glandular hyperplasia.[1,2,3]

REFERENCES

1. Pang S. Premature thelarche and premature adrenarche. Pediatr Ann 1981;10:29
2. Root AW, Shulman DI. Isosexual precocity: current concepts and recent advances. Fertil Steril 1986;45:749
3. Jabs AD, Frantz AG, Smith-Vaniz A, et al. Mammary hypertrophy is not associated with increased estrogen receptors. Plast Reconstr Surg 1990;86:64

BREAST PHYSIOLOGY

2. *Disadvantages to suction lipectomy of the breast include which of the following?*

B. Inability for precise pathologic examination of evacuated breast tissue.

Disadvantages to suction lipectomy of the beast include the inability to address breast ptosis, prolonged postoperative edema and induration, and inability to effectively send specimens for pathologic evaluation. Advantages include smaller scar, not disrupting vascular supply to nipple-areolar complex, can be performed under local or intravenous sedation easily, and not contraindicated in elderly patients.[1,2]

REFERENCES

1. Brown MH, Weinberg M, Chong N, et al. A cohort study of breast cancer risk in breast reduction patients. Plast Reconstr Surg 1999;103:1674
2. Colwell AS, Kukreja J, Breuing KH. Occult breast carcinoma in reduction mammaplasty specimens: 14-year experience. Plast Reconstr Surg 2004;113:1984

SURGICAL TECHNIQUE

3. *The inferior pedicle resection is associated with which of the following?*

D. Boxy breast appearance and high rate of bottoming out.

The inferior pedicle breast reduction provides a reliable neurovascular supply and is easily teachable. Yet, it depends on passive creation of breast shape from tailoring skin around the remaining breast parenchyma, and often creates a boxy breast and is associated with a high rate of bottoming out. The learning curve is less when compared to the superomedial or superior pedicles.[1]

REFERENCE

1. Nahai FR, Nahai F. MOCPSSM CME article: breast reduction. Plast Reconstr Surg 2008;121(1 Suppl):1

SURGICAL TECHNIQUE

4. *The superior and superomedial pedicle resections are associated with which of the following?*

C. Upper pole fullness and limited bottoming out.

Advantages to superior and superomedial pedicle breast reduction include the ability for large parenchymal resections with excision of the ptotic tissue and ability for the creation of inferior pillar support to limit bottoming out as well as superior fullness created by a superior pedicle location. Inset is more challenging with the superior or superomedial pedicle when compared to the inferior pedicle.[1]

REFERENCE

1. Nahai FR, Nahai F. MOCPSSM CME article: breast reduction. Plast Reconstr Surg 2008;121(1 Suppl):1

SURGICAL TECHNIQUE

5. *Lactation is best preserved with which of the following reduction techniques?*

B. Central pedicle.

Of the techniques listed, the central is ideal for lactation preservation due to the preservation of a majority of the ducts required for lactation.[1,2,3]

REFERENCES

1. Harris L, Morris SF, Freiberg A. Is breast feeding possible after reduction mammaplasty? Plast Reconstr Surg 1992;89:836
2. Brzozowski D, Niessen M, Evan HB, et al. Breast-feeding after inferior pedicle reduction mammaplasty. Plast Reconstr Surg 2000;105:530
3. Cruz-Korchin N, Korchin L. Breast-feeding after vertical mammaplasty with medial pedicle. Plast Reconstr Surg 2004;114:890

SURGICAL TECHNIQUE

6. *In an inferior pedicle breast reduction, what should be the typical measure of the vertical limbs?*

B. 7–8 cm.

In an inferior pedicle breast reduction, the vertical limbs should typically measure approximately 7 to 8 cm under tension. Long limbs can always be shortened on the operating table. Short limbs may result in closure under tension, which may compromise both shape and skin viability.[1]

REFERENCE

1. Hammond DC, Loffredo M. Breast reduction. Plast Reconstr Surg 2012;129:829e

SURGICAL TECHNIQUE

7. *In a superomedial pedicle breast reduction, what should be the width of the pedicle?*

C. 6–10 cm.

In a superomedial breast reduction a pedicle 6 to 10 cm in width will provide adequate perfusion to the nipple-areolar complex and allow sufficient rotation into the new nipple position. The other answer choices are either too short or too long.[1]

REFERENCE

1. Hammond DC, Loffredo M. Breast reduction. Plast Reconstr Surg 2012;129:829e

SURGICAL JUDGMENT

8. *Which of the following statements regarding the breast meridian and Pitanguy's point is correct?*

B. The breast meridian determines the new horizontal nipple position while Pitanguy's point determines the new vertical nipple position.

In marking for a breast reduction, the breast meridian determines the new horizontal nipple position. Transposition of the inframammary fold (Pitanguy's point) determines the new vertical nipple position.[1]

REFERENCE

1. Hammond DC, Loffredo M. Breast reduction. Plast Reconstr Surg 2012;129:829e

SURGICAL JUDGMENT

9. *Which is the following is the recommended surgical approach for the treatment of recurrent hypermastia in patients requiring large resections (>500 g) with unknown primary pedicle?*

E. Free-nipple graft technique.

According to the recommended algorithm for workup and treatment of recurrent mammary hypermastia (**Fig. 55.1**), a free nipple graft should be performed in a patient requiring a very large resection with an unknown primary pedicle.[1]

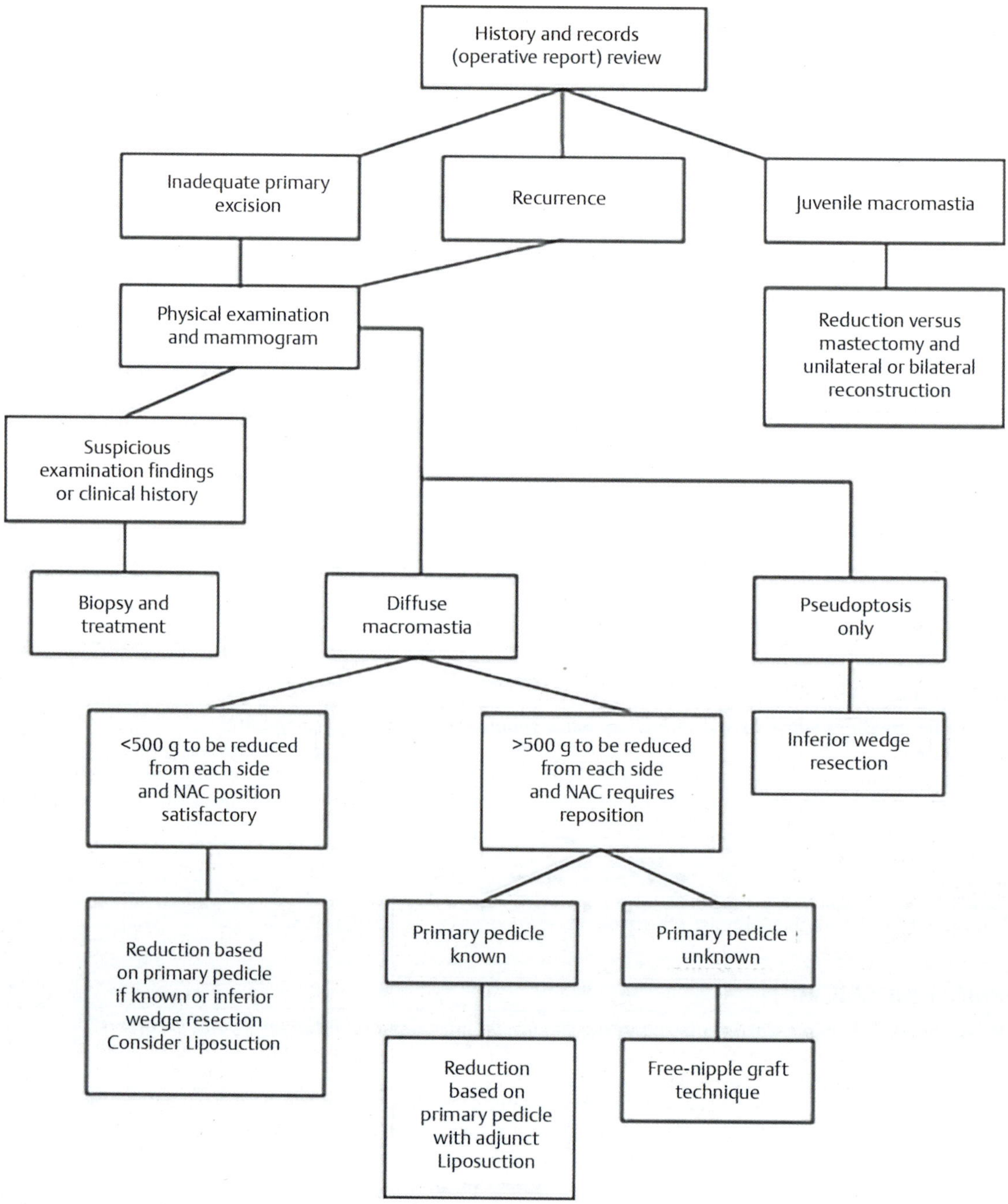

Fig. 55.1 Algorithm for workup and treatment of recurrent mammary hypermastia. (Source: Secondary breast reduction. In: Janis J, ed. Essentials of Aesthetic Surgery. 1st Edition. New York: Thieme; 2018.)

Reference

1. Hammond DC, Loffredo M. Breast reduction. Plast Reconstr Surg 2012;129:829e

SURGICAL JUDGMENT

10. *A key principle to maintaining vascularity to the nipple-areolar complex during re-reduction includes which of the following?*

B. Deepithelializing around the nipple-areolar complex.

Breast re-reduction can be performed safely and predictably, even when the previous technique is not known provided the following four key principles are followed[1]:

1. Nipple-areolar complex can be elevated by deepithelialization rather than re-creating or developing a new pedicle.
2. Breast tissue is removed where it is in excess, usually inferiorly and laterally.
3. Resection complemented with liposuction to elevate the bottomed-out inframammary fold.
4. Skin should not be excised horizontally below the inframammary fold.

REFERENCE

1. Losee JE, Cladwell EH, Serletti JM. Secondary reduction mammaplasty: is using a different pedicle safe? Plast Reconstr Surg 2000;106:1004

SURGICAL TECHNIQUE

11. *Wetting solution in breast reduction surgery should be infiltrated into which of the following areas?*

A. Retroglandular space and peri-incisional.

Two studies looked at the effects of wetting solution in breast reduction surgery. In both studies, wetting solution was infiltrated in the retroglandular space and along the incision markings. You do not want to infiltrate the wetting solution around the pedicle of choice.[1,2]

REFERENCES

1. Wilmink H, Spauwen PH, Hartman EH, et al. Preoperative injection using a diluted anesthetic/ adrenaline solution significantly reduces blood loss in reduction mammaplasty. Plast Reconstr Surg 1998;102:1913
2. Samdal F, Serra M, Skolleborg KC. The effects of infiltration with adrenaline on blood loss during reduction mammaplasty: an early survey. Scand J Plast Reconstr Hand Surg 1992;26:211

SURGICAL JUDGMENT

12. *Strategies for reducing the tension in the T region of an inverted-T skin excision breast reduction include which of the following?*

C. Leaving a small wedge of skin at the T region closure site.

Strategies to reduce tension at the T region of an inverted-T skin excision breast reduction include leaving a small wedge of skin at the T region closure site (**Fig. 55.2**), avoiding superior keyhole angles of >60 degrees, and keeping vertical limbs at least 7 cm in length.[1]

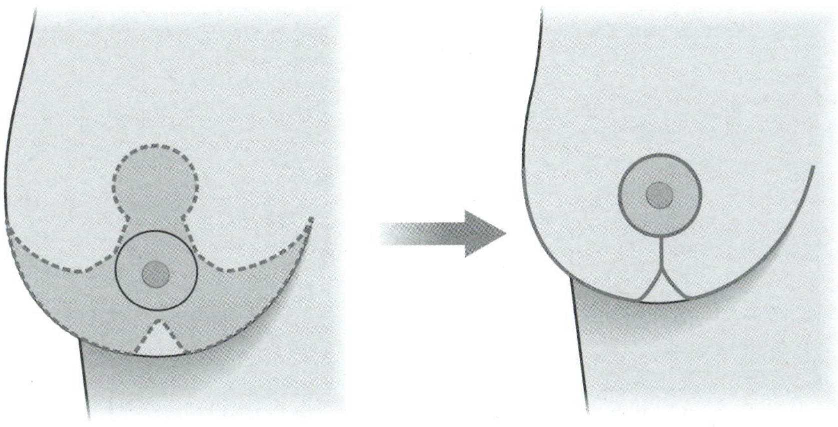

Fig. 55.2 A small wedge of skin at the site of closure limits tension at the final closure. (Source: Inverted-T skin excision. In: Janis J, ed. Essentials of Aesthetic Surgery. 1st Edition. New York: Thieme; 2018.)

Reference

1. Ribeiro L, Accorsi A, Buss A, et al. Creation and evolution of 30 years of the inferior pedicle in reduction mammaplasties. Plast Reconstr Surg 2002;110:960

SURGICAL TECHNIQUE

13. ***The use of closed suction drains in breast reductions is associated with which of the following?***

D. No difference in complications or hematomas.

Several studies have examined the use of closed suction drains in breast reduction surgeries. No study has ever demonstrated lower complication or hematoma rates with the use of drains.[1,2,3]

References

1. Wrye SW, Banducci DR, Mackay D, et al. Routine drainage is not required in reduction mammaplasty. Plast Reconstr Surg 2003;111:113
2. Corion LU, Smeulders MJ, van Zuijlen PP, et al. Draining after breast reduction: a randomized controlled inter-patient study. J Plast Reconstr Aesthet Surg 2009;62:865
3. Matarasso A, Wallach SG, Rankin M. Reevaluating the need for routine drainage in reduction mammaplasty. Plast Reconstr Surg 102:1917, 1998

SURGICAL JUDGMENT

14. ***When is pathological examination of excised breast tissue warranted?***

A. All specimens should undergo pathological examination.

The incidence of breast cancer in reduction specimens is reported at 0.6 to 1.8%; therefore, all specimens should undergo pathological examination. Additionally, a new baseline mammogram should be obtained 1 year post breast reduction.[1]

Reference

1. Lemmon JA. Reduction mammaplasty and mastopexy. Sel Read Plast Surg 2007;10(19)

56. Gynecomastia

Ira L. Savetsky
See *Essentials of Aesthetic Surgery*, pp. 789–796

INDICATIONS AND CONTRAINDICATIONS

1. ***Which of the following is true regarding neonatal and pubertal cases of gynecomastia?***
   A. Neonatal cases typically resolve within weeks while pubertal cases typically resolve within 2 years without treatment.
   B. Neonatal cases typically resolve within 2 years without treatment while pubertal cases typically resolve within weeks.
   C. Neonatal cases typically resolve within weeks while pubertal cases typically don't resolve and require treatment.
   D. Neonatal cases typically don't resolve and require treatment while pubertal cases typically resolve within 2 years without treatment.
   E. Neonatal and pubertal cases both don't resolve.

INDICATIONS AND CONTRAINDICATIONS

2. ***Patients with Klinefelter syndrome (karyotype 47, XXY) have how much of higher incidence of male breast cancer compared to XY karyotype individuals?***
   A. 2×.
   B. 10×.
   C. 25×.
   D. 50×.
   E. 75×.

INDICATIONS AND CONTRAINDICATIONS

3. ***What is the percentage of the prevalence of Klinefelter syndrome in males with breast cancer?***
   A. 2%.
   B. 7.5%.
   C. 20%.
   D. 40%.
   E. 70%.

INDICATIONS AND CONTRAINDICATIONS

4. ***A 12-year-old boy is brought in by his family for 3-month development of breast tissue. He is otherwise healthy. On examination, he has Grade 2 bilateral symmetric gynecomastia. The plan is observation. After how many months of persistent hypertrophic breast tissue is surgical treatment typically warranted?***
   A. 3 months.
   B. 6 months.
   C. 12 months.
   D. 18 months.
   E. 24 months.

INDICATIONS AND CONTRAINDICATIONS

5. ***What percentage of pubertal boys are affected with gynecomastia?***
   A. 5%.
   B. 20%.
   C. 40%.
   D. 60%.
   E. 90%.

ETIOLOGY

6. *Which of the following is the most common etiology of gynecomastia?*

A. Idiopathic.
B. Physiologic.
C. Pathological.
D. Pharmacologic.
E. Malignant.

ETIOLOGY

7. *Which of the following histologic changes are seen with gynecomastia present for more than 1 year?*

A. Florid.
B. Increased cellular stroma and ducts.
C. Intermediate.
D. Mix of florid and fibrous patterns.
E. Fibrous.

PREOPERATIVE EVALUATION

8. *Which of the following represents Grade III gynecomastia?*

A. Minimal hypertrophy (<250 g) and no ptosis.
B. Moderate hypertrophy (250–500 g) and no ptosis.
C. Severe hypertrophy (>500 g) and grade I ptosis.
D. Severe hypertrophy (>500 g) and grade II ptosis.
E. Severe hypertrophy (>500 g) and grade III ptosis.

TECHNIQUE

9. *When using ultrasound-assisted liposuction to treat gynecomastia, which of the following is the reason why the subareolar region requires more treatment?*

A. Increased adipose tissue.
B. Increased glandular tissue.
C. Increased ductal tissue.
D. Increased stromal tissue.
E. Increased fibrous tissue.

TECHNIQUE

10. *Which of the following is a treatment endpoint when using ultrasound-assisted liposuction to treat gynecomastia?*

A. Until you see skin redness.
B. Volume of lipoaspirate.
C. Loss of resistance.
D. Pinch and contour assessment.
E. Percentage power of ultrasound-assisted liposuction.

TECHNIQUE

11. *Which of the following is a treatment endpoint when using suction-assisted liposuction to treat gynecomastia?*

A. Until you see skin redness.
B. Volume of lipoaspirate.
C. Loss of resistance.
D. Pinch and contour assessment.
E. Suction power of suction-assisted liposuction in mmHg.

TECHNIQUE

12. *How long after performing ultrasound-assisted liposuction should a delayed skin excision be performed?*
   A. 4–6 weeks.
   B. 3–6 months.
   C. 6–9 months.
   D. 18 months.
   E. 2 years.

POSTOPERATIVE CARE

13. *What is the incidence of breast cancer in adolescents on pathologic examination of specimen after gynecomastia surgery?*
   A. ≤1%.
   B. 5%.
   C. 10%.
   D. 20%.
   E. 40%.

OUTCOMES

14. *What is the most common complication after an excision-only technique?*
   A. Hematoma.
   B. Seroma.
   C. Skin necrosis.
   D. Nipple necrosis.
   E. Infection.

Answers

INDICATIONS AND CONTRAINDICATIONS

1. ***Which of the following is true regarding neonatal and pubertal cases of gynecomastia?***

   A. Neonatal cases typically resolve within weeks while pubertal cases typically resolve within 2 years without treatment.

   Typically, neonatal and pubertal cases resolve with expectant management. Neonatal cases resolve within several weeks. In pubertal cases, 75% of cases resolved within 2 years without treatment.[1,2]

REFERENCES

1. Wise GJ, Roorda AK, Kalter R. Male breast disease. J Am Coll Surg 2005;200:255
2. Shulman DI, Francis GL, Palmert MR, et al; Lawson Wilkins Pediatric Endocrine Society Drug and Therapeutics Committee. Use of aromatase inhibitors in children and adolescents with disorders of growth and adolescent development. Pediatrics 2008;121:e975

INDICATIONS AND CONTRAINDICATIONS

2. ***Patients with Klinefelter syndrome (karyotype 47, XXY) have how much of higher incidence of male breast cancer compared to XY karyotype individuals?***

   D. 50×.

   Patients with Klinefelter syndrome (karyotype 47, XXY) have a 50× higher incidence of male breast cancer.[1,2]

REFERENCES

1. Hultborn R, Hanson C, Köpf I, et al. Prevalence of Klinefelter's syndrome in male breast cancer patients. Anticancer Res 1997;17:4293
2. Brinton LA. Breast cancer risk among patients with Klinefelter syndrome. Acta Paediatr 2011;100:814

INDICATIONS AND CONTRAINDICATIONS

3. ***What is the percentage of the prevalence of Klinefelter syndrome in males with breast cancer?***

   B. 7.5%.

   The prevalence of Klinefelter syndrome in males with breast cancer is 7.5%.[1,2]

REFERENCES

1. Hultborn R, Hanson C, Köpf I, et al. Prevalence of Klinefelter's syndrome in male breast cancer patients. Anticancer Res 1997;17:4293
2. Brinton LA. Breast cancer risk among patients with Klinefelter syndrome. Acta Paediatr 2011;100:814

INDICATIONS AND CONTRAINDICATIONS

4. ***A 12-year-old boy is brought in by his family for 3-month development of breast tissue. He is otherwise healthy. On examination, he has Grade 2 bilateral symmetric gynecomastia. The plan is observation. After how many months of persistent hypertrophic breast tissue is surgical treatment typically warranted?***

   C. 12 months.

   The presence of hypertrophic breast tissue for >12 months typically warrants surgical treatment because of fibrotic transformation.[1,2]

REFERENCES

1. Banyan GA, Hajdu SI. Gynecomastia: clinicopathologic study of 351 cases. Am J Clin Pathol 1972;57:431
2. Courtiss EH. Gynecomastia: analysis of 159 patients and current recommendations for treatment. Plast Reconstr Surg 1987;79(5):740–753

INDICATIONS AND CONTRAINDICATIONS

5. *What percentage of pubertal boys are affected with gynecomastia?*

D. 60%.

About 65% of pubertal boys affected (up to 75% bilateral).[1]

REFERENCES

1. Niewoehner CB, Nuttal FQ. Gynecomastia in a hospitalized male population. Am J Med 1984;77:633

ETIOLOGY

6. *Which of the following is the most common etiology of gynecomastia?*

A. Idiopathic.

Idiopathic is the most common etiology (25%). Physiologic causes include neonatal (influence of maternal estrogens), pubertal (elevated estradiol/estrogen ratio), and senile (peripheral conversion of testosterone to estrogen by aromatase). Pathologic causes include cirrhosis, kidney failure, testicular/adrenocortical/pituitary tumors, hypogonadism, hyperthyroidism, adrenal hyperplasia, and bronchogenic carcinoma. Pharmacologic causes include estrogens, gonadotropins, androgens, antiandrogens, chemotherapy agents, calcium channel blockers, ACE inhibitors, digitalis, CNS agents, antituberculosis medications, and drugs of abuse.[1,2,3]

REFERENCES

1. Banyan GA, Hajdu SI. Gynecomastia: clinicopathologic study of 351 cases. Am J Clin Pathol 1972;57:431
2. Courtiss EH. Gynecomastia: analysis of 159 patients and current recommendations for treatment. Plast Reconstr Surg 1987;79:740
3. Nuttall FQ. Gynecomastia as a physical finding in normal men. J Clin Endocrinol Metab 1979;48:338

ETIOLOGY

7. *Which of the following histologic changes are seen with gynecomastia present for more than 1 year?*

E. Fibrous.

Florid histologic pattern is seen when symptoms are present for <4 months; cellular stroma and ducts are increased. Intermediate histologic pattern is seen when symptoms are present for 4 to 12 months; there is a mix of florid and fibrous patterns. A fibrous histologic pattern is seen when gynecomastia present for >1 year; there are minimal ducts but extensive stromal fibrosis.[1]

REFERENCE

1. Banyan GA, Hajdu SI. Gynecomastia: clinicopathologic study of 351 cases. Am J Clin Pathol 1972;57:431

PREOPERATIVE EVALUATION

8. *Which of the following represents Grade III gynecomastia?*

C. Severe hypertrophy (>500 g) and grade I ptosis.

Grade I: Minimal hypertrophy (<250 g) and no ptosis. Grade II: Moderate hypertrophy (250–500 g) and no ptosis. Grade III: Severe hypertrophy (>500 g) and grade I ptosis. Grade IV: Severe hypertrophy (>500 g) and grade II or III ptosis.[1]

REFERENCE

1. Rohrich RJ, Ha RY, Kenkel JM, et al. Classification and management of gynecomastia: defining the role of ultrasound-assisted liposuction. Plast Reconstr Surg 2003;111:909

TECHNIQUE

9. *When using ultrasound-assisted liposuction to treat gynecomastia, which of the following is the reason why the subareolar region requires more treatment?*

E. Increased fibrous tissue.

When utilizing ultrasound-assisted liposuction (UAL) to address gynecomastia, the subareolar region often requires more attention and specific treatment due to the unique anatomical composition of this area, specifically because of the increased concentration of fibrous tissue.[1,2] UAL helps in liquefying and emulsifying fatty tissue, making it easier to suction out. However, the dense and fibrous nature of glandular tissue in the subareolar region can make it more challenging to treat with liposuction alone. In UAL for gynecomastia, surgeons often combine ultrasound energy with traditional liposuction techniques to address both the fatty component and the fibrous glandular tissue present in the subareolar region. This approach helps in selectively targeting the dense glandular tissue while minimizing the risk of contour irregularities or damage to surrounding structures.

REFERENCES

1. Rohrich RJ, Ha RY, Kenkel JM, et al. Classification and management of gynecomastia: defining the role of ultrasound-assisted liposuction. Plast Reconstr Surg 2003;111:909
2. Gingrass MK, Shermak MA. The treatment of gynecomastia with ultrasound-assisted lipoplasty. Semin Plast Surg 1999;12:101

TECHNIQUE

10. *Which of the following is a treatment endpoint when using ultrasound-assisted liposuction to treat gynecomastia?*

C. Loss of resistance.

The time for each treatment area is recorded. Endpoints for treatment are time and loss of resistance.[1,2] Treatment until you see skin redness or pinch test and contour assessments are not the best endpoints to determine treatment endpoints. The power level on ultrasound-assisted liposuction is not a treatment endpoint.

REFERENCES

1. Rohrich RJ, Ha RY, Kenkel JM, et al. Classification and management of gynecomastia: defining the role of ultrasound-assisted liposuction. Plast Reconstr Surg 2003;111:909
2. Gingrass MK, Shermak MA. The treatment of gynecomastia with ultrasound-assisted lipoplasty. Semin Plast Surg 1999;12:101

TECHNIQUE

11. *Which of the following is a treatment endpoint when using suction-assisted liposuction to treat gynecomastia?*

D. Pinch and contour assessment.

A bimanual technique is necessary for suction-assisted liposuction (SAL) because the nondominant hand is used to grasp and elevate the breast tissue being treated. Endpoints are determined by pinch test and contour assessment.[1] The other answer choices are not correct.

REFERENCE

1. Li CC, Fu JP, Chang SC, et al. Surgical treatment of gynecomastia: complications and outcomes. Ann Plast Surg 2012;69(5):510–515

TECHNIQUE

12. *How long after performing ultrasound-assisted liposuction should a delayed skin excision be performed?*

C. 6–9 months.

Staged skin excision is performed 6 to 9 months after ultrasound-assisted liposuction (UAL) to allow maximal skin retraction.[1]

REFERENCE

1. Rohrich RJ, Ha RY, Kenkel JM, et al. Classification and management of gynecomastia: defining the role of ultrasound-assisted liposuction. Plast Reconstr Surg 2003;111:909

POSTOPERATIVE CARE

13. *What is the incidence of breast cancer in adolescents on pathologic examination of specimen after gynecomastia surgery?*

A. ≤1%.

According to a literature review, the incidence of breast cancer risk in adolescents with gynecomastia is 1% (maximum). Some authors argue that routine histopathologic examination incurs negative productivity costs. However, the prevalence of malignancies in gynecomastia specimens increases with patient's age. Thus, histologic evaluation is recommended for all patients with pathologic gynecomastia.[1,2,3]

REFERENCES

1. Kwan D, Song DH. Discussion. Breast cancer incidence in adolescent males undergoing subcutaneous mastectomy for gynecomastia: is pathologic examination justified? A retrospective and literature review. Plast Reconstr Surg 2011;127:8
2. Senger JL, Chandran G, Kanthan R. Is routine pathological evaluation of tissue from gynecomastia necessary? A 15-year retrospective pathological and literature review. Can J Plast Surg 2014;22:112
3. Lapid O, Jolink F, Meijer SL. Pathological findings in gynecomastia: analysis of 5113 breasts. Ann Plast Surg 2015;74:163

OUTCOMES

14. *What is the most common complication after an excision-only technique?*

B. Seroma.

In a recent study with 312 consecutively treated cases who underwent subcutaneous mastectomy, there were 6 seromas (2%) and 3 hematomas (1%).[1] Given that in the excision-only technique there is an area of dead space under the skin, there tends to be a higher rate of seromas as complications in these types of cases. Without any skin removal and proper surgical technique, the rates of skin necrosis and nipple necrosis are <1% given the intact blood supply to the skin through the subdermal plexus. The rate of infections after gynecomastia surgery is 1% as well, which is in line with other plastic surgery procedures.

REFERENCE

1. Innocenti A, Melita D, Mori F, et al. Management of gynecomastia in patients with different body types: considerations on 312 consecutive treated cases. Ann Plast Surg 2017;78:492

PART IX

Body Contouring

57. Liposuction

Adam Jacoby, Simon Moradian
See *Essentials of Aesthetic Surgery*, pp. 799–817

CLINICAL CONSIDERATIONS

1. *What is the maximum safe dose of lidocaine used in tumescent solution for liposuction?*
A. 2 mg/kg.
B. 4 mg/kg.
C. 7 mg/kg.
D. 14 mg/kg.
E. 35 mg/kg.

CLINICAL CONSIDERATIONS

2. *What symptom of lidocaine toxicity is observed first, at the lowest plasma concentration of anesthetic?*
A. Tinnitus.
B. Tremors.
C. Coma.
D. Cardiac arrest.
E. Diplopia.

CLINICAL CONSIDERATIONS

3. *After patient stabilization, what is the first-line treatment for lidocaine toxicity?*
A. Flumazenil.
B. 20% lipid emulsion.
C. Methylene blue.
D. Diazepam.
E. Naloxone.

CLINICAL CONSIDERATIONS

4. *What is the minimum volume of lipoaspirate during a single operation that requires overnight monitoring?*
A. 2 liter.
B. 3 liter.
C. 4 liter.
D. 5 liter.
E. 7 liter.

CLINICAL CONSIDERATIONS

5. *Compared with suction-assisted liposuction, patient undergoing ultrasound-assisted liposuction (UAL) are at greater risk of which complication?*
A. Hematoma.
B. Seroma.
C. Thermal injury.
D. Infection.
E. Contour irregularities.

CLINICAL CONSIDERATIONS

6. ***Which wetting solution technique is defined by a 1:1 ratio of infiltrate to aspirate?***
   A. Dry.
   B. Wet.
   C. Superwet.
   D. Tumescent.
   E. Subcutaneous clysis.

CLINICAL CONSIDERATIONS

7. ***What technique can help reduce the risk of creating iatrogenic contour deformities?***
   A. Cross-hatching.
   B. Suction-assisted liposuction.
   C. Large cannula size.
   D. Superficial liposuction.
   E. Use of candy cane port configuration.

CLINICAL CONSIDERATIONS

8. ***What is considered the true endpoint of ultrasound-assisted liposuction (UAL)?***
   A. Duration of procedure.
   B. Volume of lipoaspirate.
   C. Appearance of lipoaspirate.
   D. Loss of cannula resistance.
   E. Symmetrical pinch test.

CLINICAL CONSIDERATIONS

9. ***A 36-year-old woman undergoes liposuction of the abdomen and flanks. Liposuction is performed using 2.5 liter of infiltration fluid. Each liter is mixed with 50 mL of 2% plain lidocaine and 1 mL of 1:1000 epinephrine. At which of the following times after infiltration is concentration of lidocaine in the blood expected to be the highest in this patient?***
   A. Immediately after injection.
   B. 1 hour after surgery.
   C. 3–4 hours after surgery.
   D. 8–18 hours after surgery.
   E. 20–24 hours after surgery.

CLINICAL CONSIDERATIONS

10. ***Compared with standard suction-assisted liposuction, what is a benefit of laser-assisted techniques?***
    A. Decreased postoperative ecchymosis.
    B. Decreased dermal thermal injury.
    C. Decreased operative time.
    D. Decreased surgeon fatigue.
    E. Decreased cost.

CLINICAL CONSIDERATIONS

11. ***A 43-year-old woman is requesting improved abdominal contour. She has had three children and on examination has lipodystrophy, excessive infraumbilical skin, and a moderate diastasis. Which contouring procedure would most effectively treat her complaints?***
    A. Ultrasound-assisted liposuction.
    B. Suction-assisted liposuction.
    C. Laser-assisted liposuction.
    D. Lipoabdominoplasty.
    E. Cryotherapy.

Answers

CLINICAL CONSIDERATIONS

1. *What is the maximum safe dose of lidocaine used in tumescent solution for liposuction?*

E. 35 mg/kg.

The answer is E, 35 mg/kg. The maximum safe doses for lidocaine without epinephrine and with epinephrine are 5 and 7 mg/kg, respectively. The vasoconstrictive property of epinephrine, slow infiltration, and relative avascularity of fat allow this value to be relatively higher.[1,2,3,4]

REFERENCES

1. Klein JA. Tumescent technique for local anesthesia improves safety in large-volume liposuction. Plast Reconstr Surg 1993;92:1085; discussion 1099
2. Ostad A, Kageyama N, Moy RL. Tumescent anesthesia with a lidocaine dose of 55 mg/kg is safe for liposuction. Dermatol Surg 1996;22:921
3. Lozinski A, Huq NS. Tumescent liposuction. Clin Plast Surg 2013;40:593
4. Matarasso A. Lidocaine in ultrasound-assisted lipoplasty. Clin Plast Surg 1999;26:431

CLINICAL CONSIDERATIONS

2. *What symptom of lidocaine toxicity is observed first, at the lowest plasma concentration of anesthetic?*

A. Tinnitus.

The answer is A, tinnitus, which occurs at the lowest plasma concentration of toxicity (3 µg/mL). Cardiac arrest occurs at a much higher plasma level (20 µg/mL), while tremors and coma occur between the two.[1]

REFERENCE

1. Matarasso A. Lidocaine in ultrasound-assisted lipoplasty. Clin Plast Surg 1999;26:431

CLINICAL CONSIDERATIONS

3. *After patient stabilization, what is the first-line treatment for lidocaine toxicity?*

B. 20% lipid emulsion.

The answer is B, lipid emulsion, which is bolused at a rate of 1.5 mL/g of lean body mass followed by a continuous infusion of 0.25 mL/kg/min. Flumazenil is a benzodiazepine antagonist used for overdose. Methylene blue is an antidote for methemoglobinemia and diazepam is a benzodiazepine used to treat alcohol withdrawal.[1]

REFERENCE

1. Matarasso A. Lidocaine in ultrasound-assisted lipoplasty. Clin Plast Surg 1999;26:431

CLINICAL CONSIDERATIONS

4. *What is the minimum volume of lipoaspirate during a single operation that requires overnight monitoring?*

D. 5 liter.

The answer is D, 5 liter of lipoaspirate, which is defined as large-volume liposuction. Monitoring is necessary due to fluid shifts with a higher potential of volume overload. Patients with >5 liter of liposuction are also at higher risk of lidocaine toxicity and should be monitored appropriately.[1,2,3,4]

REFERENCES

1. Iverson RE, Lynch DJ; American Society of Plastic Surgeons Committee on Patient Safety. Practice advisory on liposuction. Plast Reconstr Surg 2004;113:1478; discussion 1491
2. Weinberg GL. Lipid emulsion infusion: resuscitation for local anesthetic and other drug overdose. Anesthesiology 2012;117:180
3. Rohrich RJ, Leedy JE, Swamy R, et al. Fluid resuscitation in liposuction: a retrospective review of 89 consecutive patients. Plast Reconstr Surg 2006;117:431

4. Commons GW, Halperin B, Chang CC. Large-volume liposuction: a review of 631 consecutive cases over 12 years. Plast Reconstr Surg 2001;108:1753; discussion 1764

CLINICAL CONSIDERATIONS

5. *Compared with suction-assisted liposuction, patient undergoing ultrasound-assisted liposuction (UAL) are at greater risk of which complication?*

C. Thermal injury.

The answer is C, thermal injury, which can lead to burns. Thermal methods of liposuction lessen cannula resistance and reduce surgeon fatigue. Compared with power-assisted and suction-assisted techniques, UAL is associated with similar hematoma, seroma, and infection rates.[1,2,3]

REFERENCES

1. Rohrich RJ, Beran SJ, Kenkel JM, et al. Extending the role of liposuction in body contouring with ultrasound-assisted liposuction. Plast Reconstr Surg 1998;101:1090; discussion 1117
2. Zocchi M. Ultrasonic liposculpturing. Aesthetic Plast Surg 1992;16:287
3. Kenkel JM, Janis JE, Rohrich RJ, et al. Aesthetic body contouring: ultrasound-assisted liposuction. Oper Tech Plast Reconstr Surg 2002;8:180

CLINICAL CONSIDERATIONS

6. *Which wetting solution technique is defined by a 1:1 ratio of infiltrate to aspirate?*

C. Superwet.

The answer is C, superwet technique. "Dry" liposuction uses no infiltrate and is associated with the greatest estimated blood loss. Wet liposuction uses approximately 200 to 300 mL of wetting solution, yielding a blood loss of 4 to 30%. Superwet liposuction is the only technique defined by a 1:1 ratio of infiltrate to aspirate while tumescent liposuction is defined by 1 mL of aspirate per every 3 to 4 mL of infiltrate, yielding the lowest estimated blood loss (**Table 57.1**). Subcutaneous clysis is not a described method that is commonly used.

Infiltrate may contain lidocaine, epinephrine, and/or sodium bicarbonate, depending on surgeon's preference.[1]

Table 57.1 *Wetting Solution Infiltrate and Estimated Blood Loss by Technique*

Technique	Infiltrate	Estimated Blood Loss (as % volume)
Dry	None	20–45
Wet	200–300 mL/area	4–30
Superwet	1 mL infiltrate:1 mL aspirate	<1
Tumescent	3–4 mL infiltrate:1 mL aspirate	<1

REFERENCE

1. Iverson RE, Pao VS. MOC PS (SM) CME article: liposuction. Plast Reconstr Surg 2008;121 (4Suppl): S1

CLINICAL CONSIDERATIONS

7. *What technique can help reduce the risk of creating iatrogenic contour deformities?*

A. Cross-hatching.

The answer is A, cross-hatching. The use of multiple patient positions and multiple access incisions allows for a smooth and regular contour after liposuction. Larger cannulas suction a greater amount of fat per pass and are associated with contour deformities, as is superficial liposuction. Suction-assisted liposuction itself is not associated with creating contour deformities. Candy cane configuration is generally a more aggressive canula for liposuction and should be used in the proper plane to avoid contour deformities.[1,2,3]

REFERENCES

1. Rohrich RJ, Smith PD, Marcantonio DR, et al. The zones of adherence: role in minimizing and preventing contour deformities in liposuction. Plast Reconstr Surg 2001;107:1562
2. Neligan P, Warren RJ, eds. Plastic Surgery. Vol. 2. 3rd ed. Philadelphia: Saunders Elsevier; 2013
3. Young VL, Brandon HJ. The physics of suction-assisted lipoplasty. Aesthet Surg J 2004;24:206

CLINICAL CONSIDERATIONS

8. ***What is considered the true endpoint of ultrasound-assisted liposuction (UAL)?***

D. Loss of cannula resistance.

The answer is D, loss of resistance to probe advancement. Although the duration of the procedure and volume of liposuction are both important factors in determining a patient's fluid balance, they are not considered true endpoints. The appearance of lipoaspirate (especially if sanguinous) is often considered an accepted endpoint for standard suction-assisted liposuction. Symmetrical pinch test is considered an acceptable endpoint for suction-assisted or power-assisted liposuction.[1]

REFERENCE

1. Matarasso A. Lidocaine in ultrasound-assisted lipoplasty. Clin Plast Surg 1999;26:431

CLINICAL CONSIDERATIONS

9. ***A 36-year-old woman undergoes liposuction of the abdomen and flanks. Liposuction is performed using 2.5 liter of infiltration fluid. Each liter is mixed with 50 mL of 2% plain lidocaine and 1 mL of 1:1000 epinephrine. At which of the following times after infiltration is concentration of lidocaine in the blood expected to be the highest in this patient?***

D. 8–18 hours after surgery.

The safe dosage of lidocaine in liposuction is 35 to 55 mg/kg. Peak lidocaine levels are reported to be 8 to 18 hours after infiltration. Oftentimes, patients are discharged to home when peak levels occur.[1,2,3,4]

REFERENCES

1. Klein JA. Tumescent technique for local anesthesia improves safety in large-volume liposuction. Plast Reconstr Surg 1993;92:1085; discussion 1099
2. Ostad A, Kageyama N, Moy RL. Tumescent anesthesia with a lidocaine dose of 55 mg/kg is safe for liposuction. Dermatol Surg 1996;22:921
3. Gutowski KA. Tumescent analgesia in plastic surgery. Plast Reconstr Surg 2014;134(4 Suppl 2):50S–57S
4. Swanson E. Prospective study of lidocaine, bupivacaine, and epinephrine levels and blood loss in patients undergoing liposuction and abdominoplasty. Plast Reconstr Surg 2012;130(3):702–722

CLINICAL CONSIDERATIONS

10. ***Compared with standard suction-assisted liposuction, what is a benefit of laser-assisted techniques?***

A. Decreased postoperative ecchymosis.

The answer is A, decreased postoperative ecchymosis, as laser wavelengths can aid in photocoagulation of small vessels. Laser-assisted liposuction (LAL) is more costly and more time consuming given the addition of laser energy to the technique. Subdermal tissues are heated, leading to skin tightening but can also lead to thermal injury.[1]

REFERENCE

1. Badin AZ, Gondek LB, Garcia MJ, et al. Analysis of laser lipolysis effects on human tissue samples obtained from liposuction. Aesthetic Plast Surg 2005;29:281

CLINICAL CONSIDERATIONS

11. ***A 43-year-old woman is requesting improved abdominal contour. She has had three children and on examination has lipodystrophy, excessive infraumbilical skin, and a moderate diastasis. Which contouring procedure would most effectively treat her complaints?***

D. Lipoabdominoplasty.

The answer is D, lipoabdominoplasty, which can utilize liposuction to refine body contour after a standard abdominoplasty. Liposuction techniques alone are not appropriate as the patient has excessive skin, which will not be treated by liposuction alone. Cryotherapy may offer mild skin tightening and retraction but will not treat the patient's diastasis.[1,2]

REFERENCES

1. Iverson RE, Pao VS. MOC PS (SM) CME article: liposuction. Plast Reconstr Surg 2008;121 (4Suppl):S1
2. Saldanha OR, Azevedo SF, Delboni PS, Saldanha Filho OR, Saldanha CB, Uribe LH. Lipoabdominoplasty: the Saldanha technique. Clin Plast Surg 2010;37(3):469–481

58. Brachioplasty

Adam Jacoby
See *Essentials of Aesthetic Surgery*, pp. 818–827

SURGICAL ANATOMY

1. ***Which structure courses with the medial antebrachial cutaneous nerve, superficial to the deep fascia of the arm?***
   A. Basilic vein.
   B. Cephalic vein.
   C. Median nerve.
   D. Medial nerve.
   E. Brachial artery.

OPERATIVE SELECTION

2. ***In a patient with lipodystrophy of the upper arm, with both excess fat and skin extending on to the chest wall, what is the preferred brachioplasty technique?***
   A. Cryotherapy.
   B. Limited medial brachioplasty.
   C. Suction-assisted liposuction (SAL) alone.
   D. Ultrasound-assisted liposuction (UAL) alone.
   E. Extended brachioplasty with or without liposuction.

SURGICAL COMPLICATIONS

3. ***What is the most common patient complaint after brachioplasty?***
   A. Seroma.
   B. Hematoma.
   C. Numbness.
   D. Wound dehiscence.
   E. Scar hypertrophy.

SURGICAL TIMING

4. ***What is the minimum time between bariatric surgery and brachioplasty during which a patient should be weight stable?***
   A. 1 month.
   B. 3 months.
   C. 6 months.
   D. 12 months.
   E. 18 months.

SURGICAL ANATOMY

5. ***In a standard brachioplasty, which structure is most at risk for damage?***
   A. Posterior cord of brachial plexus.
   B. Median nerve.
   C. Medial antebrachial cutaneous nerve.
   D. Thoracic duct.
   E. Brachial artery.

PREVENTIVE COMPLICATIONS

6. ***Which of the following should be employed when brachioplasty incisions cross the axilla in order to prevent contractures?***
   A. Progressive tension sutures.
   B. Z-plasty.
   C. V-Y advancement.
   D. Drain placement.
   E. Barbed suture use.

Answers

SURGICAL ANATOMY

1. *Which structure courses with the medial antebrachial cutaneous nerve, superficial to the deep fascia of the arm?*

A. Basilic vein.

The answer is A, basilic vein, which pierces the deep fascia of the upper arm about 14 centimeters proximal to the medial epicondyle. The cephalic vein is more radial, and the median nerve/brachial artery are deeper structures, not at risk during a brachioplasty (**Fig. 58.1**).[1,2]

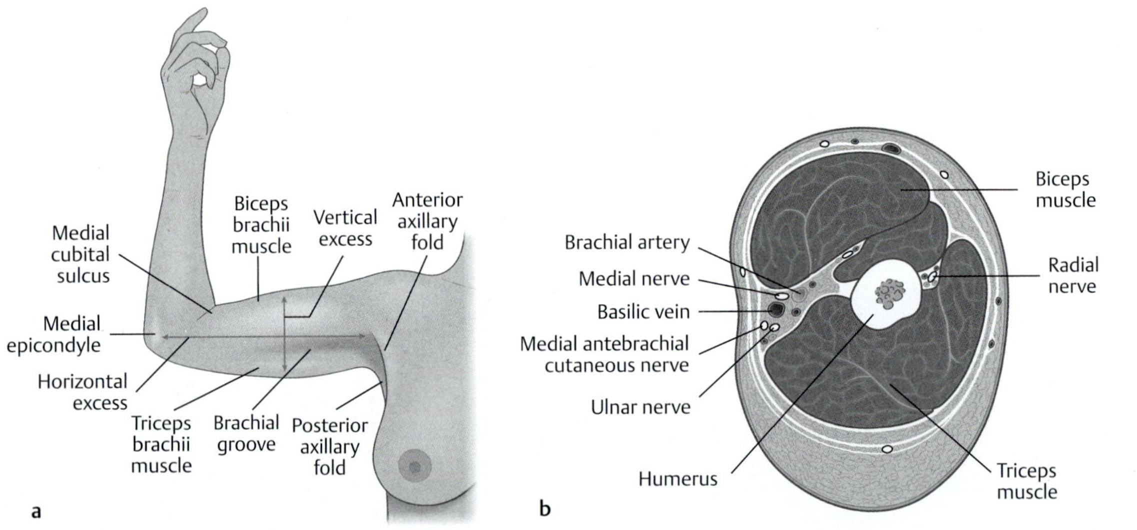

Fig. 58.1 Anatomy of the arm. **(a)** External landmarks. **(b)** Cross section. (Source: Anatomy. In: Janis J, ed. Essentials of Aesthetic Surgery. 1st Edition. New York: Thieme; 2018.)

REFERENCES

1. Cannistra C, Valero R, Benelli C, et al. Brachioplasty after massive weight loss: a simple algorithm for surgical plane. Aesthetic Plast Surg 2007;31:6
2. Knoetgen J III, Morgan SL. Long-term outcomes and complications associated with brachioplasty: as retrospective review and cadaveric study. Plast Reconstr Surg 2006;117:2219

OPERATIVE SELECTION

2. *In a patient with lipodystrophy of the upper arm, with both excess fat and skin extending on to the chest wall, what is the preferred brachioplasty technique?*

E. Extended brachioplasty with or without liposuction.

The answer is E, extended brachioplasty with or without liposuction. Limited resection techniques will not address the excess skin and subcutaneous tissue on the chest wall. Liposuction techniques alone will not address the excessive skin, which will need to be resected for an excellent result. Extended brachioplasty with extension onto the chest wall with a Z-plasty in the axilla will provide excellent contour and minimize axillary webbing or contracture. Cryotherapy may offer mild skin tightening and retraction but will not treat the level of excess skin and fat described in the above vignette.[1,2,3,4]

REFERENCES

1. Appelt EA, Janis JE, Rohrich RJ. An algorithmic approach to upper arm contouring. Plast Reconstr Surg 2006;118:237

2. Baroudi R. Body sculpturing. Clin Plast Surg 1984;11:419
3. Gusenoff JA, Coon D, Rubin JP. Brachioplasty and concomitant procedures after massive weight loss: a statistical analysis from a prospective registry. Plast Reconstr Surg 2008;122:595
4. Cannistra C, Valero R, Benelli C, et al. Brachioplasty after massive weight loss: a simple algorithm for surgical plane. Aesthetic Plast Surg 2007;31:6

SURGICAL COMPLICATIONS

3. *What is the most common patient complaint after brachioplasty?*

E. Scar hypertrophy.

The answer is D, scar hypertrophy. The other answers are possible adverse outcomes after brachioplasty but close to 10% of postoperative patients will require a scar revision. Patient counseling and preoperative discussion of scar placement are an important part of the consent process.[1,2,3]

REFERENCES

1. Samra S, Sawh-Martinez R, Liu YJ, et al. Optimal placement of brachioplasty scar: a survey evaluation. Plast Reconstr Surg 2010;126:77
2. Abramson DL. Minibrachioplasty: minimizing scars while maximizing results. Plast Reconstr Surg 2004;114:1631
3. Zomerlei TA, Neman KC, Armstrong SD, et al. Brachioplasty outcomes: a review of a multi practice cohort. Plast Reconstr Surg 2013;131:883

SURGICAL TIMING

4. *What is the minimum time between bariatric surgery and brachioplasty during which a patient should be weight stable?*

C. 6 months.

The answer is C, 6 months between bariatric surgery and brachioplasty. This allows for homeostasis of tissues and sufficient time to ensure weight stability. Fluctuations in weight place patients at a higher risk for wound healing issues. Options A and B are too short to determine weight stability.[1,2,3]

REFERENCES

1. Aly AS, ed. Body Contouring After Massive Weight Loss. New York: Thieme Publishers; 2006
2. Gusenoff JA, Coon D, Rubin JP. Brachioplasty and concomitant procedures after massive weight loss: a statistical analysis from a prospective registry. Plast Reconstr Surg 2008;122:595
3. Cannistra C, Valero R, Benelli C, et al. Brachioplasty after massive weight loss: a simple algorithm for surgical plane. Aesthetic Plast Surg 2007;31:6

SURGICAL ANATOMY

5. *In a standard brachioplasty, which structure is most at risk for damage?*

C. Medial antebrachial cutaneous nerve.

The answer is C, medial antebrachial cutaneous nerve, which arises from the medial cord of the brachial plexus, which is the most common neurovascular structure damaged during brachioplasty. Liposuction prior to resection preserve neurovascular structures and facilitates easy resection of subcutaneous tissues. The structures in all other answer choices are much deeper and should not be encountered during a brachioplasty (**Fig. 58.2**).[1,2]

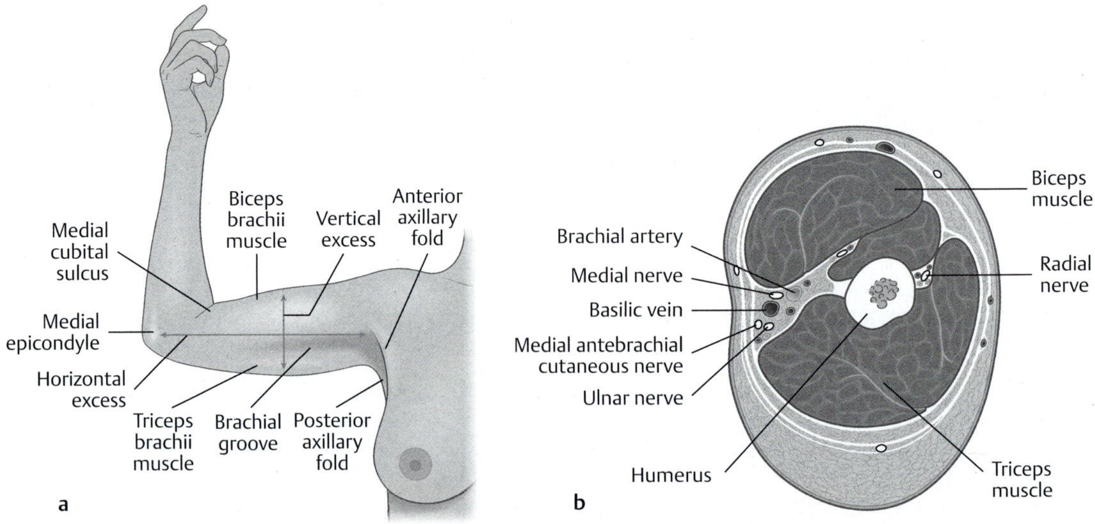

Fig. 58.2 Anatomy of the arm. **(a)** External landmarks. **(b)** Cross section. (Source: Anatomy. In: Janis J, ed. Essentials of Aesthetic Surgery. 1st Edition. New York: Thieme; 2018.)

REFERENCES

1. Cannistra C, Valero R, Benelli C, et al. Brachioplasty after massive weight loss: a simple algorithm for surgical plane. Aesthetic Plast Surg 2007;31:6
2. Knoetgen J III, Morgan SL. Long-term outcomes and complications associated with brachioplasty: as retrospective review and cadaveric study. Plast Reconstr Surg 2006;117:2219

PREVENTIVE COMPLICATIONS

6. ***Which of the following should be employed when brachioplasty incisions cross the axilla in order to prevent contractures?***

   B. Z-plasty.

   The answer is B, Z-plasty, which helps prevent contracture in the axilla. Progressive tension sutures can relieve tension on an abdominoplasty closure and are not useful in brachioplasty. Drains are often placed during brachioplasty regardless of scar position. Barbed sutures are often used in body contouring procedures to aid in efficiency but often pose problems during brachioplasty as medial arm skin is thin, interfering with wound healing, potentially leading to spitting suture (**Fig. 58.3**).[1,2,3]

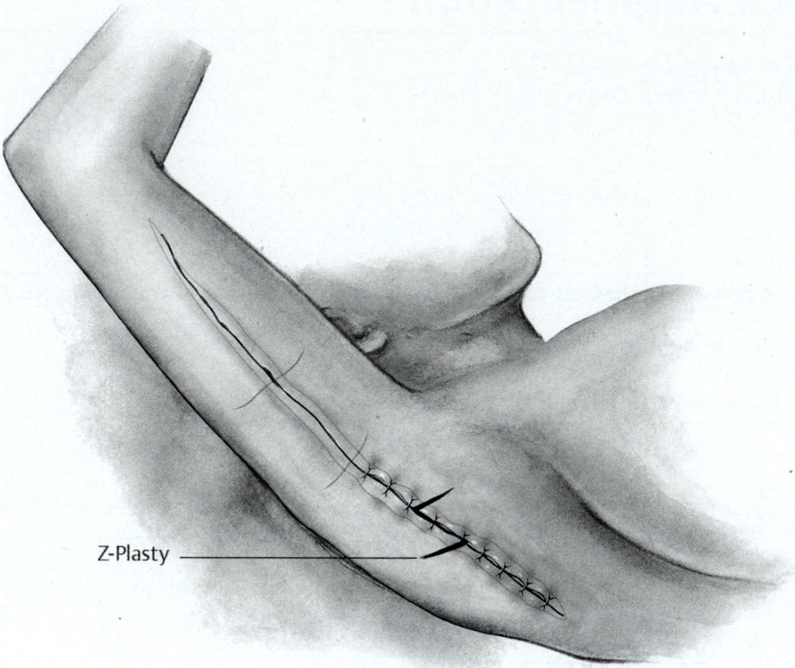

Fig. 58.3 Brachioplasty marked with vertical cross-hatches. Note the Z-plasty used to prevent contracture across the axilla. (Source: Operative Procedure. In: Janis J, ed. Essentials of Aesthetic Surgery. 1st Edition. New York: Thieme; 2018.)

References

1. Lockwood T. Brachioplasty with superficial fascial system suspension. Plast Reconstr Surg 1995;96:912
2. Samra S, Sawh-Martinez R, Liu YJ, et al. Optimal placement of brachioplasty scar: a survey evaluation. Plast Reconstr Surg 2010;126:77
3. Shermak MA, Mallalieu J, Chang D. Barbed suture impact on wound closure in body contouring. Plast Reconstr Surg 2010;126:1735

59. Buttock Augmentation

Sammy Sinno, Michael E. Nissan
See *Essentials of Aesthetic Surgery*, pp. 828–836

INDICATIONS

1. *Which of the following patients is the best candidate for gluteal augmentation via autologous fat grafting?*
A. A thin patient.
B. A slightly overweight patient.
C. A severely obese patient.
D. A massive weight loss patient.
E. A pregnant patient.

ANATOMY

2. *The gluteus maximus muscle originates at the _______ and inserts onto the _______.*
A. Medial border of the sacrum; greater trochanter of the femur.
B. Lateral border of the sacrum; lesser trochanter of the femur.
C. Posterior superior iliac spine; midshaft of the femur.
D. Posterior superior iliac spine; greater trochanter of the femur.
E. Lateral border of the sacrum; greater trochanter of the femur.

AESTHETIC ZONES

3. *Which of the following is the significance of zone 1 of the 10 gluteal aesthetic zones?*
A. For autologous fat grafting, zone 1 is targeted for lipoharvest and creates a desirable contour.
B. Zone 1 is located along the inner gluteal region and should be avoided.
C. Zone 1 is located lateral to midline and should be harvested for fat.
D. Zone 1 is located lateral to midline and should be augmented with fat.
E. Due to high density of nerves and vasculature, zone 1 should be avoided both during lipoharvest and augmentation.

LIPOHARVEST

4. *Most fat in the buttock is removed from which of the following zones?*
A. Zones 1–4.
B. Zones 5 and 6.
C. Zones 3 and 5.
D. Zones 5 and 6.
E. Zone 10.

SILICONE IMPLANTS

5. *A patient who underwent silicone implant gluteal augmentation is experiencing unilateral shooting pain down the leg. The implant will most likely be located in which of the following tissue planes?*
A. Subcutaneous.
B. Submuscular.
C. Intramuscular.
D. Subfascial.
E. Dual plane with partial subcutaneous and subfascial placement.

COMPLICATIONS

6. *Which of the following methods of augmentation has the lowest rate of complications in regard to morbidity?*

A. Autologous fat grafting.
B. Silicone implants.
C. Saline implants.
D. Autologous fat grafting with implant placement.
E. Autologous flap augmentation.

POSTOPERATIVE PERIOD

7. *After autologous fat augmentation, a patient experiences confusion, petechiae, fever, and respiratory distress. How could this complication have been avoided?*

A. Injecting into muscle.
B. Injecting near the piriformis.
C. Injecting higher volumes of fat.
D. Keeping the injection cannula perpendicular to the patient.
E. Keeping the injection cannula parallel to the patient

SILICONE IMPLANT COMPLICATIONS

8. *Which of the following complications is most likely following silicone implant augmentation?*

A. Wound dehiscence.
B. Capsular contracture.
C. Seroma.
D. Infection.
E. Paresthesias.

Answers

INDICATIONS

1. *Which of the following patients is the best candidate for gluteal augmentation via autologous fat grafting?*

B. A slightly overweight patient.

Slightly overweight patients—especially those with excess sacral, lower back, and posterior triangle fat—are excellent candidates for gluteal augmentation via autologous fat grafting. These patients typically have enough excess fat to produce a dramatic aesthetic result while not requiring additional liposuction like heavier patients would. Pregnancy is a contraindication for gluteal augmentation. Neoplasm or any other severe comorbid condition is also a contraindication.[1,2,3]

REFERENCES

1. Tardif M, de la Peña JA. Gluteal augmentation. In: Aston SJ, Steinbrech DS, Walden JL, eds. Aesthetic Plastic Surgery. Philadelphia: Saunders Elsevier; 2009
2. Cádenas-Camarena L, Arenas-Quintana R, Robles-Cervantes JA. Buttocks fat grafting: 14 years of evolution and experience. Plast Reconstr Surg 2011;128:545
3. Centeno RF, Young VL. Clinical anatomy in aesthetic gluteal body contouring surgery. Clin Plast Surg 2006;33:347

ANATOMY

2. *The gluteus maximus muscle originates at the ______ and inserts onto the ______.*

D. Posterior superior iliac spine; greater trochanter of the femur.

The gluteus maximus muscle originates along the lateral sacrum and the posterior iliac spine. It inserts into the iliotibial tract and the greater trochanter of the femur. It is the main extensor muscle of the hip and the most superficial of the gluteal muscles, responsible for the bulk and contour of the buttock region (**Fig. 59.1**).[1]

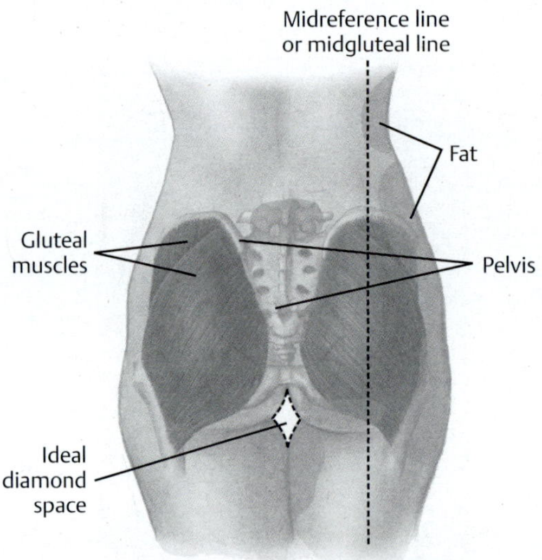

Fig. 59.1 Gluteus maximus muscle anatomy. (Source: Summary of key anatomic and aesthetic concepts. In: Aly A, ed. Body Contouring: After Massive Weight Loss. 1st Edition. New York: Thieme; 2006.)

REFERENCE

1. Centeno RF, Young VL. Clinical anatomy in aesthetic gluteal body contouring surgery. Clin Plast Surg 2006;33:347

AESTHETIC ZONES

3. *Which of the following is the significance of zone 1 of the 10 gluteal aesthetic zones?*

A. For autologous fat grafting, zone 1 is targeted for lipoharvest and creates a desirable contour.

For gluteal augmentation with autologous fat grafting, 10 zones have been defined to guide lipoharvest and augmentation (**Fig. 59.2**).[1,2,3,4,5] Zone 1, also known as the "presacral V," is defined by the superior point of the intergluteal fold and the posterior iliac dimples. This zone is ideal for lipoharvest, as it creates a desirable contour after liposuction. Zone 7 is actually the inner gluteal area and is safe to lipoharvest from.

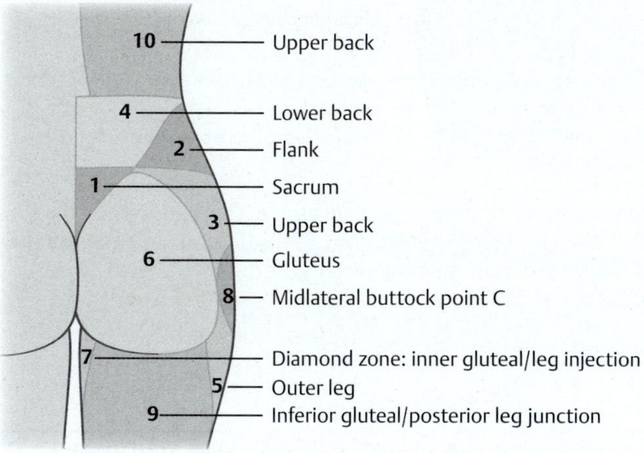

Fig. 59.2 Mendieta's 10 aesthetic units or zones. (1, Sacrum; 2, flank; 3, upper back; 4, lower back; 5, outer leg; 6, gluteus; 7, diamond zone: inner gluteal/leg injection; 8, midlateral buttock point C; 9, inferior gluteal/posterior leg junction; 10, upper back.) (Source: Autologous fat grafting (Mendieta). In: Janis J, ed. Essentials of Aesthetic Surgery. 1st Edition. New York: Thieme; 2018.)

REFERENCES

1. Mendieta CG. Classification system for gluteal evaluation. Clin Plast Surg 2006;33:333
2. Mendieta CG. Gluteal reshaping. Aesthet Surg J 2007;27:641
3. Mendieta CG. Gluteoplasty. Aesthet Surg J 2003;23:441
4. Nahai F. The Art of Aesthetic Surgery: Principles & Techniques. New York: Thieme Publishers; 2005
5. Peren PA, Gomez JB, Guerrerosantos J, et al. Gluteus augmentation with fat grafting. Aesthetic Plast Surg 2000;24:412

LIPOHARVEST

4. *Most fat in the buttock is removed from which of the following zones?*

A. Zones 1–4.

Most fat in the buttock is harvested from zones 1 to 4: sacrum, flank, upper buttock, and lower back. These regions are located superior to the gluteus muscle, often contain excess fat, and form a pleasing aesthetic contour after liposuction. Fat is harvested through a 5-millimeter cannula in the deep layers and a 4-millimeter cannula in the superficial layers (**Fig. 59.3**).[1,2,3]

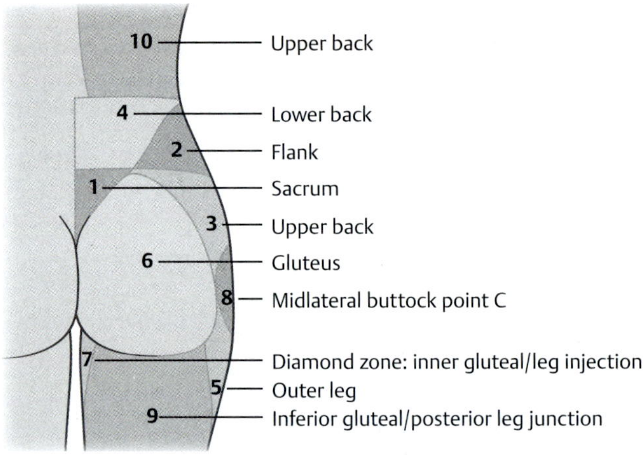

Fig. 59.3 Mendieta's 10 aesthetic units or zones. (1, Sacrum; 2, flank; 3, upper back; 4, lower back; 5, outer leg; 6, gluteus; 7, diamond zone: inner gluteal/leg injection; 8, midlateral buttock point C; 9, inferior gluteal/posterior leg junction; 10, upper back.) (Source: Autologous fat grafting (Mendieta). In: Janis J, ed. Essentials of Aesthetic Surgery. 1st Edition. New York: Thieme; 2018.)

References

1. Mendieta CG. Classification system for gluteal evaluation. Clin Plast Surg 2006;33:333
2. Nahai F. The Art of Aesthetic Surgery: Principles & Techniques. New York: Thieme Publishers; 2005
3. Peren PA, Gomez JB, Guerrerosantos J, et al. Gluteus augmentation with fat grafting. Aesthetic Plast Surg 2000;24:412

SILICONE IMPLANTS

5. *A patient who underwent silicone implant gluteal augmentation is experiencing unilateral shooting pain down the leg. The implant will most likely be located in which of the following tissue planes?*

B. Submuscular.

The patient in the vignette with unilateral, shooting leg pain in the context of silicone implant gluteal augmentation is likely experiencing symptoms related to compression of the sciatic nerve. There are four possible tissue planes for placement of a gluteal silicone implant: subcutaneous, submuscular, intramuscular, and subfascial (**Fig. 59.4**).[1,2] The submuscular approach (option A) is the most likely to cause sciatic nerve injury due to its proximity to the nerve relative to the other tissue locations. To avoid this complication, the intramuscular approach (option B) is most often used in the United States. However, the dissection is more difficult, and a seroma is more likely to form.

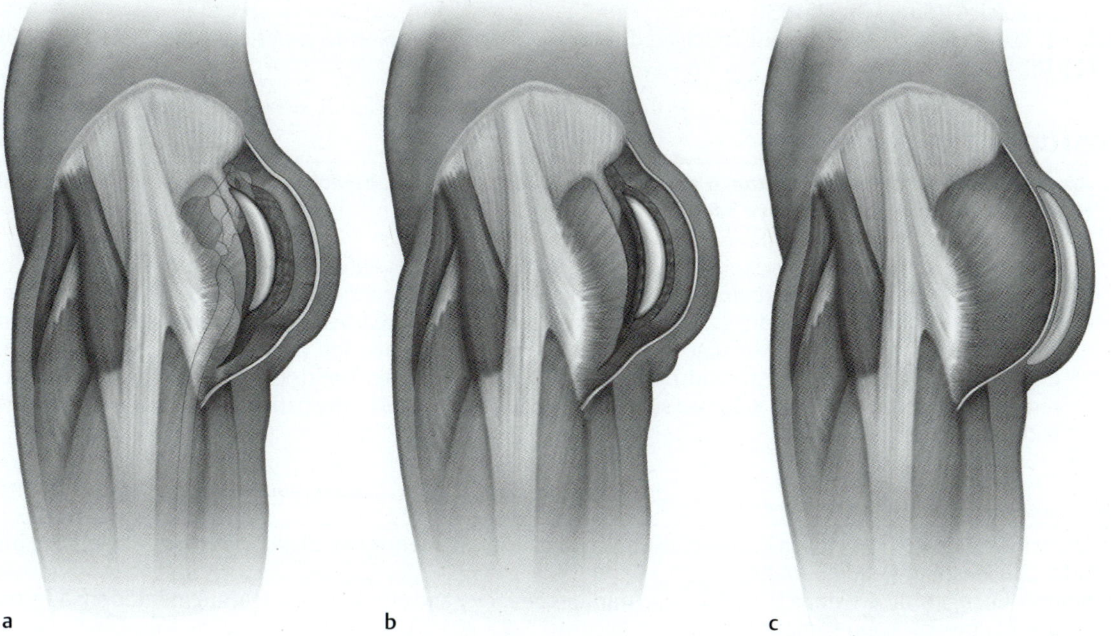

Fig. 59.4 Common locations for silicone implant placement for gluteal augmentation: **(a)** submuscular, **(b)** intramuscular, and **(c)** subfascial. (Source: Mendieta CG. The Art of Gluteal Sculpting. New York: Thieme Publishers, 2011.)

REFERENCES

1. Robles JM, Tagliapietra JC, Grandi MA. Gluteoplastia de augmento: implante submuscular. Cirplast Ibero Latinoam 1984;10:365
2. Serra F, Aboudib JH, Marques RG. Intramuscular technique for gluteal augmentation: determination and quantification of muscle atrophy and implant position by computed tomographic scan. Plast Reconstr Surg 2013;131:253e

COMPLICATIONS

6. *Which of the following methods of augmentation has the lowest rate of complications in regard to morbidity?*

A. Autologous fat grafting.

Complications that may occur after gluteal augmentation include infection, sciatica, seroma, fat resorption, oil cysts, and wound healing problems. With an overall complication rate of approximately 8%, autologous fat grafting has a lower rate of complications than other augmentation methods such as silicone implants, which are associated with a 20 to 40% complication rate. Additionally, combining methods will inherently always be associated with a slightly higher complication rate. *When discussing mortality*, according to the ASERF Task Force calculations for gluteal fat grafting, the risk of pulmonary fat emboli was 1 in 1030 (<0.08%), with a mortality risk of 1 in 3448 (0.03%). It should be noted that various centers in the South Florida area were found to have a significantlyhigher rate of mortality; however, this was ultimately attributed to the working environment, and short surgical times.[1,2,3,4]

REFERENCES

1. Bruner TW, Roberts TL, Nguyen K. Complications of buttocks augmentation: diagnosis, management, and prevention. Clin Plast Surg 2006;33:449
2. Sinno S, Chang JB, Brownstone ND, et al. Determining the safety and efficacy of gluteal augmentation: a systematic review of outcomes and complications. Plast Reconstr Surg 2016;137:1151

3. O'Neill RC, Hanson SE, Reece E, Winocour S. Safety considerations of fat grafting in buttock augmentation. Aesthet Surg J 2021;41(Suppl 1):S25–S30
4. Pat P, Onelio G. Brazilian butt lift–associated mortality: the South Florida experience. Aesthet Surg J 2023;43 (2):162–178

POSTOPERATIVE PERIOD

7. *After autologous fat augmentation, a patient experiences confusion, petechiae, fever, and respiratory distress. How could this complication have been avoided?*

E. Keeping the injection cannula parallel to the patient.

The patient in the vignette is experiencing fat embolus syndrome, a life-threatening complication that occurs when fat enters the bloodstream. The risk is increased when higher volumes of fat are injected, especially into muscle or near the piriformis due to its proximity to the gluteal vessels. Fat introduced into the inferior gluteal vein travels through the iliac veins to the inferior vena cava and then the lungs, causing respiratory distress and the unique clinical syndrome described in the vignette. The risk of fat embolus syndrome can be reduced by injecting smaller volumes subcutaneously and parallel to the patient. Adequate hydration should be maintained.[1,2]

REFERENCES

1. Bruner TW, Roberts TL, Nguyen K. Complications of buttocks augmentation: diagnosis, management, and prevention. Clin Plast Surg 2006;33:449
2. Sinno S, Chang JB, Brownstone ND, et al. Determining the safety and efficacy of gluteal augmentation: a systematic review of outcomes and complications. Plast Reconstr Surg 2016;137:1151

SILICONE IMPLANT COMPLICATIONS

8. *Which of the following complications is most likely following silicone implant augmentation?*

A. Wound dehiscence.

Silicone implant augmentation has an overall complication rate of 20 to 40%. Of the complications listed, wound dehiscence is the most likely (10%). In descending order of incidence, the other complications are seroma (5%), infection (2%), and paresthesias (1%). Implant exposure, capsular contracture, and chronic pain may also occur.[1,2,3]

REFERENCES

1. Mofid MM, Gonzalez R, de la Peña JA, Mendieta CG, et al. Buttock augmentation with silicone implants: a multicenter survey review of 2226 patients. Plast Reconstr Surg 2013;131:897
2. Bruner TW, Roberts TL, Nguyen K. Complications of buttocks augmentation: diagnosis, management, and prevention. Clin Plast Surg 2006;33:449
3. Sinno S, Chang JB, Brownstone ND, et al. Determining the safety and efficacy of gluteal augmentation: a systematic review of outcomes and complications. Plast Reconstr Surg 2016;137:1151

60. Abdominoplasty

Juan L. Rendon, Simon Moradian
See *Essentials of Aesthetic Surgery*, pp. 837–855

PERTINENT ANATOMY

1. ***Which of the follow can safely be excised in thinning of the abdominal wall flap?***
   A. The superficial fat.
   B. The deep subscarpal fat.
   C. Both the superficial and deep subscarpal fat.
   D. Thinning of the abdominal wall flap is not recommended.
   E. Deep fat should only be removed via liposuction.

PERTINENT ANATOMY

2. ***Which of the following statements describes the anterior abdominal wall anatomy?***
   A. The rectus abdominis muscles are enveloped by distinct anterior and posterior rectus sheaths along the entire muscle length.
   B. The rectus abdominis muscles are enveloped by distinct anterior and posterior rectus sheaths above the arcuate line.
   C. The rectus abdominis muscles are enveloped by distinct anterior and posterior rectus sheaths below the arcuate line.
   D. The rectus abdominus muscle does not have a distinct anterior sheath below the arcuate line but does have a posterior rectus sheath.
   E. The rectus abdominis muscles are not enveloped by distinct anterior and posterior rectus sheaths.

PERTINENT ANATOMY

3. ***Vascular zone I of the abdominal wall is supplied by which of the following?***
   A. Superior and inferior epigastric vessels.
   B. Circumflex iliac and external pudendal vessels.
   C. Circumflex iliac and intercostal vessels.
   D. Intercostal, subcostal, and lumbar vessels.
   E. Inferior epigastric and circumflex iliac vessels.

PERTINENT ANATOMY

4. ***Leaving a layer of fat over the anterior superior iliac spine helps prevent iatrogenic injury to which of the following structures?***
   A. Lateral cutaneous branches of T7–12.
   B. Anterior cutaneous branches of T7–12.
   C. Femoral nerve.
   D. Lateral femoral cutaneous nerve.
   E. Ilioinguinal nerve.

PERTINENT ANATOMY

5. ***Characteristics of an aesthetically pleasing umbilicus include which of the following?***
   A. Superior hooding, inferior retraction, round/ellipsoid shape, shallow.
   B. Superior hooding, inferior retraction, tear drop shape, deep.
   C. Inferior redundancy, superior retraction, tear drop shape, shallow.
   D. Inferior redundancy, superior retraction, round/ellipsoid shape, deep.
   E. Inferior redundancy, inferior retraction, tear drop shape, deep.

PERTINENT ANATOMY

6. *Which of the following structures contributes to the major blood supply of the umbilicus?*
A. Superior epigastric artery.
B. Deep inferior epigastric artery.
C. Median umbilical ligament.
D. Ligamentum teres.
E. Subdermal plexus.

CLINICAL CONSIDERATIONS

7. *Which of the following is an absolute contraindication to abdominoplasty?*
A. BMI >40 kg/m^2.
B. Active smoking status.
C. Body dysmorphic disorder.
D. Previous abdominal surgery with subcostal scar.
E. History of thromboembolic disease.

CLINICAL CONSIDERATIONS

8. *When should the use of sequential compression devices, which are highly recommended for the prevention of thromboembolic events, be applied/started?*
A. Prior to induction.
B. After induction but prior to incision.
C. After incision.
D. Postoperatively.
E. Sequential compression devices are not routinely needed.

CLINICAL CONSIDERATIONS

9. *In order to prevent postoperative deformity, the transverse abdominoplasty incision should be placed at least ______ from the top of the vulval commissure.*
A. 2 cm.
B. 3 cm.
C. 5 cm.
D. 8 cm.
E. 10 cm.

CLINICAL CONSIDERATIONS

10. *After removal of excess skin and subcutaneous fat, "dog-ears" can be minimized by which of the following maneuvers?*
A. Rotating the upper abdominal wall flap laterally.
B. Limiting undermining of the superior abdominoplasty flap.
C. Avoiding lateral extension of the incision.
D. Advancing the upper abdominal wall flap medially.
E. Avoiding liposuction to the flank region.

CLINICAL CONSIDERATIONS

11. *The use of progressive tension sutures results in which of the following?*
A. Increased rates of seroma and hematoma.
B. Decreased tension on the incision and decreased dead space.
C. Increased tension on the incision and prolonged need for closed suction drains.
D. Decreased tension on the increased and prolonged need for closed suction drains.
E. Decreased overall operative time.

CLINICAL CONSIDERATIONS

12. *Which of the following statements is true regarding perfusion to the abdominal wall flap in lipoabdominoplasty versus traditional abdominoplasty?*
A. Flap perfusion is equivalent in lipoabdominoplasty and traditional abdominoplasty.
B. Flap perfusion is higher in lipoabdominoplasty than in traditional abdominoplasty.

C. Flap perfusion is higher in traditional abdominoplasty than in lipoabdominoplasty.
D. Wide flap undermining and liposuction of the superior abdominoplasty flap are not associated with a decrease in flap perfusion centrally.
E. The difference in flap perfusion between lipoabdominoplasty and traditional abdominoplasty techniques is unknown.

CLINICAL CONSIDERATIONS

13. *A key surgical maneuver for preserving flap perfusion during a lipoabdominoplasty includes which of the following?*
A. Limiting undermining of the abdominal flap to zones 2 and 3.
B. Limiting undermining of the abdominal flap to zone 2 only.
C. Limiting undermining of the abdominal flap to zone 3 only.
D. Limiting undermining of the abdominal flap to the central area of zone 1 where plication will be performed.
E. Wide undermining can be performed in all zones without risk of flap perfusion.

CLINICAL CONSIDERATIONS

14. *Which of the following is true in patients undergoing a mini-abdominoplasty in which the umbilicus is transected?*
A. The umbilical stalk should never be transected during this procedure.
B. The umbilicus can be expected to move cephalad by 2 cm.
C. The umbilicus can be expected to move caudal by 2 cm.
D. The umbilicus can be expected to move up to 5 cm caudally.
E. The umbilicus should be excised from the abdominal wall flap and the defect repaired primarily.

CLINICAL CONSIDERATIONS

15. *In the Lockwood high-lateral-tension abdominoplasty, how does the oblique vector of pull result from?*
A. Uniformly excising skin centrally and laterally.
B. Excising more skin centrally than laterally.
C. Excising more skin laterally than centrally.
D. Excising skin only centrally.
E. Minimal central undermining.

CLINICAL CONSIDERATIONS

16. *In a fleur-de-lis abdominoplasty, maximal vascular supply is maintained by which of the following maneuvers?*
A. Limiting resection of excess skin and fat to the periumbilical region.
B. Addressing only horizontal excess through a vertical incision.
C. Avoidance of any liposuction.
D. Aggressively undermining the abdominal wall flaps to allow for maximal resection of excess skin and fat as well as maximal mobilization of the flaps centrally.
E. Leaving the abdominal wall flaps attached to the underlying fascia except in the areas of planned excision.

CLINICAL CONSIDERATIONS

17. *Which of the following is the best surgical plan for a patient who is seeking correction of her Grade 3 ptosis in addition to resultant epigastric skin excess and protrusion 1 year after traditional abdominoplasty?*
A. Revision traditional abdominoplasty with concurrent mastopexy using inverted-T skin excision pattern.
B. Reverse abdominoplasty with concurrent mastopexy using inverted-T skin excision pattern.
C. Liposuction of the epigastric fullness with concurrent mastopexy.
D. Reverse abdominoplasty first with staged mastopexy using an inverted-T skin excision pattern.
E. Mastopexy first using inverted-T skin excision pattern with staged reverse abdominoplasty.

CLINICAL CONSIDERATIONS

18. *Which of the following procedures carries the greatest risk of systemic complications?*
A. Abdominoplasty with liposuction of flanks.
B. Liposuction of abdomen and flanks.
C. Abdominoplasty alone.
D. Breast reduction.
E. Facelift with concurrent quad blepharoplasty.

CLINICAL CONSIDERATIONS

19. ***On postoperative day 2 following lipoabdominoplasty, a patient calls the office with persistent abdominal soreness and new shortness of breath with ambulation. The best course of action includes which of the following?***

A. Provide reassurance and instruct the patient to continue pain medications as prescribed.
B. Instruct the patient to use the incentive spirometer.
C. Provide reassurance and instruct the patient to remain on bedrest until symptoms subside.
D. Instruct the patient to go to nearest emergency room for evaluation of venous thromboembolism.
E. Instruct the patient to go to nearest emergency room for evaluation of recurrent diastasis.

Answers

PERTINENT ANATOMY

1. ***Which of the follow can safely be excised in thinning of the abdominal wall flap?***

C. Both the superficial and deep subscarpal fat.

The blood supply to the abdominal wall was initially described by Nahai and then further expanded on by Huger in 1979 with a classification system describing three zones of perfusion. The blood supply to the deeper fat (subscarpal) is distinct from the blood supply to the skin; therefore, it can be more easily excised when thinning the abdominal wall flap in an abdominoplasty. Conversely, thinning the superficial layer of fat may lead to vascular compromise of the overlying skin; however, this can be done safely using liposuction. Thinning of the deep fat can be done by direct lipectomy or via liposuction (**Fig. 60.1**). Additionally, various surgeons use a combination of direct lipectomy and liposuction to address the subscarpal and suprascarpal fat for enhanced safety during lipoabdominoplasty.[1,2,3]

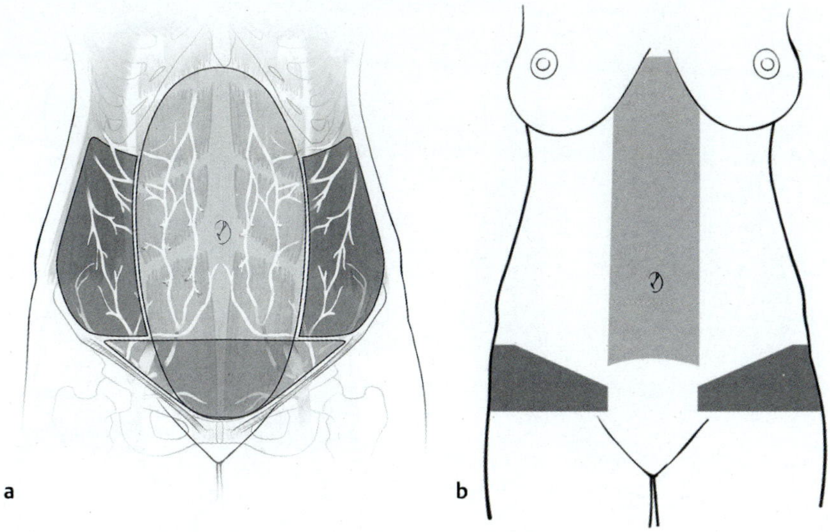

Fig. 60.1 Huger vascular zones. (Source: Vascularity of the abdominal wall. In: Janis J, ed. Essentials of Aesthetic Surgery. 1st Edition. New York: Thieme; 2018.)

REFERENCES

1. Huger WE Jr. The anatomic rationale for abdominal lipectomy. Am Surg 1979;45:612
2. Restifo RJ. Sub-Scarpa's lipectomy in abdominoplasty: an analysis of risks and rewards in 723 consecutive patients. Aesthet Surg J 2019;39(9):966–976
3. Cárdenas-Camarena L, Reyes-Herrera MF, Vargas-Flores E, López-Fabila DA, Robles-Cervantes JA. Lipoabdominoplasty: what we have implemented and what we have modified over 26 years. Plast Reconstr Surg Glob Open 2023;11(2):e4805

PERTINENT ANATOMY

2. ***Which of the following statements describes the anterior abdominal wall anatomy?***

B. The rectus abdominis muscles are enveloped by distinct anterior and posterior rectus sheaths above the arcuate line.

The arcuate line represents a transition point. Above the arcuate line, there are distinct anterior and posterior rectus sheaths. Below the arcuate line, the internal oblique and transversus abdominus join the external and internal obliques to form a single anterior rectus sheath with no posterior rectus sheath. The arcuate line is roughly halfway between the umbilicus and symphysis pubis.[1,2]

References

1. Nahai F. The Art of Aesthetic Surgery: Principles & Techniques. New York: Thieme Publishers; 2005
2. Patronella C. Redefining abdominal anatomy: 10 key elements for restoring form in abdominoplasty. Aesthet Surg J 2015;35:972

PERTINENT ANATOMY

3. *Vascular zone I of the abdominal wall is supplied by which of the following?*

A. Superior and inferior epigastric vessels.

The vascular supply to the anterior abdominal wall can be divided into three zones. Zone I is between the lateral borders of the rectus sheath from the costal margin to a horizontal line drawn between the two anterior superior iliac spines (ASISs); this area is supplied primarily by superficial branches of the superior and inferior epigastric systems. Zone II is below the horizontal line between the two ASISs to the pubic and inguinal creases; this area is supplied by the superficial branches of the circumflex iliac and external pudendal vessels. Zone III is superior to zone II and lateral to zone I; this area is supplied by intercostals, subcostals, and lumbar vessels (**Fig. 60.2**).[1]

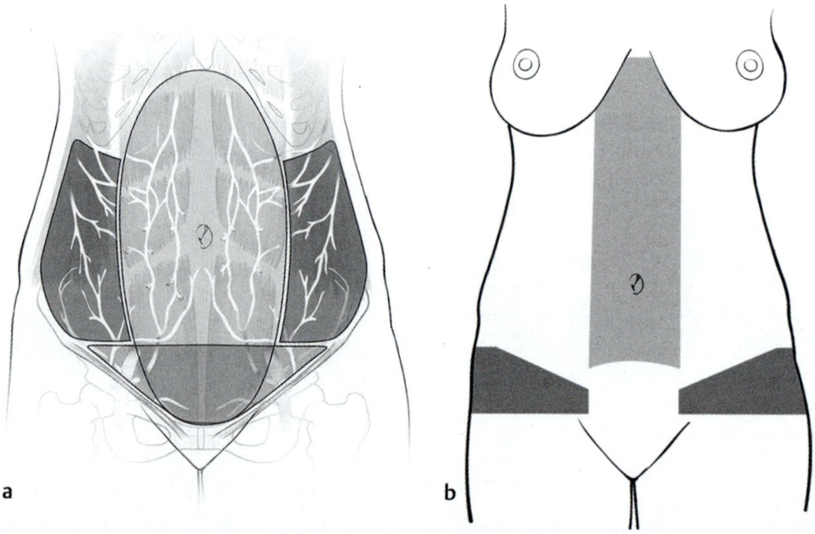

Fig. 60.2 Huger vascular zones. (Source: Vascularity of the abdominal wall. In: Janis J, ed. Essentials of Aesthetic Surgery. 1st Edition. New York: Thieme; 2018.)

Reference

1. Huger WE Jr. The anatomic rationale for abdominal lipectomy. Am Surg 1979;45:612

PERTINENT ANATOMY

4. *Leaving a layer of fat over the anterior superior iliac spine helps prevent iatrogenic injury to which of the following structures?*

D. Lateral femoral cuatenous nerve.

The lateral femoral cutanoues nerve innervates the skin in the lateral aspect of the thigh. To prevent injury, a layer of fat should be left over the anterior superior iliac spine (ASIS). Injury to this nerve can cause significant pain, numbness, and dysesthesia in the hip and medial thigh (a condition known as *meralgia paraesthetica*) (**Fig. 60.3**).[1,2]

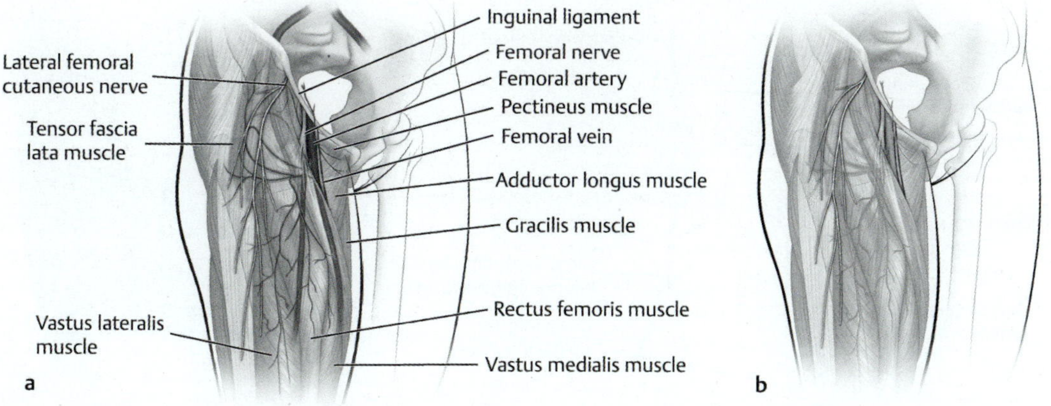

Fig. 60.3 Lateral femoral cutaneous nerve. Diagram of the nerve anatomy. (Source: Lateral femoral cutaneous nerve. In: Janis J, ed. Essentials of Aesthetic Surgery. 1st Edition. New York: Thieme; 2018.)

REFERENCES

1. Patronella C. Redefining abdominal anatomy: 10 key elements for restoring form in abdominoplasty. Aesthet Surg J 2015;35:972
2. Mandal, P, Russe E, Schwaiger K, Wechselberger G, Feigl G. Anatomical analysis of the lateral femoral cutaneous nerve and its passage beneath the inguinal ligament. Plast Reconstr Surg 2022;149(5):1147–1151

PERTINENT ANATOMY

5. *Characteristics of an aesthetically pleasing umbilicus include which of the following?*

A. Superior hooding, inferior retraction, round/ellipsoid shape, shallow.

An aesthetically pleasing umbilicus has superior hooding, inferior retraction, a round or ellipsoid shape, and is shallow.[1,2,3]

REFERENCES

1. Rohrich RJ, Sorokin ES, Brown SA, et al. Is the umbilicus truly midline? Clinical and medicolegal implications. Plast Reconstr Surg 2003;112:259
2. Nahai F. The Art of Aesthetic Surgery: Principles & Techniques. New York: Thieme Publishers; 2005
3. Hespe GE, Stepien DM, Sherif RD, et al. Umbilicoplasty in Abdominoplasty: Modifications for Improved Aesthetic Results. Aesthetic Surgery Journal Open Forum 2021;3(3):ojab025

PERTINENT ANATOMY

6. *Which of the following structures contributes to the major blood supply of the umbilicus?*

B. Deep inferior epigastric artery.

The blood supply to the umbilicus has multiple contributions from the subdermal plexus, the ligamentum teres, the median umbilical ligament, and the right and left deep inferior epigastric artery. However, the major blood supply is via the deep inferior epigastric artery system. The superior epigastric system is not a contributor to the blood supply of the umbilicus (**Fig. 60.4**).[1,2,3,4]

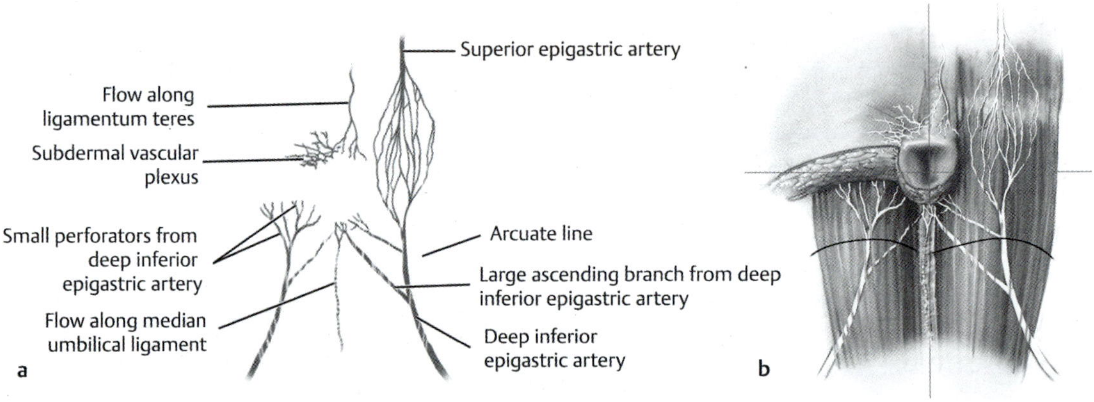

Fig. 60.4 Blood supply to the umbilicus. (Source: Lateral femoral cutaneous nerve. In: Janis J, ed. Essentials of Aesthetic Surgery. 1st Edition. New York: Thieme; 2018.)

References

1. Nahai F. The Art of Aesthetic Surgery: Principles & Techniques. New York: Thieme Publishers; 2005
2. Patronella C. Redefining abdominal anatomy: 10 key elements for restoring form in abdominoplasty. Aesthet Surg J 2015;35:972
3. Hunstad JP, Repta R. Atlas of Abdominoplasty. Philadelphia: Elsevier Health Sciences; 2008
4. Florman LD. Is the umbilicus truly midline? Correspondence and brief communications. Plast Reconstr Surg 2004;113:1089

CLINICAL CONSIDERATIONS

7. *Which of the following is an absolute contraindication to abdominoplasty?*

C. Body dysmorphic disorder.

Absolute contraindications to abdominoplasty include significant health risks, unrealistic surgical goals, and body dysmorphic disorder. Relative contraindications include: comorbid conditions (e.g., heart disease, diabetes, morbid obesity [BMI >40], cigarette smoking), plans for future pregnancy, a history of thromboembolic disease, and subcostal scars.[1,2]

References

1. Nahai F. The Art of Aesthetic Surgery: Principles & Techniques. New York: Thieme Publishers; 2005
2. Winocour J, Gupta V, Ramirez JR, et al. Abdominoplasty: risk factors, complication rates, and safety of combined procedures. Plast Reconstr Surg 2015;136:597e

CLINICAL CONSIDERATIONS

8. *When should the use of sequential compression devices, which are highly recommended for the prevention of thromboembolic events, be applied/started?*

A. Prior to induction.

For maximal benefit, sequential compression device (SCD) must be applied and started prior to induction of anesthesia. The mechanism of action of SCDs has been studied. The sequential application of external compression on the lower extremity is believed to increase pulsatile venous flow. This leads to improved emptying of the veins, thereby decreasing venous pressure resulting in an increase in arteriovenous pressure gradient and subsequent increase in arterial flow. The mechanical forces applied by the SCDs lead to shear and strain forces on the endothelial cells. This leads to enhanced antithrombotic, profibrinolytic, and vasodilatory effects, including the release of tissue plasminogen activator (tPA). The increase in tPA is believed to result from a decrease in tissue plasminogen activator inhibitor 1 (tPAI-1).[1,2,3,4,5]

References

1. Gordon RJ, Lombard FW. Perioperative venous thromboembolism: a review. Anesth Analg 2017;125(2):403–412
2. Iorio ML, Venturi ML, Davison SP. Practical guidelines for venous thromboembolism chemoprophylaxis in elective plastic surgery. Plast Reconstr Surg 2015;135(2):413–423
3. Chouhan VD, Comerota AJ, Sun L, Harada R, Gaughan JP, Rao AK. Inhibition of tissue factor pathway during intermittent pneumatic compression: a possible mechanism for antithrombotic effect. Arterioscler Thromb Vasc Biol 1999;19(11):2812–2817
4. Stewart KJ, Stewart DA, Coghlan B, et al. Complications of 278 consecutive abdominoplasties. J Plast Reconstr Aesthet Surg 2006;59:1152
5. Winocour J, Gupta V, Ramirez JR, et al. Abdominoplasty: risk factors, complication rates, and safety of combined procedures. Plast Reconstr Surg 2015;136:597e

CLINICAL CONSIDERATIONS

9. *In order to prevent postoperative deformity, the transverse abdominoplasty incision should be placed at least ______ from the top of the vulval commissure.*

C. 5 cm.

Preoperative markings begin with identification of the pubic bone and the anterior superior iliac crest. The planned incision should be marked transversely at the level of the pubic bone. At least 5 cm must be left between this incision and the top of the vulval commissure to prevent postoperative deformity. The planned incision should extend laterally below the anterior superior iliac spine (ASIS). If possible, keep the incisions low in order to prevent visibility of the scar.[1,2]

References

1. Landfair AS, Rubin JP. Applied anatomy in body contouring. In: Nahai F, ed. The Art of Aesthetic Surgery: Principles & Techniques. New York: Thieme Publishers; 2005
2. Nahai F. The Art of Aesthetic Surgery: Principles & Techniques. New York: Thieme Publishers; 2005

CLINICAL CONSIDERATIONS

10. *After removal of excess skin and subcutaneous fat, "dog-ears" can be minimized by which of the following maneuvers?*

D. Advancing the upper abdominal wall flap medially.

In order to avoid or correct "dog-ears," the abdominal wall flap should be advanced medially and if necessary, the incision should be extended laterally.[1,2]

References

1. Landfair AS, Rubin JP. Applied anatomy in body contouring. In: Nahai F, ed. The Art of Aesthetic Surgery: Principles & Techniques. New York: Thieme Publishers; 2005
2. Nahai F. The Art of Aesthetic Surgery: Principles & Techniques. New York: Thieme Publishers; 2005

CLINICAL CONSIDERATIONS

11. *The use of progressive tension sutures results in which of the following?*

B. Decreased tension on the incision and decreased dead space.

The use of progressive tension sutures helps advance the abdominal wall flap onto the musculofascia, which in turn results in progressive tension to be exerted on each suture and away from the incision. Ultimately, progressive tension sutures help decrease tension on the incision and close dead space to prevent skin necrosis, hypertrophic scaring, hematoma, and seroma formation. Additionally, placement of progressive tension sutures will increase operative time, although not usually to a significant degree.[1,2,3]

References

1. Pollock H, Pollock T. Progressive tension sutures: a technique to reduce local complications in abdominoplasty. Plast Reconstr Surg 2000;105:2583
2. Pollock T, Pollock H. Progressive tension sutures in abdominoplasty: a review of 597 consecutive cases. Aesthet Surg J 2012;32:729

3. Rosen A. Use of absorbable barbed suture and progressive tension technique in abdominoplasty: a novel approach. Plast Reconstr Surg 2010;125:1024

CLINICAL CONSIDERATIONS

12. *Which of the following statements is true regarding perfusion to the abdominal wall flap in lipoabdominoplasty versus traditional abdominoplasty?*

A. Flap perfusion is equivalent in lipoabdominoplasty and traditional abdominoplasty.

Studies demonstrate that flap perfusion is equivalent in lipoabdominoplasty compared to traditional abdominoplasty if selective undermining principles are followed. An understanding of the blood supply is key to avoiding abdominoplasty flap compromise. Saldanha et al have shown that by performing limited undermining centrally they are able to perform more lipoabdominoplasty. However, multiple strategies exist as long as care is taken to respect the dominant blood supply to the abdominoplasty flap which comes from Zone III with some minor contribution from Zone I (**Fig. 60.5**).[1,2,3]

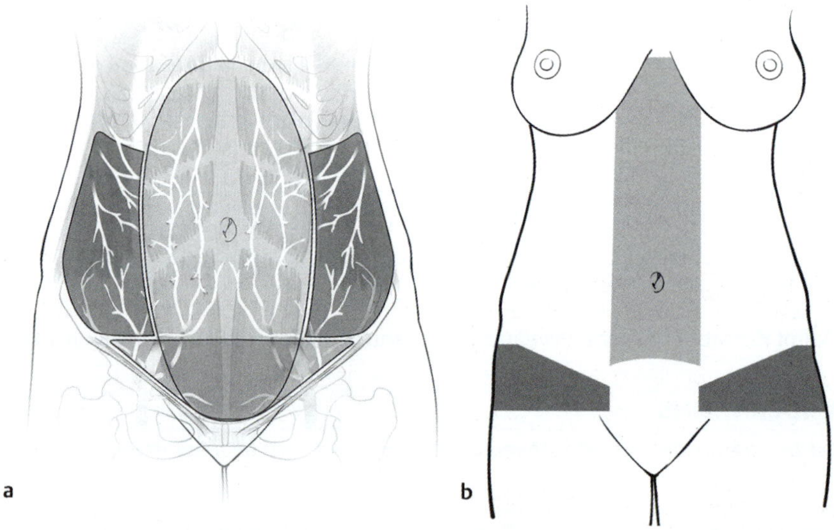

Fig. 60.5 Huger vascular zones. (Source: Vascularity of the abdominal wall. In: Janis J, ed. Essentials of Aesthetic Surgery. 1st Edition. New York: Thieme; 2018.)

REFERENCES

1. Saldanha OR, Federico R, Daher PF, et al. Lipoabdominoplasty. Plast Reconstr Surg 2009;124:934
2. Roostaeian J, Harris R, Farkas JP, et al. Comparison of limited-undermining lipoabdominoplasty and traditional abdominoplasty using laser fluorescence. Aesth Surg Journal 2014;34:741
3. Nahai F. The Art of Aesthetic Surgery: Principles & Techniques. New York: Thieme Publishers; 2005

CLINICAL CONSIDERATIONS

13. *A key surgical maneuver for preserving flap perfusion during a lipoabdominoplasty includes which of the following?*

D. Limiting undermining of the abdominal flap to the central area of zone 1 where plication will be performed.

Lipoabdominoplasty is safe if selective undermining centrally with preservation of perforators along the lateral aspects of the rectus muscles is performed. Surgical anatomical disruption of the blood supply to the abdominal wall was first considered and discussed by Nahai et al and elaborated upon by Huger, who extended these concepts to the specific case of the abdominoplasty flap. After abdominoplasty flap elevation, zone 3 vasculature remains the dominant source of blood supply to the flap; zone 1, the central abdomen, was rendered relatively underperfused.[1,2,3]

References

1. Saldanha OR, Federico R, Daher PF, et al. Lipoabdominoplasty. Plast Reconstr Surg 2009;124:934
2. Nahai F, Brown RG, Vasconez LO. Blood supply to the abdominal wall as related to planning abdominal incisions. Am Surg 1976;42(9):691–695
3. Huger WE Jr. The anatomic rationale for abdominal lipectomy. Am Surg 1979;45(9):612–617

CLINICAL CONSIDERATIONS

14. ***Which of the following is true in patients undergoing a mini-abdominoplasty in which the umbilicus is transected?***

C. The umbilicus can be expected to move caudal by 2 cm.

The mini-abdominoplasty is indicated in patients with primarily an excess of infraumbilical skin and fat. In mini-abdominoplasties, the umbilicus remains attached to the abdominal flap. If necessary, the umbilical stalk is transected at the level of the anterior rectus sheath and moved caudally (inferiorly) approximately 2 cm.[1,2]

References

1. Nahai F. The Art of Aesthetic Surgery: Principles & Techniques. New York: Thieme Publishers; 2005
2. Landfair AS, Rubin JP. Applied anatomy in body contouring. In: Nahai F, ed. The Art of Aesthetic Surgery: Principles & Techniques. New York: Thieme Publishers; 2005

CLINICAL CONSIDERATIONS

15. ***In the Lockwood high-lateral-tension abdominoplasty, how does the oblique vector of pull result from?***

C. Excising more skin laterally than centrally.

Lockwood high-lateral-tension abdominoplasty is indicated in patients with excess skin infraumbilically that is primarily vertical in nature and excess skin in the epigastric region that is primarily horizontal in nature. During the procedure, less skin is taken centrally, and more is resected laterally, resulting in an oblique vector of pull.[1]

Reference

1. Lockwood T. High-lateral-tension abdominoplasty with superficial fascial system suspension. Plast Reconstr Surg 1995;96:603

CLINICAL CONSIDERATIONS

16. ***In a fleur-de-lis abdominoplasty, maximal vascular supply is maintained by which of the following maneuvers?***

E. Leaving the abdominal wall flaps attached to the underlying fascia except in the areas of planned excision.

The fleur-de-lis abdominoplasty can address both horizontal and vertical excess. However, it is paramount to leave the skin flaps attached to the underlying fascia, except in areas contained within the fleur-de-lis excision to maximize vascularity. Liposuction can be performed concurrently.[1]

Reference

1. Dellon AL. Fleur-de-lis abdominoplasty. Aesthetic Plast Surg 1985;9:27

CLINICAL CONSIDERATIONS

17. ***Which of the following is the best surgical plan for a patient who is seeking correction of her Grade 3 ptosis in addition to resultant epigastric skin excess and protrusion 1 year after traditional abdominoplasty?***

B. Reverse abdominoplasty with concurrent mastopexy using inverted-T skin excision pattern.

The reverse abdominoplasty can safely be combined with breast procedures (e.g., a Wise pattern reduction or mastopexy) as the inframammary fold incision can be used for both the procedures. The unsightly epigastric protrusion occurs when the epigastrium bulges out against a distended lower abdomen. Epigastric protrusion occurs when plication of the muscle aponeurotic wall of the abdomen brings the epigastrium, skin, and subcutaneous tissues to the midline. After 3 to 4 months, natural loosening of the tissues may result in accommodation of the epigastrium into an unnatural shape. A revision traditional abdominoplasty would not be the best technique to address the epigastric fullness and skin excess as this would require unnecessary undermining from the pubic symphysis to the epigastric area. Liposuction of this area would not be part of an appropriate surgical treatment plan. Staging of the breast procedure and reverse abdominoplasty arenotnecessary.[1,2,3]

REFERENCES

1. Alderman AK, Collins ED, Steu R, et al. Benchmarking outcomes in plastic surgery: national complication rates for abdominoplasty and breast augmentation. Plast Reconstr Surg 2009;124:2127
2. Winocour J, Gupta V, Ramirez JR, et al. Abdominoplasty: risk factors, complication rates, and safety of combined procedures. Plast Reconstr Surg 2015;136:597e
3. Baroudi R, Keppke EM, Carvalho CG. Mammary reduction combined with reverse abdominoplasty. Ann Plast Surg 1979;2:368

CLINICAL CONSIDERATIONS

18. *Which of the following procedures carries the greatest risk of systemic complications?*

A. Abdominoplasty with liposuction of flanks.

Abdominoplasty, especially when combined with other procedures such as liposuction, has a higher systemic complication rate than any other type of routine aesthetic surgical procedure. Systemic complications can include deep vein thrombosis/pulmonary embolism, respiratory compromise, abdominal compartment syndrome, and systemic infections.[1,2]

REFERENCES

1. Alderman AK, Collins ED, Steu R, et al. Benchmarking outcomes in plastic surgery: national complication rates for abdominoplasty and breast augmentation. Plast Reconstr Surg 2009;124:2127
2. Winocour J, Gupta V, Ramirez JR, et al. Abdominoplasty: risk factors, complication rates, and safety of combined procedures. Plast Reconstr Surg 2015;136:597e

CLINICAL CONSIDERATIONS

19. *On postoperative day 2 following lipoabdominoplasty, a patient calls the office with persistent abdominal soreness and new shortness of breath with ambulation. The best course of action includes which of the following?*

D. Instruct the patient to go to nearest emergency room for evaluation of venous thromboembolism.

Any postoperative patient with shortness of breath needs to be evaluated for venous thromboembolism by venous duplex ultrasound and/or a dedicated CTPE particularly in regard to the increased potential risk of venous thromboembolism/pulmonary embolism (VTE/PE) in abdominal based procedures which may be >4 hours or in patients with a higher medical risk profile.[1,2,3]

REFERENCES

1. Spieglman J, Levine RH. abdominoplasty: a comparison of outpatient and inpatient procedures shows that it is a safe and effective procedure for outpatients in an office-based surgery clinic. Plast Reconstr Surgery 2006;118:517
2. Stewart KJ, Stewart DA, Coghlan B, et al. Complications of 278 consecutive abdominoplasties. J Plast Reconstr Aesthet Surg 2006;59:1152
3. Pannucci CJ, MacDonald JK, Ariyan S, et al. Benefits and risks of prophylaxis for deep venous thrombosis and pulmonary embolus in plastic surgery: a systematic review and meta-analysis of controlled trials and consensus conference. Plast Reconstr Surg 2016;137(2):709–730

61. Medial Thigh Lift

Ara A. Salibian
See *Essentials of Aesthetic Surgery*, pp. 856–868

ANATOMY

1. ***Which of the following structures can be utilized to anchor tissues during a medial thigh lift?***
   A. Scarpa's fascia.
   B. Colles fascia.
   C. Adductor longus tendon.
   D. Pubis.
   E. Sartorius muscle.

PREOPERATIVE EVALUATION: HISTORY AND PHYSICAL EXAMINATION

2. ***A 53-year-old female with no significant past medical history presents with complaints of excess fat and skin redundancy in bilateral thighs. Upon examination, the patient has lipodystrophy and moderate skin laxity that extends beyond the upper one-third of the thigh. What is the most appropriate surgical plan according to the classification for non-massive-weight-loss patients?***
   A. Liposuction alone.
   B. Liposuction and a horizontal skin excision only.
   C. Liposuction and a vertical skin excision only.
   D. Liposuction with a combined horizontal and vertical skin excision.
   E. Staged procedure with liposuction first then excisional thigh lift.

TECHNIQUES

3. ***A patient is undergoing a traditional medial thigh lift with crescentic excision. The surgeon marks a significant amount of skin for excision that results in some tension upon closure. What is the most likely postoperative complication in this patient?***
   A. Hematoma.
   B. Labial spreading.
   C. Infection.
   D. Complete wound dehiscence.
   E. Seroma.

TECHNIQUES

4. ***Which of the following structures is routinely encountered and should be preserved during a medial thigh lift?***
   A. Femoral artery.
   B. Sciatic nerve.
   C. Great saphenous vein.
   D. Lesser saphenous vein.
   E. Obturator nerve.

TECHNIQUES

5. ***During a medial thigh lift, the surgeon proceeds in the deep plane in the proximal portion of the excision and excises significant amount of fat between adductor longus and the sartorius muscle. Which of the following complications is most likely secondary to this technique?***
   A. Foot drop.
   B. Wound dehiscence.
   C. Paresthesias of the lateral leg.
   D. Lower extremity lymphedema.
   E. Infection.

TECHNIQUES

6. ***A massive-weight-loss patient is undergoing a medial thigh lift with a longitudinal component due to excess skin laxity in the middle and distal thigh. Which of the following muscle tendons should be used as a reference for the initial scar line during preoperative marking?***
   A. Adductor longus.
   B. Adductor magnus.
   C. Vastus medialis.
   D. Sartorius.
   E. Gracilis.

COMPLICATIONS

7. ***A 50-year-old male patient returns to the office after undergoing a medial thigh lift with a longitudinal incision complaining of pain and swelling in the right thigh. Examination reveals a large fluid collection in the mid-medial thigh with an obvious fluid wave and no overlying signs of infection. What is the best first step in management?***
   A. Return to the operating room for drainage and excision of seroma wall.
   B. Injection of a sclerosing agent.
   C. Referral to interventional radiology for closed suction drain placement.
   D. Office aspiration and compression with elastic bandage.
   E. Compression and administration of oral antibiotics.

Answers

ANATOMY

1. ***Which of the following structures can be utilized to anchor tissues during a medial thigh lift?***
   B. Colles fascia.
   The Colles fascia is a deep layer of fascia in the thigh that is contiguous with the Scarpa's fascia of the abdominal wall and attaches to the ischiopubic rami of the bony pelvis as well as the posterior border of the urogenital diaphragm. It can be recognized by its yellowish hue. It can be easily identified at the deepest and most lateral aspect of the vulvar soft tissue. Anchoring sutures should be placed to the Colles fascia in the groin to minimize labial spread and stabilize the overlying soft tissue envelope. Sutures in muscle or tendon should be avoided as these can tear through upon patient movement and ambulation.[1]

REFERENCE

1. Mathes DW, Kenkel JM. Current concepts in medial thighplasty. Clin Plast Surg 2008;35:151

PREOPERATIVE EVALUATION: HISTORY AND PHYSICAL EXAMINATION

2. ***A 53-year-old female with no significant past medical history presents with complaints of excess fat and skin redundancy in bilateral thighs. Upon examination, the patient has lipodystrophy and moderate skin laxity that extends beyond the upper one-third of the thigh. What is the most appropriate surgical plan according to the classification for non-massive-weight-loss patients?***
   D. Liposuction with a combined horizontal and vertical skin excision.
   According to the classification for non-massive-weight-loss patients, a patient with lipodystrophy and moderate skin laxity extending beyond the upper one-third of the thigh is a Type III patient. These patients benefit from both liposuction (due to the lipodystrophy) as well as a vertical component of excision added to the horizontal excision due to the increased skin laxity more distal in the thigh that will not be addressed by a crescentic excision only. Patients who are candidates for liposuction alone only have lipodystrophy without skin laxity (Type I). Those who are best suited for liposuction and a crescentic horizontal excision only have lipodystrophy and skin laxity limited to the upper one-third of the thigh (Type II). Finally, patients who have very severe skin laxity as well as lipodystrophy (Type V) may benefit from a staged procedure (**Table 61.1**).[1]

Table 61.1 *Classification and Surgical Recommendations for Non-Massive-Weight-Loss Patients*

Classification	Description	Treatment
Type I	Lipodystrophy with no sign of skin laxity	Liposuction alone
Type II	Lipodystrophy and skin laxity confined to the upper third of the thigh	Liposuction and a horizontal skin incision in the medial thigh
Type III	Lipodystrophy and moderate skin laxity that extends beyond the upper third of the thigh	Both liposuction and horizontal and vertical skin excision in the medial thigh
Type IV	Moderate skin laxity that extends the length of the thigh	Longer vertical resection than type III
Type V	Severe medial thigh skin laxity with lipodystrophy	Staged procedure: First stage: Aggressive liposuction Second stage: Excisional medial thigh lift

REFERENCE

1. Mathes DW, Kenkel JM. Current concepts in medial thighplasty. Clin Plast Surg 2008;35:151

TECHNIQUES

3. *A patient is undergoing a traditional medial thigh lift with crescentic excision. The surgeon marks a significant amount of skin for excision that results in some tension upon closure. What is the most likely postoperative complication in this patient?*

B. Labial spreading.

Labial spreading is a common complication when crescentic thigh lift patients are marked with excess excision of skin. The vulva do not tolerate much lateral tension and therefore are easily deformed with excess pull from a tight incision. Patients should be marked while they are in a frog-leg position to allow the surgeon to determine the safe amount of skin resection to prevent labial distortion when the legs are abducted. Although wound healing complications are very common with thigh lift procedures and this patient is at a higher risk of having areas of wound dehiscence secondary to tension at closure, a complete dehiscence of the entire wound is unlikely.[1,2,3]

REFERENCES

1. Lewis JR. Correction of ptosis of the thighs: the thigh lift. Plast Reconstr Surg 1966;37:494
2. Bertheuil N, Thienot S, Huguier V, et al. Medial thighplasty after massive weight loss: are there any risk factors for postoperative complications? Aesthetic Plast Surg 2013;38:63
3. Gusenoff JA, Coon D, Nayar H, et al. Medial thigh lift in the massive weight loss population: outcomes and complications. Plast Reconstr Surg 2015;135:98

TECHNIQUES

4. *Which of the following structures is routinely encountered and should be preserved during a medial thigh lift?*

C. Great saphenous vein.

The great saphenous vein is encountered in the subcutaneous tissue of the medial thigh. It runs along the posterior border of the adductor longus and will become more superficial as it travels distally, more easily encountered just posterior to the knee. Dissection should proceed in a plane superficial to the great saphenous vein and injury to the vein avoided to prevent an increased risk of lymphedema. Although the femoral artery can be encountered in the femoral triangle, this would indicate a dissection that has proceeded far too deep. The sciatic nerve resides in the posterior thigh and the lesser saphenous vein in the posterior lower leg. The obturator nerve can also be found in the medial thigh but much deeper, innervating the gracilis muscle.[1,2]t

REFERENCES

1. Lockwood TE. Maximizing aesthetics in lateral-tension abdominoplasty and body lifts. Clin Plast Surg 2004;31:523
2. Mathes DW, Kenkel JM. Current concepts in medial thighplasty. Clin Plast Surg 2008;35:151

TECHNIQUES

5. *During a medial thigh lift, the surgeon proceeds in the deep plane in the proximal portion of the excision and excises significant amount of fat between adductor longus and the sartorius muscle. Which of the following complications is most likely secondary to this technique?*

D. Lower extremity lymphedema.

The femoral triangle is bound by the adductor longus medially, the sartorius laterally, and the inguinal ligament superiorly. This triangle contains critical structure such as the femoral artery, vein, and nerve, but always houses important nodal basins and lymphatic channels. Dissection should remain superficial in this region to avoid disturbing these lymphatic channels, which can subsequently result in debilitating lymphedema of the lower extremity.[1,2,3]

REFERENCES

1. Bertheuil N, Thienot S, Huguier V, et al. Medial thighplasty after massive weight loss: are there any risk factors for postoperative complications? Aesthetic Plast Surg 2013;38:63
2. Gusenoff JA, Coon D, Nayar H, et al. Medial thigh lift in the massive weight loss population: outcomes and complications. Plast Reconstr Surg 2015;135:98
3. Moreno CH, Neto HJ, Junior AH, et al. Thighplasty after bariatric surgery: evaluation of lymphatic drainage in lower extremities. Obes Surg 2008;18:1160

TECHNIQUES

6. *A massive-weight-loss patient is undergoing a medial thigh lift with a longitudinal component due to excess skin laxity in the middle and distal thigh. Which of the following muscle tendons should be used as a reference for the initial scar line during preoperative marking?*

A. Adductor longus.

The medial thigh lift in massive-weight-loss patients often incorporates a longitudinal component extending down the medial leg to address skin laxity of the middle and distal thigh that cannot be corrected with a traditional crescentic excision. The longitudinal excision is marked by first drawing a line along the adductor longus tendon down to the knee. The skin is then displaced anteriorly and posteriorly, and points are marked along the reference line as dictated by the adductor longus tendon. Connecting these points after moving down the leg will delineate the skin excision that should place the scar in the medial thigh with the appropriate tension. Markings are checked for symmetry and rechecked in the operating room.[1,2]

REFERENCES

1. Bertheuil N, Thienot S, Huguier V, et al. Medial thighplasty after massive weight loss: are there any risk factors for postoperative complications? Aesthetic Plast Surg 2013;38:63
2. Gusenoff JA, Coon D, Nayar H, et al. Medial thigh lift in the massive weight loss population: outcomes and complications. Plast Reconstr Surg 2015;135:98

COMPLICATIONS

7. *A 50-year-old male patient returns to the office after undergoing a medial thigh lift with a longitudinal incision complaining of pain and swelling in the right thigh. Examination reveals a large fluid collection in the mid-medial thigh with an obvious fluid wave and no overlying signs of infection. What is the best first step in management?*

D. Office aspiration and compression with elastic bandage.

Seromas are relatively common complications in body-contouring procedures with incidences of around 9% cited after thigh lift in massive weight loss patients. Drains should be left in place until output is usually less than 20 to 30 cc per day; however, seromas can still form after drain removal. Initially treatment of seromas involves needle aspiration, which can be done in the office without the use of ultrasound if a palpable collection is present. Compression after aspiration helps minimize potential dead space for fluid accumulation. Secondary measures for seroma re-accumulation after aspiration include drain placement, use of sclerosing agents, or operative drainage and excise of the seroma cavity with placement of quilting sutures.[1]

REFERENCE

1. Gusenoff JA, Coon D, Nayar H, et al. Medial thigh lift in the massive weight loss population: outcomes and complications. Plast Reconstr Surg 2015;135:98

62. Body Contouring in Massive-Weight-Loss Patients

Adam Jacoby
See *Essentials of Aesthetic Surgery*, pp. 869–886

PREOPERATIVE CONSIDERATIONS

1. ***Which of the following bariatric surgery techniques is considered both a restrictive and malabsorptive procedure?***
   A. Gastric sleeve.
   B. Laparoscopic adjustable gastric band.
   C. Weight loss balloon.
   D. Roux-en-Y gastric bypass.
   E. LINX device.

PREOPERATIVE CONSIDERATIONS

2. ***After gastric bypass surgery, when should body contouring be performed?***
   A. When patient's body mass index (BMI) is >45.
   B. When the patient's body mass index (BMI) is >40.
   C. <3 months after bypass surgery.
   D. When patient's weight is fluctuating.
   E. After weight stabilization for at least 6 months.

PREOPERATIVE CONSIDERATIONS

3. ***What is the most common nutritional deficiency after bariatric surgery?***
   A. Iron deficiency anemia.
   B. Rickets.
   C. Scurvy.
   D. Pellagra.
   E. Beriberi.

OPERATIVE SELECTION

4. ***In a patient with both horizontal and vertical abdominal excess, addition of which of the following surgical techniques will improve body contour?***
   A. Progressive tension sutures.
   B. Vertical resection (fleur-de-lis).
   C. Mons lift.
   D. Circumferential body lift.
   E. Liposuction.

SURGICAL ANATOMY

5. ***In a standard brachioplasty, which structure is most at risk for damage?***
   A. Posterior cord of brachial plexus.
   B. Median nerve.
   C. Medial antebrachial cutaneous nerve.
   D. Thoracic duct.
   E. Brachial artery.

PATHOPHYSIOLOGY OF FACIAL AGING

6. ***What is the cause of premature facial aging in the massive weight loss patient?***
   A. Relaxation of the facial retaining ligaments.
   B. Subcutaneous atrophy.
   C. Skin redundancy.
   D. SMAS laxity.
   E. Osteoporotic bone loss.

POSTSURGICAL COMPLICATIONS

7. ***Early seroma after body contouring procedures is best treated first with which of the following modalities?***
   A. Compression.
   B. Aspiration.
   C. Sclerosing agent.
   D. Seroma cavity resection.
   E. Drain placement.

POSTSURGICAL COMPLICATIONS

8. ***Which of the following body contouring procedures is associated with the highest venous thromboembolism risk?***
   A. Mastopexy.
   B. Medial thigh lift.
   C. Abdominoplasty.
   D. Rhytidectomy.
   E. Brachioplasty.

SURGICAL ANATOMY

9. ***Suturing of Scarpa's fascia of the thigh to which of the following structures increases longevity of the result and decreases the risk of hypertrophic scarring?***
   A. Dartos fascia.
   B. Camper's fascia.
   C. Colles fascia.
   D. Inguinal ligament.
   E. Buck's fascia.

PATIENT SELECTION

10. ***At what body mass index (BMI) is body contouring after massive weight loss considered ideal?***
    A. <18.
    B. 25–30.
    C. 35–40.
    D. >40.
    E. >45.

Answers

PREOPERATIVE CONSIDERATIONS

1. ***Which of the following bariatric surgery techniques is considered both a restrictive and malabsorptive procedure?***

D. Roux-en-Y gastric bypass.

The answer is D, Roux-en-Y gastric bypass, which is the most common bariatric surgery procedure performed, which contains both malabsorptive and restrictive components. Body contouring procedures must be performed with caution in this patient population as vitamin, mineral, and nutritional deficiencies can be seen in up to 40% of patients. All other answer choices are considered restrictive procedures only.[1,2,3,4]

REFERENCES

1. Aly AS. Body Contouring After Massive Weight Loss. New York: Thieme Publishers; 2006
2. Rubin JP, Nguyen V, Schwentker A. Perioperative management of the post-gastric-bypass patient presenting for body contouring surgery. Clin Plast Surg 2004;31:601
3. Hamad GG. The state of the art in bariatric surgery for weight loss in the morbidly obese patient. Clin Plast Surg 2004;31:591
4. Gilbert EW, Wolfe BM. Bariatric surgery for the management of obesity: state of the field. Plast Reconstr Surg 2012;130:948

PREOPERATIVE CONSIDERATIONS

2. ***After gastric bypass surgery, when should body contouring be performed?***

E. After weight stabilization for at least 6 months.

The answer is E, after weight stabilization for at least 6 months. This usually occurs when patients' BMI is between 30 and 35, which usually occurs 12 to 18 months after surgery making answers A, B, and C incorrect. Active weight fluctuation is a contraindication to performing body contouring as rapid weight loss can interfere with wound healing and overall body contour.[1,2,3,4]

REFERENCES

1. Aly AS. Body Contouring After Massive Weight Loss. New York: Thieme Publishers; 2006
2. Rubin JP, Nguyen V, Schwentker A. Perioperative management of the post-gastric-bypass patient presenting for body contouring surgery. Clin Plast Surg 2004;31:601
3. Hamad GG. The state of the art in bariatric surgery for weight loss in the morbidly obese patient. Clin Plast Surg 2004;31:591
4. Gilbert EW, Wolfe BM. Bariatric surgery for the management of obesity: state of the field. Plast Reconstr Surg 2012;130:948

PREOPERATIVE CONSIDERATIONS

3. ***What is the most common nutritional deficiency after bariatric surgery?***

A. Iron deficiency anemia.

The answer is A, iron deficiency anemia, which is especially common after malabsorptive procedures. Rickets is caused by extreme and prolonged vitamin D deficiency which may lead to osteomalacia. Scurvy is caused by a severe lack of vitamin C (ascorbic acid) which may lead to weakness, anemia, gum disease, poor wound healing, and skin hemorrhages. Pellagra is caused by low levels of niacin (vitamin B-3) which may lead to dementia, diarrhea, and dermatitis, also known as "the three Ds." If left untreated, pellagra can be fatal. Beriberi is secondary to thiamine deficiency (vitamin B-1) which may lead to weakness, neuropathies, and pain in the limbs. All other answers may occur after weight loss surgery but are not as common as iron deficiency anemia.[1,2]

REFERENCES

1. Kenkel J. The physiological impact of bariatric surgery on the massive weight loss patient. Plast Reconstr Surg 2006;117(1 Suppl):14S; discussion 82S
2. Kenkel J. Safety considerations and avoiding complications in the massive weight loss patient. Plast Reconstr Surg 2006;117(1 Suppl):74S; discussion 82S

OPERATIVE SELECTION

4. *In a patient with both horizontal and vertical abdominal excess, addition of which of the following surgical techniques will improve body contour?*

B. Vertical resection (fleur-de-lis).

The answer is B, vertical resection resulting in a fleur-de-lis or corset abdominoplasty. Although progressive tension sutures, mons lift, and circumferential body lift may improve body contour, only addition of vertical resection will treat both vertical and horizontal excess.[1,2] **Fig. 62.1** shows markings for a fleur-de-lis abdominoplasty. Redundant vertical tissue above the umbilicus is removed as a triangle connected to the redundant skin in the lower abdomen, which is marked as a standard abdominoplasty. Points *A* and *B* will join as an inverted-T closure in the midline at the pubic symphysis (point *C*). In patients with significant mons ptosis, point *Ć* is marked 4 to 6 cm below to resect additional inferior redundancy and to elevate the mons.

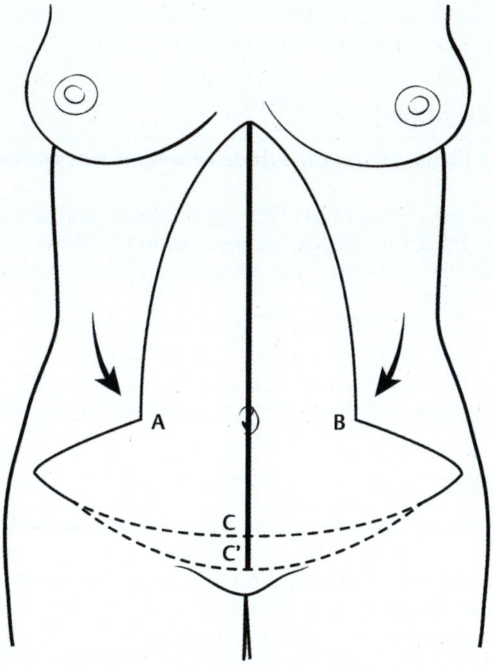

Fig. 62.1 Markings for a fleur-de-lis abdominoplasty. Redundant vertical tissue above the umbilicus is removed as a triangle connected to the redundant skin in the lower abdomen, which is marked as a standard abdominoplasty. Points A and B will join as an inverted-T closure in the midline at the pubic symphysis (point C). In patients with significant mons ptosis, point C′ is marked 4 to 6 cm below to resect additional inferior redundancy and to elevate the mons. (Source: Surgical approach to the trunk/abdomen. In: Janis J, ed. Essentials of Aesthetic Surgery. 1st Edition. New York: Thieme; 2018.)

REFERENCES

1. Kenkel J. Marking and operative techniques. Plast Reconstr Surg 2006;117(1 Suppl):45S; discussion 82S
2. Aly AS, Cram AE, Heddens C. Truncal body contouring surgery in the massive weight loss patient. Clin Plast Surg 2004;31:611

SURGICAL ANATOMY

5. *In a standard brachioplasty, which structure is most at risk for damage?*

C. Medial antebrachial cutaneous nerve.

The answer is C, medial antebrachial cutaneous nerve, which arises from the medial cord of the brachial plexus, which is the most common neurovascular structure damaged during brachioplasty. Liposuction prior to resection preserves neurovascular structures and facilitates easy resection of subcutaneous tissues. All the structures in the other answer choices are much deeper and should not be encountered during a brachioplasty.[1,2]

REFERENCES

1. Cannistra C, Valero R, Benelli C, et al. Brachioplasty after massive weight loss: a simple algorithm for surgical plane. Aesthetic Plast Surg 2007;31:6
2. Knoetgen J III, Morgan SL. Long-term outcomes and complications associated with brachioplasty: as retrospective review and cadaveric study. Plast Reconstr Surg 2006;117:2219

PATHOPHYSIOLOGY OF FACIAL AGING

6. *What is the cause of premature facial aging in the massive weight loss patient?*

C. Skin redundancy.

The answer is C, skin redundancy. Relaxation of the facial retaining ligaments can lead to tear trough deformities and jowls while superficial musculoaponeurotic system (SMAS) laxity is a common cause of facial aging in non-massive weight loss patients. Skin redundancy is the most common etiology of facial aging in the massive weight loss patient.[1]

REFERENCE

1. Sclafani AP. Restoration of the jawline and the neck after bariatric surgery. Facial Plast Surg 2005;21:28

POSTSURGICAL COMPLICATIONS

7. *Early seroma after body contouring procedures is best treated first with which of the following modalities?*

B. Aspiration.

The answer is B, aspiration, which is considered the first-line treatment for early seromas. Compression is usually ineffective as the sole modality, and sclerosing/seroma cavity resection is useful for late seromas refractory to aspiration and closed suction drain placement.[1,2]

REFERENCES

1. Kenkel J. The physiological impact of bariatric surgery on the massive weight loss patient. Plast Reconstr Surg 2006;117(1 Suppl):14S; discussion 82S
2. Kenkel J. Safety considerations and avoiding complications in the massive weight loss patient. Plast Reconstr Surg 2006;117(1 Suppl):74S; discussion 82S

POSTSURGICAL COMPLICATIONS

8. *Which of the following body contouring procedures is associated with the highest venous thromboembolism risk?*

C. Abdominoplasty.

The answer is C, abdominoplasty, which is associated with increased intraabdominal pressure leading to decreased venous return from the extremities. Although all the other options have a lower risk of venous thromboembolism (VTE), the Caprini score should be used for every patient undergoing body contouring procedures to evaluate risk and determine the best modality of prophylaxis.[1,2,3]

REFERENCES

1. Rubin JP, Nguyen V, Schwentker A. Perioperative management of the post-gastric-bypass patient presenting for body contouring surgery. Clin Plast Surg 2004;31:601

2. Kenkel J. Safety considerations and avoiding complications in the massive weight loss patient. Plast Reconstr Surg 2006;117(1 Suppl):74S; discussion 82S
3. Moran MC. Benefits of epidural anesthesia over general anesthesia in the prevention of deep vein thrombosis following total hip arthroplasty. J Arthroplasty 1995;10:405

SURGICAL ANATOMY

9. *Suturing of Scarpa's fascia of the thigh to which of the following structures increases longevity of the result and decreases the risk of hypertrophic scarring?*

C. Colles fascia.

The answer is C, Colles fascia, also known as the superficial perineal fascia. Securing the superficial fascial system of the thigh to Colles fascia prevents scar migration and widening. Dartos fascia is present in the penis and therefore incorrect. Camper's fascia is ill-defined, superficial, and would not provide a lasting result. Suturing the superficial fascial system to the inguinal ligament would not provide the correct vector of pull and place neurovascular structures at unnecessary risk.[1,2]

REFERENCES

1. Kenkel J. Marking and operative techniques. Plast Reconstr Surg 2006;117(1 Suppl):45S; discussion 82S
2. Aly AS, Cram AE, Heddens C. Truncal body contouring surgery in the massive weight loss patient. Clin Plast Surg 2004;31:611

PATIENT SELECTION

10. *At what body mass index (BMI) is body contouring after massive weight loss considered ideal?*

B. 25–30.

The answer is B, 25 to 30, as the risk of surgical complications dramatically decreases as patients approach their ideal body weight. A body mass index (BMI) of <18 after weight loss surgery may suggest malnutrition while obese patients (BMI >30) may still be losing weight and are at higher risk of postoperative complications and dissatisfaction.[1,2,3,4]

REFERENCES

1. Aly AS. Body Contouring After Massive Weight Loss. New York: Thieme Publishers; 2006
2. Rubin JP, Nguyen V, Schwentker A. Perioperative management of the post-gastric-bypass patient presenting for body contouring surgery. Clin Plast Surg 2004;31:601
3. Hamad GG. The state of the art in bariatric surgery for weight loss in the morbidly obese patient. Clin Plast Surg 2004;31:591
4. Gilbert EW, Wolfe BM. Bariatric surgery for the management of obesity: state of the field. Plast Reconstr Surg 2012;130:948

63. Female Aesthetic Genital Surgery

Sammy Sinno, Jeremie Oliver Piña
See *Essentials of Aesthetic Surgery*, pp. 887–926

VULVOVAGINAL AESTHETIC SURGERY

1. *Which of the following vulvovaginal plastic surgery procedures is the most commonly requested?*

A. Clitoral hood reduction.
B. Perineoplasty.
C. Vaginal tightening.
D. Labiaplasty.
E. Labia majora reduction.

VULVOVAGINAL AESTHETIC SURGERY

2. *What is the most widely accepted upper limit of normal length of labia minora, measured from the labial base to the labial edge?*

A. 2 cm.
B. 3 cm.
C. 5 cm.
D. 7 cm.
E. Has not been defined.

VULVOVAGINAL AESTHETIC SURGERY

3. *What is the most common reason for patients to request revision vulvovaginal plastic surgery?*

A. Reduced sensation.
B. Vaginal laxity.
C. Clitoral hood redundancy.
D. Irritation with form-fitting clothes.
E. Perforated labia minora skin.

VULVOVAGINAL AESTHETIC SURGERY

4. *What is the most appropriate treatment method for a patient presenting with enlarged mons fat?*

A. Nutrition consult.
B. Encouraging 6 to 12 months of diet and exercise.
C. Cryotherapy.
D. Liposuction.
E. Surgical resection.

VULVOVAGINAL AESTHETIC SURGERY

5. *Addressing which of the following structures will most effectively correct ptosis of the anterior vaginal commissure?*

A. Clitoral hood.
B. Clitoral body.
C. Introitus.
D. Labia majora.
E. Mons pubis.

VULVOVAGINAL AESTHETIC SURGERY

6. ***Which of the following preoperative assessment approaches can help in preventing postoperative vaginal splaying?***
   A. Adduction/abduction of patient's legs.
   B. Use of mirror while pointing out areas of concern.
   C. Examination in both standing and lithotomy positions.
   D. Hip flexion/extension.
   E. Ultrasound imaging.

VULVOVAGINAL AESTHETIC SURGERY

7. ***All labiaplasty procedures are performed with the patient in which position?***
   A. Prone.
   B. Reverse Trendelenburg.
   C. Supine.
   D. Lithotomy.
   E. Left-side fetal.

VULVOVAGINAL AESTHETIC SURGERY

8. ***When combining clitoral hood and labiaplasty procedures, what is the proper order in which to address these multiple concerns?***
   A. Clitoral hood first.
   B. Labiaplasty first.
   C. Both simultaneously.
   D. Refer to gynecologist for recommendation.
   E. Defer treatment if multiple concerns.

VULVOVAGINAL AESTHETIC SURGERY

9. ***In which vulvovaginal procedure should a plastic surgeon most strongly consider the involvement of a urologist?***
   A. Labiaplasty.
   B. Perineoplasty.
   C. Monspexy.
   D. Clitoropexy.
   E. Labia majora direct excision.

VULVOVAGINAL AESTHETIC SURGERY

10. ***What is a potential result of labia majora direct excision/reduction?***
    A. Decreased sensation to clitoris.
    B. Pelvic organ prolapse.
    C. Perceived decreased prominence of the clitoral hood or labia minora.
    D. Friction discomfort on ambulation with clothing.
    E. Decreased contrast of skin color and hair pattern.

Answers

VULVOVAGINAL AESTHETIC SURGERY

1. ***Which of the following vulvovaginal plastic surgery procedures is the most commonly requested?***
   D. Labiaplasty.
   Defined as a reduction of the labia minora, labiaplasty has become the cornerstone of vulvovaginal plastic surgery. Multiple factors are suspected to be driving this trend, including aesthetic concerns (particularly in Western cultures) through the media, Brazilian waxing, and some functional issues such as rubbing or hygiene.[1]

REFERENCE

1. Koning M, Zeijlmans IA, Bouman TK, et al. Female attitudes regarding labia minora appearance and reduction with consideration of media influence. Aesthet Surg J 2009;29:65

VULVOVAGINAL AESTHETIC SURGERY

2. ***What is the most widely accepted upper limit of normal length of labia minora, measured from the labial base to the labial edge?***
   C. 5 cm.
   In evaluating labia minora enlargement and hypertrophy from baseline, most providers feel that 5 cm in length, measured from the base of the minora to the labial edge, is the upper limit of normal.[1] This would be in the range of Felicio classification type III.[2]

REFERENCES

1. Tepper OM, Wulkan M, Matarasso A. Labioplasty: anatomy, etiology, and a new surgical approach. Aesthet Surg J 2011;31:551
2. Felicio Yde A. Labial surgery. Aesthet Surg J 2007;27:322

VULVOVAGINAL AESTHETIC SURGERY

3. ***What is the most common reason for patients to request revision vulvovaginal plastic surgery?***
   C. Clitoral hood redundancy.
   Clitoral hood redundancy often becomes noticeable following a labiaplasty that does not address the clitoral hood concomitantly or after overly aggressive trimming of the labia minora. It often presents with apparent hypertrophy of hood after aggressive edge trim labiaplasty.[1] Hood redundancy is the most common reason patients seek revision vulvovaginal plastic surgery.[2]

REFERENCES

1. Hunter JG. Commentary on: Labioplasty: anatomy, etiology, and a new surgical approach. Aesthet Surg J 2011;31:519
2. Alter GJ. Labia minora reconstruction using clitoral hood flaps, wedge excisions, and YV advancement flaps. Plast Reconstr Surg 2011;127:2356

VULVOVAGINAL AESTHETIC SURGERY

4. ***What is the most appropriate treatment method for a patient presenting with enlarged mons fat?***
   E. Surgical resection.
   Enlarged mons fat is typically associated with labia majora hypertrophy as a result of fat excess and stretched skin. Unfortunately, these are rarely ever addressed by diet and exercise. Often times, this fat needs to be resected as a part of an abdominal contouring procedure. Liposuction may be of limited use given the excess skin laxity described above which would result in a suboptimal aesthetic outcome.[1,2,3]

REFERENCES

1. Mirzabeigi JN, Jandali S, Mettel RK, et al. The nomenclature of "vaginal rejuvenation" and elective vulvovaginal plastic surgery. Aesthet Surg J 2011;31:723
2. Alter GJ. Aesthetic labia minora and clitoral hood reduction using extended central wedge resection. Plast Reconstr Surg 2008;122:1780
3. Moore KL, Dalley AF. Clinically Oriented Anatomy. 4th ed. Philadelphia: Lippincott Williams & Wilkins; 1999

VULVOVAGINAL AESTHETIC SURGERY

5. *Addressing which of the following structures will most effectively correct ptosis of the anterior vaginal commissure?*

E. Mons pubis.

By lifting and tightening the mons pubis, the anterior commissure is effectively elevated from its previous ptotic position.[1,2,3]

REFERENCES

1. Mirzabeigi JN, Jandali S, Mettel RK, et al. The nomenclature of "vaginal rejuvenation" and elective vulvovaginal plastic surgery. Aesthet Surg J 2011;31:723
2. Alter GJ. Aesthetic labia minora and clitoral hood reduction using extended central wedge resection. Plast Reconstr Surg 2008;122:1780
3. Moore KL, Dalley AF. Clinically Oriented Anatomy. 4th ed. Philadelphia: Lippincott Williams & Wilkins; 1999

VULVOVAGINAL AESTHETIC SURGERY

6. *Which of the following preoperative assessment approaches can help in preventing postoperative vaginal splaying?*

A. Adduction/abduction of patient's legs.

Evaluating the labia majora with the legs abducted and adducted is critical, as the relationship of the labia to the inner thighs is distinguishable in this maneuver. Recognizing this preoperatively helps to prevent possible overresection of the labia majora and secondary tethering of skin, a complication which can often lead to vaginal splaying.[1,2,3]

REFERENCES

1. Alter G. Female genital aesthetic surgery. In: Nahai F, ed. The Art of Aesthetic Surgery: Principles and Technique. 2rd ed. New York: Thieme Publishers; 2011
2. Mirzabeigi JN, Jandali S, Mettel RK, et al. The nomenclature of "vaginal rejuvenation" and elective vulvovaginal plastic surgery. Aesthet Surg J 2011;31:723
3. Felicio Yde A. Labial surgery. Aesthet Surg J 2007;27:322

VULVOVAGINAL AESTHETIC SURGERY

7. *All labiaplasty procedures are performed with the patient in which position?*

D. Lithotomy.

All techniques are performed with patients in the lithotomy position under local anesthesia. Additionally, positioning the stirrups so that the hips flex at 90 degrees in the lithotomy position will help maximize venous drainage. However, in the initial evaluation, the patient should be examined in both standing and lithotomy positions. An examination chair with retractable stirrups facilitates visualization and promotes patient comfort. In the standing position, the labia minora are noted for the degree of projection beyond the labia majora, and the labia majora are noted for ptosis, volume, and fullness.[1,2,3]

REFERENCES

1. Dobbleleir JM, Van Landuyt KV, Monstrey SJ. Aesthetic surgery of the female genitalia. Semin Plast Surg 2011;25:130
2. Alter G. Female genital aesthetic surgery. In: Nahai F, ed. The Art of Aesthetic Surgery: Principles and Technique. 2nd ed. New York: Thieme Publishers; 2011
3. Gelder C, McCallum AL, Macfarlane AJR, Anderson JH. A systematic review of mechanical thromboprophylaxis in the lithotomy position. Surgeon 2018;16(6):365–371

VULVOVAGINAL AESTHETIC SURGERY

8. *When combining clitoral hood and labiaplasty procedures, what is the proper order in which to address these multiple concerns?*

B. Labiaplasty first.

When clitoral hood reduction procedures are coupled with labia minora procedures, the labia must be addressed first. This enables the surgeon to avoid overexposing the gland in aggressive clitoral hood reduction. Excess folds of the clitoral hood are addressed after the labia minora are treated.[1,2]

REFERENCES

1. Hunter JG. Commentary on: Labioplasty: anatomy, etiology, and a new surgical approach. Aesthet Surg J 2011;31:519
2. Alter GJ. Labia minora reconstruction using clitoral hood flaps, wedge excisions, and YV advancement flaps. Plast Reconstr Surg 2011;127:2356

VULVOVAGINAL AESTHETIC SURGERY

9. *In which vulvovaginal procedure should a plastic surgeon most strongly consider the involvement of a urologist?*

D. Clitoropexy.

Given the technical difficulty of the clitoropexy operation, it is not uncommon to result in malposition of the clitoris. Thus, strong consideration should be given to collaboration with a urologist.[1,2,3]

REFERENCES

1. Alter GJ. Labia minora reconstruction using clitoral hood flaps, wedge excisions, and YV advancement flaps. Plast Reconstr Surg 2011;127:2356
2. Alter GJ. Pubic contouring after massive weight loss in men and women: correction of hidden penis, mons ptosis, and labia majora enlargement. Plast Reconstr Surg 2012;130:936
3. Alter GJ. Aesthetic labia minora and clitoral hood reduction using extended central wedge resection. Plast Reconstr Surg 2008;122:1780

VULVOVAGINAL AESTHETIC SURGERY

10. *What is a potential result of labia majora direct excision/reduction?*

D. Friction discomfort on ambulation with clothing.

Overresection of labia majora fat and skin in direct excision/reduction procedures may cause a gaping introitus leading to vaginal dryness, discomfort with clothing, discomfort with activity, and an inability to completely abduct the legs. Also, a perceived increased prominence of the clitoral hood or labia minora, as well as a contrast of skin color and hair pattern may occur. These potential results of surgery should be discussed in the preoperative consultation and informed consent.[1,2,3,4]

REFERENCES

1. Tepper OM, Wulkan M, Matarasso A. Labioplasty: anatomy, etiology, and a new surgical approach. Aesthet Surg J 2011;31:551
2. Felicio Yde A. Labial surgery. Aesthet Surg J 2007;27:322
3. Hodgkinson DJ, Hait G. Aesthetic vaginal labioplasty. Plast Reconstr Surg 1984;74:414
4. Alter G. Female genital aesthetic surgery. In: Nahai F, ed. The Art of Aesthetic Surgery: Principles and Technique. 2rd ed. New York: Thieme Publishers; 2011

64. Noninvasive Body Contouring

Stelios C. Wilson
See *Essentials of Aesthetic Surgery*, pp. 927–933

PREOPERATIVE EVALUATION

1. *Which of the following patients would be an appropriate candidate for noninvasive body contouring?*
A. A 45-year-old man with BMI of 32 who has recently undergone a 100 lb weight loss.
B. A 32-year-old female with a BMI of 23 with small areas of stubborn flank lipodystrophy but who otherwise was unwilling to undergo a surgical procedure.
C. A 37-year-old female with a BMI of 36 with a large area of concern of anterior abdominal wall, flank, and back lipodystrophy.
D. A 41-year-old woman, mother of three children, with rectus diastasis looking for improvement in abdominal contour but unwilling to undergo a surgical procedure.
E. A 48-year-old man with a BMI of 29 and actively losing weight following laparoscopic sleeve gastrectomy.

INFORMED CONSENT

2. *Which of the following should be counseled to the patient when describing noninvasive body contouring procedures?*
A. There will be no procedural discomfort.
B. There will be minimal to no postprocedural erythema/edema.
C. There is no risk of temporary sensory deficits.
D. No guarantee of final aesthetic outcome.
E. Most noninvasive procedures require only one treatment.

METHODS

3. *Which of the following would be considered to be invasive body contouring?*
A. Cryolipolysis.
B. High-intensity focused ultrasound (HIFU).
C. Low-level laser therapy.
D. Radiofrequency energy.
E. Power-assisted liposuction.

CRYOLIPOLYSIS

4. *What is the mechanism of action of cryolipolysis that occurs by placing cooling panels to a localized area?*
A. Allow vasoconstriction of the peripheral blood supply that perfuse the local adipocytes.
B. Cause apoptosis-mediated cell death and subsequent inflammatory response.
C. Decrease volume by limiting edema and improving the egress of lymphatic fluid.
D. Tighten the skin and subcutaneous tissue through myofibroblast activation.
E. Tighten the skin and subcutaneous tissue through heating via low frequency electromagnetic waves.

CRYOLIPOLYSIS

5. *Which of the following medical problems is a contraindication to cryolipolysis?*
A. Sickle cell anemia.
B. Factor V Leiden.
C. Cold-induced dermatologic syndromes.
D. Protein C deficiency.
E. Thalassemia.

CRYOLIPOLYSIS

6. *What is the incidence of localized erythema and edema following cryolipolysis?*
A. <1%.
B. 5%.
C. 15%.
D. 50%.
E. 100%.

CRYOLIPOLYSIS

7. *What is the incidence of paradoxical adipose hyperplasia following cryolipolysis?*
A. <1%.
B. 5%.
C. 15%.
D. 50%.
E. 100%.

HIGH-INTENSITY FOCUSED ULTRASOUND (HIFU)

8. *What is the mechanism of action of high-intensity focused ultrasound (HIFU)?*
A. Thermal ablation of subcutaneous tissue with induction of neocollagenesis.
B. Increased peripheral blood flow leading to greater metabolic demand.
C. Decreased volume by limiting edema and improving the egress of lymphatic fluid.
D. Tightening the skin and subcutaneous tissue through myofibroblast activation.
E. Tightening the skin and subcutaneous tissue through heating via low frequency electromagnetic waves.

HIGH-INTENSITY FOCUSED ULTRASOUND (HIFU)

9. *Generally, what is the focal depth of high-intensity focused ultrasound (HIFU)?*
A. <5 mm.
B. 5–10 mm.
C. 11–16 mm.
D. 20–30 mm.
E. >30 mm.

HIGH-INTENSITY FOCUSED ULTRASOUND (HIFU)

10. *What is the incidence of minor complications following high-intensity focused ultrasound (HIFU)?*
A. <1%.
B. 5%.
C. 15%.
D. 50%.
E. 100%.

HIGH-INTENSITY FOCUSED ULTRASOUND (HIFU)

11. *At what time point will results be typically seen following treatment with high-intensity focused ultrasound (HIFU)?*
A. Immediate.
B. 1 week.
C. 2–4 weeks.
D. 8–12 weeks.
E. 6 months.

LOW-LEVEL LASER THERAPY (LLLT)

12. *What is the mechanism of action of low-level laser therapy (LLLT)?*
A. Thermal ablation of subcutaneous tissue with induction of neocollagenesis.
B. Increased peripheral blood flow leading to greater metabolic demand.
C. Induction of a transitory pore into an adipocyte resulting in the release of lipids and adipocyte deflation.
D. Tightening the skin and subcutaneous tissue through myofibroblast activation.
E. Tightening the skin and subcutaneous tissue through heating via low frequency electromagnetic waves.

LOW-LEVEL LASER THERAPY (LLLT)

13. *At what distance should the diode be from the skin for low-level laser therapy (LLLT)?*
A. Directly on the skin.
B. Several millimeters above the skin with ultrasound jelly on the skin.
C. 2 cm above the skin.
D. 10 cm above the skin.
E. 15 cm above the skin.

LOW-LEVEL LASER THERAPY (LLLT)

14. *Which of the following is a very rare and unexpected risk following low-level laser therapy (LLLT)?*
A. Mild warming during the procedure.
B. Erythema.
C. Intermittent paresthesias after first treatment.
D. Potential skin ulceration.
E. Paroxysmal hypertrophy of subcutaneous tissue.

LOW-LEVEL LASER THERAPY (LLLT)

15. *What is the incidence of skin ulceration from low-level laser therapy (LLLT)?*
A. <1%.
B. 3%.
C. 12%.
D. 20%.
E. 33%.

NONINVASIVE BODY CONTOURING

16. *Which of the following is accurate regarding the use of noninvasive body contouring procedures?*
A. The number of noninvasive body contouring procedures performed in the United States each year is growing quickly.
B. Noninvasive body contouring typically has a prolonged patient downtime.
C. Noninvasive body contouring often requires only 1 to 2 treatments to achieve excellent results.
D. Noninvasive body contouring modalities can be considered as replacement for liposuction, healthy lifestyle, or a treatment to lose weight.
E. Noninvasive body contouring results are usually seen within 1 to 2 weeks after treatment.

Answers

PREOPERATIVE EVALUATION

1. ***Which of the following patients would be an appropriate candidate for noninvasive body contouring?***

 B. A 32-year-old female with a BMI of 23 with small areas of stubborn flank lipodystrophy but who otherwise was unwilling to undergo a surgical procedure.

 Of the candidates described, the best candidate for noninvasive body contouring would be choice B. In general, this is a thin woman with localized areas of concern. Noninvasive body contouring would not be good for the massive weight loss patient with excess skin, those who are actively losing weight, or for the correction of a rectus diastasis. In addition, noninvasive body contouring modalities are not a replacement for liposuction, healthy lifestyle, or a treatment to lose weight. In addition, noninvasive modalities often require multiple treatments to achieve modest results.[1,2,3]

REFERENCES

1. Manstein D, Laubach H, Watanabe K, et al. Selective cryolysis: a novel method of non-invasive fat removal. Lasers Surg Med 2008;40:595
2. Zelickson B, Egbert BM, Preciado J, et al. Cryolipolysis for noninvasive fat cell destruction: initial results from a pig model. Dermatol Surg 2009;35:1462
3. Ingargiola MJ, Motakef S, Chung MT, et al. Cryolipolysis for fat reduction and body contouring: safety and efficacy of current treatment paradigms. Plast Reconstr Surg 2015;135:1581

INFORMED CONSENT

2. ***Which of the following should be counseled to the patient when describing noninvasive body contouring procedures?***

 D. No guarantee of final aesthetic outcome.

 Although generally well tolerated, almost all modalities will have some component of discomfort during the procedure. This is generally followed by a few days to a week of erythema/edema. With some modalities, there is a risk of peripheral nerve paresthesias or hyperesthesias. Most importantly, there is no guarantee of aesthetic outcome and results are largely dependent on an individual's response to these energy devices.[1,2,3,4,5]

REFERENCES

1. Ingargiola MJ, Motakef S, Chung MT, et al. Cryolipolysis for fat reduction and body contouring: safety and efficacy of current treatment paradigms. Plast Reconstr Surg 2015;135:1581
2. Coleman SR, Sachdeva K, Egbert B, et al. Clinical efficacy of noninvasive cryolipolysis and its effects on peripheral nerves. Aesthetic Plast Surg 2009;33:482
3. Jewell ML, Baxter RA, Cox SE, et al. Randomized sham-controlled trial to evaluate the safety and effectiveness of a high-intensity focused ultrasound device for noninvasive body sculpting. Plast Reconstr Surg 2011;128:253
4. Robinson DM, Kaminer MS, Baumann L, et al. High-intensity focused ultrasound for the reduction of subcutaneous adipose tissue using multiple treatment techniques. Dermatol Surg 2014;40:641
5. Neira R, Arroyave J, Ramirez H, et al. Fat liquefaction: effect of low-level laser energy on adipose tissue. Plast Reconstr Surg 2002;110:912; discussion 923

METHODS

3. ***Which of the following would be considered to be invasive body contouring?***

 E. Power-assisted liposuction.

 Power-assisted liposuction requires incisions and is not considered a noninvasive body contouring method. The other options are all technologies currently used for noninvasive body contouring.[1,2,3,4]

REFERENCES

1. Ingargiola MJ, Motakef S, Chung MT, et al. Cryolipolysis for fat reduction and body contouring: safety and efficacy of current treatment paradigms. Plast Reconstr Surg 2015;135:1581
2. Robinson DM, Kaminer MS, Baumann L, et al. High-intensity focused ultrasound for the reduction of subcutaneous adipose tissue using multiple treatment techniques. Dermatol Surg 2014;40:641
3. Friedmann DP. A review of the aesthetic treatment of abdominal subcutaneous adipose tissue: background, implications, and therapeutic options. Dermatol Surg 2015;41:18
4. Jackson RF, Stern FA, Neira R, et al. Application of low-level laser therapy for noninvasive body contouring. Lasers Surg Med 2012;44:211

CRYOLIPOLYSIS

4. *What is the mechanism of action of cryolipolysis that occurs by placing cooling panels to a localized area?*

B. Cause apoptosis-mediated cell death and subsequent inflammatory response.

The proposed mechanism of cryolipolysis is through an apoptosis-mediated cell death and subsequent inflammatory response to the subcutaneous fat. The panels act to cool the tissue in a controlled manner. The subcutaneous tissue is more susceptible to damage than the skin, thus causing a hypotrophy of the subcutaneous tissue. The other mechanisms are not supported by the current body of literature.[1,2,3]

REFERENCES

1. Manstein D, Laubach H, Watanabe K, et al. Selective cryolysis: a novel method of non-invasive fat removal. Lasers Surg Med 2008;40:595
2. Zelickson B, Egbert BM, Preciado J, et al. Cryolipolysis for noninvasive fat cell destruction: initial results from a pig model. Dermatol Surg 2009;35:1462
3. Ingargiola MJ, Motakef S, Chung MT, et al. Cryolipolysis for fat reduction and body contouring: safety and efficacy of current treatment paradigms. Plast Reconstr Surg 2015;135:1581

CRYOLIPOLYSIS

5. *Which of the following medical problems is a contraindication to cryolipolysis?*

C. Cold-induced dermatologic syndromes.

Patients are contraindicated for cryolipolysis if they pregnant or have a history of cold-induced dermatologic syndromes (e.g., cryoglobulinemia, paroxysmal cold hemoglobinuria, or cold urticaria). Clotting deficiencies and other hematology disorders are not generally thought of as contraindications to cryolipolysis. Other relative contraindications are those with excessive skin laxity and large-volume weight loss in obese patients.[1,2,3]

REFERENCES

1. Manstein D, Laubach H, Watanabe K, et al. Selective cryolysis: a novel method of non-invasive fat removal. Lasers Surg Med 2008;40:595
2. Zelickson B, Egbert BM, Preciado J, et al. Cryolipolysis for noninvasive fat cell destruction: initial results from a pig model. Dermatol Surg 2009;35:1462
3. Ingargiola MJ, Motakef S, Chung MT, et al. Cryolipolysis for fat reduction and body contouring: safety and efficacy of current treatment paradigms. Plast Reconstr Surg 2015;135:1581

CRYOLIPOLYSIS

6. *What is the incidence of localized erythema and edema following cryolipolysis?*

E. 100%.

All patients should expect localized erythema immediately following the treatment. The patient should understand that this could last up to 7 days. In addition, patients should know that there is a 67% incidence of developing postprocedural sensory deficits in the treated area. These deficits generally self-resolve by 2 months.[1,2]

References

1. Ingargiola MJ, Motakef S, Chung MT, et al. Cryolipolysis for fat reduction and body contouring: safety and efficacy of current treatment paradigms. Plast Reconstr Surg 2015;135:1581
2. Coleman SR, Sachdeva K, Egbert B, et al. Clinical efficacy of noninvasive cryolipolysis and its effects on peripheral nerves. Aesthetic Plast Surg 2009;33:482

CRYOLIPOLYSIS

7. *What is the incidence of paradoxical adipose hyperplasia following cryolipolysis?*

A. <1%.

Paradoxical adipose hyperplasia is a rare but potential side effect of cryolipolysis. Specifically, rates have been quoted at approximately 0.52%. There have been no reports of spontaneous resolution. Liposuction is the preferred method of treatment but some cases require surgical excision.[1,2]

References

1. Ingargiola MJ, Motakef S, Chung MT, et al. Cryolipolysis for fat reduction and body contouring: safety and efficacy of current treatment paradigms. Plast Reconstr Surg 2015;135:1581
2. Karcher C, Katz B, Sadick N. Paradoxical hyperplasia post cryolipolysis and management. Dermatol Surg 2017;43:467

HIGH-INTENSITY FOCUSED ULTRASOUND (HIFU)

8. *What is the mechanism of action of high-intensity focused ultrasound (HIFU)?*

A. Thermal ablation of subcutaneous tissue with induction of neocollagenesis.

The mechanism of action of HIFU is thought to be thermal ablation of subcutaneous tissue with induction of new collagen formation. HIFU increases the local temperature in the midlamellar fat layer leading to a coagulative necrosis of adipocytes and a reduction of the fat layer. The other mechanisms have not been proposed or defended based on the current body of literature.[1,2,3,4]

References

1. Fatemi A. High-intensity focused ultrasound effectively reduces adipose tissue. Semin Cutan Med Surg 2009;28:257
2. Fatemi A, Kane MA. High-intensity focused ultrasound effectively reduces waist circumference by ablating adipose tissue from the abdomen and flanks: a retrospective case series. Aesthetic Plast Surg 2010;34:577
3. Jewell ML, Baxter RA, Cox SE, et al. Randomized sham-controlled trial to evaluate the safety and effectiveness of a high-intensity focused ultrasound device for noninvasive body sculpting. Plast Reconstr Surg 2011;128:253
4. Robinson DM, Kaminer MS, Baumann L, et al. High-intensity focused ultrasound for the reduction of subcutaneous adipose tissue using multiple treatment techniques. Dermatol Surg 2014;40:641

HIGH-INTENSITY FOCUSED ULTRASOUND (HIFU)

9. *Generally, what is the focal depth of high-intensity focused ultrasound (HIFU)?*

C. 11–16 mm.

The focal depth of HIFU is generally considered to be between 1.1 and 1.6 cm. The focal depth is determined by the thickness of adipose tissues being treated (**Fig. 64.1**). The total energy dose is 100 to 150 J/cm^2. Multiple passes are made with the HIFU transducer to deliver the appropriate amount of energy with treatment durations typically lasting <1 hour.[1,2,3,4]

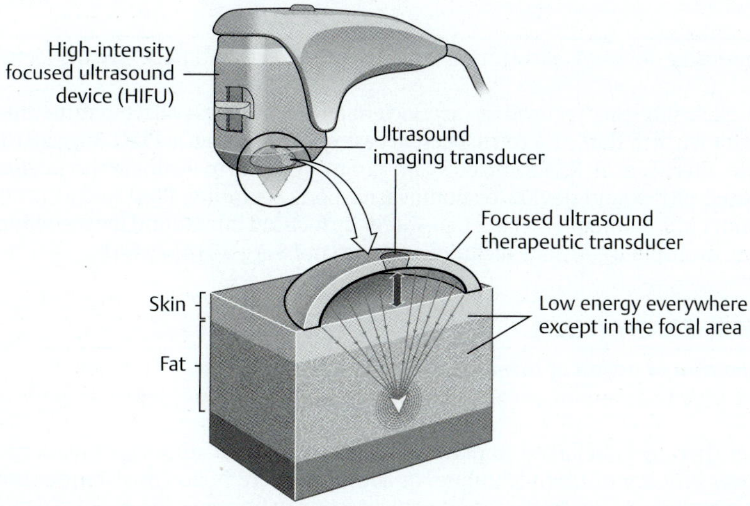

Fig. 64.1 The HIFU transducer focally delivers the beam to the treatment nodes to thermally ablate fat. The low-energy beams pass through skin over a wider area (with minimal damage) to converge at a focal depth within the fat. (Source: Technique. In: Janis J, ed. Essentials of Aesthetic Surgery. 1st Edition. New York: Thieme; 2018.)

References

1. Fatemi A. High-intensity focused ultrasound effectively reduces adipose tissue. Semin Cutan Med Surg 2009;28:257
2. Fatemi A, Kane MA. High-intensity focused ultrasound effectively reduces waist circumference by ablating adipose tissue from the abdomen and flanks: a retrospective case series. Aesthetic Plast Surg 2010;34:577
3. Jewell ML, Baxter RA, Cox SE, et al. Randomized sham-controlled trial to evaluate the safety and effectiveness of a high-intensity focused ultrasound device for noninvasive body sculpting. Plast Reconstr Surg 2011;128:253
4. Robinson DM, Kaminer MS, Baumann L, et al. High-intensity focused ultrasound for the reduction of subcutaneous adipose tissue using multiple treatment techniques. Dermatol Surg 2014;40:641

HIGH-INTENSITY FOCUSED ULTRASOUND (HIFU)

10. ***What is the incidence of minor complications following high-intensity focused ultrasound (HIFU)?***

C. 15%.

The incidence of minor complications from HIFU is 10 to 15%, which have been shown to resolve on their own over 1 to 2 weeks. These included tenderness, edema, ecchymosis, and hard lumps in the treated areas. Pain is adequately controlled with topical or oral analgesics. All complications are self-limited.[1]

Reference

1. Jewell ML, Baxter RA, Cox SE, et al. Randomized sham-controlled trial to evaluate the safety and effectiveness of a high-intensity focused ultrasound device for noninvasive body sculpting. Plast Reconstr Surg 2011;128:253

HIGH-INTENSITY FOCUSED ULTRASOUND (HIFU)

11. ***At what time point will results be typically seen following treatment with high-intensity focused ultrasound (HIFU)?***

D. 8–12 weeks.

The results of HIFU are not immediate. Instead, results are typically seen 8 to 12 weeks after treatment. This is important when counseling potential patients and when seeing early postprocedural patients.[1,2,3,4]

References

1. Fatemi A. High-intensity focused ultrasound effectively reduces adipose tissue. Semin Cutan Med Surg 2009;28:257
2. Fatemi A, Kane MA. High-intensity focused ultrasound effectively reduces waist circumference by ablating adipose tissue from the abdomen and flanks: a retrospective case series. Aesthetic Plast Surg 2010;34:577
3. Jewell ML, Baxter RA, Cox SE, et al. Randomized sham-controlled trial to evaluate the safety and effectiveness of a high-intensity focused ultrasound device for noninvasive body sculpting. Plast Reconstr Surg 2011;128:253
4. Robinson DM, Kaminer MS, Baumann L, et al. High-intensity focused ultrasound for the reduction of subcutaneous adipose tissue using multiple treatment techniques. Dermatol Surg 2014;40:641

LOW-LEVEL LASER THERAPY (LLLT)

12. *What is the mechanism of action of low-level laser therapy (LLLT)?*

C. Induction of a transitory pore into an adipocyte resulting in the release of lipids and adipocyte deflation.

Low-level laser therapy is believed to place transient pores into adipocytes leading to deflation. There is controversy over efficacy of this technique. In addition, there is no consistent observations of adipocyte disruption on histology or electron-scanning microscopy in human cells or animal models. That being said, there were several studies that report decrease in circumference measurements following LLLT. It should be noted that these studies have low sample size, no postprocedural body mass index (BMI) control, and encouraged patients to undergo diet and exercise regiments after treatments.[1,2,3]

References

1. Neira R, Arroyave J, Ramirez H, et al. Fat liquefaction: effect of low-level laser energy on adipose tissue. Plast Reconstr Surg 2002;110:912; discussion 923
2. Friedmann DP. A review of the aesthetic treatment of abdominal subcutaneous adipose tissue: background, implications, and therapeutic options. Dermatol Surg 2015;41:18
3. Brown SA, Rohrich RJ, Kenkel J, et al. Effect of low-level laser therapy on abdominal adipocytes before lipoplasty procedures. Plast Reconstr Surg 2004;113:1796

LOW-LEVEL LASER THERAPY (LLLT)

13. *At what distance should the diode be from the skin for low-level laser therapy (LLLT)?*

E. 15 cm above the skin.

For LLLT, the diode modules are suspended approximately 15 cm above the anterior and then the posterior aspect of the treatment area. A 635 nm laser is used for transdermal delivery of energy. That being said, specific distances, wattage, wavelength, and delivery duration vary depending on the device used.[1,2,3]

References

1. Neira R, Arroyave J, Ramirez H, et al. Fat liquefaction: effect of low-level laser energy on adipose tissue. Plast Reconstr Surg 2002;110:912; discussion 923
2. Friedmann DP. A review of the aesthetic treatment of abdominal subcutaneous adipose tissue: background, implications, and therapeutic options. Dermatol Surg 2015;41:18
3. Brown SA, Rohrich RJ, Kenkel J, et al. Effect of low-level laser therapy on abdominal adipocytes before lipoplasty procedures. Plast Reconstr Surg 2004;113:1796

LOW-LEVEL LASER THERAPY (LLLT)

14. *Which of the following is a very rare and unexpected risk following low-level laser therapy (LLLT)?*

E. Paroxysmal hypertrophy of subcutaneous tissue.

Following low-level laser therapy (LLLT), mild warming of the skin during the procedure is likely followed by the potential for prolonged erythema (>24 hours). Skin ulceration is a potential complication. Although most complications are self-limited, prolonged erythema and skin ulceration have been shown in 12% of cases. Patients should be counseled on these risks before electing to undergo these procedures. Paroxysmal hypertrophy is a rare risk related to cryolipolysis.[1,2,3,4,5]

References

1. Jackson RF, Dedo DD, Roche GC, et al. Low-level laser therapy as a non-invasive approach for body contouring: a randomized, controlled study. Lasers Surg Med 2009;41:799
2. Jackson RF, Stern FA, Neira R, et al. Application of low-level laser therapy for noninvasive body contouring. Lasers Surg Med 2012;44:211
3. Nestor MS, Zarraga MB, Park H. Effect of 635nm low-level laser therapy on upper arm circumference reduction. J Clin Aesthet Dermatol 2012;5:42
4. Thornfeldt CR, Thaxton PM, Hornfeldt CS. A six-week low-level laser therapy protocol is effective for reducing waist, hip, thigh, and upper abdomen circumference. J Clin Aesthet Dermatol 2016;9:31
5. Jankowski M, Gawrych M, Adamska U, et al. Low-level laser therapy (LLLT) does not reduce subcutaneous adipose tissue by local adipocyte injury but rather by modulation of systemic lipid metabolism. Lasers Med Sci 2017;32:475

LOW-LEVEL LASER THERAPY (LLLT)

15. *What is the incidence of skin ulceration from low-level laser therapy (LLLT)?*

C. 12%.

The rate of skin ulceration from low-level laser therapy (LLLT) has been shown to be as high as 12%. This is also true of prolonged erythema. Patients must understand this risk prior to electing to undergo LLLT.[1,2,3,4,5]

References

1. Jackson RF, Dedo DD, Roche GC, et al. Low-level laser therapy as a non-invasive approach for body contouring: a randomized, controlled study. Lasers Surg Med 2009;41:799
2. Jackson RF, Stern FA, Neira R, et al. Application of low-level laser therapy for noninvasive body contouring. Lasers Surg Med 2012;44:211
3. Nestor MS, Zarraga MB, Park H. Effect of 635nm low-level laser therapy on upper arm circumference reduction. J Clin Aesthet Dermatol 2012;5:42
4. Thornfeldt CR, Thaxton PM, Hornfeldt CS. A six-week low-level laser therapy protocol is effective for reducing waist, hip, thigh, and upper abdomen circumference. J Clin Aesthet Dermatol 2016;9:31
5. Jankowski M, Gawrych M, Adamska U, et al. Low-level laser therapy (LLLT) does not reduce subcutaneous adipose tissue by local adipocyte injury but rather by modulation of systemic lipid metabolism. Lasers Med Sci 2017;32:475

NONINVASIVE BODY CONTOURING

16. *Which of the following is accurate regarding the use of noninvasive body contouring procedures?*

A. The number of noninvasive body contouring procedures performed in the United States each year is growing quickly.

The number of noninvasive body contouring procedures performed in the United States each year is growing quickly. Noninvasive body contouring typically has a limited patient downtime. Additionally, it often requires multiple treatments to achieve even modest results. Noninvasive body contouring modalities are not considered a replacement for liposuction, healthy lifestyle, or a treatment to lose weight. Noninvasive body contouring results are usually seen 2 months after treatment. This is a growing field and should not be overlooked as potential adjunct or precursor to surgery for selected patients. That being said, patients must understand the risk and limitations of these modalities.[1,2,3,4,5,6,7,8,9]

References

1. Ingargiola MJ, Motakef S, Chung MT, et al. Cryolipolysis for fat reduction and body contouring: safety and efficacy of current treatment paradigms. Plast Reconstr Surg 2015;135:1581
2. Fatemi A. High-intensity focused ultrasound effectively reduces adipose tissue. Semin Cutan Med Surg 2009;28:257
3. Fatemi A, Kane MA. High-intensity focused ultrasound effectively reduces waist circumference by ablating adipose tissue from the abdomen and flanks: a retrospective case series. Aesthetic Plast Surg 2010;34:577
4. Robinson DM, Kaminer MS, Baumann L, et al. High-intensity focused ultrasound for the reduction of subcutaneous adipose tissue using multiple treatment techniques. Dermatol Surg 2014;40:641

5. Friedmann DP. A review of the aesthetic treatment of abdominal subcutaneous adipose tissue: background, implications, and therapeutic options. Dermatol Surg 2015;41:18
6. Brown SA, Rohrich RJ, Kenkel J, et al. Effect of low-level laser therapy on abdominal adipocytes before lipoplasty procedures. Plast Reconstr Surg 2004;113:1796
7. Jackson RF, Stern FA, Neira R, et al. Application of low-level laser therapy for noninvasive body contouring. Lasers Surg Med 2012;44:211
8. Nestor MS, Zarraga MB, Park H. Effect of 635 nm low-level laser therapy on upper arm circumference reduction. J Clin Aesthet Dermatol 2012;5:42
9. American Society of Plastic Surgeons. National Clearinghouse of Plastic Surgery Statistics: 2010 Report of the 2009 Statistics. Arlington Heights, IL: American Society of Plastic Surgeons, 2010

65. Aesthetics of Gender Affirmation Surgery

Juan L. Rendon
See *Essentials of Aesthetic Surgery*, pp. 934–956

ANATOMIC CONSIDERATIONS

1. *Which of the following statements is an accurate description regarding the female face relative to male face?*

A. The upper female craniofacial skeleton is characterized by greater bone volume relative to males.
B. The female nose tends to be larger because of increased volume of bone and cartilage.
C. In females, the mandibular angle tends to be squared with well-defined corners.
D. Females have a greater concentration of fat in the middle third of the face while males tend to have greater malar bone volume.
E. Males have a greater concentration of fat in the middle third of the face while females tend to have greater malar bone volume.

ANATOMIC CONSIDERATIONS

2. *Which of the following is an accurate description and consideration when evaluating the hairline?*

A. Females tend to have an M-shaped hairline while males have a rounded hairline.
B. Both females and males tend to have M-shaped hairlines.
C. Both females and males tend to have rounded hairlines.
D. Females tend to have a rounded hairline while males have an M-shaped hairline.
E. Females tend to have a rounded hairline that extends slightly lower in the center than in men.

ANATOMIC CONSIDERATIONS

3. *A transgender female patient wishes to undergo facial feminization surgery. CT scan demonstrates that the anterior table of her frontal sinus is 2 mm in thickness. Which of the following approaches is appropriate?*

A. A combination of frontal bone set back and burring of the anterior table of the frontal sinus is necessary for optimal results.
B. Frontal bone set back with osteotomy and repositioning of the anterior wall of the frontal sinus alone.
C. Burring of the anterior table of the frontal sinus is necessary for optimal results.
D. Placement of an alloplastic implant will achieve similar results.
E. The patient is a not a candidate for feminizing forehead surgery.

ANATOMIC CONSIDERATIONS

4. *During facial feminization surgery, hair transplantation should ______________.*

A. Be performed before androgenic alopecia stabilizes.
B. Be performed after androgenic alopecia stabilizes.
C. Be performed to create an M-shaped hairline.
D. Be performed to create a rounded hairline.
E. Not be performed, as there is no difference between male and female hairlines.

ANATOMIC CONSIDERATIONS

5. *Which is the following is a potential reason to be cautious if performing an upper lip lift in conjunction with an open rhinoplasty in the same stage?*

A. Unpredictable aesthetic result.
B. Higher rates of infection.
C. Concern for skin necrosis between the intervening segment of skin between the two incisions.
D. Higher incidence of abnormal scarring and narrowing of the alar base.
E. Higher rates of hematomas.

ANATOMIC CONSIDERATIONS

6. ***Which of the following is an appropriate technique for addressing the upper lip in the facial feminization process?***
   A. An indirect lip lift through a modified bullhorn technique.
   B. An indirect lip lift through a modified bullhorn performed in conjunction with open rhinoplasty.
   C. Temporarily lengthening the upper lip with Botox injection.
   D. A direct lip lift through a gullwing lip lift to decrease the vertical dimension of the upper lip.
   E. A direct lip lift through a gullwing lip lift to increase the vertical dimension of the upper lip.

ANATOMIC CONSIDERATIONS

7. ***In order to obtain optimal results when addressing the thyroid cartilage during facial feminization surgery which of the following strategies should be employed?***
   A. Wide exposure through a 3-cm incision placed as caudally as possible with aggressive sculpting in the area of the vocal cords.
   B. Wide exposure through a 3-cm incision placed as cephalad as possible with aggressive sculpting in the area of the vocal cords.
   C. Wide exposure through a 3-cm incision placed as cephalad as possible with minimal sculpting in the area of the vocal cords.
   D. Concealing scar by keeping incision to <2 cm placed as caudally as possible with aggressive sculpting in the area of the vocal cords.
   E. Concealing scar by keeping incision to <2 cm placed as cephalad as possible with minimal sculpting in the area of the vocal cords.

ANATOMIC CONSIDERATIONS

8. ***When should breast augmentation in a transgender man be performed?***
   A. After receiving one letter from a mental health provider recommending the patient undergo the procedure but before initiation of feminizing hormone therapy.
   B. After receiving one letter from a mental health provider recommending the patient undergo the procedure but within 6 months of initiation of feminizing hormone therapy.
   C. After receiving one letter from a mental health provider recommending the patient undergo the procedure but after a minimum of 1 year of feminizing hormone therapy.
   D. After receiving one letter from a mental health provider recommending the patient undergo the procedure; feminizing hormone therapy has no bearing on the timing of breast augmentation.
   E. After receiving two letters from a mental health provider recommending the patient undergo the procedure but after a minimum of 1 year of feminizing hormone therapy.

ANATOMIC CONSIDERATIONS

9. ***Which of the following techniques is likely to yield an acceptable aesthetic result after breast augmentation in a transgender female?***
   A. Inframammary incision marked lower than the preoperative inframammary fold with the nipple-areolar complex placed centrally on the implant.
   B. Inframammary incision marked higher than the preoperative inframammary fold with the nipple-areolar complex placed centrally on the implant.
   C. Inframammary incision marked lower than the preoperative inframammary fold with the implant placed as medially as possible to maximize medial fullness.
   D. Inframammary incision marked higher than the preoperative inframammary fold with the implant placed as medially as possible.
   E. Implant placement through a periareolar incision marked lower than the preoperative inframammary fold with the implant placed as medially as possible.

ANATOMIC CONSIDERATIONS

10. ***In female to male top surgery, the goals of subcutaneous mastectomy include which of the following?***
    A. Expansion of the nipple-areolar complex to better match the size of a male nipple-areolar complex.
    B. Removal of breast tissue and excess skin.
    C. Moving the inframammary fold inferiorly.
    D. Moving the inframammary fold superiorly.
    E. Addressing secondary effects of testosterone hormone therapy.

ANATOMIC CONSIDERATIONS

11. ***The surgical technique for female to male top surgery is best decided based on which of the following?***
A. Breast volume.
B. Breast skin excess and breast volume.
C. Breast skin excess and skin elasticity.
D. Breast skin laxity and breast volume.
E. Breast skin laxity.

ANATOMIC CONSIDERATIONS

12. ***Which of the following is the most commonly performed female to male subcutaneous mastectomy technique?***
A. Semicircular.
B. Transareolar.
C. Concentric circle.
D. Nipple-sparing mastectomy.
E. Double incision mastectomy with free nipple grafts.

ANATOMIC CONSIDERATIONS

13. ***In a double incision mastectomy with free nipple grafts, which of the following locations is an appropriate placement for the new nipple position?***
A. Along the breast meridian (vertical nipple line), 2 to 3 cm above the lower level of the pectoralis major.
B. Lateral to the breast meridian (vertical nipple line), 4 cm lateral to the lower level of the pectoralis major.
C. Along the breast meridian (vertical nipple line), at the lower level of the pectoralis major.
D. Medial to the breast meridian (vertical nipple line), 2 to 3 cm above the lower level of the pectoralis major.
E. Medial to the breast meridian (vertical nipple line), at the lower level of the pectoralis major.

ANATOMIC CONSIDERATIONS

14. ***In marking for a double incision mastectomy with free nipple grafts, where should the horizontal incisions be placed?***
A. 1 to 2 cm above the inframammary fold, medially the incision should cross midline to connect with the contralateral side.
B. 1 to 2 cm below the inframammary fold, medially the incision should not cross midline.
C. 2 to 4 cm below the inframammary fold, medially the incision should not cross midline.
D. 1 to 2 cm above the inframammary fold, medially the incision should not cross midline.
E. At the inframammary fold, medially the incision should cross midline to connect with the contralateral side.

ANATOMIC CONSIDERATIONS

15. ***Maneuvers for achieving good aesthetic results and minimizing complications after double incision mastectomy with free nipple grafts include which of the following?***
A. Preserving subcutaneous fat on the skin flaps, preserving the pectoralis fascia, using closed suction drains.
B. Preserving subcutaneous fat on the skin flaps, resecting the pectoralis fascia, avoiding the use of closed suction drains.
C. Preserving subcutaneous fat on the skin flaps, using closed suction drains and progressive tension sutures.
D. Resection of subcutaneous fat on the skin flaps, preserving the pectoralis fascia, using closed suction drains or progressive tension sutures.
E. Resection of subcutaneous fat on the skin flaps, preserving the pectoralis fascia, avoiding the use of closed suction drains or progressive tension sutures.

ANATOMIC CONSIDERATIONS

16. ***As compared to the colon vaginoplasty approach, the penile skin-flap vaginoplasty carries which of the following advantages?***
A. This technique obviates the need for dilation.
B. The neovagina is self-lubricating.
C. The penile skin-flap vaginoplasty always results in vaginal cavity of sufficient length for sexual penetration.
D. This technique may preserve local innervation for sensibility of the neovagina.
E. The neovagina commonly has hair remnants.

ANATOMIC CONSIDERATIONS

17. ***During dissection of the penile skin flap, which of the following best describes appropriate management of the subcutaneous tissue?***

A. The subcutaneous tissue should be preserved for added bulk.
B. The subcutaneous tissue should be resected to allow for full mobilization of the long skin flap.
C. The subcutaneous tissue should be preserved to ensure adequate vascularity to the skin flap.
D. The subcutaneous tissue should be resected to help create a better contour.
E. The subcutaneous tissue should be preserved to ensure moisture postoperatively.

ANATOMIC CONSIDERATIONS

18. ***Which of the following comorbidities would still allow a patient to undergo a sigmoid colon vaginoplasty with an acceptable complication rate?***

A. Inflammatory bowel disease.
B. HIV positive status.
C. Active smoking status.
D. Body mass index of >30 kg/m^2.
E. Intestinal malignancy.

ANATOMIC CONSIDERATIONS

19. ***Which of the following conditions is an inappropriate indication for a sigmoid colon vaginoplasty?***

A. Outstretched phallus length of 4.5 inches.
B. Body mass index of 28 kg/m^2.
C. Stenosis of primary vaginoplasty.
D. A patient who refuses daily dilation.
E. A patient who wishes to have sexual intercourse without the use of lubrication.

ANATOMIC CONSIDERATIONS

20. ***As compared to the phalloplasty surgery, a metoidioplasty __________.***

A. Is often a multistage procedure.
B. Is associated with significant donor site scar morbidity.
C. Can provide a neophallus 12 cm in length.
D. Offers the ability to retain reproductive potential.
E. Results in the ability for standing micturition in all patients.

ANATOMIC CONSIDERATIONS

21. ***Relative to a metoidioplasty, phalloplasty surgery is associated with increased rates of which of the following?***

A. Inability for standing micturition.
B. Inability to accommodate penile prosthesis for penetrative intercourse.
C. Urethrocutaneous fistulas and urinary stricture rate of 90 to 100%.
D. Urethrocutaneous fistula and urinary stricture rate of 41 to 80%.
E. Orgasmic ability after surgery.

Answers

ANATOMIC CONSIDERATIONS

1. *Which of the following statements is an accurate description regarding the female face relative to male face?*

D. Females have a greater concentration of fat in the middle third of the face while males tend to have greater malar bone volume.

In the upper third of the face, males tend to have greater bone volume than females. In the middle third, the male nose is generally larger, and males have greater malar bone volume, resulting in well-defined cheeks. Females also have a greater concentration of fat in middle third of the face, giving them prominent round cheeks. In males, the distance between the upper lip and nose is longer than in females. In the lower third, males have squared mandibular angles with well-defined corners.[1]

REFERENCE

1. Wan D, Amirlak B, Rohrich R, et al. The clinical importance of the fat compartments in midfacial aging. Plast Reconstr Surg Glob Open 2014;1:e92

ANATOMIC CONSIDERATIONS

2. *Which of the following is an accurate description and consideration when evaluating the hairline?*

D. Females tend to have a rounded hairline while males have an M-shaped hairline.

Males have M-shaped hairline with recession at temples, which may be affected by androgenic alopecia; females usually have rounded hairline that extends slightly higher in the center than in men (**Fig. 65.1**).[1,2] Based on the hairline analysis of transgender patients treated to date ($N = 492$) for any facial feminization procedure by our team, both treatments, namely, simultaneous hair transplant (SHT) (follicular unit strip surgery technique) and hairline lowering surgery (HLS), are performed in combination with a forehead reconstruction during the same surgery. A deferred hair transplant (DHT) treatment (follicular unit strip surgery or follicular unit extraction technique) is performed alone in a second session.

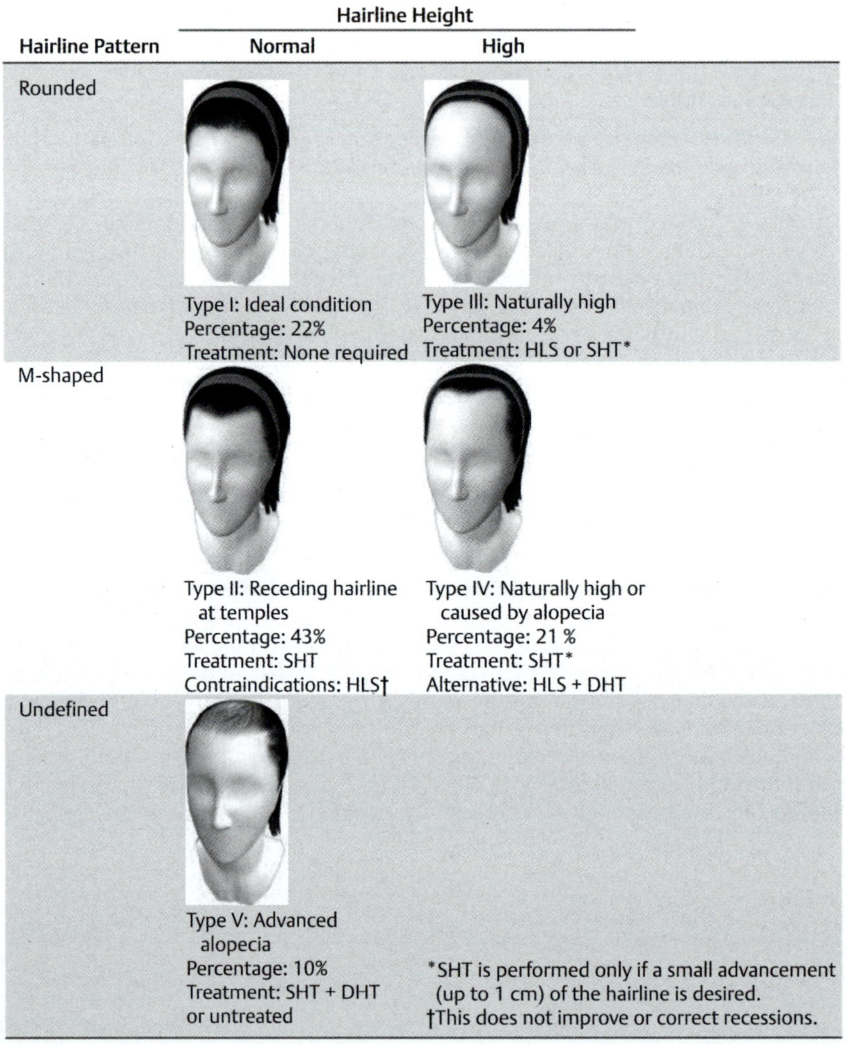

Fig. 65.1 Hairline variations and possible treatments in male-to-female transgender patients. Based on the hairline analysis of transgender patients treated to date (N = 492) for any facial feminization procedure by our team. Both treatments, SHT (follicular unit strip surgery technique) and HLS, are performed in combination with a forehead reconstruction during the same surgery. A DHT treatment (follicular unit strip surgery or follicular unit extraction technique) is performed alone in a second session. (DHT, Deferred hair transplant; HLS, hairline lowering surgery; SHT, simultaneous hair transplant.) (Source: Reprinted with permission from Capitán L, Simon D, Meyer T, et al. Facial feminization surgery: simultaneous hair transplant during forehead reconstruction. Plast Reconstr Surg 139:573, 2017.)

References

1. Norwood OT. Male pattern baldness: classification and incidence. South Med J 1975;68:1359
2. Nusbaum BP, Fuentefria S. Naturally occurring female hairline patterns. Dermatol Surg 2009;35:907

ANATOMIC CONSIDERATIONS

3. *A transgender female patient wishes to undergo facial feminization surgery. CT scan demonstrates that the anterior table of her frontal sinus is 2 mm in thickness. Which of the following approaches is appropriate?*

B. Frontal bone set back with osteotomy and repositioning of the anterior wall of the frontal sinus alone.

Osteotomy and repositioning of the anterior wall of the frontal sinus or burring of the anterior table of the frontal sinus are both well accepted procedures to soften this region during facial feminization surgery. However, if the anterior table thickness is 3 mm or less, osteotomy and repositioning is the recommended technique. In the setting of attaining a more feminine forehead contour with a more pronounced supraorbital rim with projection past the cornea, placement of an alloplastic implant could provide a very aesthetically pleasing result. However, in the above scenario, this is a transgender female and oftentimes this involves a reduction of a more pronounced forehead which typically would be better treated with burring and/or a formal set back.[1,2]

REFERENCES

1. Capitá L, Simon D, Kaye K, et al. Facial feminization surgery: the forehead. Surgical techniques and analysis of results. Plast Reconstr Surg 2014;134:609
2. Capitán L, Simon D, Meyer T, et al. Facial feminization surgery: simultaneous hair transplant during forehead reconstruction. Plast Reconstr Surg 2017;139:573

ANATOMIC CONSIDERATIONS

4. *During facial feminization surgery, hair transplantation should ______________.*

B. Be performed after androgenic alopecia stabilizes.

Males have M-shaped hairline with recession at temples, while females usually have rounded hairline that extends slightly higher in the center. The goal of hair transplantation in transgender females is to address the recessed corners of the hairline. Hair transplantation should be delayed until androgenic alopecia stabilizes (**Fig. 65.2**).[1,2,3]

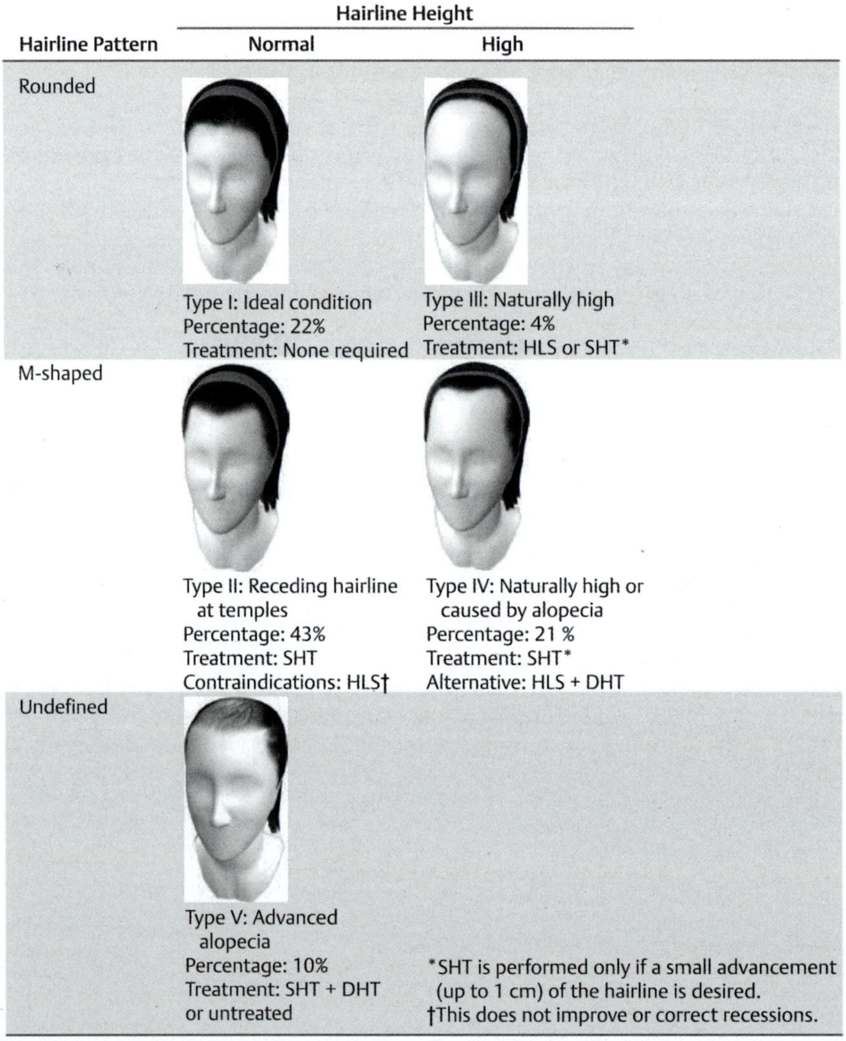

Fig. 65.2 Hairline variations and possible treatments in male-to-female transgender patients. Based on the hairline analysis of transgender patients treated to date (*N* = 492) for any facial feminization procedure by our team. Both treatments, SHT (follicular unit strip surgery technique) and HLS, are performed in combination with a forehead reconstruction during the same surgery. A DHT treatment (follicular unit strip surgery or follicular unit extraction technique) is performed alone in a second session. (DHT, Deferred hair transplant; HLS, hairline lowering surgery; SHT, simultaneous hair transplant.) (Source: Reprinted with permission from Capitán L, Simon D, Meyer T, et al. Facial feminization surgery: simultaneous hair transplant during forehead reconstruction. Plast Reconstr Surg 139:573, 2017.)

References

1. Norwood OT. Male pattern baldness: classification and incidence. South Med J 1975;68:1359
2. Nusbaum BP, Fuentefria S. Naturally occurring female hairline patterns. Dermatol Surg 2009;35:907
3. Hembree WC, Cohen-Kettenis P, Delemarre-van de Waal HA, et al; Endocrine Society. Endocrine treatment of transsexual persons: an Endocrine Society clinical practice guideline. J Clin Endocrinol Metab 2009;94:3132

ANATOMIC CONSIDERATIONS

5. ***Which is the following is a potential reason to be cautious if performing an upper lip lift in conjunction with an open rhinoplasty in the same stage?***

   C. Concern for skin necrosis between the intervening segment of skin between the two incisions.

   Although many surgeons perform simultaneous lip lifts in conjunction with an open rhinoplasty with a satisfactory result, some prefer to perform this in separate stages in order to avoid potential skin necrosis along the columella. There is no evidence to suggest that there are any higher rates of infection or hematoma. Additionally, the potential sequelae of abnormal scarring can occur; however, this occurs in conjunction with widening of the alar base, not narrowing.[1,2]

REFERENCES

1. Talei B. The modified upper lip lift: advanced approach with deep-plane release and secure suspension: 823-patient series. Facial Plast Surg Clin North Am 2019;27(3):385–398
2. Salgado CJ, Monstrey SJ, Djordjevic ML, eds. Gender Affirmation Medical & Surgical Perspectives. Stuttgart, Germany: Thieme Publishers; 2017

ANATOMIC CONSIDERATIONS

6. ***Which of the following is an appropriate technique for addressing the upper lip in the facial feminization process?***

   A. An indirect lip lift through a modified bullhorn technique.

   Males have a longer vertical length between the nose and the upper lip vermillion, so the goal is to reduce the vertical dimension between the upper lip and nose. A modified bullhorn technique is the preferred technique to remove a strip of skin and subcutaneous tissue without violating the orbicularis oris to shorten the cutaneous upper lip. Additionally, a direct lip lift through a gullwing technique would violate the orbicularis oris. This should NOT be performed at the same time as an open rhinoplasty as this may lead to necrosis of the skin between the upper lip and the nose along the inferior columella.[1,2,3]

REFERENCES

1. Capitá L, Simon D, Kaye K, et al. Facial feminization surgery: the forehead. Surgical techniques and analysis of results. Plast Reconstr Surg 2014;134:609
2. Capitán L, Simon D, Meyer T, et al. Facial feminization surgery: simultaneous hair transplant during forehead reconstruction. Plast Reconstr Surg 2017;139:573
3. Salgado CJ, Monstrey SJ, Djordjevic ML, eds. Gender Affirmation Medical & Surgical Perspectives. Stuttgart, Germany: Thieme Publishers; 2017

ANATOMIC CONSIDERATIONS

7. ***In order to obtain optimal results when addressing the thyroid cartilage during facial feminization surgery which of the following strategies should be employed?***

   E. Concealing scar by keeping incision to <2 cm placed as cephalad as possible with minimal sculpting in the area of the vocal cords.

   Addressing the thyroid cartilage during facial feminization surgery should be done through a maximal 2 cm incision placed as cephalad as possible in the area of the cervicomental fold for concealment. Additionally, sculpting should not be done near the vocal cords.[1,2,3]

REFERENCES

1. Capitán L, Simon D, Kaye K, et al. Facial feminization surgery: the forehead. Surgical techniques and analysis of results. Plast Reconstr Surg 2014;134:609
2. Capitán L, Simon D, Meyer T, et al. Facial feminization surgery: simultaneous hair transplant during forehead reconstruction. Plast Reconstr Surg 2017;139:573
3. Salgado CJ, Monstrey SJ, Djordjevic ML, eds. Gender Affirmation Medical & Surgical Perspectives. Stuttgart, Germany: Thieme Publishers; 2017

ANATOMIC CONSIDERATIONS

8. *When should breast augmentation in a transgender man be performed?*

C. After receiving one letter from a mental health provider recommending the patient undergo the procedure but after a minimum of 1 year of feminizing hormone therapy.

All "top" surgical procedures require one letter from a mental health provider recommending the patient undergo the procedure. Hormone therapy promotes mammogenesis, which follows a pattern similar to female pubertal mammogenesis; therefore, transgender females should undergo feminizing hormone therapy for a minimum of 1 year before breast augmentation surgery.[1,2,3]

REFERENCES

1. Hage JJ, van Kesteren PJ. Chest-wall contouring in female-to-male transsexuals: basic considerations and review of the literature. Plast Reconstr Surg 1995;96:386
2. Hage JJ, Bloem JJ. Chest wall contouring for female-to-male transsexuals: Amsterdam experience. Ann Plast Surg 1995;34:59
3. Monstrey S, Selvaggi G, Ceulemans P, et al. Chest-wall contouring surgery in female-to-male transsexuals: a new algorithm. Plast Reconstr Surg 2008;121:849

ANATOMIC CONSIDERATIONS

9. *Which of the following techniques is likely to yield an acceptable aesthetic result after breast augmentation in a transgender female?*

A. Inframammary incision marked lower than the preoperative inframammary fold with the nipple-areolar complex placed centrally on the implant.

Males tend to have a wider chest, stronger pectoral fascia, more developed pectoralis muscles, and smaller nipple-areolar complex. In order to achieve good aesthetic results after breast augmentation, the nipple-areolar complex should always overlie the implant centrally though this may result in wide cleavage between breasts. Additionally, the inframammary incision is preferred and should be designed lower than preoperative inframammary fold because the inferior areolar margin and inframammary fold will expand after augmentation.[1]

REFERENCE

1. Bekeny JC, Zolper EG, Fan KL, Del Corral G. Breast augmentation for transfeminine patients: methods, complications, and outcomes. Gland Surg 2020;9(3):788–796

ANATOMIC CONSIDERATIONS

10. *In female to male top surgery, the goals of subcutaneous mastectomy include which of the following?*

B. Removal of breast tissue and excess skin.

The goals of subcutaneous mastectomy in female to male top surgery include: removal of breast tissue and excess skin, reduction and proper positioning of the nipple-areolar complex, obliteration of the inframammary fold, and minimization of chest wall scars to achieve aesthetically pleasing male chest.[1,2,3]

REFERENCES

1. Hage JJ, van Kesteren PJ. Chest-wall contouring in female-to-male transsexuals: basic considerations and review of the literature. Plast Reconstr Surg 1995;96:386
2. Hage JJ, Bloem JJ. Chest wall contouring for female-to-male transsexuals: Amsterdam experience. Ann Plast Surg 1995;34:59
3. Monstrey S, Selvaggi G, Ceulemans P, et al. Chest-wall contouring surgery in female-to-male transsexuals: a new algorithm. Plast Reconstr Surg 2008;121:849

ANATOMIC CONSIDERATIONS

11. *The surgical technique for female to male top surgery is best decided based on which of the following?*

C. Breast skin excess and skin elasticity.

According to the algorithm for choosing the appropriate subcutaneous mastectomy technique (**Fig. 65.3**), the technique is determined by the amount of excess skin and skin elasticity, not by breast volume.[1,2]

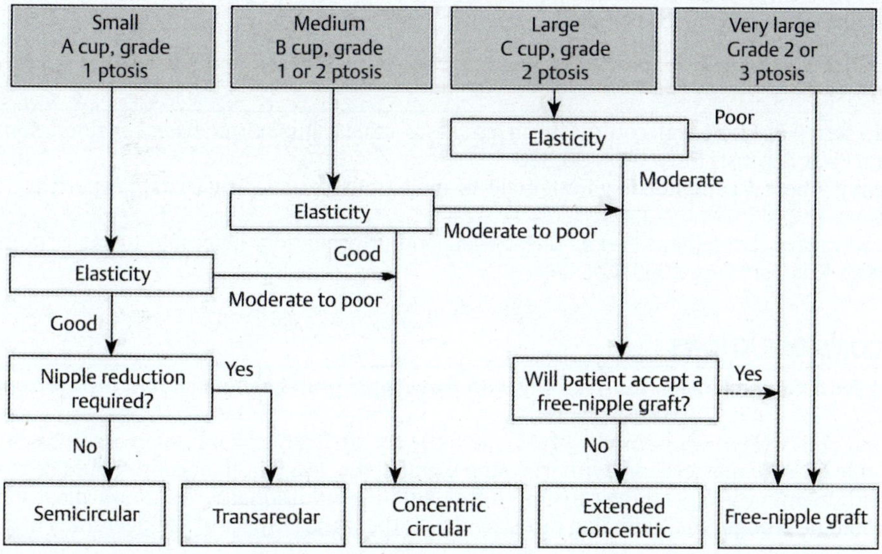

Fig. 65.3 Algorithm for choosing the appropriate subcutaneous mastectomy technique. (Source: Sex reassignment surgery in the femaleto-male transsexual. Semin Plast Surg 25:229, 2011.)

REFERENCES

1. Salgado CJ, Monstrey SJ, Djordjevic ML, eds. Gender Affirmation Medical & Surgical Perspectives. Stuttgart, Germany: Thieme Publishers; 2017
2. Hage JJ, Bloem JJ. Chest wall contouring for female-to-male transsexuals: Amsterdam experience. Ann Plast Surg 1995;34:59

ANATOMIC CONSIDERATIONS

12. ***Which of the following is the most commonly performed female to male subcutaneous mastectomy technique?***

D. Nipple-sparing mastectomy.

The most commonly performed top surgery for transgender males is the double incision mastectomy with free nipple grafts. The semicircular and transareolar techniques are limited to patients with small breasts and are technically challenging given the small operative window. The concentric circular technique is limited to patients with small or medium breasts with poor skin elasticity but can result in scar widening necessitating revision.[1,2,3]

REFERENCES

1. Hage JJ, van Kesteren PJ. Chest-wall contouring in female-to-male transsexuals: basic considerations and review of the literature. Plast Reconstr Surg 1995;96:386
2. Hage JJ, Bloem JJ. Chest wall contouring for female-to-male transsexuals: Amsterdam experience. Ann Plast Surg 1995;34:59
3. Monstrey S, Selvaggi G, Ceulemans P, et al. Chest-wall contouring surgery in female-to-male transsexuals: a new algorithm. Plast Reconstr Surg 2008;121:849

ANATOMIC CONSIDERATIONS

13. ***In a double incision mastectomy with free nipple grafts, which of the following locations is an appropriate placement for the new nipple position?***

A. Along the breast meridian (vertical nipple line), 2 to 3 cm above the lower level of the pectoralis major.

In a double incision mastectomy with free nipple grafts, the new nipple position should be placed along the existing vertical nipple line, approximately 2 to 3 cm above the lower border of pectoralis major (usually at fourth or fifth intercostal segment). The patient should always be positioned upright intraoperatively to confirm acceptable nipple position.[1,2,3]

REFERENCES

1. Hage JJ, van Kesteren PJ. Chest-wall contouring in female-to-male transsexuals: basic considerations and review of the literature. Plast Reconstr Surg 1995;96:386
2. Hage JJ, Bloem JJ. Chest wall contouring for female-to-male transsexuals: Amsterdam experience. Ann Plast Surg 1995;34:59
3. Monstrey S, Selvaggi G, Ceulemans P, et al. Chest-wall contouring surgery in female-to-male transsexuals: a new algorithm. Plast Reconstr Surg 2008;121:849

ANATOMIC CONSIDERATIONS

14. ***In marking for a double incision mastectomy with free nipple grafts, where should the horizontal incisions be placed?***

D. 1 to 2 cm above the inframammary fold, medially the incision should not cross midline.

In a double incision mastectomy with free nipple grafts, the horizontal incision should be marked 1 to 2 cm above inframammary fold, taking care not to cross midline. Additionally, the lateral-most aspect of the incision should be brought in a cephalad direction along the lateral aspect of the pectoralis major muscle (**Fig. 65.4**).[1,2,3]

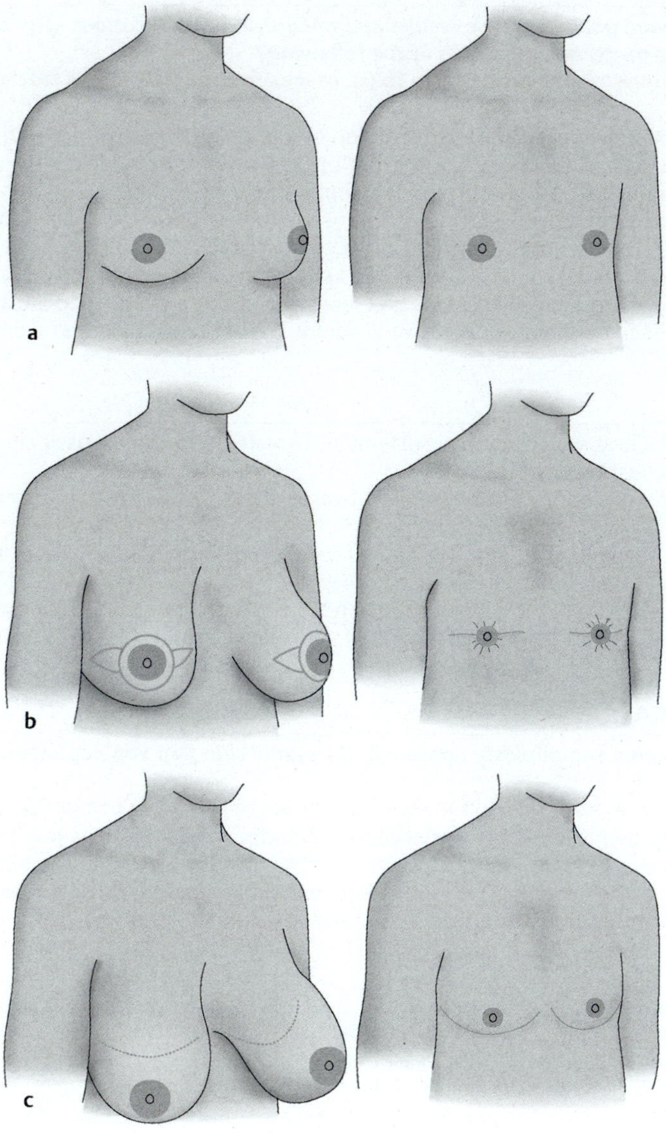

Fig. 65.4 (a–c) Monstrey's schematic for choosing the appropriate SCM technique. (Source: Sex reassignment surgery in the femaleto-male transsexual. Semin Plast Surg 25:229, 2011.)

References

1. Hage JJ, van Kesteren PJ. Chest-wall contouring in female-to-male transsexuals: basic considerations and review of the literature. Plast Reconstr Surg 1995;96:386
2. Hage JJ, Bloem JJ. Chest wall contouring for female-to-male transsexuals: Amsterdam experience. Ann Plast Surg 1995;34:59
3. Monstrey S, Selvaggi G, Ceulemans P, et al. Chest-wall contouring surgery in female-to-male transsexuals: a new algorithm. Plast Reconstr Surg 2008;121:849

ANATOMIC CONSIDERATIONS

15. *Maneuvers for achieving good aesthetic results and minimizing complications after double incision mastectomy with free nipple grafts include which of the following?*

A. Preserving subcutaneous fat on the skin flaps, preserving the pectoralis fascia, using closed suction drains.

Preserving all subcutaneous fat during dissection of glandular tissue from skin flaps and pectoralis fascia and during dissection of glandular tissue from chest wall will prevent tethering of flaps to chest wall. Closed suction drains are usually placed intraoperatively and removed at the first postoperative visit. Additionally, progressive tension sutures can be used; however, they have been shown to increase surgical time, reduce drain outputs, and have the same clinical and ultrasound seroma frequency as the use of drains alone. The combination of both methods simultaneously does not add any advantages. However, complications and interventions increase if at least one of them is not used. Postoperatively, a circumferential elastic bandage or chest compressive garment should be applied and worn for 4 to 6 weeks.[1,2,3,4]

REFERENCES

1. Hage JJ, van Kesteren PJ. Chest-wall contouring in female-to-male transsexuals: basic considerations and review of the literature. Plast Reconstr Surg 1995;96:386
2. Hage JJ, Bloem JJ. Chest wall contouring for female-to-male transsexuals: Amsterdam experience. Ann Plast Surg 1995;34:59
3. Monstrey S, Selvaggi G, Ceulemans P, et al. Chest-wall contouring surgery in female-to-male transsexuals: a new algorithm. Plast Reconstr Surg 2008;121:849
4. Andrades P, Prado A, Danilla S, et al. Progressive tension sutures in the prevention of postabdominoplasty seroma: a prospective, randomized, double-blind clinical trial. Plast Reconstr Surg 2007;120(4):935–946

ANATOMIC CONSIDERATIONS

16. *As compared to the colon vaginoplasty approach, the penile skin-flap vaginoplasty carries which of the following advantages?*

D. This technique may preserve local innervation for sensibility of the neovagina.

Advantages to the penile skin-flap vaginoplasty include: penile skin has less tendency to contract, this technique may preserve local innervation for sensibility of the neovagina as well as result in a relatively hairless neovagina. The advantages to the colon vaginoplasty are that it provides a neovagina with sufficient vaginal depth that is self-lubricating and has less tendency to shrink.[1,2]

REFERENCES

1. Karim RB, Hage JJ, Mulder JW. Neovaginoplasty in male transsexuals: review of surgical techniques and recommendations regarding eligibility. Ann Plast Surg 1996;37:669
2. Selvaggi G, Ceulemans P, De Cuypere G, et al. Gender identity disorder: general overview and surgical treatment for vaginoplasty in male-to-female transsexuals. Plast Reconstr Surg 2005;116:135e

ANATOMIC CONSIDERATIONS

17. *During dissection of the penile skin flap, which of the following best describes appropriate management of the subcutaneous tissue?*

C. The subcutaneous tissue should be preserved to ensure adequate vascularity to the skin flap.

During dissection of the penile skin flap, preservation of the subcutaneous tissue is essential for formation of a long, vascularized pedicle. Resection of the subcutaneous tissue may compromise vascularity and is not necessary for flap mobilization.[1,2]

REFERENCES

1. Garaffa G, Christopher NA, Ralph DJ. Total phallic reconstruction in female-to-male transsexuals. Eur Urol 2010;57:715
2. Hu ZQ, Hyakusoku H, Gao JH, et al. Penis reconstruction using three different operative methods. Br J Plast Surg 2005;58:487

ANATOMIC CONSIDERATIONS

18. *Which of the following comorbidities would still allow a patient to undergo a sigmoid colon vaginoplasty with an acceptable complication rate?*

B. HIV positive status.

Contraindications to the sigmoid colon vaginoplasty include intestinal malignancy, inflammatory bowel disease, previous extensive abdominal surgery, active smoking, and BMI >30 kg/m^2. Positive HIV status is not a contraindication to sigmoid colon vaginoplasty but patients must have adequate CD4 count and undetectable viral load to avoid complications.[1,2]

REFERENCES

1. Karim RB, Hage JJ, Mulder JW. Neovaginoplasty in male transsexuals: review of surgical techniques and recommendations regarding eligibility. Ann Plast Surg 1996;37:669
2. Selvaggi G, Ceulemans P, De Cuypere G, et al. Gender identity disorder: general overview and surgical treatment for vaginoplasty in male-to-female transsexuals. Plast Reconstr Surg 2005;116:135e

ANATOMIC CONSIDERATIONS

19. *Which of the following conditions is an inappropriate indication for a sigmoid colon vaginoplasty?*

A. Outstretched phallus length of 4.5 inches.

Preference is given to a colon vaginoplasty in patients who desire less vaginal dilation and vaginal penetration without lubrication and who have an outstretched phallus length of ≤3.5 inches and have had no prior abdominal surgery.[1,2]

REFERENCES

1. Karim RB, Hage JJ, Mulder JW. Neovaginoplasty in male transsexuals: review of surgical techniques and recommendations regarding eligibility. Ann Plast Surg 1996;37:669
2. Selvaggi G, Ceulemans P, De Cuypere G, et al. Gender identity disorder: general overview and surgical treatment for vaginoplasty in male-to-female transsexuals. Plast Reconstr Surg 2005;116:135e

ANATOMIC CONSIDERATIONS

20. *As compared to the phalloplasty surgery, a metoidioplasty ________.*

D. Offers the ability to retain reproductive potential.

Metoidioplasty is a single-stage surgery that provides a 3- to 8-cm long microphallus capable of engorgement with erotic sensation. Metoidioplasty is the only female-to-male bottom surgery that offers the ability to retain reproductive potential. However, standing micturition is not possible in all patients who undergo metoidioplasty.[1,2]

REFERENCES

1. Selvaggi G, Ceulemans P, De Cuypere G, et al. Gender identity disorder: general overview and surgical treatment for vaginoplasty in male-to-female transsexuals. Plast Reconstr Surg 2005;116:135e
2. Djordjevic ML, Bizic M, Stanojevic D, et al. Urethral lengthening in metoidioplasty (female- to-male sex reassignment surgery) by combined buccal mucosa graft and labia minora flap. Urology 2009;74:349

ANATOMIC CONSIDERATIONS

21. *Relative to a metoidioplasty, phalloplasty surgery is associated with increased rates of which of the following?*

C. Urethrocutaneous fistulas and urinary stricture rate of 90 to 100%.

Phalloplasty is associated with a high (41–80%) rate of urinary complications, including urethrocutaneous fistulas and urinary stricture.[1,2]

REFERENCES

1. Selvaggi G, Ceulemans P, De Cuypere G, et al. Gender identity disorder: general overview and surgical treatment for vaginoplasty in male-to-female transsexuals. Plast Reconstr Surg 2005;116:135e
2. Djordjevic ML, Bizic M, Stanojevic D, et al. Urethral lengthening in metoidioplasty (female- to-male sex reassignment surgery) by combined buccal mucosa graft and labia minora flap. Urology 2009;74:349

Index

Note: Page numbers set **bold** or *italic* indicate headings or figures/tables, respectively.